AIDS UPDATE
2003

An Annual Overview of
Acquired Immune Deficiency Syndrome

GERALD J. STINE, PH.D.

University of North Florida, Jacksonville

Prentice
Hall

Prentice Hall
Upper Saddle River, New Jersey 07458

AIDS IS A WAR THAT NO ONE WANTS TO LOSE
BUT NO ONE YET KNOWS HOW TO WIN

• • • • • •

This book, as with my eleven other HIV/AIDS college-level textbooks,
is also dedicated to
those who have died of AIDS,
those who have HIV disease,
and to those who must prevent the spread of this plague—

EVERYONE, EVERYWHERE.

Senior Editor: *Halee Dinsey*
Executive Managing Editor: *Kathleen Schiaparelli*
Assistant Managing Editor: *Beth Sturla*
Assistant Manufacturing Manager: *Michael Bell*
Manufacturing Buyer: *Lynda Castillo*
Director of Marketing, ESM: *John Tweeddale*
Art Director: *Jayne Conte*
Cover Designer: *Bruce Kenselaar*
Production Supervision/Composition: *WestWords, Inc.*
Editorial Assistant: *Susan Zeigler*
Cover: Three-dimensional model of HIV created by Louis E. Henderson, PhD, is reproduced with permission from *The PRN Notebook*™, June 2002. Published by Physicians' Research Network, Inc. ®, New York, NY, USA. All rights reserved. © June 2002. For further information visit www.prn.org.

©2003 by Pearson Education, Inc.
Upper Saddle River, New Jersey 07458

This book is an alternate version of *Acquired Immune Deficiency Syndrome: Biological, Medical, Social, and Legal Issues, 3rd edition* by Gerald J. Stine, ©1998 by Prentice Hall.

Printed in the United States of America

10 9 8 7 6 5 4 3 2

ISBN 0-13-047546-7

Pearson Education Ltd., *London*
Pearson Education Australia Pty. Ltd., *Sydney*
Pearson Education Singapore, Pte. Ltd.
Pearson Education North Asia Ltd., *Hong Kong*
Pearson Education Canada, Inc., *Toronto*
Pearson Educación de Mexico, S.A. de C.V.
Pearson Education—Japan, *Tokyo*
Pearson Education Malaysia, Pte. Ltd.
Pearson Education, Inc., *Upper Saddle River, New Jersey*

AIDS UPDATE 2003

WHY DO I WRITE ABOUT HIV/AIDS?

I began writing about a new disease, later called AIDS, in 1981 shortly after the Centers for Disease Control and Prevention issued the first of its reports. These writings were limited in scope because not much was known at the time. My writing then was for classroom use. Little did I know at the time the passion that I would develop about this disease. As the number of infected people and their deaths continued to rise, fear and discrimination reared its ugly head because in some cases people are what they are, and in other cases, because of the lack of available nonbiased educational material. At the time, in the mid-1980s, I felt a need to write, to help educate people about this disease, hopefully to answer questions and reduce the blatant discrimination occurring against those who already had the overwhelming burden of HIV disease. So, I began—I created a college-level HIV/AIDS course, taught it for several years, constantly shaping and reshaping the information necessary to help others learn the facts about this pandemic, and to destroy destructive myths. After I felt I had set the record straight in my classroom, I began writing HIV/AIDS college-level textbooks so that information on this pandemic could be shared more broadly.

There are many reasons I have not stopped writing about HIV/AIDS. **First,** because as Yogi Berra supposedly said, "It ain't over till it's over," and it "ain't" near over yet! **Second,** AIDS summons up the greatest themes in literature, among them sex, faith, and death—themes that are universal and unexpectedly permanent. Anyone who has lost a loved one to death, untimely or by nature, can read about AIDS and understand the emotional forces that take place. Anyone who has taken care of someone who has been ill understands the need for compassion. Anyone who has faced death from a prolonged or life-threatening illness should be able to identify with those who suffer with AIDS. Anyone interested in uncovering acts of human kindness or conversely acts of despicable behavior can find them in writings about this disease.

But more than any of these reasons, my writing about AIDS is fueled by a need to do something, anything, to help. For the millions of people who are in pain and dying, I have little to offer except my writing. Although my only known risk factor was a blood transfusion in the mid-1970s, I cannot help but feel lucky that so far neither AIDS nor any other serious disease threatens my life. Is there a reason that I have been spared to my present age when so many others have died? I write about AIDS, not just because I live but because it is part of our history. The AIDS pandemic has changed my feelings and attitudes toward people. I find myself more sensitive to others. AIDS has changed the world in some way for most everyone and, at least some of the information about this disease—its impact and repercussions—needs telling. So, I write about AIDS because someone needs to tell the story.

—The Author

INTO THE NEW MILLENNIUM

The war on AIDS is still closer to the **beginning** than it is to the **end** but I have never been more positive about the future for those who are HIV-infected in the United States and other developed nations. The use of anti-HIV drugs in combination has led to a dramatic reduction in HIV-infected babies and AIDS-related deaths, as well as a significant reduction in new AIDS cases and reductions in opportunistic infections. These events, along with new insight into the biology and pathology of HIV may lead to a preventive vaccine and provide a shining light against a stark history of the first 22 years of a pandemic first reported in the United States in 1981.

Unfortunately, the high cost of anti-HIV drugs makes them unavailable for widespread distribution in underdeveloped nations. But hope and help must begin somewhere—someone must first benefit before others can. **Let us pull together so that help, not just hope, will be available to all who need it!**

—Gerald Stine, Ph.D.

The information on HIV/AIDS within this text goes where the pandemic has taken us over the last 22 years. This information is not designed to replace the relationship that exists between you and your doctor or other health advisor. For all medical events, consult with your physician.

Contents

**11 Prevalence of HIV Infection
and AIDS Cases Among Women,
Children, and Teenagers in the
United States 356**

**12 Testing for Human
Immunodeficiency Virus 396**

Features

Chapter 6

Chapter 7

Chapter 8

Chapter 9

Chapter 10

Chapter 13

Preface

THE GREAT PARADOX

I hope that as you read this edition of AIDS UP-DATE 2003, you will gain a clearer perspective on the ways in which the issue of HIV/AIDS is paradoxically at the center of controversy and, at the same time, sidelined by the silence about its causes and prevention. The edition of AIDS UPDATE also presents information on how the terrorist attack on September 11th, 2001, on the World Trade Center towers in New York and on the Pentagon in Washington, D.C., impacted financial donations and behaviors with respect to the needs of the global HIV/AIDS pandemic. This attack has had ripple effects that altered the lives of so many people worldwide. It has caused people to re-evaluate their personal goals and shifted public awareness away from long-term problem solving to anxious anticipation of preparedness for the next attack. Regardless, the AIDS crisis in not nearly over—the hardest parts of dealing with this disease are in progress.

—The Author

THE AIDS PANDEMIC IN PERSPECTIVE

To place the HIV/AIDS pandemic in perspective, consider Michael Crichton's *The Andromeda Strain.* The essence of this story revolves around the release of an unidentified and untreatable lethal strain of bacteria into the human population. With a few changes—substituting HIV for bacterium, adjusting the time of death after infection, and describing how one dies from the disease—Crichton could have been writing about HIV/AIDS. But with HIV/AIDS, the onset of a real human tragedy, we are learning about our social contradictions, our strengths and our weaknesses, and we are questioning whether this is a morally acceptable disease. How long will it take for this to become a socially acceptable disease?

AIDS: THE WORST-CASE SCENARIO

As presented in this book, the reader will note the ability of HIV to cause a slow, progressive, and permanent disease. Thus, with no recovery, no loss of infectivity, no development of either individual or group immunity, there is at present no known biological mechanism that can stop the continuing expansion of the disease unless an effective vaccine were to come about, and at present there is no feasible design for such an effective vaccine. The progressive increase in the pool of HIV can, in theory, only lead to an exponential increase in the number of individuals who will become infected until eventually the majority of the sexually active population will be infected unless interventions are at least moderately successful.

It is **because** this scenario may become reality and **because** people worldwide are becoming HIV-infected every few seconds and dying of AIDS each minute, and **because** together we must try to prevent the further spread of HIV, that this text continues to be updated.

This text reviews important aspects of HIV infection, HIV disease, and the acquired immune deficiency syndrome. **It presents a balanced review of factual information about the biological, medical, social, economic, and legal aspects of this modern-day pandemic.**

The intricacy of the HIV/AIDS pandemic has unfolded over the last 22 years. Many of the details of basic research, applied biology, medicine, and social unrest are presented in an attempt to convey the few victories and many setbacks within this ongoing saga. Medical and social anecdotes help to convey a sense of the HIV/AIDS tragedy worldwide. The history of the disease describes how the virus is and is not transmitted. Throughout the text there is a special focus on risk behaviors and risk situations involved in HIV transmission and the means to prevent its transmission. The number of social issues raised by this disease are mind-boggling. Many of these issues are presented—some as open-ended questions for class discussions. Such questions help the student reflect on what he or she has read.

PURPOSE

The purpose of this text is to present an understandable scientific explanation of what has been learned about HIV/AIDS over the last 22 years. In addition, it is particularly important to provide students with a conceptual framework of the issues raised by the HIV/AIDS pandemic so that they will be better able to deal with the challenges posed by this disease. Clearly, this pandemic poses new and unforeseen problems with no quick biological solutions. Only through reason can we respond in a socially acceptable fashion.

Because there is a constant stream of new information to be interpreted and shared, a new edition will be published every year. What has been learned and what must still be learned to bring HIV infection, HIV disease, and AIDS under control is valuable information to most, if not all, of us.

TEXT USE

This text is intended for use in college-level courses on AIDS and as a supplemental HIV/AIDS resource in medical and nursing schools, in colleges of allied health sciences, in psychology department courses on human sexuality and human behavior, in courses on sexually transmitted diseases, in summer teachers programs, in the training of AIDS counselors, in state-mandated AIDS education courses for health care workers, and for physicians who need a ready source of information on how to prevent HIV infection, HIV disease, and its progression to AIDS, and types of therapy available. This text is suitable in those cases where information and education about the various aspects of HIV infection, disease, and AIDS are either wanted or required.

During the 22 years since HIV/AIDS was defined as a new disease, more manpower and money has been poured into HIV/AIDS research than into any other disease in history. Information on the virus that causes AIDS has accumulated at an unprecedented pace. Since the discovery of this virus in 1982–1983, scientists have learned much about how it functions and how it affects the immune system. More was learned about the virus in the first six years after its discovery than had been

learned about the polio virus in the first 40 years of the polio epidemic. During the first six years of AIDS research, the virus's genetic material was cloned, its structure ascertained, and individual viral genes identified. In fact, so many billions of dollars have been spent on HIV/AIDS that many now believe HIV/AIDS research has taken away much-needed resources from other diseases that kill many times more people per year than does AIDS.

TEXT OVERVIEW

Because so much of the HIV/AIDS pandemic has been based on the manipulation of distorted scientific fact, it is necessary to counter these distortions and myths by presenting the most consistent, reproducible, and scientifically acceptable facts as possible. Therefore, this text offers answers to questions many people have about HIV and how their immune systems are affected by it. Covered herein are the activity of the immune system with respect to HIV disease, where the virus might have come from, how it is transmitted, who is most likely to become infected, viral prevalence (geographical distribution of the number of people infected and those expressing HIV disease and AIDS), possible means of preventing infection, signs and symptoms of HIV disease and AIDS, chronological definitions of AIDS, the opportunistic infections most often associated with AIDS, FDA-approved and nonapproved drugs and their effectiveness, the potential for a vaccine to HIV, the tests available to detect HIV infection, the accuracy of these tests, their cost, availability, and confidentiality. The last chapter deals with the fear of HIV infection and the social reaction of the uninfected toward the HIV-infected.

The majority of references herein are dated between 1988 and year 2002. Every state in the United States has HIV-infected people and reported people diagnosed with AIDS. The World Health Organization (WHO) reports that of 209 countries reporting to it, 194 have reported diagnosed cases of AIDS through year 2002. The virus is truly pandemic and now threatens most of the human population. Yet it is a preventable disorder, and the steps to prevention are presented in Chapter 9.

ORGANIZATION OF THE TEXT

The Introduction, a **must read**, presents examples of fear and ignorance that surrounded previous global pandemics and now AIDS! Also presented is an overview of the HIV/AIDS pandemic—its place in the history of pandemics and some of the ways groups and organizations have reacted to this new disease: the 14th World International AIDS Conference, the making of the AIDS quilt, and the founding of World's AIDS Day every December 1. There are photographs of people who, through their deaths from AIDS, brought a focus to this disease that was not there before. Ending the Introduction is a list of national toll-free AIDS hotlines and very timely and useful internet addresses.

Chapter 1 presents information on the discovery of the disease and naming of the illness. Chapter 2 discusses the cause of AIDS and the possible origin of the AIDS virus. Chapter 3 presents the biological characteristics of the virus. Chapter 4 presents current retroviral therapy, and its problems using those drugs to prevent HIV reproduction. Chapter 5 discusses the human immune system as it relates to HIV disease and the loss of the immune system's function. Chapter 6 presents the various opportunistic diseases, how they are affected by the use of retroviral therapy, and forms of cancer associated with HIV disease and AIDS. Chapter 7 discusses the clinical profile of biological indicators of HIV disease and AIDS. Chapter 8 presents the means by which HIV is most efficiently transmitted among humans. Chapter 9 details the most effective means to date of preventing HIV infection and the possibilities for a vaccine. Chapter 10 gives the incidence of HIV infections, HIV disease, and AIDS cases among selected behavioral at-risk persons for HIV infection **worldwide and in the United States.** Also, this chapter presents more detailed information on AIDS in Africa because no other place on Earth has been so devastated by this disease. Chapter 11 presents the prevalence and problems of HIV disease in women, children, and teenagers. Chapter 12 presents those tests most often used to detect the presence of HIV, biological shortcomings of the tests, the confidentiality or lack of confidentiality before and after test results, and costs. Chapter 13 offers insight to the many social ramifications of having HIV disease or AIDS, human attitudes, and behaviors. This chapter offers a section on the AIDS industry. It presents the billions of dollars spent on this disease by the federal government and private industry over the first 22 years of this pandemic. There is also a new section on financial waste and fraud. There is also a glossary of terms and index and a list of telephone numbers to federal, state, and other groups that offer information and help with all aspects of the HIV/AIDS pandemic.

SPECIAL FEATURES

Each chapter contains chapter concepts, a summary, review questions, and references. Answers to questions appear at the back of the book. Chapters also contain definitions for new terms as they are introduced, illustrations, photographs, and tables. All 13 chapters contain boxed information. **All of the chapters contain either highlighted points of view, points of information, cases in point, sidebars, side issues, looking back features, points to ponder and pro and con discussions.** They illustrate and emphasize important events and information about HIV infection, HIV disease, and AIDS. At certain places in the text, there are sets of class discussion statements and class questions. Instructors may wish to challenge the class in these areas.

ACCESS TO INFORMATION

Internet addresses, state HIV/AIDS hotlines, toll-free national HIV/AIDS information on prevention, therapy, health care providers, local and state programs relating to specific areas of research and funding, access to information on women, children, and teenage HIV/AIDS programs, and information on where to access materials on what HIV-infected parents may want to tell their children about their condition and the disease in general, can be found within and at the ends of most chapters.

TO THE EDUCATORS

As educators, it is our job to expose our students to the new concepts in biology that are shaping humanity's future. To do that, we must expose them to new vocabulary, new methodologies, new information and new ideas. It is my hope that this text will help in this endeavor.

IN APPRECIATION

The help of the following organizations or people is most deeply appreciated: The Centers for Disease Control and Prevention (CDC) Atlanta, for use of slides and literature produced in their *National Surveillance Report* and the *Morbidity and Mortality Weekly Report;* Mara Lavitt and *The New Haven*

Register for information on William Bluette; from the *Sun Sentinel* of Ft. Lauderdale, Florida, Director of photography, Jerry Lower, and photo archivist, Britt Head, for photographs out of the Caribbean; from the CDC, Richard Salik and Patricia Sweeney (Surveillance Branch); Robin Moseley, Patricia Fleming, Todd Webber (Division of HIV/AIDS Prevention); Barry Bennett, head of Retroviral Testing Services, for his permission and guidance on photographing HIV testing procedures at the Florida Health and Rehabilitation Office of Laboratories Services, Jacksonville, Florida; Denise Reddington, Department of Health and Human Services, Washington, DC; and PANOS Institute for their help in obtaining data on the economics of HIV/AIDS worldwide; personnel of the National Institute for Allergy and Infectious Diseases, the National Center for Health Statistics, Brookwood Center for Children with AIDS in New York; the George Washington AIDS Policy Center in Washington, DC; the National Institutes for Health; Hoffman-LaRoche Co., Abbott Laboratories, the Pharmaceutical Mfg. Association; the National Cancer Institute; Pan American Health Organization; and the Office of Technological Assessment; Teresa M. St. John, University of North Florida for illustrations; the individuals who have contributed photographs; the text reviewers whose work has been greatly appreciated; a special thank you to Rhonda Varner and Gilbertine Yadao who word processed the updated material; Guy Selander, M.D. and Jack Giddings, M.D., who, over the years, have shared their medical journals with me; James Alderman, Eileen Brady, Mary Davis, Signe Evans, Paul Mosley, Sarah Philips, Barbara Tuck, and Joe Tusing—reference/research librarians at the University of North Florida; and to my wife Delores who helped with proofreading and demonstrated a great deal of patience and understanding and gave up family weekends so the text could be completed on time.

This book has benefited from the critical evaluation of the following reviewers:

- ◆ Dr. Paul R. Elliott, Florida State University
- ◆ Dr. Robert Fulton, University of Minnesota
- ◆ Dr. Robert M. Kitchin, University of Wyoming
- ◆ Dr. Richard J. McCloskey, Boise State University
- ◆ Dr. William H. Fenn, Western Michigan University
- ◆ Dr. Michael Sulzinski, University of Scranton
- ◆ Dr. Judy Kaufman, Monroe Community College
- ◆ Dr. Seth Pincus, Montana State University
- ◆ Dr. Wayne B. Merkley, Drake University
- ◆ Dr. Linda L. Williford Pifer, University of Tennessee
- ◆ Dr. Bernard P. Sagik, Drexel University
- ◆ Professor James D. Slack, Cleveland State University
- ◆ Dr. Carl F. Ware, University of California, Riverside
- ◆ Dr. Phyllis K. Williams, Sinclair Community College
- ◆ Dr. Charles Wood, University of Kansas

Gerald J. Stine, Ph.D.
904-641-8979

"THE FACE OF AIDS"

The face AIDS wears is both many and one. The face of AIDS is women and men, children, youth, and adults. It is our sons and daughters, brothers and sisters, husbands and wives, mothers and fathers. Sometimes the face AIDS wears is that of a person without a home or a person in prison. Other times it's the face of a pregnant woman who is fearful she will pass HIV to her unborn child. Sometimes it's a baby or child who has no caregiver and little hope of adoption or being placed in foster care.

The faces of AIDS come from all walks of life. They represent all racial and ethnic groups, religious backgrounds, and countries of the world.

It is two boys, ages 10 and 12, caring for their mother, who is dying from AIDS. The boys get themselves off to school in the morning, make dinner for their mother after school, carry her to the tub to bathe her, softly towel dry her body, which is covered with sores, then help her into bed. How do you go to school and compete academically when your mother is home dying, your family is broke, and you are afraid to tell anyone about the problem?

It is a young gay man in Orange County, California, who is having difficulty breathing. At the local hospital, he is diagnosed with pneumocystic carinii pneumonia (one of the characteristic infections afflicting people with AIDS) and is told, "We don't take care of this kind of pneumonia here." Packed into a car for a six-hour drive to San Francisco, he's given an oxygen tank—only the oxygen runs out after four hours. Arriving at the emergency room at 2 A.M., in a city with no friends or family, he can barely breathe. Three months later he is dead.

It is a young woman who is knitting a scarf for her 2-year-old daughter. She said "I want to leave some legacy for her." She did not yet know her daughter was HIV positive and most likely would not live long enough to understand the legacy. Most likely the daughter would die before her mother.

It is an HIV-infected child born to a woman who is an injection drug user. With parents unable to care for her, hospitals too crowded to board her, and foster agencies unable to place her, no one knows where or how this child will endure what promises to be a brief, sickly life.

It is Maria, 26 and pregnant, who found out that she had AIDS while on a respirator for PCP. She died still muted by the plastic tubing that was her last lifeline. Or John, an artist, who had his life choked out of him by tonsilar lymphoma from one end, while intractable isospora diarrhea drained it away from the other. Or Kathy, who clung desperately to life in order to continue caring for her two children, the children who helplessly watched their mother waste away and die.

It is about a 25-year-old male who looks 40 less than a year after his AIDS diagnosis. When he first tested HIV positive, he decided to kill himself when his T4 cell count dropped to 100. When it did, he prepared his last meal, said goodbye to close friends, and bought a handgun. After dinner he put on his favorite cassette, raised the gun—but could not end his life. "What now" he asks. "This was my ace in the hole!"

It is a young man who lives in Miami, and he's not ready to come home. He wants to remain independent. Eventually he will come home. His family must be prepared to care for him and to deal with all the issues they will face. His mother is a high school teacher, but she has never told anyone about her son. She says that when he comes home it will be impossible to hide the fact that he has AIDS. "I am not sure how the community and our friends are going to respond."

The Face of AIDS Is Aging. In the United States about 13% of AIDS cases are among people over age 50. Beginning year 2003 that's about 110,000 people—30,000 are between ages 60 and 69 and about 5,000 are age 70 and older.

The Face of AIDS Is Changing. For 1997 through the year 2003 and beyond, the Face of AIDS, due to the successful use of AIDS drug cocktail therapy, takes on new and different looks—those of rejuvenation and of GUILT. Many who have recovered, even from their deathbeds, and feel "new" again, feel guilty because many are still dying and many do not have access to these drugs.

It is about establishing new relationships, giving up disability insurance, finding employment, and experiencing a life they thought they had lost.

It is THE FEAR THAT ALL THIS MAY BE JUST SHORT TERM—THAT THE VIRUS WILL WIN IN

THE END!—This is a Face of AIDS made possible because science has provided new drug therapies!

The Face of AIDS is surely around us. It is a disease that invites commentary, requires research, and demands intervention. Inevitably linking sex and death, passion and politics, it continues to generate controversy. Appearing as a new and lethal infectious disease, at a time when the biomedical establishment in the United States has shifted its focus to chronic disease, AIDS has called into question many of the premises of the biomedical profession.

TWENTIETH ANNIVERSARY OF AIDS PLUS TWO, JUNE 6, 2003

The AIDS crisis is not over, it has just begun. The statistics over the last 22 years numb one beyond comprehension. Who can understand the meaning of 43 million people throughout the world carrying the virus? Or that the rate of infection continues to explode throughout much of the world? It is only when people realize that by this anniversary 25 million people have died of AIDS or, that a 15-year old in South Africa has a 50:50 chance of dying of AIDS before the age of 30, that the horror begins to take on a human scale. The American perception of AIDS has gone through a cycle of meanings over the last two decades. In the early days there was no name for the disease; today we continue to ask how to cure it. In the early days there were major protests against the FDA and the medical and pharmaceutical companies. Today, there is quiet acceptance. The early demonstrators influenced basic research, the federal drug approval process, and the massive federal funding for a single disease. This disease as no other before it has changed the way people interact with their physicians, demand medical services, and take control of their own treatments regardless of illness. An entire generation has now been born that has never known an AIDS-free world. The disease has changed the personal as well as the political—how we think and how we love, what we teach our children and what words we say in public. More than anything else, AIDS has changed the way we view the threat of emerging diseases. Until AIDS, most of us thought of catastrophic plagues, like the Black Death and the Spanish flu epidemic of 1918, as things of the past. We lost sight of the fact that every once in awhile a new disease will emerge. It happened with HIV/AIDS and it can happen again. AIDS also changed what it means to be a patient. People with AIDS stormed scientific conferences, banded together in ways no other patients ever had, helped revolutionize the process of testing experimental drugs, and inspired others. There is no question that breast cancer activism started because of AIDS activism. Those with cancer saw its success and decided to emulate it, deploying thousands of people to lobby for increased research funding.

AIDS also changed what it means to be gay in America. The images of gay men dying of this disease rendered them objects of sympathy and opened the doors to compassion. In the eyes of straight America, death gave gay men a humanity they had long been denied. Homophobia, and attacks on gays, became a little less acceptable. Although some argue that AIDS divided gays—positives from negatives—it seems more likely that a united gay community was forged in the crucible of AIDS. People facing mortality responded courageously and seized the chance to proclaim their identity. And it forced society's institutions—from hospitals that barred gay men from seeing their dying lovers to employers that denied them bereavement leave—to recognize gay relationships. On June 25, 2001, the United Nations General Assembly convened a session on HIV/AIDS, the first ever devoted to a public health crisis. Delegates tried to agree on a global action plan, and grapple with how to fund it: $7 billion to $10 billion a year is needed to fight the spread of HIV. If lucky with prevention, treatment, and a vaccine, by 2021 AIDS will be killing 5 million people a year. If not, the toll could be 12 million. AIDS is 22 years young. The worst plague in modern history is far from finished with us. While searching for a vaccine, people die from AIDS or the drugs intended to treat it.

Introduction: Histories of Global Pandemics, World AIDS Conferences, Overview of HIV/AIDS, and the AIDS Quilt

THE NEW MILLENNIUM

Now into the third decade of AIDS, the disease HIV/AIDS remains a great challenge to public health, human rights, development, and national security. This is the first plague in the era of globalization! The figures are truly alarming—over the last four years, 1999 through 2003, about 25 million people became infected with HIV, bringing the total number of infections to about 70 million since the outbreak of this pandemic. While 95% of the cases are concentrated in developing countries, industrialized countries are experiencing about 90,000 new infections each year. Ending 2003, about 26 million people will have died from AIDS worldwide.

HIV/AIDS is devastating for the individual who may be infected, and its impact on communities and society at large is enormous. This disease disproportionately affects those population groups that are already vulnerable: children, women, the poor, the destitute, and millions of others whose life situations are further degraded by the denial of basic human rights. The majority of those infected are unable to afford the cost of effective health care. Individuals and communities are denied the opportunity to discuss the difficult issues surrounding HIV/AIDS, to organize themselves into self-help groups, and to take the necessary measures for protection from HIV infection. In an environment where human rights are not fully respected, the likelihood of vulnerability to infection and further exclusion increase dramatically. Clearly, political and economic solutions must be found if millions of lives are to be saved. Of all the promises the new millennium holds, of all the secrets it will tell, the cure for HIV disease will surely unfold among them.

DÉJÀ VU: A TIME OF AIDS

It was the best of times, it was the worst of times, it was the age of wisdom, it was the age of foolishness, it was the epoch of belief, it was the epoch of incredulity, it was the season of Light, it was the season of Darkness, it was the spring of hope, it was the winter of despair . . .

Charles Dickens, *A Tale of Two Cities*

Nothing in recent history has so challenged our reliance on modern science nor emphasized our vulnerability before nature. We have lived with the Acquired Immune Deficiency Syndrome (**AIDS**) epidemic, witnessing its paradoxes every day. People living with the Human Immunodeficiency Virus (**HIV**) live with the fear, pain, and uncertainty of the disease; they also endure prejudice, scorn, rejection, and despair. **This must change!**

HISTORY OF GLOBAL EPIDEMICS

There has never been a time in human history when disease did not exist. The history of epidemics dates at least as far back as 1157 BC to the

---

LOOKING BACK I.1

June 1981—Twenty years ago, a report written by UCLA scientist **Michael Gottlieb** and published by the Center for Disease Control and Prevention alerted physicians to an unusual constellation of fungal infections and pneumonia in otherwise healthy young gay men. The condition was later named the Acquired Immune Deficiency Syndrome (AIDS). Activists took to the streets and convinced a skeptical public that AIDS was a deadly crisis.

INFECTIOUS DISEASE PARADIGM

WARS

Although death in battle is the most obvious form of war-related mortality, in many eras the deadliest killer was not the opposing army but epidemics. Throughout history where armies go disease has followed. Much of military history is actually the story of how battles and campaigns correlated with diseases occurring in both the military and the civilian populations. Indeed, medieval and early modern history is a continuing chronicle of the cycle of invasions and epidemics. In the late 18th and early 19th centuries, Napoleon faced his greatest resistance not from the British navy but from microorganisms. French forces were routed in Syria and Egypt by plague. Of Napoleon's wars, his Russian campaign stands out as a classic example of devastation by disease. Of the 600,000 soldiers who left France, 70% succumbed to typhus before they reached Moscow. Russian delaying tactics allowed typhus to ravage the remainder. Thus, Napoleon was left with only 50,000 soldiers to occupy Russia. After the winter killed still more troops, only 3,000 returned to France. During the American Civil War (1861–1865), the vast majority of deaths on both sides were due to disease. Prison camps like Andersonville were notorious for the prevalence of disease; incarceration was a virtual death sentence.

SOCIETY IN GENERAL

Most new infections are **not** caused by truly new pathogens. They are caused by microorganisms (bacteria, fungi, protozoa, and helminths) and viruses that have been present for hundreds or thousands of years, but they are newly recognized and named because of recently developed techniques to identify them. Human activities drive the emergence of disease and a variety of social, economic, political, cultural, climatic, technological, and environmental factors can shape the pattern of a disease and influence its emergence into populations. For example, travel can greatly affect the emergence of disease and human migrations have been the main source of epidemics throughout history. Trade caravans, religious pilgrimages, and military campaigns facilitated the speed of plague, smallpox, cholera, and now AIDS. Global travel is a fact of modern life and, equally so, the continued evolution of microorganisms and viruses; therefore, seemingly new infections will continue to emerge, and known infections will change in distribution, frequency, and severity.

DISEASES CAUSED BY VIRUSES AND MICROORGANISMS HAVE HAD 3 BILLION YEARS TO EVOLVE—WE SHOULD NOT EXPECT TO CONQUER THEM EASILY!

death of the Egyptian pharaoh, Ramses V, from smallpox. Over the centuries, this extraordinarily contagious virus spread around the world, changing the course of history time and again. It killed 2000 Romans a day in the 2nd century AD, more than 2 million Aztecs during the 1520 conquest by Cortez, and some 600,000 Europeans a year from the 16th through the 18th centuries. Three out of four people who survived the high fever, convulsions, and painful rash were left deeply scarred and sometimes blind. Because victims' skin looked as if it had been scalded, smallpox was known as the **"invisible fire."** Even now, malaria in underdeveloped countries afflicts 300 million people, killing between 2 and 3 million each year. The problem is compounded by development of drug-resistant malarial strains of protozoa. **Thus**

epidemics are not new to humankind, but the fear they impose on each generation is.

Major recorded pandemics (global) and epidemics (regional) that have devastated large populations are described in Table I-1.

EMERGING DISEASES

The 1970s witnessed the emergence of Lyme disease (1975), Legionnaires disease (1976), and Toxic Shock Syndrome (1978). In the 1980s, HIV and three new human herpes viruses (HHV 6, 7, and 8) were identified. In 1994, a physician in Gallup, New Mexico, was called to care for a man who had collapsed at a funeral. Soon, several others in New Mexico had also suffered from sudden respiratory failure.

Table I-1   Plagues in History[1]

Disease	Dates	Place	Number Killed		Causative Organism	Time to Prevention/Cure (in years)
Measles	from 430 BC	Greece/Rome/World	Millions		Paramyxovirus	1,712
Plague	542–1894	Europe/Asia/Africa	7100 million		Yersinia pestis	580
Cholera	1826–1837	New Jersey	900,000		Vibrio cholerae	75
	1849	United Kingdom	53,293			
	1947	Egypt	11,755			
Tuberculosis	1930–1949	United States	1,000,000		Mycobacterium tuberculosis	85
	1954–1970		150,000			
Malaria	1847–1875	Africa/India	20 million+		Plasmodia	100
Scarlet Fever	1861–1870	United Kingdom	972 per million people		Streptococcus pyogenes	45–44
Polio	1921–1970	North America	37,000		Polio viruses Types I, II, III	30–50
Typhus	1917–1921	Russia	2,500,000		Rickettsias	25
Influenza	1918–1919	U.S./Europe	21,640,000		Influenza virus	57
Smallpox	from 1122 BC	Europe (middle ages)	Hundreds of millions		Smallpox virus	3,050
	1926–1930	India	423,000			
Gonorrhea	from 590 BC				Neisseria gonorrhoeae	1,832
	1921–1992	United States	57,477			
Yellow Fever	from AD				Arbovirus	488
	1986–1988	Nigeria	10,000			
HIV/AIDS[2]			*Deaths*	*HIV Infections*	Human	Treatments but no cure
	1981–2003	United States (estimated)[3]	495,000	1,445,000	Immunodeficiency Virus	
	1981–2003	Global (estimated)	26,000,000	70,000,000		

1. Historical time line on first suspected cases of the above diseases are: Plague, 11th century BC; Cholera, 1781; Tuberculosis, 451 BC; Malaria, 1748; Scarlet Fever, 1735; Polio, 1894; Typhus, 1083; Influenza, 1580; Smallpox, 429 BC; Gonorrhea, 1768; Yellow Fever, 1647; HIV/AIDS, United States in the 1970s; in Africa, 1959.

2. Total AIDS data estimated through year 2003. Living in some state of HIV disease (10 million living with AIDS + 34 million with HIV disease = 44 million people living with HIV infection + 26 million dead = 70 million total HIV infections worldwide).

3. United States: of the estimated HIV infections, about 34% or 495,000 will have died through 2003.

As victims contracted the disease, they went from seemingly perfect health to flu-like symptoms, to a horrific state where their lungs began to fill with blood. Most of them died.

Within a few weeks, the Centers for Disease Control and Prevention identified this killer: **hantavirus**—a rodent-borne organism that had infected many GIs during the Korean War and killed hundreds. But the Korean type of hantavirus causes death through kidney failure. Somehow the hantavirus had found its way to the United States and mutated (changed) into a virus that invades the lungs.

The outbreak of hantavirus in America occurred in May 1993, first in Arizona, Colorado, New Mexico, and Utah. Beginning year 2003, 336 people have been infected in 31 states with the rodent-borne deermouse virus and 124 of these people have died of acute respiratory distress. (There is no vaccine for this virus.) In mid-1994 there was an outbreak of **necrotizing fasciitis** (fash-e-i-tis)—tissue destruction caused by a tissue-invasive strain of Group A streptococcus, a bacterium. This bacterium is a deadly variant strain of the Group A streptococcus that causes strep throat. The infected may die from bacterial shock, disseminated blood coagulation (clotting), or respiratory or renal (kidney) failure. Also, in September of 1994, health authorities in Brisbane, Australia, were suddenly confronted with 11 dead horses and the death of their trainer. The killing agent was identified within two weeks. It is a new virus called **equine morbillivirus** that causes a fatal respiratory disease. Although nonhuman morbilliviruses have been associated with new and emerging animal diseases, no new human morbillivirus has been reported since the 10th century, when measles was described [Cause of fatal outbreak in horses and humans traced. (1995). *Science*, 268 (32): 94–97]. Overall the virus has killed 13 of 25 infected horses and one of the two humans who became infected. This outbreak is an isolated event; no additional infections have been identified. The virus in this case was eliminated by the death of the infected. **But where did the virus come from? Where will it show up next and under what conditions?** The natural host of the virus has not been identified. This virus causes the cells lining the blood vessels to clump, creating holes in the vessel walls that allow fluid leakage into the lungs. The horses and the human drowned in their own fluids.

Although emerging viruses may contain new mutations or represent gradual evolution, more often they emerge because of changes in human behavior or the environment whereby they are introduced to a new host. Viruses that are pathogenic in human and nonhuman hosts include Marburg and Ebola viruses; hantaviruses; human immunodeficiency virus; Lassa virus; dolphin, porpoise, and seal morbilliviruses; feline immunodeficiency virus; and bovine spongiform encephalopathy agent, which from 1996 through 2001 has threatened the possible destruction of the entire cow population of Europe causing economic loss of billions of dollars and a major unemployment problem. And, there are the **rotaviruses.** Rotaviruses are detected in 20% to 70% of fecal specimens from children hospitalized with acute diarrhea, and in developing countries they cause about 870,000 deaths each year. Even in the United States, rotavirus is associated with 3% of all hospitalizations of children younger than 5 years old, which translates to 55,000 to 70,000 hospitalizations per year, with medical and indirect costs in excess of $1 billion. Efforts to prevent disease by improving water or sanitation seem unlikely to succeed because all children in developed and developing countries become infected with rotavirus in the first three to five years of life.

Some 30 newly identified disease-causing agents have emerged over the past 25 years, and six old diseases are reemerging: TB, diphtheria, cholera, dengue fever, yellow fever, and bubonic plague.

Cases of **dengue** or **breakbone** fever have been recognized for over 200 years. Diseases caused by the dengue virus, such as dengue and dengue hemorrhagic fever (DHF), are a greater burden to human health than **any other mosquito-borne viral disease.** About two-thirds of the world's population live in environments where DHF is either endemic or epidemic, **and an estimated 80 million persons are infected with dengue virus each year.** The nature of dengue epidemics has changed considerably during this century. Where classic dengue was once the norm, we are now witnessing epidemics that affect larger numbers of people and produce more severe symptoms of the disease. This is particularly evident in the Americas, where the disease has made dramatic inroads during the past two decades. In contrast, the virus that causes **hepatitis C** (HCV) was identified in 1989. An effective blood screen for it was in use by 1992. It is estimated that 4 million Americans, 9 million Europeans, and about 200 million people worldwide are infected with hepatitis C, marking an epidemic much larger than HIV. About 70% of infected people eventually develop a chronic liver disease. There are an estimated 30,000 new infections annually in the United States, with 10,000 **deaths** attributed to the virus. These numbers are expected to triple over the next 10 years. **Hepatitis C is an incurable, bloodborne virus that can cause irreparable liver damage—it is the leading cause for liver transplant in America.** It has an extended latency period, and symptoms are not manifested until the disease has advanced, making treatment difficult. Currently, the only treatment for HVC infection is the use of interferon, which has many side effects, although clinical trials are underway for other possible treatments.

The fact that so many infectious diseases remain out of control represents a shared failure—of individuals, health care providers, communities, industry, and governments worldwide.

The world is not becoming a safer place in which to live. More people are crowding into cities and humans continue to intrude into once remote areas. Clearly some diseases are more lethal than others and AIDS may be the most lethal of all "new" diseases to strike humans in the 20th and 21st centuries.

SILENT TRAVELERS

First Recognition of an Infectious Disease

In 1773, Charles White, an English surgeon and obstetrician, published his "Treatise on the Management of Pregnant and Lying-In Women." In it he appealed for surgical cleanliness to combat childbed or puerperal fever. (**Puerperal fever** is an acute life threatening condition that may follow childbirth. Its cause, at this time in history, was unknown.) In 1795, Alexander Gordon, a Scottish obstetrician, published his "Treatise on the Epidemic Puerperal Fever of Aberdeen," which demonstrated for the first time that the disease was contagious. In 1843, Oliver Wendell Holmes, a noted American physician, published a paper entitled "On the Contagiousness of Puerperal Fever." In the paper he appealed for surgical cleanliness to stop the spread of this disease.

However, the first person to realize that a pathogen could be transmitted from one person to another was the Hungarian physician Ignaz Phillip Semmelweis. Between 1847 and 1849, Semmelweis observed that women who had their babies at the hospital with the help of the medical staff were four times more likely to contract puerperal fever than those who gave birth with the help of midwives outside the hospital. He concluded that the physicians were infecting women with material remaining on their hands after autopsies and other hospital activities. Semmelweis thus began washing his hands with a calcium chloride solution before examining patients or delivering babies. This simple procedure of hand washing led to a dramatic decrease in the number of cases of puerperal fever and saved the lives of many women. Hand washing remains basic to medical procedures in medical establishments and restaurants in developed nations.

The Importance of Infectious Diseases: Up Then Down and Up Again

In the early 1900s there were thousands of typhoid fever cases, and many people died of the disease. Most of these cases arose when people drank water contaminated with sewage or ate food handled by or prepared by individuals who were, unknowingly, shedding the typhoid fever bacterium, *Salmonella typhi*. An interesting case of one person spreading typhoid fever occurred between 1896 and 1906 in New York City. Mary Mallon was infected but did not become ill—she just carried and shed the bacterium. She worked as a cook in seven homes in New York City. Twenty-eight cases of typhoid fever occurred in these homes while she worked in them. As a result, the New York City Health Department had Mary arrested and admitted to an isolation hospital on North Brother Island in New York's East River. Examination of Mary's stools showed that she was shedding large numbers of the typhoid bacteria. An article published in 1908 in the *Journal of the American Medical Association* referred to her as "Typhoid Mary," an epithet by which she is still known today. Upon being released, she pledged not to cook for others or serve food to them, but Mary changed her name and began to work as a cook again. For five years she managed to avoid capture while continuing to spread typhoid fever.

Eventually the authorities tracked her down. She was held in custody for 23 years until she died in 1938. As a lifetime carrier, Mary was positively linked with 10 outbreaks of typhoid fever, 53 cases, and 3 deaths.

In 1962, Sir MacFarlane Burnet, the 1960 Nobel Prize recipient for his work on immunological tolerance, wrote, ". . . one can think of the middle of the 20th century as the end of one of the most important social events in history, **THE VIRTUAL ELIMINATION OF THE INFECTIOUS DISEASE AS A SIGNIFICANT FACTOR IN SOCIAL LIFE.**" This statement represents the complacency that developed in the United States and some other countries in regard to threats to the human race posed by the microbial world. More recently, Joshua Lederberg, president of the Rockefeller University from 1978 to 1990, wrote, "The ravaging epidemic of AIDS has shocked the world . . . **We will face similar catastrophes again** . . . We have too many illusions that we can . . . govern the remaining vital kingdoms, the microbes, that remain our competitors of last resort for domination of the planet." This statement represents a more realistic assessment of the current situation, by recognizing the fact that improvements in sanitation and introduction of antimicrobial agents and vaccines **have failed to eliminate the health risks from exposure to infectious agents.**

Infectious disease, meanwhile, has climbed to the third leading cause of death in the United States. Worldwide, infectious diseases account for 25% of the 54 million global deaths per year and are the leading cause of death among children.

Since the 1980s, we have come to view infectious diseases with a humbler eye. The victories of a quarter century ago ring hollow as AIDS ravages, disease-causing bacteria become resistant to all standard treatments, and the once easily treated pneumococcus demonstrates antimicrobial drug resistance. Unknown diseases develop with uncomforting frequency, and the Ebola virus has been identified outside the confines of Zaire. Once considered unique and isolated, these events penetrate every corner of the globe. As was recognized in 1892 when the first international sanitary convention on cholera was adopted, infectious diseases cannot be observed, battled, or understood street by street or country by country. A global approach is necessary [WINKER, M.A., et al. (1996). Infectious diseases: a global approach to a global problem. *JAMA*, 275:245–246].

Far from being invulnerable, humans are in fact at the mercy of innumerable microscopic agents that can erupt at any time by mutating (changing) into a virulent form, crossing a species barrier, escaping from an environmental niche, or from bioterrorism.

There have been some great achievements in the battle against these microbes. Yet the only complete victory over any infectious disease so far has been the eradication of smallpox. However, one of the achievements of this millennium will be the global eradication of poliomyelitis by the end of the year 2002, a new target date set by the World Health Organization.

VIRUS ASSOCIATED WITH CANCERS AND OTHER KNOWN DISEASES

In the mid- to late 1980s, numerous correlations were discovered between viruses and various types of cancers. For example, Epstein-Barr virus was associated with nasopharyngeal carcinoma and B-cell lymphoma, hepatitis B virus with liver cancer, and human papillomavirus with cervical cancer. Now, a decade later, scientists are finding out that viruses may also play a role in an array of other diseases, like atherosclerosis, diabetes, certain cancers, Alzheimer's disease, and even neuropsychiatric disorders such as schizophrenia. Additional connections will be made between viruses and many types of diseases in the future because virologists are turning their attention more and more to diseases to which there is no known cause.

FEAR AND IGNORANCE ABOUT AIDS AND OTHER PANDEMICS

The Black Plague during its most destructive time killed over 500 people a day. Instead of being concerned about providing care to the victims, people spent their time deciding how deep to dig the graves so that none of the horrid fumes would come up and infect others. It was determined that a grave should be six feet deep; and that is exactly how deep it is today. Plague victims were herded together into cathedrals to die or to pray for faith healing to save them. In 14th century Germany and Switzerland, the Christians blamed the Jews for the outbreak of bubonic plague, believing that the Jews were poisoning

BOX I.1

OTHER LETHAL VIRUSES IN OUR TIME

Richard Preston, in his 1994 book *The Hot Zone* describes the progression of illness as the Ebola virus kills humans:

Ebola . . . triggers a creeping, spotty necrosis that spreads through all the internal organs. The liver bulges up and turns yellow, begins to liquefy, and then it cracks apart. . . . The kidneys become jammed with blood clots and dead cells, and cease functioning. As the kidneys fail, the blood becomes toxic with urine. The spleen turns into a single huge, hard blood clot the size of a baseball. The intestines may fill completely with blood. The lining of the gut dies and sloughs off into the bowels and is defecated along with large amounts of blood.

The Ebola virus resists all drug therapy to date and kills up to 80% or more of those infected within one to three weeks after infection. (HIV kills over 90%—it is slower but more lethal.)

HISTORY

There have been nine confirmed outbreaks of Ebola. The first was in 1976 when Belgian doctors discovered the virus at a hospital in northern Zaire; it was named Ebola Zaire after the Zairian river flowing through the region. In December 2001, it struck in Gabon and in the Republic of Congo. Each time the virus quickly ran its course of human destruction and disappeared. Beginning 2003, there were 1443 confirmed cases of Ebola infection that have caused 750 deaths. In 1989, a strain of Ebola virus appeared in Reston, Virginia, just a short distance from Washington, DC. One hundred monkeys had arrived at the Reston Primate Quarantine Unit from the coastal forests of the Philippines on October 4. Two monkeys were dead on arrival and 10 more died during the next few days. Their tests proved positive for Ebola Zaire. The investigation quickly became a potentially volatile political crisis. The quarantine unit was a hot zone containing an organism classified as "biosafety level four": one for which no cure or vaccine existed.

In what has to be considered as an EXTRAORDINARY PIECE OF LUCK, this strain of Ebola virus, even though it appeared identical to the lethal form of Ebola Zaire, was harmless to humans. Because the viruses appeared to be spread among the monkeys via the air, if that virus was the lethal form of Ebola, the consequences for this heavily populated area of the Eastern Coast would have been unimaginably horrific.

Class Discussion: In what ways would the entire United States and other countries have been affected?

SOME OTHER LETHAL VIRUSES THAT INFECT HUMANS

Ebola is just one of a number of viruses to have emerged from the jungle in the past few decades; others include **Lassa** and **Marburg** viruses in Africa; **Sabía, Junin,** and **Machupo** viruses in South America. In 1995 a virus, yet to be named, was found, in Brazil, to cause lung destruction and death. HIV probably originated in Africa, but unlike Ebola, it is ideally suited to spread around the globe. The HIV-infected can remain symptom-free for years, which provides the opportunity for them to infect others.

WEST NILE VIRUS A virus never seen before in America, the **West Nile-like encephalitis (brain inflammation) virus**, was identified after infecting 61 humans and causing the deaths of seven people and about two-thirds of the crows in and around New York City during the summer of 1999. This virus has now been found in over 40 mosquito species and in some 120 species of birds ranging from robins to broad-winged hawks that migrate long distances. An outbreak of this virus has occurred simultaneously in Russia. Reasons for the spread of this virus out of Africa are unknown at this time. From 1999 through the year of 2002, the virus spread from Canada down the East coast to the Florida Keys, from the Atlantic coast going West passing the Rocky Mountains. Through 2002, the virus had spread to 44 states and Washington D.C., killing at least 140 more people and newly infecting about 3,000. Twenty-three states have registered one or more deaths due to this virus. In 2002, the state of Louisiana had 14 deaths and 316 infected, Mississippi had 46 newly infected, and Texas had 33. Twenty-seven died and 466 were infected in Illinois. These four states had a total of at least 800 newly-infected people in 2002. For about 30% of the infected, the virus offers a life-threatening experience. This virus is expected to cross the United States by year 2004.

BOX I.1 *(continued)*

Are there other viruses as dangerous as HIV— or even more dangerous—lurking on the edge of civilization? That is the question that haunts public health officials. Scientists have identified over 200 viruses capable of causing human disease at some level and they believe there may be 5 to 10 times that many still to be identified!

[HORTON, RICHARD. (1995). *Infection: The Global Threat.* New York: Reviews April 6, 24–28.]

CLASS QUESTION: Should the public be informed about the dangers of research on viruses lethal to humans before it is allowed to begin? to continue?

the water—the very same water that the Jews were drinking. As a result, entire communities of Jews were slaughtered. In the 1400s and 1500s, when syphilis was spreading across the world killing thousands, the Italians called it the French disease. Of course, the French called it the Italian disease. In the 1930s, cholera was considered a punishment for people unwilling to change their lives—the poor and the immoral. In New York the Irish were blamed. In the early 20th century, polio in America was believed to be caused by Italian immigrants.

The history of epidemics teaches us, again and again, that blame is a central component of these events, whether it is cast upon socially ostracized groups of people, water supplies, politics, or religious or cultural beliefs. The 16th-century rise of Protestantism, especially Calvinism, increased public intolerance toward the ill. Victims of syphilis were condemned as targets of God's wrath and were ignored by many medical and charitable institutions. Religious artists often depicted Jesus striking down the unjust, raining murderous arrows down from heaven upon syphilis and those who suffered from bubonic plague. It was during this early modern period that the notion of "guilty" and "innocent" victims of disease arose.

The fear of HIV infection and the ignorance about its causes have also created bizarre behavior and at times barbaric practices, strange rituals, and attempts to isolate those afflicted.

Deaths from Disease

Measles, Plague, Smallpox, Polio, Influenza, Tuberculosis, Hepatitis B, and Malaria— These diseases are responsible for many hundreds of millions of human deaths throughout history.

The population of the indigenous Indians of Central and South America dropped from an estimated 130 million to about 1.6 million, more as a result of measles and plague than from war. In the 19th century measles has been held responsible for the total annihilation of the Indian population of the island of Tierra del Fuego. Plague swept through Europe in the 14th century destroying a quarter of Europe's population. Between 1600 and 1650 the population of Italy actually fell from 13.1 million to 11.4 million. In Venice, an average of 600 bodies were collected daily on barges. More than 50,000 Venetians died in the plague of 1630–1631, leaving a population smaller than at any time during the 15th century. Recent outbreaks of bubonic plague occurred in India in August of 1994, in Mozambique in June of 1997 and in Uganda in November 1998.

The smallpox and polio viruses may well go back to the early beginnings of humans but would have mostly been concealed by the enhanced susceptibility of those infected to more common (or more recognizable) infections. Childhood leukemia, apparently newly emergent in the 1950s, was similarly an artifact of the widespread use of antibiotics for the treatment of the infections from which leukemic people previously died.

Worldwide, smallpox killed over 100 million people by 1725. **Smallpox is the only viral disease ever eradicated.** The smallpox death of Egyptian pharaoh Ramses V in 1157 BC is the first known. Invading armies then spread smallpox through Africa and Europe. The Spanish brought it to Mexico. Edward Jenner used a cowpox pustular material from a cow named **Blossom** to create a vaccine against small pox in the 1870s. Only humans got smallpox. It disappeared after a global vaccination campaign in the 1960s. The last known natural case was in Somalia in 1977.

AMERICA ATTACKED BY TERRORISTS

Shortly after foreign terrorists destroyed the World Trade Center towers in New York City on September 11, 2001, the United States Postal Service, a newspaper office in Florida, and several government buildings in Washington, D.C., received Bacillus anthracis-(which causes anthrax) laden mail from bioterrorists. Eleven infected people were placed on antibiotics, but five died of anthrax, and several buildings were quarantined and had to be disinfected. The loss of life this time was limited to four people. Vaccine production against Bacillus anthracis received a high priority. What infectious agent may be used next time? The overwhelming choice, according to medical bioterrorism experts, is the dissemination of the smallpox virus. Sufficient smallpox virus vaccine is being produced to inoculate every person in the United States should it become necessary. Problem: telling bioterrorists we now have sufficient vaccine against smallpox only means they will select another infectious agent. And as discussed in this introduction, there are many to choose from.

Influenza— Each year as winter approaches, about 70 million shots of influenza (flu) vaccine are given, mainly to people who are especially susceptible to the virus (the very young, the elderly, asthmatics, and diabetics). Each year in the United States, from 20 million to 50 million people contract the flu, and between 10,000 and 40,000 (in a bad year) die from it! The vaccine is a cocktail of recent influenza A and B strains and affords some protection against genetic changes in these strains. Nevertheless, in recent history many thousands have died from influenza infection; in the 1957–1958 epidemic, for instance, 1 in 300 over age 65 died. Influenza was first described by Hippocrates in 412 BC. The first well-described flu pandemic occurred in 1580. Thirty-one flu pandemics have occured since then. In 1890, in China, the duck-borne flu virus crossed over into swine, then into humans, causing thousands of deaths. This epidemic was followed by **severe flu pandemics** in 1900, 1918 (the Spanish flu), 1957 (the Asian flu), 1968 (the Hong Kong flu), and in 1977 (the Russian flu). The flu pandemic of 1918 has recently been estimated to have caused about 100 million deaths worldwide. (See *Flu: The Story of the Great Influenza Pandemic of 1918*, Gina Kolata, 1999.) This virus was antigenically similar to the swine virus and it appears to have disappeared from the human population following the 1918–1919 pandemic. This virus is, however, still carried in the swine population with an occasional crossover into humans without person-to-person transmission. Why such widespread transmission of the swine virus among humans has not reoccurred is not known—and that in itself is fearful! It could happen again, even though there is a vaccine. The current theory from the Armed Forces Institute of Pathology on where the 1918 flu virus originated is: The virus most likely traveled **back and forth** between pigs and people until there was a single mutation or a sufficient number of lesser mutations that allowed the virus to cause a serious disease in humans and pigs!

UNITED STATES 1918, America was caught up in the last year of World War I. Deadly influenza, the so-called "Spanish flu," was sweeping the country, spreading terror everywhere. The first documented deaths were in Boston. Explanations were offered, but in fact no one had an answer. Viruses were still largely unknown. That particular strain of flu virus is still one of the mysteries of the 1918 pandemic. Once started, the disease moved west in lethal waves that appeared to follow railroad lines. The speed with which it killed was appalling, the loss of life unimaginable. The pandemic took 675,000 lives in just a few months! It would be as if today, with our present population, more than 1,400,000 people were to die in a sudden outbreak for which there was no explanation and no known cure. It was said every family lost someone. **Time wise,** this is the worst epidemic/pandemic America has ever known. It killed more Americans than all the wars of this century combined. There were so many people dying from the flu that communities nationwide were running out of caskets.

WHERE DID THE FLU PANDEMIC BEGIN? Some people believe that 1918 pandemic began in the spring of 1918, when soldiers at Fort Riley, Kansas, burned tons of manure. A gale kicked up. A choking dust storm swept out over the land—a stinging, stinking yellow haze. The sun went black in Kansas. Two days later—on March 11, 1918—an Army private reported to the camp hospital before breakfast. He had a fever, sore throat, headache—nothing serious. A minute later, another soldier showed up. By noon, the hospital had over 100 cases; in a week, 500. That spring, 48 soldiers died at Fort Riley. The cause of death was listed as pneumonia. The sickness then seemed to disappear—leaving as quickly as it had come. That same summer and fall, over 1.5 million Americans crossed the Atlantic for war. Some of those soldiers came from Kansas, and it is believed that they carried the virus with them. Almost immediately, the Kansas sickness resurfaced in Europe. American, English, French, and German soldiers became ill. As the sickness spread, it appeared to get worse. By the time the disease came back to America, it was a deadly killer.

On a rainy day in September, Dr. Victor Vaughan, acting Surgeon General of the Army, received urgent orders: Proceed to a base near Boston called Camp Devens. On the day that Vaughan arrived, 63 men died at Camp Devens. An autopsy revealed lungs that were swollen, filled with fluid, and strangely blue. Doctors were stunned. When the strange new disease was finally identified, it turned out to be a very old and familiar one: influenza, the flu. But, it was unlike any flu that anyone had ever seen.

During the epidemic of 1918, all San Francisco citizens were required to wear masks. One form of therapy was "cabbage baths." People did not jump into a tub with some cooked cabbage; they ate the cabbage and urinated into the tub. The flu victims then got into the tub. There may have been a positive side to the bath because once you got out, a distance was created between you and other people. In this way, the baths may have helped stop person-to-person transmission. [Researchers seek new weapon against flu. (1997). *Science*, 275:756; Influenza 1994–1995: Now's the time to prepare. (1994). *J. Resp. Dis.*, 15: 675].

In 1998, over 1 million chickens, ducks, and geese were gassed to death in the first week of January in Hong Kong in an effort to stop the "bird flu" virus before it spread beyond the boundary of Hong Kong. The new strain of influenza type A virus was isolated from a dead three-year-old boy in Hong Kong in May 1997. CDC scientists are investigating how this virus made the huge species jump from chickens into humans. By the end of January 1998, 21 cases were confirmed and 6 people died of this flu.

Tuberculosis, Hepatitis B, and Malaria— In 1937, 112,000 Americans contracted tuberculosis and 70,000 died. About **1 billion** people worldwide have died from Mycobacterium tuberculosis (a bacterium 1/25,000th of an inch long) since 1770. **Over 100 million people will have died of TB from 1990 through the year 2002!** One in three people worldwide carry this organism! Currently, about 10 million people in the United States are infected with TB, but only 5% develop the disease. In 1997, over 2 million adults worldwide died of hepatitis B and of the 44 million children who contracted measles, 1.5 million died. Five to six thousand people die every day from malaria. **Despite over 50 years of global experience in malaria control, more people are dying of malaria now than when malaria control campaigns began! Malaria, like all of the major infectious diseases, is a disease of poverty.** Parents and children quietly cope; the ill were and are served, not shunned—that is, until the HIV/AIDS epidemic.

AIDS: ITS PLACE IN HISTORY

As the statistics on AIDS cases mounted, its identity as an inescapable plague seemed confirmed. It appeared to mimic the frightening epidemics of the past: cholera, yellow fever, leprosy, syphilis, and the plague or Black Death. The history of AIDS—the history that seemed relevant to understanding the new pandemic—would be the history of the epidemics of the past. Medical history suddenly gained new social relevance; policy analysts, lawyers, and journalists all wanted to know whether past epidemics could provide some clues to the current crisis. How had societies attempted to deal with epidemics in the past? The contemporary meaning of past plagues is read in the face of AIDS.

THE AIDS PANDEMIC IS CERTAINLY ONE OF THE DEFINING EVENTS OF OUR TIME. There are stories to be told from it, stories of the people infected and affected by it—the well, the ill, the dying, and the survivors. There are the stories of scientific discovery, of HIV and viral mechanisms, and of genetic mysteries being understood. Then there are stories of scientific politics, claims and counterclaims, and the manipulating that goes on in the stratosphere of high-level science.

"A third of the world died," wrote Jean Froissart at the end of the 14th century, when medieval medicine had little to offer against the Black Death. Now, at the beginning of the 21st century, we see modern science registering its progress about a plague of our own time.

AIDS was identified on planet earth just 22 years ago and it is now the leading killer among all known infectious diseases. AIDS is ranked fourth among all microbial causes of death.

AIDS is the most dramatic, pervasive, and tragic pandemic in recent history. So deep an impression has the AIDS epidemic made on public perceptions that according to a recent Louis Harris poll, almost 30% of the population believes that the "greatest threat to human life" is AIDS or some other kind of plague.

THE HIV/AIDS PANDEMIC CONSISTS OF TWO PARTS: ONE MEDICAL, THE OTHER SOCIAL. HIV/AIDS infection has provoked a reassessment of society's approaches to public health strategy, health care resource allocation, medical research, and sexual behavior. Fear and discrimination have affected virtually every aspect of our culture. Both the medical challenge and, in particular, the social challenge will continue in the foreseeable future. **Arthur Ashe,** a world-class tennis player, so feared discrimination against himself and family that he lived with AIDS for 3 1/2 years before he was forced to reveal he had the disease (Figure I-1).

OVERVIEW ON HIV/AIDS

AIDS: A Big Disease with a Little Name

The global numbers of people who are HIV infected along with those who have died from AIDS is almost incomprehensible and very difficult to express. The numbers are too large to grasp and the implications too terrifying to contemplate. In addition, at this time the future appears grim: **First,** there is no near-term prospect of a vaccine. **Second,** existing drug therapies, though relatively effective, are too expensive for the vast majority of those infected, and **third,** those preventive interventions that can be effective in reducing the numbers of people becoming infected annually are not in place, in countries most in need, because the majority of the infected are undereducated and their countries still lack the infrastructure to deal with many infectious diseases including AIDS!

FIGURE I-1 Arthur Ashe—Winner of Two U.S. Tennis Championships. On April 8, 1992, Ashe announced that he had AIDS. He died on February 6, 1993, at age 49. He became infected with HIV from a blood transfusion during heart bypass surgery in 1983. In 1988, his right hand suddenly became numb. Brain surgery revealed a brain abscess caused by toxoplasmosis. He asked two questions, **"Why do bad things happen to good people?"** and **"Is the world a friendly place?"** Ashe was the U.S. Davis Cup Captain for five years and supported the NCAA Proposition 42 academic requirements for athletes. In 1975 he became the first black to win a Wimbledon men's title. After learning that he had AIDS, Ashe completed his third book, *A Road to Glory*, a three-volume history of black athletes in the United States. *(Photograph courtesy of AP/Wide World Photos)*

What Is AIDS?

AIDS is defined primarily by severe immune deficiency, and is distinguished from virtually every other disease in history by the fact that it has no constant, specific symptoms. Once the immune system has begun to malfunction, a broad spectrum of health complications can set in. AIDS is an umbrella term for any or all of some 27 known diseases and symptoms. When a person has any of these diseases or has a CD4 or T4 lymphocyte count of less than $200/\mu L$ (microliter) of blood and also tests positive for antibodies to HIV, an AIDS diagnosis is given.

AIDS: A Human Affair

The history of AIDS is a human affair and is part of a cultural process of attempting to come to terms with a new and often terrifying series of events—of young people dying before their time, of the intermingling of sex and death—in a period in which the world itself is changing before our eyes.

The social meaning of the history of AIDS intimately touches upon ideas about sexuality, social responsibility, individual privacy, health, and the prospect of living a normal life span. Understanding how to respond to AIDS and how to think about this pandemic is important not only for what it reveals about the ways in which health policy is created in the United States and elsewhere, but also for what it implies about the human ability to meet the challenge of future emerging diseases and long-standing public health problems. The HIV/AIDS pandemic is a current and long-term public health problem worldwide.

AIDS is reversing decades of public health progress, lowering life expectancy, and significantly affecting international businesses. Lost productivity and profitability, the cost of sickness and death benefits, and the decline in a skilled workforce in the developing world will have economic effects worldwide. AIDS is affecting the military capabilities of some countries as well as international peacekeeping forces.

Lessons Learned

From the lessons of history it is difficult to conceptualize how the AIDS epidemic will be halted, let alone reversed, in the absence of a **cheap curative drug or a cheap and effective preventative vaccine.** The syphilis epidemic at the early part of the century displayed a similar kind of epidemiology to the present-day AIDS epidemic. The campaigns that were initiated then closely paralleled those in place at present for AIDS. There were vigorous educational programs to reduce sexual high-risk behavior, which were targeted at brothels and prostitutes as well as at military recruits to the U. S. Army. **Scare tactics** were spread through the use of posters, pamphlets, and radio—today it is television. Serological testing became mandatory before marriages could be licensed in certain states. However, these measures had little appreciable effect on the expansion of the syphilis epidemic. It was only the advent of a cheap, safe, and effective drug, penicillin, that eventually brought the epidemic under control. The bacterium (a spirochete) that causes syphilis does not change or mutate as rapidly as the virus that causes AIDS. There are mutant HIV in the human population for drugs that have yet to be tested and a highly effective preventive vaccine may not be a reality for HIV!

One lesson learned from HIV/AIDS is that any disease that is occurring in a distant part of the globe may be in the United States, in your state, or in your town, tomorrow. Twenty or even fifteen years ago one would not have expected to read that statement.

The advent of miracle drugs and vaccines that conquered the plagues of polio, smallpox, and measles led many people—including scientists—to believe that the age of killer diseases was coming to an end.

The AIDS epidemic changed that perception, and the best-selling nonfiction book *The Hot Zone* graphically illustrates how an exotic killer called the Ebola virus—carried into Virginia in 1989 by 450 imported research monkeys—came close to breaking loose in this country. In the hit film *Outbreak*, Dustin Hoffman plays a doctor battling a deadly virus that neither medicine nor the U.S. government can handle. Today, the Centers for Disease Control and Prevention are rethinking their position on the possibility of new plagues occurring in our lifetimes!

Who Are the Most Likely To Become HIV-Infected?

When all things are held equal, the most important identifying variable is **income.** Regardless of race, orientation, or language, those in the lower economic brackets are more likely to become HIV-infected. As the pandemic spreads, it is becoming more of a disease that can affect any person regardless of sexual preference or race, but in particular it is becoming more of a disease of the poor, the group within any society that has inadequate access to health care. As the pandemic increases globally, it is becoming more of a disease of the underdeveloped nations. **Where HIV is becoming more a disease of heterosexuals, it is also becoming a disease of women because transmission to women from heterosexual contact is easier than for men** (see Chapter 11). Also, remember that women are disproportionately represented among those living in poverty anywhere in the world.

AIDS: A UNIQUE DISEASE

The impact of this pandemic is unique. Unlike malaria or polio, previous modern pandemics, it mostly affects young and middle-aged adults. This is not only the sexually most active years for individuals, but also their prime productive and reproductive years. Thus the impact of HIV/AIDS is demographic, economic, political, and social. HIV/AIDS is a disease of human groups and its demographic and social impacts multiply from the infected individual to the group. In the most affected areas, infant, child, and adult mortality is rising and life expectancy at birth is declining rapidly. The cost of medical care for each infected person overwhelms individuals and households.

AIDS: A CAUSE OF DEATH

Peter Piot, (Figure I-2) executive director of the United Nations Program on HIV/AIDS, speaking at the 37th Interscience Conference on Antimicrobial Agents and Chemotherapy said that "HIV has transformed the world joining tuberculosis and malaria as a major cause of death worldwide. This epidemic won't be under control in any country until it is brought under control everywhere."

AIDS is now the seventh leading cause of death among 1- to 4-year-olds, sixth among 15- to 24-year-olds, and second among 25- to 44-year-olds in the United States.

There is the expectation that parents will die before their children. Because of the HIV/AIDS epidemic, it is not working out that way for many thousands of parents. They are watching their children die in the prime of life.

FIGURE I-2 Peter Piot, executive director of the Joint United Nations Program on HIV/AIDS (UNAIDS). He is a Belgian physician, microbiologist, and codiscoverer of the Ebola virus in 1976. He is the world's leading advocate for HIV/AIDS control and prevention. *(Photograph courtesy of UNAIDS/Yoshi Shimizu)*

The facts on HIV infection, disease, and AIDS that are presented in the following chapters, when understood, clearly place the responsibility for avoiding HIV infection on *YOU*. You must assess your lifestyle; if you choose not to be abstinent, you must know about your sexual partner and you must practice safer sex. **NEVER THINK THAT YOU ARE IMMUNE TO HIV INFECTION.**

ANOTHER ANNIVERSARY

June 5, 2003, will mark the beginning of the 22nd year of the AIDS pandemic. No cure has been found and, although AIDS is now called a "manageable illness," people who are sick must make endless compromises to this disease. The AIDS pandemic forces people to face their mortality daily, for months and years.

FIRST REPORTS ON AIDS CASES IN THE UNITED STATES

In January 1981, while Ronald Reagan was taking his first oath of office as president, doctors around the country were just discovering the pattern of symptoms and infections in patients that was to become a very new disease.

Initially, AIDS appeared among homosexual males; most frequently those who had many sex partners. Further study of the gay population led to the conclusion that the agent responsible for AIDS was being transmitted through sexual activities. In July of 1982, cases of AIDS were reported among hemophiliacs, people who had received blood transfusions, and injection drug users. These reports all had one thing in common—**an exchange of body fluids.** In particular, blood or semen was involved. In January 1983, the first cases of AIDS in heterosexuals were documented. Two females, both sexual partners of injection-drug users (IDUs), became AIDS patients. This was clear evidence that the infectious agent could be transmitted from male to female as well as from male to male. Later in 1983, cases of AIDS were reported in Central Africa, but with a difference. The vast majority of African AIDS cases were among heterosexuals **who did *not* use injection drugs.** These data supported the earlier findings from the American homosexual population: that AIDS is primarily a sexually transmitted disease. Also, the risk for contracting AIDS increased with the number of sex partners one had and the sexual behaviors of those partners. Early empirical observations on which kinds of social behavior placed one at greatest risk of acquiring AIDS were later supported by surveillance surveys, testing, and analysis.

FIRST REACTION TO AIDS: DENIAL

When the disease that would eventually be called AIDS first emerged in 1981, a few officials within agencies like the Centers for Disease Control and Prevention realized that a new infectious agent was at work and that it could well be spreading rapidly. They most cautiously tried to sound the

---

LOOKING BACK I.2

SILENCE = DEATH: SILENCE AND STIGMA

The silence comes because we are talking about sex, we are talking about needles and injection drug use—things we are not good at talking about as a community. But silence is also perpetuating this pandemic, and it must be talked about everywhere, by everyone! By the time former president Ronald Reagan gave his first speech on the AIDS crisis in America, hundreds of thousands of Americans were HIV-infected, 36,000 men, women, and children had been diagnosed with AIDS, and over 25,000 had died of AIDS—the year, 1987!

---

alarm, but the nation was not ready to talk about subjects like **anal sex, needles**, and **condoms.** Among those most heavily in denial were gay men, who were most at risk. They were still enjoying sexual liberation won in the 1970s, and nobody was in a mood to call the party off, even as close friends and sexual partners began dying.

New York playwright Larry Kramer attempted to break through this denial in early 1983 with an article in a widely read gay magazine. Headlined **"1,112 and Counting"** Kramer warned: "If this article doesn't rouse you to anger, fury, rage and action, gay men have no future on this Earth."

As they turned their fears into political engagement, the activists confronted a Washington that resisted action. Blood banks denied that any extra precautions were needed to prevent transmission. AIDS was buried deep inside newspapers and seldom mentioned on television. **The death of movie star Rock Hudson in 1985 finally put AIDS on the front pages.** But still, three young hemophiliacs, Ricky, Robert, and Randy Ray, were firebombed out of their Florida home when their neighbors learned they were HIV positive two years later. While there was already convincing evidence that AIDS could not be transmitted by casual contact, people were nevertheless fired from their jobs across the country because of fears that they posed a threat to coworkers.

THE EDUCATIONAL COMMUNITY

Like most complex problems, the AIDS epidemic poses special problems for educators.

WHY ALL THE FUSS ABOUT HIV/AIDS?

Why has the U.S. federal government spent over $100 billion over the past 13 years (1989–2002) on just this one disease? More money has been spent on HIV/AIDS in its relatively short history than on any other human disease in our history! In addition, the public/private sector has spent a sum equal to or greater than the government over the same time period. (See Chapter 13 for a breakdown of the $200 billion plus spent on this one disease.)

First, over the past years, AIDS has been killing over 2.5 million people each year worldwide. Through 2003, an estimated 26 million people will have died of AIDS worldwide. Malaria, TB, heart disease, cancer: No other disease is spreading or growing at this rate. In spite of HIV/AIDS campaigns in most countries, there is little evidence so far of any slowdown in the spread of the epidemic. By the end of 2003, about 70 million people are expected to have been infected by HIV.

Second, this virus is mainly transmitted during sexual intercourse. Since few human societies talk openly and honestly about sex, this makes this disease difficult to discuss; and since sex is a very private activity, it makes the transmission of HIV very difficult to control.

Third, it has an extraordinary capacity for change and rapid global spread.

Fourth, there is a long asymptomatic period between infection and illness. On average, it takes about 10 to 12 years for someone infected with HIV to develop AIDS. During this time, the HIV-infected will show few if any recognizable symptoms, but they are able to infect other people.

This long asymptomatic period is **rare in human infectious diseases.** People dying today represent those infected 10 to 20 years ago; the results of anything we do now to reduce transmission will not be apparent until sometime in the new millennium.

Fifth, HIV/AIDS is more serious than many more common diseases **because of the age groups it attacks.** Some diseases—measles and diarrhoea, for example—affect mainly infants and children; others, such as heart disease and cancer, affect mainly the old. But because HIV is predominantly transmitted sexually, AIDS mainly kills people in **their 20s through their 40s.** A major increase in deaths among these age groups, society's most productive group, presents a much greater impact socially and economically than deaths that occur among children or old people would have.

Sixth, in the past, plagues were often marked by their lack of discrimination, by the way in which they killed large numbers of people with little regard for race, wealth, sex, or religion. **But AIDS was different from the beginning.** It immediately presented a political as much as a public health problem. Homosexuals, who until this pandemic had been mostly closeted in the United States, were suddenly at the heart of a health crisis as profound as any in modern American history.

Seventh, with respect to therapy, HIV disease/AIDS requires the use of some of the most **expensive** and **toxic drugs** in medical history.

Eighth, it is a disease that has severely stigmatized those who have it.

Ninth, it is a disease that has parents burying their children!

Tenth, and lastly, this virus means there are other viruses in waiting—this has awakened our most primal fear: dying a horrible death by an unknown agent, for example, the **West Nile encephalitis virus** that struck the New York City metropolitan area in the summer and fall of 1999!

So why all the fuss about HIV/AIDS? It is caused by a **unique virus** that **changes itself faster** than a rumor making the gossip column of a tabloid. It is lethal, it is transmitted, most often sexually, it affects people in their reproductive and most productive years, it is exceptionally expensive to treat, it defies our best scientists who are working to create a vaccine for preventing infection and transmission, and it is a disease that has severely stigmatized those who have it.

HIV HAS BUT ONE REQUIREMENT TO CONTINUE ITS PRESENCE ON EARTH: A HUMAN HOST!

One of the most disturbing is discrimination against the HIV-infected. People worldwide have from the very beginning of the AIDS pandemic learned to **categorize, rationalize, stigmatize,** and **"persecutize"** those with HIV disease and AIDS. Perhaps the worst display of stigmatization and discrimination occurs against children, especially those of school age. Guidelines from the U.S. Surgeon General, federal and state health officials, and the medical community have not calmed the fears of misinformed parents. Many stories have made headlines and television news concerning children who have been barred from attending school. **While the courts can order admission, they cannot assure peer and adult acceptance.** Persuasion must come through a better understanding of the disease. Parents can be reassured through reminders that HIV/AIDS is not transmitted by casual contact. Students must also be educated about HIV/AIDS.

The U.S. Department of Health and Human Services report in their "Healthy People 2000 Review—1998–1999" that 41.4% of America's college students received information on HIV/AIDS at their respective college campuses. The year 2000 target was to raise the number of college students receiving HIV/AIDS information on their campuses to 90%. **It failed!**

WORLD INTERNATIONAL AIDS CONFERENCES

The World International AIDS Conference is believed to be the single most important meeting on AIDS.

The International AIDS Conference has been the timepiece of the pandemic. The venue, content, style, and mood of each meeting temporarily freezes in time the state of the worldwide HIV/AIDS pandemic. (Figure I-3)

In 1983, there were relatively so few groups involved with HIV/AIDS research that they could

FIGURE I-3 David Ho, 11th International HIV/AIDS Conference, Vancouver, BC, July 11, 1996. Ho, a leading AIDS researcher from the Diamond AIDS Research Centre in New York is speaking about the recent success in reducing viral load using protease inhibitors and combination drug therapy. His pioneering efforts using new HIV/AIDS drugs, have helped lift a death sentence—for a few years at least, and perhaps longer—on tens of thousands of AIDS sufferers. He asked the question, **"Can HIV be eradicated from the body?"** With this single question based on his research, he **galvanized** the AIDS community. David Ho was *Time's* **MAN OF THE YEAR FOR 1996.** In January 2001 David Ho received the Presidential Citizens Medal From President Clinton for his work using antiretroviral drugs. In mid-2002, David Ho agreed to establish and head an HIV/AIDS center at the University of Hong Kong. The new institute, whose opening date and budget have not been announced, will seek to develop an AIDS vaccine and to provide advice to Asian nations, particularly China. *(Photograph courtesy of REUTERS/Jeff Vinnick/Archive Photos)*

TWO INTERESTING DETAILS FROM THE FIRST INTERNATIONAL AIDS CONFERENCE

First, in the exhibit area there was a huge map of the United States which said on the top: **"The Problem: AIDS. The Solution: Banish All Homosexuals."** It had little pushpins on all the major cities of the United States indicating how many homosexuals lived in each. **Second,** then-Vice President George Bush addressed the assembly. As soon as he started to talk, he was shouted down. (Remember, this was seven years into the Reagan administration and it would be another year before Reagan uttered the word AIDS.) When people started to boo and shout, Bush stepped back from the podium a bit, turned around and said to the Secret Service agent standing behind him (thinking he was turned away from the microphone), "It must be a gay group." The words reverberated throughout the auditorium of the Washington Hilton.

stay in contact by telephone. As the virus spread many countries became involved in HIV/AIDS research and clinical care. International, national, and state meetings were formed as a way to exchange new information. The international meetings continue to receive the most press coverage. Since the **first** international AIDS conference in 1985, the conferences have grown in size to the point that scientists questioned their usefulness. As of 1994, the International Conference on AIDS is held every two years (Table I-2). The year 2000 13th International AIDS Conference was held in an underdeveloped nation for the first time. It was held in Durban, South Africa, a country where a significant proportion of the population has HIV/AIDS. Over 12,000 people attended this conference. The International AIDS Conferences are usually grim, but the 13th International AIDS Conference was the grimmest yet, reporting death and infection rates that carry near-apocalyptic implications for the Third World, and particularly Africa.

The theme for this conference was **"Breaking the Silence"** but it is likely the conference will be

Table I-2 International AIDS Conferences[1]

Presented is a list of past International AIDS Conferences by month, year, and location. The number of **reported** AIDS cases and deaths are accumulative by year in the United States.

Number	Month	Year	Location	AIDS Cases[2]	Deaths
1st	June	1985	Atlanta, Georgia	17,000	18,000
2nd	June	1986	Paris, France	36,000	19,000
3rd	June	1987	Washington, DC	65,000	33,000
4th	June	1988	Stockholm, Sweden	100,000	55,000
5th	June	1989	Montreal, Canada	143,000	83,000
6th	June	1990	San Francisco, California	191,000	116,000
7th	June	1991	Florence, Italy	249,000	147,000
8th	July	1992	Amsterdam, Netherlands	327,000	192,000
9th	June	1993	Berlin, Germany	432,000	259,000
10th	August	1994	Yokohama, Japan	502,000	286,000
11th	July	1996	Vancouver, Canada	624,000	378,000
12th	June	1998	Geneva, Switzerland	683,000[3]	410,000
13th	July	2000	Durban, South Africa	775,000	440,000
14th	July	2002	Barcelona, Spain	855,000	473,000
15th	July	2004	Bangkok, Thailand	936,000	510,000

1. Based on UNAIDS data, during the six days of the 13th conference, about 100,000 new HIV infections occurred and 43,000 people died of AIDS worldwide.

2. AIDS cases and deaths are minimum estimates for the United States, based on reported data to the CDC and updated data accumulative for 2002 and 2004 are estimated.

3. UNAIDS Executive Director Peter Piot reported that between the 10th 1996 AIDS Conference and the 12th in 1998, 10 million people were infected with HIV! This, he said "represents a collective failure of the world." The rate of over 5 million new infections per year continues!

remembered for the "Durban Declaration," a document signed by over 5,000 physicians and scientists testifying to their belief that HIV causes AIDS (for clarification see Box 2.2).

The XIV International AIDS Conference was held in Barcelona, Spain. The theme of this Conference was "Knowledge and Commitment for Action," reflecting a focus on translating the knowledge gained from science and experience from all nations, particularly the most affected areas of the world—sub-Saharan Africa, South and Southeast Asia, Eastern Europe and Latin America—into prevention action at all levels.

THE AIDS MEMORIAL QUILT

Conception of the Quilt

The quilt was the idea of Cleve Jones, of San Francisco, who in 1985 feared AIDS would become known for the number of people it killed. He wanted a way of remembering the people, who were, in many cases, his friends.

During the eighth candlelight march in San Francisco, Jones asked fellow marchers to write on placards the names of friends and loved ones who died of AIDS. At the end of the march, Jones and others stood on ladders, above the sea of candlelight, taping these placards to the walls of the San Francisco Federal Building. The walls of names looked to Jones like a patchwork quilt.

The purpose of the quilt is to educate. The "AIDS Quilt" is made up of individual fabric panels, each the size of a grave, measuring three feet by six feet, stitched together into 12 foot × 12 foot sections. In October 1987, the AIDS Quilt was first put on display on the mall in Washington, DC. At that time it contained 1,920 panels and covered an area larger than two football fields. It took less than two hours to read all the names. In 1992 it took 60 hours. By mid-1994, the quilt contained over 28,000 panels bearing over 40,000 names, required over 30 acres to lay out and weighed 28 tons. As of mid-2003 the quilt weighed 55 tons with 47,000 panels of about 85,000 names. Displayed in its entirety, it will cover over 45 football fields. **It is the largest piece of folk art in the world and continues to increase in size daily.** There are about 50 miles of seams and 26 miles of canvas edging. There are panels from each of the 50 states and Washington DC. Each day new panels arrive from across the United States and 37 foreign countries to be added to the quilt (Figure I-4). For those left behind, the panels represent an expression of love and a sign of grief—a part of the healing process. A few of the well-known people who have died of AIDS are seen in Figures I-5 and I-6.

Portions of the quilt tour in major cities. About 14 million people have visited the quilt at thousands of displays around the world. Dona-

FIGURE I-4 World AIDS Day, December 1, 2000. A member of the New Hope Church AIDS Quilt Committee helps spread out AIDS quilt panels at their church in Delray, Florida. Their program included songs, prayer, and candle lighting. *(Photo by Scott Fisher/South Florida Sun-Sentinel)*

FIGURE I-6 Randy Shilts, author of "And The Band Played On" (Viking Penguin Press, 1987), died of AIDS February 17, 1994, at the age of 42. *(Photograph courtesy of AP/Wide World Photos)*

FIGURE I-5 Rock Hudson, movie and television star. A Hollywood legend and undisclosed homosexual. He was the first major public figure to reveal he had AIDS. The conventional wisdom, expressed by journalist Randy Shilts in 1987 (Figure I-6) is **"that there were two clear phases to the disease in the United States: there was AIDS before Rock Hudson and AIDS after."** This common observation has been confirmed by others who also note that Hudson's July 1985 disclosure that he was suffering from AIDS led to a permanent increase in media attention to the disease. Over 6,000 Americans had already died of AIDS, but now with Hudson's famous face on the front page, the AIDS epidemic suddenly counted. The press developed an instant passion to cover AIDS. Hudson died in 1985 at age 59. *(Photograph courtesy of AP/Wide World Photos)*

tions made for viewing the quilt are being used to support local Names Project chapters and their staffs.

Each panel has its own story. The stories are told by those who make the panels for their lost friends, lovers, parents, and children. The complete quilt was displayed in Washington, DC, October 11–13, 1996, for the last time—it is too large to view again as a whole. It took 10 boxcars and a freight train to transport this work of art to the nation's capital.

Beginning year 2003, about 480,000 Americans have died from AIDS. If each of their names made up a separate panel, imagine the size of the quilt. If a name is read every 10 seconds, it would take over seven weeks of calling names, 24 hours a day!

Remembrance

People nationwide will celebrate the 15th anniversary of the AIDS Quilt on July 21, 2002. In mid-2001, The AIDS Quit was moved from San Francisco to Atlanta where it will be housed in a climate-controlled warehouse.

For more information about the Names Project's AIDS Memorial Quilt, call (415) 882–5569, ext. 375, e-mail: chapters@aidsquilt.org.

For information about your state chapter, contact the Names Project coordinator at (201) 888–1790.

CANDLELIGHT MEMORIAL

The **first** candlelight march occurred in San Francisco in November 1978 as a response to the killing of Harvey Milk, a city superintendent. The fact that he was gay was reported to be a primary motive for his death. The **first** candlelight march for AIDS occurred in 1981. The memorial march is now international. The International AIDS Candlelight Memorial honors the memory of those lost to AIDS, shows support for those living with HIV and AIDS, raises community awareness of HIV/AIDS, and mobilizes community involvement in the fight against HIV/AIDS. In 2002, the Candlelight Memorial was observed in about 1000 locations in 70 nations on every continent but Antarctica. The Candlelight march takes place on the 3rd Sunday of May. The theme was, "Share Your Vision for a Brighter Tomorrow." For 2003, the theme is "Remembering the Cause, Renewing our Commitment". (For additional information contact Matthew Matassa, email: candlelight@globalhealth.org or visit the website: http://www.globalhealth.org.)

WORLD AIDS DAY

December 1, 1988, was the first acclaimed *World AIDS Day* (WAD). The theme was **"Join the Worldwide Effort."** World AIDS Day is a day set aside to pay tribute to those who have AIDS and to those who have died of AIDS. Its purpose is to increase our awareness of AIDS. The first WAD did not attract much attention outside the gay community. In 1989, the theme was **"Our Lives, Our World—Lets Take Care of Each Other."** Artists got together and held the first annual *Day Without Art* to coincide with World AIDS Day. For the second annual Day Without Art/World AIDS Day on December 1, 1990, at least 3,000 art organizations in the United States were involved. They included the Smithsonian Institution as well as small American art galleries and art galleries in Canada, England, France, and The Netherlands.

The second annual Day Without Art/World AIDS Day was commemorated by shrouded sculptures, darkened marquees, and exhibits depicting the loss of life to HIV infection and AIDS. At 8 PM on December 1, 1990, the Manhattan and San Francisco skylines were dimmed for 15 minutes. On Broadway, the marquees were darkened for 1 minute and 23 cable TV stations as well as broadcasts in England, Canada, and Australia were interrupted with a 1-minute announcement about AIDS. (Theme was **"Women and AIDS"**)

The third annual Day Without Art/World AIDS Day, 1991, was the largest AIDS event ever. The theme was **"Sharing the Challenge."** It was intended to underline the global nature of the pandemic and to foster awareness that only by pooling efforts, resources, and imagination can hope prevail against the common threat. Many more people, businesses, and industries became involved for the first time. World AIDS Day 1992 adopted the theme **"A Community Commitment."** The theme for World AIDS Day 1993 was **"A Time to Act."** The theme for 1994 was **"The Global Challenge; AIDS and the Family."** World AIDS Day 1995 carried the theme **"Shared Rights, Shared Responsibilities."** For 1996, the theme was **"One World. One Hope."** For 1997, the theme was **"Children Living in a World with AIDS."** For 1998 the theme was **"Force for Change: World AIDS Campaign with Young People."** For 1999 the theme was **"Listen, Learn, Live! Challenges for Latin America and the Caribbean."** For the years 2000 and 2001 there is an **"AIDS and Men"** theme. For year 2000 it was **"Men Can Make a Difference."** For 2001 the theme was **"I Care. Do You?"** For 2002 it was **"Stigma and Discrimination."** For information on World AIDS Day 2003, write 108 Leonard Street, 13th Floor, New York, NY 10013 or call (212) 513-0303, or World AIDS Day Public Information Office, WHO-GPA, 1211 Geneva 27, Switzerland.

THE WORLD HEALTH ORGANIZATION

In May 1998 Gro Harlem Brundtland, a former prime minister of Norway was elected to a five-year term as director-general of the World Health Organization (WHO).

The WHO has established a global program on HIV infection and AIDS. The program has three objectives: to prevent new HIV infections, to provide support and care to those already infected, and to link international efforts in the fight against HIV infection and AIDS.

In 1995, the United Nations Secretary-General chose Peter Piot to begin a Joint United Nations Program on HIV/AIDS (UNAIDS). Piot's job is to coordinate actions and reduce duplication among the eight cosponsors of UNAIDS: United Nations Children's Fund (UNICEF), the United Nations Development Programme (UNDP), the United Nations Educational, Scientific and Cultural Organization (UNESCO), the United Nations Population Fund (UNFPA), the United Nations Drug Control Program (UNDCP), the World Health Organization (WHO), the World Bank, and the International Labor Organization.

THE FUTURE

The history of HIV/AIDS is one of remarkable scientific achievement. Never in the history of humans has so much been learned about so complex an illness in so short a time. We moved into the new millennium, the third decade of AIDS, with hope and the determination to find better therapies and a vaccine. The task is formidable but it has to be done and it will be accomplished. The evolving story of the HIV/AIDS epidemic has been one of the major medical news events of the past 22 years. It is getting hard to imagine medicine or society without HIV/AIDS.

HIV/AIDS is a truly persistent global pandemic and will require a proportionate response to bring it to heel. It is the plague of our lifetimes—and probably that of our children's lives as well. **We already have people age 21 and younger who don't know what an HIV-free world is. They were born into this recognized pandemic (1980).** To survive this pandemic, society must prevent the face of AIDS from becoming faceless. The chapters on HIV infection, HIV disease, and AIDS in this book will help bring widespread information on the virus into focus. The information within these chapters should also help eliminate many of the myths and irrational fears, or FRAID (**fear of AIDS**), generated by this disease. There is much work to be done by both scientists and society.

Perhaps a borrowed anecdote says it best:

> **As the old man walked the beach at dawn, he noticed a young woman ahead of him picking up starfish and flinging them into the sea. Finally catching up with the youth, he asked her why she was doing this. The answer was that the stranded starfish would die if left to the morning sun.**
>
> **"But the beach goes on for miles and there are millions of starfish," countered the old man. "How can your effort make any difference?"**
>
> **The young woman looked at the starfish in her hand and threw it to safety in the waves. "It makes a difference to this one," she said.**

(Adapted from *The Unexpected Universe* by Loren Eiseley. Copyright 1969, Harcourt Brace, New York)

Too easily we can become overwhelmed by the enormity of the AIDS pandemic. The numbers of patients and their constant needs have caused many to become paralyzed into inactivity and lulled into indifference. Like the old man, many ask "Why bother?"

For the sake of every individual living with HIV, we must focus on what each one of us can do. Each person can make a difference. Believing this, we are empowered to cope with the larger whole. **WE MUST NOT LET AIDS DICTATE THAT 49 IS OLD AGE AND AGE 39 OUR LIFE EXPECTANCY.**

TOLL-FREE NATIONAL AIDS HOTLINE ───────────

- For the English-language service (open 24 hours a day, 7 days a week), call 1-800-342-AIDS (2437).
- The Spanish service (open from 8 AM to 2 AM, 7 days a week) can be reached at 1-800-344-SIDA (7432).
- A TTY service for the hearing impaired is available from 10 AM to 10 PM Monday through Friday at 1-800-243-7889.
- National Prevention Information Network, 1-800-458-5231.

- National HIV Telephone Consultation Service for Health Care Professionals, (800) 933–3413, San Francisco General Hospital, Bldg. 80, Ward 83, Room 314, San Francisco, CA 94110.
- HIV/AIDS Treatment Information Service, (800) HIV-0440 (448-0440), 9 AM to 7 PM Eastern time, Monday-Friday. (800) 243–7012 Teletype number for the hearing-impaired, 9 AM to 5 PM Eastern

time, Monday-Friday, Box 6303, Rockville, MD 20849-6303.

♦ AIDS Clinical Trials Information Service, (800) TRIALS-A 874–2572, 9 AM to 7 PM Eastern time, Monday-Friday. Information on clinical trials of AIDS therapies.

♦ National Gay and Lesbian Task Force AIDS Information Hotline (800)221–7044.

♦ Gay Men's Health Crisis AIDS Hot Line, (212) 807–6655.

♦ National HIV/AIDS Education & Training Centers Program, (301)443–6364, Fax: (301) 443–9887.

♦ AIDS National Interfaith Network, (202) 546–0807, Fax: (202) 546–5103, 110 Maryland Ave., NE, Room 504, Washington, DC 20002.

♦ National Hemophilia Foundation, (212) 219–8180, 110 Greene St., Suite 303, New York, NY 10012.

♦ Pediatric AIDS Foundation, (310) 395–9051.

♦ National Pediatric HIV Resource Center, 1(800) 362–0071.

♦ AIDSLINE via the National Library of Medicine. Free access via Grateful Med, obtained from NLM at (888) 346–3656.

♦ National Institute on Drug Abuse Hotline, (800) 662-HELP (4357).

♦ National Sexually Transmitted Diseases Hotline (800) 227–8922.

♦ American Civil Liberties Union Guide to local chapters, 202-544-1076.

♦ AIDS Policy and Law, (215) 784–0860.

♦ National Conference of State Legislatures HIV, STD and Adolescent Health Project, (303) 830–2200.

♦ United States Conference of Mayors, (202)293–2352.

♦ Centers for Disease Control and Prevention, Public Inquiry, (404) 639–3534.

♦ Food and Drug Administration, Office of Public Affairs, (301) 443–3285.

♦ American Red Cross, Office of HIV/AIDS Education, 1(800) 375–2040.

♦ World Health Organization, (202) 861–4354.

USEFUL INTERNET ADDRESSES

♦ AIDS Treatment Data Network, (800) 734–7104, 611 Broadway, Suite 613, New York, NY 10012. http://health.nyam.org:8000/public_html/network/index:html, e-mail: AIDS-TreatD@AOL.COM. A home page on the internet for people with AIDS and their caregivers, it provides information on approved and experimental treatments for AIDS-related conditions. It also publishes a quarterly directory of clinical trials on HIV and AIDS in English and Spanish.

♦ AMA HIV/AIDS Information Center, World Wide Web site (http://www.ama-assn.org) offers clinical updates, news, and information on social and policy questions. Cosponsored by Glaxo Wellcome Inc.

♦ Gay Men's Health Crisis (GMHC), Site on the World Wide Web (http://www.gmhc.org) provides online forums hosted by GMHC representatives.

For additional help you may wish to consult with your college or community library. They may have access to the following AIDS-related data bases:

♦ AEGIS (AIDS Education Global Information System): http://www.aegis.org

♦ HIV Info Web: http://www.infoweb.org

♦ Kaiser Daily Global HIV/AIDS information: www.kaisernetwork.org

♦ Southern Africa AIDS Information Dissemination Service: www.safaids.org.zw

♦ Immunet: http://www.immunet.org

♦ Project Inform: http://www.projinf.org

♦ The Body: http://www.thebody.com/cgi/treatans.html

♦ HIVInSite: http://www.hivinsite.ucsf.edu/medical/tx-guidelines

♦ Search AIDSLINE, MEDLINE: http://www.igm.nim.nih.gov

♦ Vaccines: http://www.avi.org

♦ Women, children, health care workers, hemophiliacs, blind, deaf, and other affected groups: http://beaconclinic.org/website/groups

♦ AIDS/HIV statistics: http://www.avert.org/statindx.htm

♦ http://www.healthcg.com/hiv/links.html (provides linkage to nine major US Guidelines for HIV Testing, OIs, Treatment etc.)

♦ The *Centers for Disease Control and Prevention's (CDC) National Prevention Information Network (NPIN) Links*: http://www.cdcnac.org/hivlink. html and http://www.cdcnac.org/daynews.html

♦ National Institute of Allergy and Infectious Diseases (NIAID) online at: http://www.niaid.nih. gov.

♦ *Critical Path AIDS Project* a Philadelphia organization for people with HIV disease, provides another online source for the latest news in HIV disease prevention, research, clinical trials, and treatments. The publication's hot link leads to a directory of AIDS-related publications: (http://www.critpath.org)

- UNAIDS Global HIV/AIDS Information www.unaids.org
- AIDS MAP Global HIV/AIDS information www.aidsmap.com
- *Managing Desire: HIV Prevention Counseling for the 21st Century* targets the HIV test counseling community as well as the general consumer. The site is produced by Nicholas Sheon, the Prevention Editor of the *HIV Inside* web site of the UCSF Center for AIDS Prevention Studies (http://hivsinsite.ucsf.edu) and an HIV test counselor at the Berkeley Free Clinic: (http://www.managingdesire.org)
- *AIDS* offers abstracts from recent issues: (http://www.aidsonline.com)
- *AIDS Weekly Plus* contains more than 35,000 articles on health-related topics. Full access is available by subscription: (http://www.newsfile.com)
- *AIDS Treatment News* posts the contents of every issue since the publication began in 1986: (http://www.immunet.org/immunet/atn.nsf/homepage)
- The *Bulletin of Experimental Treatment on AIDS (BETA)* published by the San Francisco AIDS Foundation, is free online: (http://www.sfaf.org/beta.html)
- *Treatment Issues* published by the Gay Men's Health Crisis, provides free access to issues dating back to 1995: (http://www.gmhc.org/aidslib/ti/ti.html)
- *Project Inform* e-mail (INFO@projinf.org), website, established in 1985 as a national, nonprofit, community-based HIV/AIDS treatment information and advocacy organization, serves HIV-infected individuals, their caregivers, and their health care and service providers through its national, toll-free treatment hotline: (http://www.projinf.org)
- Western Canada's largest AIDS group (in Vancouver, BC) has launched its redesigned website featuring online publications, a map of provincial resources, and links to over 100 AIDS websites. The website, published by the British Columbia Persons with AIDS Society, is one of the most popular sites in Canada and has operated for two years. The site carries information about:
  - *Treatments* http://www.bcpwa.org/treat.htm;
  - *AIDS news* http://www.bcpwa.org/news.htm;
  - *Organizational activities* http://www.bcpwa.org/AboutBCPWA/board.htm; and
  - *Links* http://www.bcpwa.org/Resources/links.ht.
  - For more information: Pierre Beaulne, Developer, Communications and Marketing, British Columbia Persons With AIDS Society, mail to: pierreb@parc.org.

The following is a sampling of general internet resources for community research and HIV/AIDS information in Canada:

- The Community-Based HIV/AIDS Research Program National Health Research and Development Program, Health Canada http://www.hc-sc.gr.ca/hppb/nhrdp/cdr.htm
- The HIV/AIDS Aboriginal Research Program National Health Research and Development Program, Health Canada http://www.hc-sc.gr.ca/hppb/nhrdp/abrfp.htm
- Community-University Research Alliances (CURAs), Social Sciences and Humanities Research Council of Canada http://www.sshrc.ca/english/programinfo/grantsguide/cura.html
- Canadian Strategy on HIV/AIDS http://www.hc-sc.gc.ca/hppb/hiv aids/
- Canadian HIV/AIDS Clearinghouse http://www.cpha.ca/clearinghouse e.htm
- Canadian AIDS Society http://www.cdnaids.ca/
- Canadian Aboriginal AIDS Network http://www.caan.ca/
- Community AIDS Treatment Information Exchange http://www.catie.ca/
- Canadian HIV/AIDS Legal Network http://www.aidslaw.ca/
- Bureau of HIV/AIDS, STD and TB, Health Canada http://www.hc-sc.gc.ca/hpb/lcdc/bah/epi/epi e.html
- Global Network of People Living with HIV/AIDS (GNP+) e-mail: gnp@gn.apc.org.

Global AIDS Directory 2000: It contains a comprehensive listing of 250 agencies—a "who's who" among groups working globally on HIV/AIDS. Copies of Global AIDS Directory 2000 are US$50 each, US$25 for Global Health Council members. For shipping and handling in the United States, please include US$5; for international orders, please include US$15. To order a copy of Global AIDS Directory 2000, send your name and address with a check drawn on a U.S. bank, a U.S. postal money order, U.S. traveler's check or credit card information to: The Global Health Council, c/o First Union National Bank, Dept. 5100, Washington, DC, 20061-5100, USA. VISA, MasterCard and American Express credit card orders are accepted and should include account numbers, expiration date and signature. If you are unable to afford Global AIDS Directory 2000 or have further questions, please contact: William Craig, Information Officer, Tel: +1-802-649-1340 or email: wcraig@globalhealth.org.

ACQUIRED IMMUNE DEFICIENCY SYNDROME
AIDS

What do we know about AIDS? The next 13 chapters will present the many faces of the AIDS pandemic in the United States and other countries. Unlike people, the AIDS virus (HIV) does not discriminate; and it appears that most humans are susceptible to HIV infection, its suppression of the human immune system, and the consequences that follow. The viral infection that leads to AIDS is the most lethal, the most feared, and the most socially isolating of all the sexually transmitted diseases. **We must, as a people, fight against AIDS, not against each other** (Figure P-1).

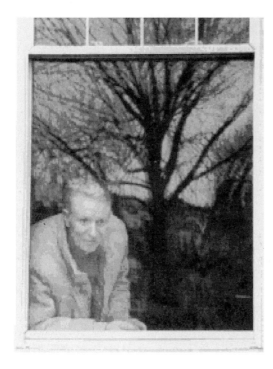

FIGURE P-1   The Loneliness of AIDS. Skip Bluette, diagnosed with AIDS July 1986, died July 1988. He suffered the indignity of having to lie to a dentist to get treatment. He suffered the ignorance of nurses afraid to touch him. He suffered the loss of his greatest pleasures—discos, gourmet meals, movies, and sex with men. Family was vital to Skip. So vital that on July 17, the day he died, their presence was his final wish. Skip Bluette wanted his story told. Photographer Mara Lavitt interviewed and photographed him during the last eight months of his life. Portions of Lavitt's article, which appeared in *The New Haven Register*, are presented in the following chapters. *(By permission of Mara Lavitt and* The New Haven Register*)*

Discovering AIDS, Naming the Disease

CHAPTER CONCEPTS

♦ The letters A, I, D, S (AIDS) are an acronym for Acquired Immune Deficiency Syndrome.
♦ AIDS is a syndrome, not a single disease.
♦ The first cases of AIDS-related *Pneumocystis carinii* pneumonia (PCP) were reported by the Centers for Disease Control and Prevention (CDC) in June of 1981; the first case of Kaposi's sarcoma in July 1981.
♦ Luc Montagnier discovered the AIDS virus in 1983.
♦ The first CDC definition of AIDS was presented in 1982 and expanded in 1983, 1985, and 1987, and again on January 1, 1993.

A = acquired = a virus received from someone else
I = immune = an individual's natural protection against disease-causing microorganisms
D = deficiency = a deterioration of the immune system
S = syndrome = a group of signs and symptoms that together define AIDS as a human disease

---

AIDS: A DISEASE OR A SYNDROME?

AIDS has been presented in journals, nonscience magazines, newspaper articles, and on television as a disease. However, a disease is a pathological condition with a single identifiable cause. As we learned from the days of Louis Pasteur and Robert Koch, there is a single identifiable organism or agent for each infectious disease.

AIDS patients may have many diseases. Most AIDS patients have more than one disease at any given time. Each disease produces its own signs and symptoms. Collectively, the diseases that are expressed in an AIDS patient are referred to as a **syndrome**. The number of different diseases an AIDS patient has and the severity of their expression reflects the functioning of that person's immune system.

WHAT CAUSES AIDS?

In the Beginning, 1980, 1981, 1982

There were very few facts, but many plausible theories about the causes of AIDS. Perhaps the cytomegalovirus had mutated to cause a more severe illness. Maybe the illness was related to

"poppers" (amyl and butyl nitrite) and other drugs popular among gay men for enhancing sexual pleasure. Some researchers thought the other sexually transmitted infections that many gay men contracted somehow overwhelmed the immune system to cause the mysterious disease. Government researchers suggested that sperm in the male bowel caused the disease, a theory that made little sense because homosexuality is probably as old as society. One thing few doctors considered was the possibility of a new infectious agent. Prior to the outbreak of this strange disease, infectious disease scientists, quite arrogantly, believed that virtually all diseases were known. It was just that many things were unknown about the individual diseases. In fact, an editorial in *The New England Journal of Medicine* in December 1981 on possible causes of AIDS, omitted the whole idea that AIDS might be caused by an unknown infectious agent!

Early in 1983, the agent that destroys an essential portion of the human immune system was identified by French scientists as a virus. From that point on there was a specific infectious agent associated with the cause of AIDS. The symptoms of viral-induced AIDS can begin **only** after one has been infected with a specific virus. This virus is now called the **Human Immunodeficiency Virus (HIV)**. The specific viral induced disease is referred to specifically as HIV/AIDS because there are other reasons for a suppressed immune system, like congenital inherited immune deficiencies, exposure to radiation, alkylating agents, corticosteroids, certain forms of cancer, and cancer chemotherapy that also produce AIDS-like symptoms. (Stadtmauer et al. 1997) *Because individuals can express AIDS for reasons other than becoming HIV-infected, unless stated otherwise all information herein will refer only to AIDS caused by HIV and be referred to as HIV/AIDS.*

HOW DOES HIV CAUSE AIDS?

Over time, HIV depletes a subset of lymphocytes called **T4 helper cells**, or CD4+ cells, that are essential in the proliferation of cells necessary to cell-mediated immunity and in the production of antibodies (Figure 1-1). Thus, cell-mediated immunity and antibodies are critical components of the human immune system. Without the ability to produce a sufficient number of immune specific cells and immune specific antibodies, the body is vulnerable to a large variety of infections caused by organisms and viruses that normally do not cause human disease. It is these infections that create the symptoms and progression of illnesses that eventually kill AIDS patients. Thus AIDS begins with HIV infection. Technically it can be called **HIV disease, HIV T4 helper cell or CD4+ cell disease**, but the popular press, scientists, and others still refer to HIV disease as AIDS. AIDS is the end stage of chronic HIV infection. **AIDS IS NOT TRANSMITTED, THE VIRUS IS.** People do not die of AIDS per se. They die of opportunistic infections, cancers, and organ failures brought on by the results of a failed immune system.

It is believed that eventually almost everyone who is **correctly** diagnosed with HIV/AIDS will die from AIDS. But all who become HIV-infected may not progress to AIDS. Estimates are that some 5% of the HIV-infected population will not progress to AIDS. This implies that there is a percentage of the population that is resistant to HIV-associated immune system suppression. Since mid-1996, several genes

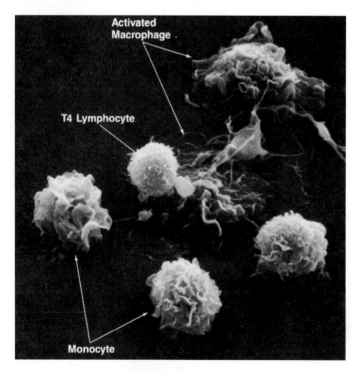

FIGURE 1-1 Normal Human T4 Lymphocytes, Monocytes, and Macrophages. Scanning electron micrograph of monocytes, macrophages, and a T4 or CD4+ lymphocyte, magnified 9,000 times. These white blood cells are the targets of HIV infection. Note that the T4 lymphocyte (round cell, at the center) is adhered to a flattened macrophage. *(Photograph courtesy of Dr. M. A. Gonda)*

that offer resistance to HIV infection have been identified (See Chapter 4.)

Naming the Disease

Early in 1981, practically coincident with the report of the first cases of a new disease in the male homosexual community in the United States, there were reports of 34 cases of a new disease among Haitian immigrants to the United States and 12 cases of a disease previously unrecognized in **Haiti**—an aggressive form of **Kaposi's sarcoma**. Michael Gottlieb, who had identified the new disease that seemed to target gay men, found that although each of the cases was different, **all had one thing in common: whatever was making the men sick had singled out the T lymphocyte cells for destruction.** Eventually the body's battered defenses couldn't shake off even the most harmless microbial intruder. The men were dying from what doctors termed opportunistic infections,

such as **Pneumocystis pneumonia**, which attacks the lungs, and **toxoplasmosis**, which often ravages the brain.

THE CENTERS FOR DISEASE CONTROL AND PREVENTION REPORTS

In June 1981, the Centers for Disease Control and Prevention (CDC) first reported on diseases occurring in gay men that previously had only been found to occur in people whose immune systems were suppressed by drugs or disease [*Morbidity and Mortality Weekly Report (MMWR)*, 1981].

The report stated that five young men in Los Angeles had been diagnosed with *Pneumocystis carinii* pneumonia (PCP) in three different hospitals. Because cases of PCP occurred almost exclusively in immune-suppressed patients, five new cases in one city at one time were termed by the

---

LOOKING BACK 1.1

THE NEW YORK TIMES AND A.I.D.S., AUGUST 8, 1982

An article, "A Disease's Spread Provokes Anxiety," alerted its readers to the growing health crisis in the homosexual community that was baffling medical science. While the *Times* had previously reported on a disease causing opportunistic infections in gay men, this was the first time the term acquired immune deficiency syndrome or A.I.D.S. (the punctuation had not been dropped) appeared in the nation's newspaper of record. Later in 1982, the *Washington Post* joined the *Times* in reporting on the death of an infant who had received a blood transfusion from an AIDS-afflicted donor. With that, a second major national newspaper was officially in the business of covering the AIDS story.

The Centers for Disease Control (CDC): 1982/1983

Regardless that this new disease was increasing rapidly and killing all those who displayed the strange set of symptoms, the epidemiologists at the CDC in 1982 had other things to worry about; President Ronald Reagan was moving to reduce the size of the federal government and CDC staff members were facing dismissal. Harold W. Jaffe, who lost seniority as he scurried

to stay employed, later went on to become chief epidemiologist for the center's AIDS team. Progress was also impeded by scientists who withheld information from health officials because they were competing against one another to be first to publish articles in medical journals that demanded exclusive information. Communication to the public was also poor. People had misplaced fears and misconceptions about the disease even after epidemiologists found, by late 1982, that this disease was transmitted through sex, blood transfusions, injecting drugs with contaminated needles and syringes, and from mother to child. Because health officials and journalists used the phrase "bodily fluids" instead of specifying semen, blood, and vaginal secretions, many people feared that they could contract AIDS from toilet seats or drinking fountains, or by eating at restaurants or going to school.

At a meeting of the World Health Organization (WHO) in Geneva in November 1983, it was clear that AIDS was a global health problem and that cases were occurring in many countries that had officially denied it. But these warning signs were disregarded.

---

report as unusual. The report also suggested "an association between some aspects of homosexual life-style or disease acquired through sexual contact and PCP in this population. Based on clinical examination of each of these cases, the possibility of a cellular immune dysfunction related to a common exposure might also be involved."

In July 1981, the CDC (*MMWR*, 1981) reported that an uncommon cancer, Kaposi's sarcoma (KS), had been diagnosed in 26 gay men who lived in New York City and California. This was also an unusual finding because KS, when it occurred, was usually found in **older** men of Jewish or Italian ancestry. The sudden and dramatic increase in pneumonia cases, all of which were caused by a widespread but generally harmless fungus, *P. carinii*, and KS cases indicated that an infectious form of immune deficiency was on the increase. This immune deficiency disease, initially called **GRID** for **Gay-Related Immune Deficiency**, was noted to be quickly spreading in the homosexual community, among users of injection drugs, and among blood transfusion recipients. This new mysterious and lethal illness appeared to be associated with one's lifestyle. These early cases of immune deficiency heralded the beginning of an epidemic of a previously unknown illness. By 1982 and 1983, the disease was reported in hemophiliacs, adult heterosexuals, and children. Because a *cellular deficiency of the human immune system* was found in every AIDS patient, along with an assortment of other signs and symptoms of disease, and because the infection was *acquired* from the action of some environmental agent, it was named **AIDS** for **Acquired Immune Deficiency Syndrome**.

DISCOVERY OF THE AIDS VIRUS

There was no shortage of ideas on what caused AIDS. It was believed by some to be an act of God, a religious curse or penalty against the homosexual for practicing a biblically unacceptable lifestyle that included drugs, alcohol, and sexual promiscuity. The reverend Billy Graham said "**AIDS is a judgment of God.**" Jerry Falwell stated that AIDS is God's punishment, the scripture is clear, "**we do reap it in our flesh when we violate the laws of God.**" Some believed AIDS was due to sperm exposure to amyl nitrate, a stimulant used to heighten sexual pleasure (Gallo, 1987). Others believed there was no specific infectious agent. They believed that certain people who *excessively stressed their immune systems* experienced immune system failure, and before it could recover other infections killed them. But many scientists who had expertise in analyzing the sudden onset of **new** human diseases thought the cause of this form of human immune deficiency was an infectious agent. They believed that the agent was transmitted through sexual intercourse, blood, or blood products and from mother to fetus. They also believed that this agent, which led to the loss of T4 or CD4+ cells, was smaller than a bacterium or fungus because it passed through a filter normally used to remove those microorganisms. This agent fit the profile of a virus.

In January 1983, **Luc Montagnier** (Montan-ya) and colleagues at the Pasteur Institute in Paris isolated the virus that causes AIDS. (Hobson et al., 1991). In May of that year, they published the first report on a T cell retrovirus found in a patient with **lymphadenopathy** (lim-fad-eh-nop-ah-thee), or swollen lymph glands. Lymphadenopathy is one of the early signs in patients progressing toward AIDS. The French scientist (Figure 1-2) named this virus **lymphadenopathy-associated virus** (LAV) (Barre-Sinoussi et al., 1983).

Naming the Viruses That Cause AIDS: HIV-1, HIV-2

During the search for the AIDS virus, several investigators isolated the virus but gave it different names. For example, Robert Gallo (Figure 1-3) named the virus HTLV III (For the Third Human T Cell Lymphotropic Virus). Because the collection of names given this virus created some confusion, the Human Retrovirus Sub-committee of the Committee on the Taxonomy of Viruses reduced all of the names to one: **Human Immunodeficiency Virus** or **HIV.** This term is now used worldwide.

In 1985, a second type of HIV was discovered in West African prostitutes. It was named HIV type 2 or **HIV-2.** The first confirmed case of HIV-2 infection in the United States was reported in late 1987 in a West African woman with AIDS. By December 1990, 16 additional cases of HIV-2 infection were reported to the CDC (*MMWR*, 1990). Beginning year 2003, a total of 94 HIV-2 infections have been reported from 22 states of the United States and the District of Columbia. Of the 94 infected persons, 70 are black and 54 are male. Sixty-six were born in West Africa, 13 in the

FIGURE 1-2 Luc Montagnier, from the Pasteur Institute in Paris. He and colleagues discovered the human immunodeficiency virus (HIV), the cause of AIDS. In October 1997, he moved to the United States. He accepted an endowed professorship at Queens College, New York, to run a new AIDS research institute. *(Photograph courtesy of AP/Wide World Photos)*

FIGURE 1-3 Robert Gallo, Director, Institute of Human Virology. *(Photograph courtesy of AP/Wide World Photos)*

United States (including 3 infants born to mothers of unspecified nationality), 2 in India and 3 in Europe. The region of origin was not identified for 10 of the persons. Seventeen have developed AIDS-defining conditions and 10 have died. These case counts represent minimal estimates because completeness of reporting has not been assessed; reporting varies from state to state according to state policy.

First Reported Case of HIV-2 Infection

The earliest evidence to date of an individual exposed to HIV-2 comes from a case report on an infection most likely occurring in Guinea Bissau in the 1960s. Earlier extensive serosurveys in West Africa are rare or nonexistent. In genetic terms,

HIV-2 is much more closely related to SIV, a group of monkey viruses, than to HIV-1. Both HIV-2 and HIV-1 are said to have been derived from ancestral SIV variants that were from distinct regions and species and do not appear to be direct genetic descendants of each other (Marlink, 1996; Hahn et al. 2000). Clinically, what has been learned about HIV-1 appears to apply to HIV-2, except that HIV-2 appears to be less harmful (cytopathic) to the cells of the immune system and it reproduces more slowly than HIV-1. There is the question of why is there no HIV-2 epidemic or pandemic. According to scientists working with HIV-2, most likely an epidemic has not occurred because of different behaviors of HIV-2 in relation to viral load. Based on surveys in West Africa, it was found that HIV-2 never reaches a high viral load in the blood as found with HIV-1. Thus, it is reasoned that fewer HIV-2 means there are less to transmit to other people and fewer virus to attack the immune system.

UNLESS STATED OTHERWISE, ALL REFERENCES TO HIV IN THIS BOOK REFER TO HIV-1.

DEFINING THE ILLNESS: AIDS SURVEILLANCE

The CDC reported that through 1983 there were 3,068 AIDS cases in the United States and 1,478 of these had died (48%). All demonstrated a loss of CD4+ or T4 lymphocytes, and all died with severe opportunistic infections. Opportunistic infections are caused by organisms and viruses that are normally present but do **not** cause disease unless the immune system is damaged. Clearly there was an immediate need for a name and definition for this disease so that a rational surveillance program could begin.

Definitions of AIDS for Surveillance Purposes

The initial objective of AIDS surveillance was to describe the epidemic in terms of time, place, and individuals and to recognize immediately changes in rate and pattern in the spread of AIDS.

In order to establish surveillance, a system for monitoring where and when AIDS cases occurred, a workable definition had to be developed. The definition had to be *sensitive* enough to detect every possible AIDS patient, while at the same time *specific* enough to exclude those who may have AIDS-like symptoms, but were not infected by HIV.

In 1982, there was no *single characteristic* of AIDS that would allow for a useful definition for surveillance purposes. And so, the first AIDS surveillance definition was based on the **clinical description** of symptoms. The **first** of many criteria for the diagnosis of AIDS were: (**1**) the presence of a reliably diagnosed disease at least moderately predictive of cellular immune deficiency; and (**2**) the absence of an underlying cause for the immune deficiency or for reduced resistance to the disease (*MMWR*, 1982). Because the symptoms varied greatly among individuals, **this was a poor first definition.**

AIDS Definition Modified

The initial definition of AIDS was thus an arbitrary one, reflecting the partial knowledge of the clinical consequences that prevailed at the time. Various systems for classifying HIV-related illnesses have been devised since 1982 to take into account increasing knowledge about the spectrum of those illnesses. Had the whole picture of HIV infection and its clinical consequences been known in 1982, the term **"AIDS"** would not have been used. Instead, it would have been called **"HIV disease"** (or perhaps, following an older tradition, "Gottlieb's disease," after Mike Gottlieb, who first described it).

The 1982 definition was modified in 1983 to include new diseases then found in AIDS patients. With this modification, AIDS became reportable to the Centers for Disease Control and Prevention (CDC) in every state. In 1985, additional diseases were included in the AIDS case definition (Table 1-1).

Broadly speaking, the term **AIDS** may be understood as referring to the onset of life-threatening illnesses as a result of HIV disease that results from an HIV infection. AIDS is the end stage of a disease process that may have been developing for 5, 10, 15 or more years, for most of which time the infected person will have been well and quite possibly unaware that he or she has been infected.

Thus the number of AIDS cases reported from 1987 through 1992 reflects the revisions of the initial surveillance case definitions.

Problems with AIDS Definitions, 1981–1992

One major drawback to all of the CDC AIDS definitions is the fact that through 1992, the Social Security Administration (SSA) used the CDC AIDS definition to determine disability. But all the definitions were primarily based on symptoms and opportunistic infections in men. Therefore, about 65% of women with HIV/AIDS symptoms were excluded from Supplemental Securily Income (SSI) benefits. They were excluded because of failure to be diagnosed with AIDS by the CDC AIDS definition (Sprecher, 1991).

AIDS Redefined in 1993: The Impact!

On January 1, 1993, the newest definition of AIDS was put into the surveillance network. The reason for the new CDC definition was that epidemiologists felt the 1987 definition failed to reflect the true magnitude of the pandemic. In particular, it failed to address AIDS in women. In addition, those with T4 counts under 200/μL of blood are

Table 1-1 1987 CDC Definition of AIDS

ADULT

A. Without laboratory evidence for HIV infection:
   - Lymphoma of brain (<60 years of age)
   - Lymphoid interstitial pneumonitis (<13 years of age)
B. With laboratory evidence for HIV infection:
   - Disseminated coccidioidomycosis
   - HIV encephalopathy
   - Isosporiasis (persisting >1 month)
   - Lymphoma of brain (any age)
   - Non-Hodgkin's lymphoma (B cell or undifferentiated)
   - Recurrent Salmonella septicemia
   - Extrapulmonary tuberculosis
   - HIV-wasting syndrome
   - Recurrent bacterial infections (<13 years of age)
   - Disseminated histoplasmosis

PEDIATRIC

Children with AIDS may have infectious diseases that are not covered by the adult CDC AIDS definitions. Thus children under 15 months are classified separately from older children because passive maternal antibodies may be present.

To Be HIV-Infected, Children Under 15 Months Must:

1. Show HIV in blood and tissues.
2. Show evidence of humoral and acquired immune deficiency and have one or more opportunistic infections associated with AIDS.
3. Show other symptoms meeting the CDC definition of AIDS.

To be HIV-infected, children between 16 months and 12 years must:

1. Show 1 and 3 above.
2. Show HIV antibodies.

This definition was updated on January 1, 1993, to include all persons with a T4 cell count of less than 200/μL of blood. See text for additional details.

(Adapted from Roger J. Pomerantz, M.D., "The Chameleon Called AIDS," Harvard Medical School, 1988.)

most likely to be severely ill or disabled and in greatest need of medical and social services. With the new AIDS definition, these people are eligible earlier in their illness for federal and state medical and social assistance programs.

CDC revised the classification system for HIV infection to emphasize the clinical importance of the T4 lymphocyte count in the categorization of HIV-related clinical conditions. Consistent with this revised classification system, **CDC expanded the AIDS surveillance case definition to include all HIV-infected persons who have less than 200 T4 lymphocytes/μL of blood, or a T4 lymphocyte percent less than 14% of total lymphocytes.** In addition to retaining the 23 clinical conditions in the 1987 AIDS surveillance case definition, the expanded definition includes (**1**) pulmonary tuberculosis, (**2**) invasive cervical cancer, and (**3**) recurrent pneumonia. The **objectives** of these changes are to simplify the classification of HIV infection and the AIDS case reporting process, to be consistent with standards of medical care for HIV-infected persons, to better categorize HIV related morbidity, and to reflect more accurately the number of persons with severe HIV-related immunosuppression who are at highest risk for severe HIV-related morbidity and most in need of close medical follow-up.

The expanded AIDS surveillance case definition had a substantial impact on the number of reported cases in 1993 (*MMWR*, 1993).

Of the 106,618 Adult/Adolescent AIDS cases reported in 1993, 57,574 (54%) were reported based on conditions added to the definition in 1993; and 49,044 (46%) were reported based on pre-1993 defined conditions. A substantial increase in the number of reported AIDS cases occurred in all regions of the United States.

When compared to 1992 data the increase in reported cases in 1993 was greater among females (151%) than among males (105%). Proportionate increases were greater among blacks and Hispanics than among whites. The largest increases in case reporting occurred among persons aged 13–19 years and 20–24 years; in these age groups, a greater proportion of cases were reported among women (35% and 29%, respectively) and were attributed to heterosexual transmission (22% and 18%, respectively).

Compared with homosexual/bisexual men, proportionate increases in case reporting were greater among heterosexual injecting-drug users (IDUs) and among persons reportedly infected through heterosexual contact.

The pediatric AIDS surveillance case definition was not changed in 1993. During 1993, 990 children aged <13 years were reported with AIDS, an increase of 21% compared with the 783 cases reported in 1992. In 1994, for the first time, pediatric AIDS cases exceeded 1,000 (1,090). By year 2000, that number decreased to less than 200 cases per year. Collectively, since 1990, 50% were female, and most were either black (55%) or Hispanic (27%) and were infected through perinatal HIV transmission (93%). New York, Puerto Rico, and Florida reported 51% of the pediatric AIDS cases.

If all of the approximately 1 million persons in the United States with HIV infection were diagnosed and their immune status known, it is estimated that 120,000–190,000 persons who do not have AIDS-indicator diseases would be found to have T4 lymphocyte counts $<200/\mu L$. However, since not all of these persons are aware of their HIV infection status, and of those who are, not all have had an immunological evaluation, the immediate impact on the number of AIDS cases will be considerably less. Under the 1987 AIDS surveillance criteria, approximately 49,106 AIDS cases were reported in 1992, but 106,618 were reported for 1993. In 1994, there were 80,691 new AIDS cases. For 1995, the number of new cases was 74,180; about 43,000 for 2002.

Revised AIDS Definition Creates Backlog

The effects of the expanded surveillance definition was greatest in 1993 because of the backlog in number of persons who fit the new AIDS definition. Once most of these cases were reported through 1998, the yearly incidence dropped off to less than 50,000 cases a year.

Problems Stemming from Changing the AIDS Definition for Surveillance Purposes

Each time the definition of AIDS has been altered by the CDC, it has led to an increase in the number of AIDS cases. In 1985, the change in definition led to a 2% increase over what would have been diagnosed prior to the change. The 1987 change led to a 35% increase in new AIDS cases per year over that expected using the 1985 definition. The 1993 change resulted in a 52% increase in AIDS cases over that expected for 1993. Such rapid changes alter the baseline from which future predictions are made and make the interpretations of trends in incidence and characteristic of cases difficult to process. **For the first time because of the 1993 AIDS definition, one could be diagnosed with AIDS and remain symptom-free for years (become HIV positive and have a T4 or CD4+ cell count of less than 200).**

SUMMARY

Much continues to be written about HIV/ AIDS. Some of it, especially in lay articles, has been less than accurate and has led to public confusion and fear. **HIV infection is not AIDS. HIV infection is now referred to as HIV disease. AIDS is a syndrome of many diseases,** each resulting from an opportunistic agent or cancer cell that multiplies in humans who are immunosuppressed. The new 1993 CDC AIDS definition will allow, over the long term, earlier access to federal and state medical and social services for HIV-infected individuals.

REVIEW QUESTIONS

(Answers to the Review Questions are on page 489.)

1. The letters A, I, D, and S are an acronym for?

2. Is AIDS a single disease? Explain.

3. When was the AIDS virus discovered and by whom?

4. In what year did CDC first report on a strange new disease that later was named AIDS?

5. Name one different acronym for HIV.

6. How many times has CDC changed and expanded the definition of AIDS? In what years?

7. Why did the CDC do away with the ARC definition?

8. What is one major advantage of the new CDC AIDS definition for the HIV-infected?

What Causes AIDS: Origin of the AIDS Virus

2

CHAPTER CONCEPTS

♦ President Thabo Mbeki of South Africa says AIDS is not caused by HIV infection.
♦ AIDS scientists say AIDS is caused by HIV infection.
♦ An unbroken chain of HIV transmission has been established between those infected and the newly infected.
♦ HIV is believed to have crossed into humans from chimpanzees.
♦ A third new HIV strain is found.
♦ The earliest AIDS case to date is reported in 1959.
♦ Precursor HIV may have entered humans 300 years ago.

THE CAUSE OF AIDS: THE HUMAN IMMUNODEFICIENCY VIRUS

The unexpected appearance and accelerated spread of an unknown lethal disease soon raised several important questions: **What** is causing the disease? **Where** did it come from? **How** does the causative agent function? These three questions will be answered.

This section has a subtitle that states that AIDS is the result of HIV infection. There are a relatively small number of scientists and non-scientists as of this writing who claim that HIV does **not** cause AIDS. For a balanced HIV/AIDS presentation, this claim will be presented first.

HIV Does Not Cause AIDS: A Minority Point of View

Fronted locally by ACT UP/San Francisco, a renegade chapter long ago disowned by the rest of the AIDS activist movement (and not to be confused with ACT UP/Golden Gate, which respects most conventional AIDS research), members have repeatedly plastered the Castro district with stickers reading, "AIDS Is Over," and "Don't Buy the HIV Lie." In May and June 1999, the Los Angeles-based dissident group Alive & Well ran a series of full-page ads in several gay/lesbian and alternative papers, including the *Bay Area Reporter*, *Bay Times*, and *Bay Guardian*, arguing that AIDS is not contagious, HIV is harmless, and that HIV/AIDS

drugs are the real danger. The first of the ads states that, "What we have experienced for 20 years is not a sexually transmitted epidemic but a tragic medical mistake. Contrary to popular beliefs, AIDS is not a new disease, AIDS is a new name given by the Centers for Disease Control (CDC) to a collection of 29 old illnesses and conditions. . . . These illnesses and conditions are called AIDS only when they occur in persons who also have certain protective, disease-fighting proteins called antibodies in their blood." In her book, **"What If Everything You Thought You Knew About AIDS Was Wrong?"** Christine Maggiore elaborates, "None of these diseases appear exclusively in those who test (HIV) positive. . . . All 29 indicator diseases have established causes and treatments unrelated to HIV." AIDS, in other words, isn't an epidemic at all; it's a phony construct. Maggiore, who tested HIV positive in 1992, and remains relatively symptom-free, believes that those who have died of AIDS actually died from prescription or recreational drugs, or fear. Her explanations for the global AIDS pandemic: In Africa, people are dying at the same rate as before; in America, people are victims of the prescription drugs.

Disbelieving Scientists

Scientist Peter Duesberg is perhaps the most vocal in his concern that the scientific community is investigating the wrong causative agent. Duesberg is a molecular biologist at the University of California at Berkeley and a member of the National Academy of Sciences. Duesberg has advanced his anti-HIV/AIDS hypothesis at great expense to himself. He states that "I have been excommunicated by the retrovirus-AIDS community with noninvitations to meetings, noncitations in the literature and nonrenewals of my research grants, which is the highest price an experimental scientist can pay for his convictions."

Duesberg's financial and laboratory problems reflect his lonely battle with HIV/AIDS investigations and drug companies who, he believes, have invested so much in the HIV/AIDS theory that they cannot afford to entertain an alternative theory.

In 1971 at age 33, Duesberg codiscovered cancer-causing genes in viruses. In the March 1987 issue of *Cancer Research*, he published "Retro-viruses as Carcinogens and Pathogens: Expectations and Reality." The article provoked wide-based scientific discussion and received a lot of popular press coverage. In the article **Duesberg argues that there is no evidence that HIV causes AIDS.** He has published additional articles in *Science* (1988) and in the *Proceedings of the National Academy of Sciences* (1989) stating that HIV is not the cause of AIDS. In May 1992, Duesberg was the featured speaker at an alternative AIDS conference, "AIDS: A Different View," promoted by homeopathic physician Martien Brands. The week of meetings was spent giving new interpretations to some of the data used to establish HIV as the causative agent of AIDS. In short, Duesberg suggests that there is no single causative agent, that the disease is due to one's **"lifestyle."** He marshals arguments to support his theory that, in the United States and probably in Europe, AIDS is a collection of noninfectious deficiencies predominantly associated with drug use, malnutrition, parasitic infections, and other specific risks. To read more on Duesberg, see the Wayt Gibbs article, "Dissident or Don Quixote?" in the August 2001 *Scientific American*.

Duesberg believes the tests that detect HIV antibodies are useless. In the June 1988 issue of *Discovery* he said, "If somebody told me today that I was antibody positive, I wouldn't worry one second. I wouldn't take Valium. I wouldn't write my will. All I would say is that my immune system seems to work. I have antibodies to a virus. I am protected."

In June 1990, Weiss and Jaffe wrote a critical refutation of Duesberg's theory that HIV cannot be the cause of AIDS. Duesberg's response suggested that he was unaware of published data that clearly answer the questions he raises concerning HIV involvement in AIDS. For example, one of Duesberg's major points is that no one has yet shown that hemophiliacs infected with HIV progress to AIDS. The data on matched groups of homosexual males and hemophiliacs, which show that *only*

BOX 2.1

SEX AND HIV DO NOT CAUSE AIDS!

Medical Doctor Puts His Life on the Line To Prove It.

On October 28, 1993, Robert Willner held a press conference at a North Carolina hotel, during which he jabbed his finger with a bloody needle he had just stuck into a man **who said he was infected with HIV.** Willner was a physician who had his medical license revoked in Florida for, among other infractions, claiming to have cured an AIDS patient with ozone infusions. He is also the author of a book, *Deadly Deception: The Proof that SEX and HIV Absolutely DO NOT CAUSE AIDS.* He insists that jabbing himself with the bloody needle, which he describes as "an act of intelligence," was not meant to sell books. "I'm interested in proving to people that there isn't one shred of scientific evidence that HIV causes any disease."

On October 3, 1994, *USA Today* carried a full-page advertisement promoting Willner's book. If carried nationally, a full-page ad in the newspaper, regardless of location, then cost $57,500. **Question for class discussion:** Did *USA Today* management provide socially responsible advertisement or did money talk and responsibility walk? What is the potential medical downside of this advertisement?

The scientific journal *Science* (1994; 226: 1642–1649) presented a series of six articles by Jon Cohen concerning the *question* of whether HIV causes AIDS. The articles are a balanced review of the scientific facts as they relate to the question.

Robert Willner died April 15, 1995, from an apparent heart attack.

---

those infected with HIV develop AIDS, have been available for a number of years. (Weiss et al., 1990).

Duesberg's arguments and disagreements with the vast majority of prominent scientists who have researched the causal agent of AIDS are many. But they pale when placed next to the overwhelming evidence that leaves no doubt in the opinion of most scientists that HIV causes AIDS (see Andrews, 1995; Cohen, 1995; Moore, 1996).

Based on an August 1992 report in *Newsweek,* a father discussed his decision, based on Duesberg's claims, to counsel his infected hemophiliac son to avoid zidovudine (ZDV) treatment. This situation is similar to what happened when desperate cancer patients followed the advice of a credentialed academician who recommended vitamin therapy as the cure for cancer. Based on such advice, some people failed to undergo truly effective therapy.

CLASS QUESTIONS: Is Duesberg's opinion on this issue inadvertently harmful to humans? To the scientific process? Will the use of his idea, that HIV does not cause AIDS, provide a course of action that will stop the Acquired Immune Deficiency Syndrome?

Duesberg's Belief that HIV Does Not Cause AIDS Continues

In 1996, Duesberg's book, **Inventing the AIDS Virus,** was published and in 1998 he and David Rasnick published a paper, **"The AIDS Dilemma: drug diseases blamed on a passenger virus."** Through year 2002, Duesberg still insisted that HIV does not cause AIDS. He believes that HIV is just another opportunistic agent like those that cause other opportunistic diseases (Duesberg, 1993, 1995a, 1995b; Moore, 1996). With each new scientific report, it becomes more difficult for Duesberg to maintain his position. However, he remains unconvinced that HIV causes AIDS regardless of the reports that newborn infants with HIV got HIV **only** from HIV-infected mothers and progress to AIDS while noninfected newborns from the same mothers do not progress to AIDS and that some 50% of HIV-infected hemophiliacs have developed AIDS yet **no** HIV-negative hemophiliac has ever developed AIDS (Darby et al., 1995; Levy, 1995; Sullivan et al., 1995). In addition, Duesberg claims that the drug AZT (Zidovudine) causes AIDS. What does he make of the AIDS Clinical Trials Group (ACTG) Protocol 076 that demonstrated AZT treatment of women during pregnancy and delivery reduced

transmission from mother to infant from 25% in the placebo-treated mothers to 8% in those who received AZT (Connor et al., 1994)?

For those who wish to know more on the rebuttal of Duesberg's arguments, read the study reporting on the death rate among HIV-positive and HIV-negative British hemophilia patients (Baum, 1995; Darby et al., 1995; Editorial, 1995). For more by Duesberg see his web page, **www.duesberg.com.**

In Defense of Duesberg

In defense of Duesberg, Buianoukas (1995) writes that "We at HEAL (Health Education AIDS Liaison) maintain that what is called AIDS is no more complicated than a recreational drug–fear–medical drug disease syndrome which, with the exception of acute medical care, is out of the purview of orthodox medicine." Robert Root-Bernstein authored "Rethinking AIDS" in 1993. This book attempts to support Duesberg's hypothesis that there is no link between HIV and AIDS. His main thesis is that scientists do not have the necessary information to conclude that HIV causes AIDS. He believes, first, that the right studies on the cause of immunosuppression have not been done and, second, that there need not be a common thread (such as the virus) associated with this new disease, no common denominator such as a causative transmissible agent. On the other hand he does not rule out the case for a single infectious organism that has yet to be identified.

In 1993, Britain's *Sunday Times* took the Duesberg claim that HIV does not cause AIDS to a new level by running a series of articles disclaiming HIV as the cause of AIDS. The *Sunday Times* continued to run these articles throughout 1994 (Dickson, 1994; Karpas, 1994). In mid-1994, Kary Mullis (recipient of the Nobel Prize in chemistry for his invention of the polymerase chain reaction—see Chapter 12 for explanation) joined Duesberg and the *Sunday Times* by saying, "The idea that HIV was the 'probable cause of AIDS' was not a scientifically proven fact, nor, indeed, was there any clear evidence that AIDS was spread through sexual contact. I think we [spread] retroviruses by our lungs, not by our genitals." Mullis continued by saying, "it is not a scientific fact, or even a supposed fact, that HIV is the probable cause of AIDS." Mullis is unrepentant in the face of those who complained his ideas were undermining the activities of AIDS health workers around the world. Critics of Mullis state that he has limited knowledge of HIV/AIDS and no scientific authority to speak on the cause of AIDS (Dickson, 1994).

Mullis himself appeared unfazed by such criticisms. His main concern was that the efforts of "a lot of talented people in the medical profession had been diverted" by misconceptions about HIV. Opinions about Mullis are as mixed as opinions about HEAL. He is famous for taking intellectual risks, sometimes wild ones. His book *Dancing Naked in the Mind Field* (published by Pantheon in August 1998) covers his **disbelief** that HIV causes AIDS and, among other things, his passion for hallucinogenic drugs and his belief in flying saucers.

UPDATE 2002

David Rasnick, an American chemist, is a leader of the HIV/AIDS dissidents in the United States. He is also the person who is thought to be, at least partially, responsible for South African President Mbeki's belief that HIV does not cause AIDS. In February 2002, Rasnick and South African computer science professor Philip Machanick, who believes that HIV causes AIDS and that the antiretroviral drugs are not as toxic as Rasnick says, have agreed, after a heated exchange of letters, to a challenge. The date, at this time, has not been set. But should this bizarre game of chicken occur, the scenario will go something like this. Rasnick will intentionally infect himself with HIV to prove that it does not cause disease, and Machanick will take drugs to prove they are not toxic. Under the agreement, Rasnick will inject himself with HIV on television and the two will meet annually to compare health status. It is doubtful that the action of this challenge will ever occur. Machanick is never going to get a doctor to prescribe him medication for a disease he doesn't have and Rasnick stipulated that he be injected with a highly purified virus, a condition that is impossible to meet. Results, if any, will be offered after they occur.

BOX 2.2

SCIENCE TAKES BACKSEAT TO POLITICS: SOUTH AFRICAN PRESIDENT THABO MBEKI SAYS HIS GOVERNMENT HAS A RIGHT/OBLIGATION TO DOUBT WHETHER HIV CAUSES AIDS

Beginning in March of 2000, two tragedies began unfolding simultaneously in South Africa. The **first** is epidemiological, with millions of men, women, and children infected with HIV destined to develop AIDS. The **second** is political, with President Thabo Mbeki (Figure 2-1) seriously entertaining a discredited view that challenges the role of HIV as the cause of AIDS. Together, the tragedies may well increase the AIDS pandemic in South Africa. The outcome can only be measured in untold suffering, death, and orphans.

The International Expert Panel—In early April, Mbeki's minister of health put together a 36-member panel of HIV/AIDS experts and HIV/AIDS dissidents to seek the truth as to whether HIV causes AIDS. The panel met on May 6 and 7 in Pretoria. At least 14 of the 36-member panel are known HIV/AIDS dissidents. The panel members were first given six weeks to contact each other via the internet and then provide Mbeki with their conclusions on whether HIV causes AIDS.

On April 4, 2001, the expert panel presented Mbeki with their conclusions. Nothing had changed. The dissidents did not move the believers in HIV and vice versa. The result, the panel did not offer Mbeki scientific grounds to depart from his belief that HIV does not cause AIDS. Further, after reading the panels' conclusions, Mbeki refused to take an HIV test because he said, "It would send a message that he supported a particular scientific viewpoint."

The Controversy—Why Now?

Why is a respected world leader embracing the dissidents' anti-HIV/AIDS doctrine now? Some say by refusing to allow the purchase or distribution of AZT to pregnant women, Mbeki is making a statement against the power of Western drug companies. After all, if HIV does not cause AIDS, why use AZT at all? Parallel to saying AZT is too toxic to use, Mbeki noted it was too expensive to buy. His minister of health said that to treat the 4 million people who need AZT would cost $47 billion—10 times the annual health de-

BOX 2.2 *(continued)*

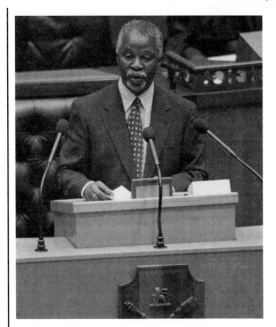

FIGURE 2-1   South African President Thabo Mbeki making his first address to the country's parliament, June 25, 1999. *(Photograph courtesy of Archive Photos)*

partment budget. Perhaps on a deeper level, Mbeki fears that high-priced AIDS treatment will derail economic development in a country finally emerging from oppression. Faced with a choice of AIDS drugs or new water systems, AIDS drugs or housing, AIDS drugs or health clinics, schools, and highways, the drugs fall short. Mbeki's loyal aides say there are too many unanswered questions about the disease and the current drugs to treat it.

DENIAL THAT HIV CAUSES AIDS

President Thabo Mbeki appears to be actively flirting with a new form of denial, one that claims that HIV is harmless, AIDS is a phony epidemic, and the only thing endangering the health of Africans is the same set of poverty-related health issues the continent has long faced. To the chagrin of doctors and scientists in his own country and around the world, Mbeki has tried to turn this into an issue of free speech rather than one of science.

Mbeki and other HIV dissidents believe that if HIV exists it does **not** cause AIDS. The disease

AIDS does not exist. There is no epidemic nor are there deaths from AIDS. There is just mass hysteria caused by a conspiracy among pharmaceutical multinationals, aided and abetted by political and medical self-interest. The views of the dissidents—or rethinkers as some like to call themselves—appear to be backed by an impressive range of scientific citations from reputable journals and leading scientists, including at least one Nobel Prize winner. But close examination of the sources dissidents cite often reveals extremely selective quotations from articles, or use of research that is outdated.

Orthodoxy—People who believe HIV causes AIDS have demonstrated a rapidly expanding foundation of scientific and medical understanding that rests upon a detectable virus, and have documented evidence of the impact of this virus on the human immune system. There is an impressive array of leading scientific names—the signatories to the Durban Declaration include many Nobel laureates. (See following.) **Yes,** there are still many gray areas, things about HIV and this disease that are still unknown, but that too is in the nature of science when it addresses new issues and a new virus. It is impossible to be absolute about medicine because of the complexity of the human body. Imperfect understanding means doctors and scientists sometimes encounter exceptional cases. For example, human cancers sometimes regress spontaneously for no understandable reason, even though the vast majority of people with the same kind of tumor die. To find a handful of people who are not detectably HIV-positive but who appear to have AIDS does not outweigh the millions of people who have AIDS where the only common link is HIV.

Believing in the orthodox position suggests that things can be done to prevent people from becoming HIV infected and dying of AIDS. These include abstinence, using condoms, preventing mother-to-child HIV transmission, being careful about blood transfusions and using antiretroviral drugs to help the immune systems of HIV-positive people delay the progression to AIDS.

Belief in the dissident view tends to suggest that because HIV does not cause AIDS, there is no epidemic; nothing needs to be done. People are dying of diseases exacerbated by poverty, as they have always done. It is simply that these are being recorded more often. There is **no** infectious

BOX 2.2 *(continued)*

agent at work, in South Africa or in the world, causing a new and different disease!

HIV either causes AIDS or it does not, and the answer must come from science—not politics!—The reasons supporting HIV as the cause of AIDS are too numerous to list here—but many of those reasons are found in this chapter and in Chapter 10 (see HIV/AIDS statistics for Africa). Nelson Mandela, (Figure 2-2) past president of South Africa said, "Mbeki is a man of great intellect who takes scientific thinking very seriously, while on the other hand the scientific community was committed to freedom of inquiry, unencumbered by undue political interference. Let us get on with what we know works!"

Update 2001—First: President Mbeki approved some pilot programs to provide free antiretroviral drugs to HIV-positive pregnant women. **Second:** in early 2001, 39 of the largest pharmaceutical companies in the world backed down on their claim that South Africa should not be allowed to manufacture generic (cheaper) versions of their antiretroviral drugs or to import them from other countries. Providing a highly visual court trial in Pretoria, South Africa, top American and foreign drug companies have offered their antiretroviral drugs to Africa at greatly reduced prices. However, South Africa's minister of health, Manto

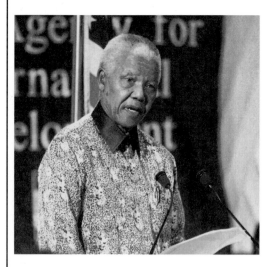

FIGURE 2-2 Former South Africa President Nelson Mandela holding a news conference at the 13th International AIDS Conference. He believes that HIV causes AIDS. *(Photograph courtesy of AP/Wide World Photos)*

Tshabalala-Msimang, declared in mid-2001 that she is opposed to the use of antiretrovirals in the public health sector. She said UNAIDS Director Peter Piot, the executive director of UNAIDS, and the manufactures of these medicines all now apparently share the belief that antiretrovirals are too complicated to use, too toxic, and have too severe side effects for use in Africa.

In November 2001 and in early February 2002, President Mbeki again defended his government's refusal to make antiretroviral drugs available through the public health system. He told a British Broadcasting Network reporter that crime was killing more South Africans aged 16 to 45 than this so called AIDS. And using the World Health Organization 1995 data, he told his minister of health that AIDS is not the main killer of South Africans and recommended new priorities in health spending—not that spending on AIDS received spending priority in South Africa. In October 2001, the South African Medical Council presented a shocking report on AIDS, "The Impact of HIV/AIDS on Adult Mortality in South Africa." The report stated that AIDS was the largest killer of people, that seven million would be dead from AIDS by 2010, and predicted that millions more will continue to die from AIDS. The government tried to suppress, then discredit, the report. Still, President Mbeki stands fast on his position and beliefs.

Update 2002—In April, President Mbeki began to distance himself from the AIDS dissidents. Mbeki has decided to cut informal contact with them and communicate with them only when the advisory panel meets. The President has instructed the Health Ministry to write to the dissidents telling them to stop using Mbeki's name when signing their correspondence. Several dissident members of Mbeki's AIDS Advisory Panel, among them Americans David Rasnick and Peter Duesberg, have taken to using this designation when writing documents and signing letters to newspapers. They have also been using Mbeki's name at international platforms when questioning the link between HIV and AIDS.

In May 2002, in a major departure from his controversial stance on AIDS, Mbeki's government made the dramatic announcement that it was to put in place a plan for a universal rollout of antiretroviral drugs for HIV-positive pregnant women, rape survivors, and people infected through needle stick injuries, beginning January 2003.

BOX 2.2 *(continued)*

SUMMARY

HIV/AIDS dissidents not only reject the evidence that HIV causes AIDS, most even reject the idea that the term **AIDS** describes a unique medical condition. The dissidents include a handful of scientists who had substantial credentials but have done little or no research with actual HIV/AIDS patients. Although members of this movement don't agree completely, most reject virtually all accepted HIV/AIDS medical treatment, as well as the use of condoms and safer sex to prevent HIV infection.

The current political and scientific furor in South Africa fueled largely by dissidents' theories on HIV/AIDS and the seeming support of President Mbeki has much broader implications for South Africa and South Africans than some are prepared to admit. The current controversy is undermining the constructive public health messages this government has put in place. It is sending mixed messages to all those who have dedicated themselves to the alleviation and eradication of this epidemic and is having a negative impact on the morale of affected patients and families. The undermining of scientists and the scientific method is especially dangerous in a developing country still in the process of establishing a strong scientific research base. Furthermore, it may erode investor confidence in the country, causing dire consequences.

The Durban Declaration—a statement signed by over 5,000 HIV/AIDS scientists and physicians from 50 countries and 5 continents was released to the press on July 1, 2000 (www. nature.com). Their statement that HIV causes AIDS is their answer to those who believe otherwise. They believe the evidence that HIV causes AIDS is clear, concise, exhaustive, and unambiguous! To conquer AIDS, everyone must understand that HIV is the enemy. (The Durban Declaration can be found at http:// www.eurakalert.org/releases/hte-uncc063000.html. The evidence that HIV causes AIDS can be found at http://www.thebody.com/niaid/hivcauseaids. html.)

In short, the vast majority of HIV/AIDS scientists and medical personnel feel as **George Orwell** stated in his book *1984*, **"What can you do against the lunatic . . . who gives your arguments a fair hearing and then simply persists in his lunacy?"** HIV DOES CAUSE AIDS!

CLASS QUESTION: What if you were president of a country in which 1 in 9 people were infected with a virus that you were told would kill them unless they were treated with exceptionally expensive medications that will always be outside the range of your health care system finances? Add to that a mandate from your country's constitution guaranteeing each citizen the right to health care. What would you do? Might you search for a way to deny that HIV is a major factor in AIDS? Offer pro/con discussion.

NEWSWEEK MAGAZINE AGAIN!

On December 2, 1996, the magazine cover read "The End of AIDS?" in large bold letters. In August 2000, the magazine ran a 3.5-page article complete with anti-HIV scare photographs entitled, **"The HIV Disbeliever."** Although the article attempted to be balanced between what science offers and what the HIV dissidents believe, the article left the readers in doubt as to who was right on the question—**does HIV cause AIDS?** In terms of balance the article presents much more about those who **do not believe.** The article presents personal testimonies from those who were told they where HIV positive, but after years of living with the virus and refusing antiviral therapy, remain very healthy. In short, the article states that the dissidents believe that "HIV is a lie! It's the toxic pills that made them die." A brief counter to the dissidents' arguments occupied two brief paragraphs of 49 words. A Boston college psychology professor who has studied holocaust deniers and AIDS dissenters believes that the dissidents gain "the basis of denial as a need to escape something that is terribly uncomfortable. If something is horrific, I might want to pretend it doesn't exists."

Question: Knowing that the article advocates, through the dissidents' beliefs, that people stop taking anti-HIV medications and stop worrying about catching the virus, is this article irresponsible? The CDC says that over 450,000 American deaths have been caused by HIV/AIDS, but the dissidents ask you to believe they died from the HIV drugs or recreational drugs, or perhaps succumbed to a profound fear of AIDS itself.

WHAT DO YOU BELIEVE AND WHY?

Question: Should freedom of the press be permitted when that freedom permits the delivery of information judged by global experts on the subject to be harmful to the public at large? Your response is (pro/con).

A Member of the U.S. Government Enters the Dispute

In March 1995, a letter was sent to eight government scientists and officials who influence AIDS research and policies, in which freshman Representative Gil Gutknecht (R-MN) questions the "HIV=AIDS hypothesis and its inability or effective treatment." His query echoes the arguments of Peter Duesberg. Gutknecht's initial inquiry asks whether recreational drug use and anti-HIV drugs might be the true cause of AIDS and questions whether AIDS is contagious.

Gutknecht's staffers think the federal AIDS effort—based on the conclusion that HIV causes AIDS—"will be seen as the greatest scandal in American history and will make Watergate look like a no-fault divorce" (Stone, 1995).

Talk Show Host Claims AIDS Is a Myth—October 1996, Fort Lauderdale, Florida—A talk show host and two medical professionals proclaimed over the airwaves on Miami's WLQY-AM, probably South Florida's most popular Haitian radio station, that AIDS is a myth, and urged an estimated 155,000 Haitian listeners to discontinue medication and refuse treatment.

The commentators told the Fort Lauderdale *Sun-Sentinel* that they had ample proof that AIDS does not exist and that the health care industry made it up to increase business. People should stop taking AIDS drugs and wearing condoms, they said in interviews for the article.

"We are not spreading lies. What we are saying are facts," said Henri-Claude Saint-Fleur, a North Miami Beach psychologist who was educated in France. "I'm happy to tell people the truth. I know lots of people who stopped taking their AIDS medication and are living well."

HIV/AIDS counselors say Haitian patients from at least four treatment centers stopped seeing doctors because of the show.

Class Discussion: Comment on the radio station's right to provide air time to promote this theme "AIDS IS A MYTH." Do the commentators have a right to tell people to stop taking their medications? Are they liable for such advice? Should they be liable?

Evidence That HIV Causes AIDS

It has been firmly established that there is a high correlation between HIV infection and the development of AIDS. With respect to establishing HIV as the causative agent of AIDS, look at some of the evidence:

1. The one common denominator is the presence of HIV within the entire range of people with this particular disease. That is, individuals who are HIV positive and have symptoms of HIV disease; and in individuals who are HIV positive but appear to be healthy.

2. The virus has been identified by electron microscopy inside and on the surface of T4 cells only in HIV-positive and AIDS patients (Figure 2-3 A, B).

3. Recent work of Bruce Patterson and Steven Wolinsky has shown that the genetic material of HIV (HIV-DNA) can be found in as many as 1 in 10 blood lymphocytes of persons with HIV disease (Cohen, 1993).

4. Antibodies against the virus, viral antigens, and HIV RNA have been found in HIV-positive and AIDS patients.

5. There is an absolute chronological association between the emergence of AIDS and the appearance of HIV in humans worldwide.

6. There is a chronological association of HIV-positive individuals who progress to AIDS. People who are truly HIV negative, and without the need for chemotherapy or radiation treatments, do not demonstrate HIV antibodies and never demonstrate AIDS. For example, people with hemophilia, unlike homosexual men, represent a well-defined group with long-term documentable changes in morbidity and mortality, since they had been well studied as a group before the era of AIDS. This research shows that people with hemophilia began to die of dramatically different things starting about 1982. Looking back shows little evidence of a special incidence of opportunistic diseases in people with hemophilia in the United States from the turn of the century up to 1979. Significantly, however, in the years before AIDS, people with hemophilia had never been noted to be particularly susceptible to the more obvious fungal infections, such as candida esophagitis, common to

FIGURE 2-3 Viral Replication in Human Lymphocytes. Scanning electron micrograph of HIV-infected human T4 lymphocyte. **A.** A single cell infected with HIV showing virus particles and microvilli on the cell surface (magnified 7,000 times). **B.** Enlargement of a portion of the mountain-like cell surface in **(A.)** showing multiple virus particles budding out of the cell surface (magnified 20,000 times). As each HIV exits the cell, it leaves a hole in the cell membrane. *(Photograph courtesy of K. Nagashima, Program Resources, Inc., NCI-Frederick Cancer Research and Development Center)*

AIDS patients and others with low-lymphocyte type immune deficiency. After 1984, this type of AIDS-associated opportunistic infection and immune failure rapidly became the single most common cause of death in people with hemophilia in America.

The rise in total mortality in people with hemophilia was sudden: Death in this population, which had been stable in 1982 and 1983, suddenly increased by a factor of approximately 900% in the first quarter of 1984. This increase in numbers of deaths was consistent with an epidemic, or some new very toxic contamination of the clotting factor supply. Mortality figures in hemophilia patients also showed something else important, which was that the new deaths of the late-1980s, by virtue of all being diagnosed with AIDS, demonstrated that most or all of them occurred in people with hemophilia who were HIV positive. Since these deaths accounted for almost the entire new increase in mortality, it could be inferred that the mortality rate for HIV-negative people with hemophilia did not increase much in the 1980s, if at all (Harris, 1998).

7. Hemophiliacs from low- and high-risk behavior groups were equally infected from HIV-contaminated blood factor VIII concentrates.

8. With the exception of persons who had their immune systems suppressed due to genetic causes or by drug therapy, prior to the appearance of the virus, there were no known AIDS-like cases. The virus has been isolated worldwide—but only where there are HIV-positive people and AIDS patients.

9. An HIV-positive identical twin born to an HIV-positive mother developed AIDS, but the HIV-negative twin did not.

10. Only HIV-positive mothers transmit HIV into their fetuses and only these HIV-positive newborns progress to AIDS. HIV-negative newborns from HIV-positive mothers **DO NOT** get AIDS!

11. Drugs developed specifically to inhibit the replication and/or maturation of HIV, thereby lowering the level of HIV found in HIV-infected people, have delayed the onset of HIV disease and, for HIV-infected pregnant women, have **decreased** the birth of HIV infected infants by 66%.

12. If HIV does not cause AIDS, how do HIV dissenters explain the positive effects of drugs used to affect the early and late stages in the life cycle of HIV that have lowered viral load to unmeasurable levels in the blood of those with HIV disease and AIDS and have virtually restored life for those at death's door

and who are now back at work? Or, how do they explain the positive effects offered by HIV phenotype- and genotype-resistant drug testing?

13. Finally, there have been numerous reports in the literature on HIV-infected individuals (homosexual, bisexual, and heterosexual) transmitting the virus to their sexual partners, both eventually dying of AIDS. *The unbroken chain of HIV transmission between prostitutes and their customers, between injection drug users sharing the same syringe, from infected mothers to their unborn fetuses, and so on all lead to the inescapable conclusion that HIV does cause AIDS.*

In short, Koch's Postulates have been satisfied: HIV disease meets all four criteria!

1. The causative agent must be found in all cases of the disease. (**It is.**)
2. It must be isolated from the host and grown in pure culture. (**It was.**)
3. It must reproduce the original disease when introduced into a susceptible host. (**It does.**)
4. It must be found in the experimental host so infected. (**It is.**)

In summary, HIV is the singular common factor that is shared between AIDS cases in gay men in San Francisco, well-nourished young women in Uganda, hemophiliacs in Japan, and children in Romanian orphanages. The identification of HIV as the causative agent of AIDS is now firmly accepted by scientists worldwide.

Class Discussion: You have just read some of the evidence for and against HIV being the cause of AIDS. Assuming you agree with the vast majority of HIV/AIDS investigators worldwide that HIV does cause AIDS, do you think there comes a time at which dissenters forfeit their right to make claims on other people's time and trouble by the poverty of their arguments and by the wasted effort and exasperation they have caused?
NOW discuss the value of the dissenter.
NOW discuss the danger of the dissenter's information or claims.

ORIGIN OF HIV: THE AIDS VIRUS

Clarification of the term "Origin of HIV." Scientists are searching for the **source** of HIV or HIV-like ancestor. Finding this source will give us the **Origin of HIV** as it pertains to where and in which animal the virus was housed prior to entering humans. But it does not mean the beginning of the virus per se—that will most likely never be known.

Tracking the origins and early history of a newly recognized disease is more than just an academic exercise. Unless we understand where HIV came from we run the risk of new emergencies, and unless we understand the ecology that allowed it to spread, we will be unable to control newly identified diseases. A classic example of tracking a source of a disease and the local epidemic it caused is **John Snow's** investigation of the cholera epidemic in Golden Square, London, in 1854; his removal of the handle of the Board Street pump contained the outbreak.

More than virtually any other disease, AIDS has generated myths and far-fetched theories about its origin, its causes, and even its very existence. These are probably linked to fear and denial prompted by a virus that is fatal, incurable, and sexually transmitted—and can infect people for years before they show any signs of illness.

Why Do Scientists Want to Know Where HIV Originated?

The object of determining the origin of the AIDS virus is to gain insight into how the virus may have evolved the unique set of characteristics that enable it to destroy the human immune system. Such information will offer valuable clues as to how rapidly the virus is evolving and how to combat it and perhaps help prevent future viral plagues.

If, for example, HIV is a new virus, say less than 30 years old, the many different varieties of HIV now infecting people worldwide probably evolved from a common ancestor sometime after World War II. New varieties can be expected to continue evolving at a frightening pace for several more decades, possibly producing new strains of the virus that are even more dangerous than those now infecting people. This could mean that vaccines now being developed based on current virus strains may not be useful in 10 to 20 years. But, should the known strains of the virus prove to be hundreds or thousands of years old, it might be possible that the current types of HIVs are in a state of global balance and they would not be expected to offer scientists any shocking evolutionary surprises in the future.

THE CAUSE AND EFFECT OF DISEASES: THE UNBROKEN CHAIN

For more than a century, four postulates set down by the German microbiologist Robert Koch have guided the hunt for disease-causing microbes. Koch argued in 1890 that to prove an organism causes a disease, microbiologists must (a) show that the organism occurs in every case of the disease; (b) that it is never found as a harmless parasite associated with another disease; (c) the organism must be isolated from the body and grown in laboratory culture; and (d) it must be introduced into a new host and produce the disease again.

Koch's criteria for cause and effect with respect to identifying a disease-causing agent **(bacterium)** are now being swept aside by new technology. Many of the microbes isolated in recent years by molecular techniques that pull segments of their DNA or RNA directly out of infected tissues **cannot be grown in culture.** That makes it impossible to fulfill all of Koch's postulates. As a result, many biologists are modifying Koch's strict requirements. Researchers can now build a convincing case against a microbe by examining a wide variety of molecular circumstantial evidence, such as how tightly the suspect microbe is associated with infected tissues and how closely the time course of the disease correlates with the amount of microbial genetic material present. But, as with Koch's methodology, the newer methodology for microbe identification with a specific disease also has its pitfalls.

Ideas on the Origin of HIV: UFOs, Biological Warfare, and Cats

Fear stimulates the imagination. Out of human fear have come some rather strange explanations for the origin of the AIDS virus. Early reports had unidentified flying objects (UFOs) crashing to Earth and releasing a "new organism" that would wipe out humanity.

There were frequent reports in the Soviet press linking AIDS with American biological warfare research. The Soviets agreed in August 1987 to stop these reports (Holder, 1988). There are also reports of extremism, as in the case of Illinois State Representative Douglas Huff of Chicago who told the *Los Angeles Times* that he gave over $500 from his office allowance fund to a local official of the Black Hebrew sect to help the group investigate its claim that Israel and South Africa created the AIDS virus in a laboratory in South Africa. Huff said AIDS is **"clearly an ethnic weapon, a biological weapon"** designed specifically to attack nonwhites (*CDC Weekly*, 1988).

Still another myth to surface is that the AIDS virus came from domestic cats. Because of its similarities to human AIDS, feline immunodeficiency virus has been called "feline AIDS." The cat retrovirus may damage cats' immune systems leaving the animals vulnerable to opportunistic infections *or* it may cause feline leukemia. However, the cat virus has never been shown to cause a disease in humans.

The origin of HIV has been attributed to HIV-contaminated polio, smallpox, hepatitis, and tetanus vaccines; the African green monkey; African people; their cattle, pigs, and sheep—and the United States CIA. With respect to the use of HIV-contaminated vaccines, a number of articles suggest that early monkey kidney cultures used to produce the polio vaccine carried HIV. Review of the literature offers *no* evidence that this occurred. The argument for the safety of the polio vaccine lies in the absence of any AIDS-related diseases among the hundreds of millions of persons vaccinated worldwide (Koprowski, 1992).

Now 22 years (1981–2003) into the AIDS epidemic, researchers are still baffled by the question: Where did HIV come from? AIDS is now known to be caused by two human immunodeficiency viruses, HIV-1 and HIV-2. The former, the cause of most AIDS cases worldwide, **appears to have spread from Central Africa, while the latter has so far been confined mainly to West Africa and the islands off its coast.** Several theories have been proposed to explain the origins of the AIDS pandemic. Most have been speculative rather than verifiable, and several have caused offense, particularly those that refer to sexual practices with monkey blood (Gilks, 1991). Charles Gilks (1992) states that HIV may have entered the human population by the direct inoculation of malaria-HIV-infected blood into human prisoner-volunteers. **The problem with this theory is that it is not testable so it, like** others, will remain an unproven theory proposed to explain the origin of HIV/AIDS.

Other Ideas on the Origin of HIV

Vanessa Hirsch and colleagues (1995) presented evidence that a virus isolated from a species of West African monkey, the Sooty Mangabey (an ash-colored monkey), may have infected humans 20 to 30 years ago. They believe this virus subsequently *evolved into HIV-2*. Hirsch et al. studied a virus known as the simian immunodeficiency virus (SIVsm) that infects both wild and captive sooty mangabey monkeys. They molecularly cloned and sequenced the DNA of the virus and constructed an evolutionary tree of the several known primate immunodeficiency viruses. This tree showed SIVsm to be more closely related to HIV-2 than to HIV-1.

Gerald Meyers of Los Alamos National Laboratory states that SIVsm and HIV are so closely related that when HIV-2 is found in a human, it may be the sooty mangabey virus. However, HIV-1, which causes AIDS, does not sufficiently resemble HIV-2 or SIVsm, thus HIV-1 probably did not evolve from SIVsm/HIV-2. **The prevailing theory is that humans were first infected through direct contact with HIV-infected primates. The primate to human scenario is easier to accept than humans infecting primates.**

Be a Virus, See the World

Albert Osterhaus of Erasmus University Rotterdam, The Netherlands, believes that **all** human viral infectious diseases ultimately have an animal origin, and natural transfer of these infections is a common event in animal populations.

Humans have hunted, handled, and even eaten primates for thousands of years. Recent laboratory accidents have shown that SIV can infect humans. Even though at the moment, no identifiable disease has been associated with the SIV/human infections, such accidents have demonstrated the potential for cross-species or zoonotic transmission of HIV-related viruses. Why not believe the same for the origin of HIV-1?

The possibility remains that HIV has been present but remained an obscure virus in the human population for a long time before it changed into a lethal agent.

The first recorded AIDS case in America was that of a 15-year-old male prostitute who demonstrated Kaposi's sarcoma and died in 1969. Frozen tissue samples contained HIV antibodies. These findings were reported at the 11th International Congress of Virology in August 1999.

The first documented case of AIDS in Europe was seen in a Danish surgeon who had worked in Zaire. She died in 1976.

POINT OF INFORMATION 2.1

SCIENTISTS REPORT ON EARLIEST AIDS CASE

Scientists have pinpointed what is believed to be the earliest known case of AIDS—an African man who died in 1959. The scientists looked for signs of HIV in 1,213 blood samples that were gathered in Africa between 1959 and 1982. They found clear signs of the virus in one taken from a Bantu man who lived in Leopoldville, Belgian Congo—what is now Kinshasa, Republic of Congo—in 1959. Scientists compared the genes from the 39-year-old sample of HIV with current versions of HIV. They realized that if they had an old sequence of HIV genes it would serve as a yardstick to measure the evolution of the current HIV. HIV has mutated over the years to form 11 distinct subtypes, lettered A through K. One of these, subtype B, is the dominant strain in the United States and Europe, while subtype D is most common in Africa. The family tree of HIV looks like a bush

with the various subtypes forming the limbs. Scientists believe the 1959 HIV is near the trunk, around the point where the subtypes B and D branch off and that this virus is an ancestor to B and D. These data suggest that all HIV subtypes evolved from one introduction of HIV into people, rather than from many crossovers from animals to humans, as some have speculated.

However, the question scientists are trying to answer is why the disease took so long to start manifesting itself, ultimately hitting the homosexual and hemophiliac populations in the United States in the late 1970s. Current thinking is that HIV probably first infected rural areas of Africa, slowly moving into the cities and around the world until it hit homosexual communities where conditions were sufficient for rapid transmission of the disease.

The first documented case of AIDS in Africa occurred in 1959 (see Point of Information 2.1).

The Current Theory on HIV Origin: A Chimpanzee

Beatrice Hahn and colleagues (1999; 2000) from the University of Alabama at Birmingham feel that they have gathered sufficient evidence to believe the origin of HIV-1 in humans to be cross-species transmission from a particular subspecies of chimpanzee—meaning that a simian virus **closely related to HIV** jumped from monkeys to humans, and later mutated into its current form, following one of many interspecies transmissions. (Figure 2-4)

Hahn presented three lines of evidence in support of their thesis. **First,** the genes of all four **SIVcpz** isolates cluster on evolutionary trees according to their subspecies or origin, either *Pan troglodytes troglodytes* from West Africa or *Pan troglodytes scheinfurthii* in East Africa. By sequencing parts of the virus' genetic material, the scientists found that more segments of the simian and human virus overlapped than had been identified in three previous simian viruses isolated in recent years from other chimpanzees. The investigation revealed that the other previously studied simian viruses were more closely related to very rare forms of HIV that don't account for most of the infections in the world.

Second, all known HIV-1 strains, including the M group that accounts for about 99% of all HIV-1 infections, as well as the O group and the N group, form a genetic cluster with the West African chimpanzee viruses. This clustering is also geographic and consistent with the likely equatorial Central African origin of HIV-1. (Figure 2-5) Hahn said she had initially been equally ready to accept the idea that chimps had gotten HIV from humans, rather than vice versa. However, a **third** line of evidence convinced her that HIV-1 was introduced into the human population from at least three cross-species transmission from chimpanzee—she found evidence of genetic recombination among the SIVcpz strains of the **troglodytes'** lineage.

UPDATE 2002 Two reports at the Eighth Annual Retrovirus Conference (2001) show that several monkey species carry HIV-like viruses. Eric Delacorte of the University of Montpelier, France, took blood samples from various West

FIGURE 2-4 Photograph of *Pan troglodytes troglodytes*. This photograph was taken in the Gabon region of Africa where the sole species of Pan troglodytes is found. Their numbers are declining rapidly due to the "bush meat" trade—the slaughter and selling of their body parts. *(Photograph courtesy of Karl Ammann, wildlife photographer)*

African monkey species that were sold as bush meat (meat from the African wilderness), as well as blood from animals kept as pets. Laboratory analyses of the viruses in those animals showed that about 17% of the specimens harbored SIVcpz strains, including four strains not seen before. In addition, scientists in the United States found evidence in chimpanzees that SIVcpz is found in animals in East Africa as well as West Africa, suggesting that not only is the virus widely distributed in Africa, but that continued hunting of the species for food and keeping the animals as pets could result in another outbreak of an AIDS-like disease. These data document, for the first time, that humans are continuously

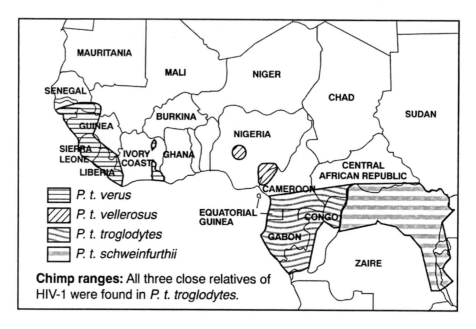

FIGURE 2-5 Geographic Ranges of Four Subspecies of Chimpanzee *Pan troglodytes.* All three close relatives of HIV-1, as determined by genetic sequencing of their genetic material, were found in Pan troglodytes troglodytes. *(Adapted from Hahn, 1999)*

exposed to an unprecedented variety of SIVs through the consumption of bush meat. (Santiago et al., 2002; Peeters et al., 2002)

Is the Search for the Origin of HIV Over?

It is nice to think that the issue of HIV origin has been solved. However, time will tell if Hahn's current effort will be the final word on the subject. Some questions still remain. Why, for example, does HIV-1 appear to be so benign in chimpanzees (as has been shown in numerous infection experiments over the years). Most interesting perhaps will be to learn what insight this history of HIV might provide for predicting the ultimate evolutionary accommodation between HIV and humans. For scientists, the new chimpanzee finding is just as much a beginning as an end. Although researchers may have the best evidence so far that HIV came from chimpanzees, no one can yet say how the virus became lethal to humans, and when. Chimpanzees share over 98 percent of the genes that exist in humans, yet they don't get AIDS. So which of the remaining genes protect chimpanzees from an infection that has turned

out to be almost universally fatal in people? Also, researchers are still investigating how, after taking root in just a few people, HIV gradually traveled all over the world.

Researchers now believe that AIDS-like viruses jumped from chimp to human more than once, creating different strains of HIV. This means a vaccine against one strain of HIV may not control a new epidemic. As it turned out, **Pan troglodytes troglodytes** lives in the region of Africa where HIV-1 was first recognized. Since there are three separate kinds of HIV-1, the scientists believe that HIV-1 crossed into people from chimps at least three times. Hahn said that SIV appears to have dwelled in primates for hundreds of thousands of years before turning into the deadly human virus, HIV. Hahn believes hunting, which exposes people to excessive amounts of blood during slaughter, allowed precursor HIV to infect humans.

UPDATE 2002 With regard to the question of why chimpanzees resist HIV infection, in late 2002, Dutch investigators presented a theory that an AIDS-like epidemic killed large populations of chimps about 2 million years ago. The survivors of this viral (SIVcpz-like?) eradication were selected for survival because they carried the genes necessary to resist the viral infection. Over the years, this genetic selection gave rise to chimpanzees that are resistant to viruses that are closely related to HIV, for example SIVcpz and HIV itself.

Where did HIV Begin to Circulate Among Humans?—

According to Nicole Vidal and colleagues (2000), because of the unprecedented degree of HIV-1 group M genetic diversity found in the Democratic Republic of Congo (9 of the 11 different group M subtypes), the HIV-1 pandemic must have originated in Central Africa.

Daniel Vangroenweghe (2001) states that the earliest cases of HIV infection and AIDS in the 1960s and 1970s occurred in Congo-Kinshasa (Zaire), Rwanda, and Burundi. These countries appear to be the source of HIV group M epidemic, which then spread outwards to neighboring Tanzania and Uganda in the East, and Congo-Brazzaville in the West. Further spread to Haiti and onwards to the United States can be explained by the hundreds of single men from Haiti who participated in the UNESCO educational program in the Congo between 1960 and 1975.

When did HIV Begin to Circulate Among Humans?—

Scientists do have some idea when the virus began to circulate among people. From looking at samples of HIV taken at different times and in different parts of the world, researchers have constructed a type of genetic clock for HIV-1. The speed of the clock is determined by how much the virus changes over time. A key to setting this clock came with the discovery of the oldest known HIV infection, found in the man who lived in what is now Congo in 1959. That year, he was one of 1,200 Africans who had given a blood sample as part of a study of the immune system. After the AIDS epidemic began, the frozen samples were thawed and screened.

Timing the Crossover

By comparing HIV-1 samples taken over time, Steven Wolinsky and his colleagues determined that HIV began to spread within decades before the 1959 sample was drawn (Balter, 1998; Korber et al. 1998). The estimate is based on the assumption that the rate of change for HIV has remained about the same. This would place the crossover into humans

around 1924 to 1946. Studies have also indicated that HIV-2 began to spread about the same time.

From the 7th Conference on Retrovirus and Opportunistic Infections—February 2000, **Bette Korber** from Los Alamos National Laboratory presented data attempting an exact estimate as to when the virus SIVcpz from **Pantroglodytes** crossed into humans. Summarizing months of work involving incredibly complicated mathematical modeling of thousands of primate lentivirus gene sequences on a Los Alamos supercomputer that can perform 1 trillion computations/second, Korber made two new and important take-home points. **First,** the timing of the origin of the HIV-1 (M) group (from which all other HIV species have evolved) is near 1930, with the 95% CIs (confidence intervals) spanning from 1910 to 1950. **Second,** although she could not disprove with certainty the possibility that HIV-1 was introduced into humans by the polio vaccine trials in Africa in the 1950s and 1960s, she did state that this event had very low probability. Her computer analysis of gene sequences traces back to a single viral ancestor—**a viral EVE** (after the EVE, common female ancestor of modern humans who migrated out of Africa between 100,000 and 200,000 years ago)—that emerged around 1930. That is, this pandemic got started when the precursor SIVcpz crossed into one or a small group of humans at that time. More recently Korber and colleagues reported that the best estimate for the date when the common ancestor of HIV-1 M group came into existence was between 1915 and 1941. Molecular clock analysis provided the date of 1931 (Korber et al., 2000). This report states that the HIV-1 M group had a **single origin**—from one animal. The most common form of HIV in America, M **subgroup B** is believed to have evolved between 1960 and 1971 with 1967 being the most likely year.

UPDATE 2001 Marco Salemi and colleagues (2000) reported that by using new computerized dating methods based on virus genetic data, their group found that HIV-1 group M and its closest related simian virus SIVcpz, isolated from chimpanzees, shared a common ancestor about 300 years ago, around 1675. According to the Belgian investigators, the virus jumped from chimpanzees to humans somewhere between 1675 and the early 1990s. They placed the emergence of HIV in humans between the 1920s and 1930s. This means that HIV was in humans and beginning to evolve, diverge, accumulate, and spread.

Twice This Century!

Preston Marx of the Aaron Diamond AIDS Research Center said, "Never before in thousands of years of exposure to SIV did these viruses cross over to cause (widespread) disease in people, and yet it happened twice this century.... Not only did this happen in chimpanzees, it happened in sooty mangabeys 1,000 miles away." Many scientists have speculated about why the virus might have become amplified in post-World War II Africa. Among the possibilities: the exploding population of urban centers; social upheaval and commerce that led to migration across the continent; and widespread vaccination campaigns that could have reused needles. In the end, HIV's early accomplices aren't known for sure. Nor is it clear how AIDS came to the United States.

Continued Evolution of HIV in Humans?— Possible *good* news (?) is that HIV will, after killing millions of humans, become a harmless passenger as most likely its precursor SIV did thousands of years ago in chimpanzees. The **bad** news would be that HIV is evolving into a virus that is more easily spread and/or that it becomes more lethal. Time will tell.

HIV Is Stigmatizing Africa

Discussion of the African origins of HIV has caused controversy. Some African governments protested suggestions that Africa was "responsible" for the AIDS epidemic, and even denied that AIDS was a problem in their countries. For most of the 1980s, the military government of Zaire would not allow outsiders to investigate the spread of AIDS and did not report AIDS cases to the World Health Organization. Some Africans denounced "racist" Western media for reporting AIDS as an African plague. Carr states that "by 1990, when it was obvious to all that HIV infection was tragically widespread in central, southern, and eastern Africa, this controversy had largely ended. HIV infection is far too widespread in Africa to be the result of recent importation from outside; the African epidemic clearly precedes the Western one." **Regardless, where HIV/AIDS arose is irrelevant to medical science—when and how HIV entered the human population is relevant.**

SUMMARY ON THE ORIGIN OF HIV

In summary, there are at least three ideas on the possible origins of the AIDS virus: (1) it is a human-made virus, perhaps from a germ warfare laboratory; (2) it originated in the animal world and crossed over into humans; and (3) HIV has existed in small isolated human populations for a long time and, given the right set of conditions, it escaped into the larger population. Computer modeling of DNA sequence in HIV and SIVsm and the recent work of Beatrice Hahn and colleagues and Marco Salemi and colleagues suggests that HIV evolved within the last 100 to 300 years. So for now, the question remains: Is AIDS a new disease or an old disease that was late being recognized—so late that we will never know its true source of origin, the origin of HIV? Continued investigations may answer these questions.

Has HIV Always Caused a Lethal Disease—AIDS?

An additional question to where HIV came from is whether it has always caused disease. From the study of human history, as it relates to human disease, scientists have numerous examples that show that as human habits change, new diseases emerge. Regardless of whether HIV is old or new, history will show that social changes, however small or sudden, have most likely hastened the spread of HIV. Increased rounds of HIV replication presented humans with new HIV mutations, some of which were to become lethal. In the 1960s, war, tourism, and commercial trucking forced the outside world on Africa's once isolated villages. At the same time, drought and industrialization prompted mass migrations from the countryside into newly teeming cities. Western monogamy had never been common in Africa, but as the French medical historian Mirko Grmek notes in his book, *History of AIDS* (1990), urbanization shattered social structures that had long contained sexual behavior. Prostitution exploded, and venereal diseases flourished. Hypodermic needles came into wide use during the same period, creating yet another mode of infection. Did these trends actually turn a chronic but relatively benign infection into a killer? The evidence is circumstantial, but it's hard to discount.

BOX 2.4

ORIGIN OF HIV IN HUMANS: A COMPETING HYPOTHESIS

After years of speculation, most scientists now agree that the HIV/AIDS pandemic began when an AIDS-like virus from a chimpanzee, probably in west-central Africa, jumped species and infected a human being sometime in the first half of this century. The mystery, however, is exactly how that cross-species jump from chimpanzee into humans occurred. The most popular theory in scientific circles is that the chimp virus entered the human race when an African hunter in a remote area butchered a chimpanzee for food and accidentally cut himself, exposing his own blood to infected chimpanzee blood. But there's a competing hypothesis: The chimp virus, the one that causes AIDS, may have been unwittingly introduced into humans when scientists from Philadelphia's Wistar Institute conducted mass human trials of an experimental polio vaccine in the former Belgian Congo and nearby countries during the late 1950s.

HOW WAS THE POLIO VACCINE MADE IN THE 1950S?

Oral polio vaccines are made from viruses that have been weakened so that they don't cause disease. In the 1950s, scientists grew live polio vaccines in monkey kidneys that had been cut into tiny pieces and placed in a jar filled with fluid. Cells would grow out of the minced pieces of tissue and form an underwater film of cells on the bottom of the dish. A few drops of a solution containing a weak vaccine strain of polio virus would be added to the dish; the virus would reproduce inside the cells, and after a week or so the fluid would contain many billions of polio vaccine viruses. The fluid was filtered, diluted, and then given to people. Their immune systems would learn to destroy the vaccine virus, and when vaccinated people encountered the real virus later on, their previously alerted immune system would produce antibody quickly and destroy the virus. The hypothesis that the early polio vaccines were contaminated with HIV has been kicking around the edges of mainstream science for more than a decade and is the subject of a new book, **The River: A Journey to the Source of HIV and AIDS,** (1999) by British journalist Edward Hooper. The 1070-page work has received mixed reviews in academic medical journals and has drawn the interest of AIDS activists.

Hooper collected volumes of circumstantial evidence gathered in hundreds of interviews and from thousands of medical papers. Hooper says that some batches of Wistar's polio vaccine were accidentally tainted with the chimp form of the AIDS virus, known as SIVcpz, picked up in the polio vaccine manufacturing process, which used monkey kidney cells not chimp cells, to produce the polio virus for the polio vaccines in the 1950s. But Hooper states that Wistar and its Belgian colleagues established a chimpanzee colony, the Lindi Camp, just outside the present-day Kisangani in central Congo, headquarters of the polio campaign. Hooper alleges the camp not only provided chimps on which to test the vaccine, but also supplied the scientists with chimp kidneys to grow the vaccine virus back in Philadelphia and possibly in Belgium and Congo as well. Hooper says that between 1957 and 1960, a million people, mostly children, in what is now Congo, Rwanda, and Burundi received that polio vaccine. He suggests that a few children likely became infected with the chimp form of AIDS when contaminated polio vaccine was squirted into their mouths. The AIDS-like virus might have been taken up by cells on the tonsils and gotten into the bloodstream. As these infected children grew up they could have passed the virus on to others through sexual contact. Of the 39 confirmed cases of HIV-positive blood collected in Africa before 1981, 87% came from towns where polio vaccine was administered. Hooper says that all HIV-positive blood samples came from places within 100 miles of the vaccination sites.

Hooper's theory caused such an uproar that the Wistar Institute asked three independent laboratories to examine samples of the 40-year-old vaccine for signs of HIV, SIV, and chimpanzee mitochondrial DNA.

Tests performed by three independent laboratories on 1950s-era polio vaccine samples from the Wistar Institute in Philadelphia failed to find any traces of SIV, HIV-1, or DNA indicating that chimpanzee cells were NOT used to prepare the vaccine, according to the scientist who coordinated the testing.

The results of the tests were announced at the September 2000 meeting of the Royal Society of London. But at the Royal Society meeting, Hooper immediately dismissed the tests as irrelevant

BOX 2.4 *(continued)*

because, he said, the key batches of vaccine that he claims were produced with chimp kidney tissue no longer exist.

In the meantime, investigations on the origin of HIV in humans by Beatrice Hahn and Bette Korber show that the chimpanzee virus, the precursor to HIV, is located in west-central Africa—not in the Congo—and that it entered humans in the 1930s, long before a polio vaccine was made. In addition, both researchers point out that if the polio vaccine were at fault, it would have had to contain at least 11 genetically separate viral strains from different chimpanzees. Anne-Mieke Vandamme of the Riga Institute in Belgium along with colleagues in France, Germany, and Ireland believe HIV was derived from SIVcpz between 1675 and 1700! If true, why did HIV remain invisible for 300 years? Clearly the case for the origin of HIV in humans has not yet been closed.

STATEMENT/QUESTION

After reading the preceding information, there remain a few nagging questions. Placed in perspective, the problem is the earliest confirmed AIDS case to date occurred in Kinshasa, Africa, in 1959. But how did its precursor HIV enter humans? We know that HIV does not survive well outside the body and the most effective means of transmission is via blood. The going theory as put forth by Beatrice Hahn and others before her is that the blood of an infected monkey entered humans during killing and eating rituals or perhaps through a monkey bite.

Question: Most bothersome is that these events are ancient rituals passed down for a thousand years, so why did it take until the 1930s or 1950s to enter humans? And until the 1980s to become recognized? Perhaps Beatrice Hahn, Bette Korber, and others are wrong about how HIV entered humans. Does it make Edward Hooper right? NO, but what then? Hypotheses continue.

Another hypothesis—In March 2002, German investigators offered a new theory on how

the precursor virus to HIV entered humans. Gerhard Brandner and Werner Kloft of the University of Bonn, and Mangred Eigen of the Max Planck Institute for Biophysical Chemistry in Goettingen, suggest that bloodsucking flies may have unleashed the world's AIDS pandemic by transmitting an HIV-like virus from chimpanzees to humans. They believe the stable fly, a blood feeding fly that regularly swarm over bloody carcasses, could have taken up the virus and passed it on to humans. The stable fly, unlike mosquitoes and other biting insects, stores the ingested blood that it later regurgitates, in an enzyme-free environment. Therefore, HIV in such blood would not be destroyed. And the theories go on!

GENERAL STATEMENT CONCERNING ANIMALS, THEIR DISEASES, AND HUMANS

In our efforts to make things better for ourselves, we sometimes make things worse. If HIV entered human populations through new medical technologies such as needles, blood transfusions, and through vaccines, it will not be the first time that a microbe has flourished in the wake of scientific advancement. HIV is not the first disease-causing agent to cross over into humans. Smallpox, brucellosis, anthrax, and tuberculosis are all cattle diseases; influenza comes from hogs; leprosy from the water buffalo; the common cold from horses; and measles, rabies, and hydatid cysts from dogs. All these diseases probably first affected human beings after these animals were domesticated and when the density of human populations increased sufficiently to permit these microbes to propagate. Epidemics of polio only emerged in the nineteenth century with improvements in sanitation. Animal husbandry and sanitation have saved generations from malnutrition, dysentery, cholera, and many other plagues. Now we find some of the old and new emerging together!

Can Humans Be Creating Scenarios for the Introduction of New Diseases?

Whatever the forces are that brought us HIV and AIDS, they can surely bring other diseases. By encroaching on rain forests and wilderness areas, humans are placing themselves in ever- **closer contact with animal species and their deadly parasites.** Activities, from irrigation to the construction of dams and cities, can expose humans to new diseases by expanding the range of the rodents or insects that carry them. Stephen Morse, a Rockefeller virologist, studies the movement of microbes among populations and species. He worries that human activities are speeding the flow of viral traffic. More than a dozen new diseases have shown up in humans since the 1960s, nearly all of them the result of once-exotic parasites exploiting new opportunities. (Certain of these new disease-causing agents, for example, the Ebola virus, are discussed in Box I.1 on page 6.)

SUMMARY

The AIDS virus was discovered and reported by Luc Montagnier of France in 1983. Identifying the virus that caused the immunosuppression that caused AIDS allowed for AIDS surveillance definitions that began in 1982. The recent recognition of non-HIV AIDS cases is not unexpected and can be explained. **Presently, there is no new threat of another AIDS-causing biological agent.**

The recent work of Beatrice Hahn and colleagues may have pinpointed the reservoir of a precursor, HIV-like virus in the chimpanzee, *Pan troglodytes troglodytes*. The work of Bette Korber and colleagues may have set the time frame in which precursor HIV crossed into humans.

REVIEW QUESTIONS

(Answers to the Review Questions are on page 489.)

1. What may be the strongest nonlaboratory evidence for saying that AIDS is caused by an environmental agent?

2. Where might HIV have originated and where did the first HIV infections appear?

Biological Characteristics of the AIDS Virus

3

CHAPTER CONCEPTS

- ◆ Retroviruses are grouped into three families: oncoviruses, lentiviruses, and foamy viruses.
- ◆ HIV is a lentivirus.
- ◆ HIV contains **nine genes**; its three major structural genes are GAG-POL-ENV.
- ◆ HIV contains 9749 nucleotides, its genetic code.
- ◆ Six HIV genes regulate HIV reproduction and at least one gene directly influences infection.
- ◆ HIV RNA produces HIV DNA, which integrates into the host cell to become **proviral** DNA.
- ◆ HIV undergoes rapid genetic changes within infected people.
- ◆ The reverse transcriptase enzyme is very error prone.
- ◆ HIV causes immunological suppression by destroying T4 helper cells or CD4+ cells.
- ◆ HIV is classified into major (M), outlier (O), and type (N) genetic subtypes. Type M is responsible for 99% of the HIV infections worldwide.

VIRUSES NEED HELP

Viruses are microscopic particles of biological material, so small that they can be seen only with electron microscopes. A virus consists solely of a strip of genetic material (nucleic acid) within a protein coat.

Viral genomes (DNA and RNA that contain the genetic information to replicate) are very small and contain few genes compared to living cells. With their limited coding capacity, viruses must borrow

---

SIDEBAR 3.1

HOW HIV ESCAPES THE INFECTED CELL

This is a primary example of how a virus, in this case HIV, uses living cells to achieve its mission—to infect, replicate, or exit a cell. In October 2001, Jennifer Garrus and colleagues reported on how HIV takes over the human cells normal processes in order to leave a cell. This discovery could lead to new drugs to control HIV disease in those who are HIV infected. In a key part of their study, the scientists crippled the cells machinery by silencing a gene that normally makes the protein (Tsg101) necessary for HIV to escape or bud out of the cell. Thus, clusters of connected HIV particles were stuck at the cell membrane and could not get out. The researchers already knew that a part of HIV known as the GAG protein is essential for HIV to bud out from the cell. The new study showed the Tsg101 protein within cells acts as a key link to the budding process. One part of Tsg101 protein connects to the HIV GAG protein. Another part of the Tsg101 protein links to other proteins within a cell—proteins the cell normally uses to exit the cell. Shutting down the means by which HIV leaves the cell means that the infection of other susceptible cells will not become infected. Blocking Tsg101 protein after a person becomes infected could keep the virus from spreading to other cells. These scientists speculate that many other viruses may use the same exit pathway. After 22 years, scientists still do not know just how HIV kills cells bearing a CD4 protein and scientists still do not know why T4 or CD4+ cells fall from 1000 per microliter of blood to less than 100 per microliter of blood over a 10-year period while viral loads may remain constant or show an enormous increase over a short time interval. And in many people, the relationship of viral load to the rate of their disease progression is questionable at best.

or hijack host or cell proteins to complete their replication. The interactions between a virus and its host have been shaped by long stretches of coevolution, and the borrowed proteins do not necessarily serve the same function in viral replication as they serve in the host. Indentification of these borrowed host proteins, which perform essential functions during viral replications, is important for understanding virus-host interactions, which influence the host range and virulence of the virus.

VIRUSES ARE PARASITES

Viruses are parasitic agents; they live inside the cells of their host animal or plant, and **can reproduce themselves only by forcing the host cell to make viral copies.** The new virus leaves the host cell and infects other similar cells. By damaging or killing these cells, some viruses cause diseases in the host animal or plant. Genetically, viruses are the simplest forms of **"life-like agents"**; the genetic blueprint for the structure of the **human immunodeficiency virus (HIV)** is 100,000 times smaller than that contained in a human cell. The complete sequence of 9749 nucleotides that form the genetic code for HIV have been identified and their arrangement sequenced (mapped).

Scientists have produced a great deal of information about HIV over a relatively short time. The immediate involvement of so many scientists followed by the rapid identification of the causative agent of AIDS is unequaled in the history of medical science. More is known about HIV than about the viruses that cause such long-standing human diseases as polio, measles, yellow fever, hepatitis, flu, and the common cold. Humankind is fortunate that HIV began spreading through the human population as a pathogen in the mid- to late-1970s. By then scientists had discovered and begun to exploit the molecular aspects of biology. Molecular methodologies necessary to begin the immediate molecular study of HIV were in place to define and refine our knowledge of viruses and, in particular, to learn about HIV.

RETROVIRUSES

Viruses that belong to the Retroviridae family have a Janus-like relationship with modern medicine.

POINT OF INFORMATION 3.1

VIRAL SPECIFICITY

1. **Viruses are very specific with regard to the types of cells they can enter/reproduce.** Not all viruses can attach to or enter all cells. Humans survive in a world full of viruses that **only** enter or reproduce in a variety of bacteria, protozoa, fungi, and higher forms of plant and animal life. It appears that most of these viruses are harmless to humans—if they enter the body they cannot reproduce in human cells—they do not cause human damage. For those viruses that do enter human bodies from animals such as pigs, chickens, rabbits, mice, cows, monkeys, etc. that cause a human disease, most are very specific as to which cells in a human body they can enter/reproduce and cause damage. For example, the flu virus enters the human respiratory tract cells. Epstein-Barr virus infects cells in the nose and throat. The hepatitis viruses enter liver cells, but each of the hepatitis viruses causes a different degree of human cell damage over time. Some cause a more immediate disease—for example, hepatitis A virus—while hepatitis B or hepatitis C may

not cause significant cell damage for years. Polio virus enters cells of the human nervous system that are different from those cells of the nervous system that herpes virus invades. HIV enters and reproduces in cells of the human immune system.

2. **Why do different viruses enter specific cell types?** Each of the viruses that cause human disease do so by finding a cell type that carries a receptor molecule (a protein or a protein attached to a sugar molecule) that **fits** with a projection of a surface molecule of a given virus—much like the key to a lock. That's why specific viruses are known to be associated with certain types of human tissue. For example, there are viruses that attach only to the receptors of heart, gut, eyes, throat, liver, and other specific human cell type tissues. Find a way to block either the human cell receptors (CD4, CXCKR4, and CCKR5—to which HIV attaches), without harming the cell or block the given viral receptor (in HIV its gp120) and one has a therapy for the given viral disease.

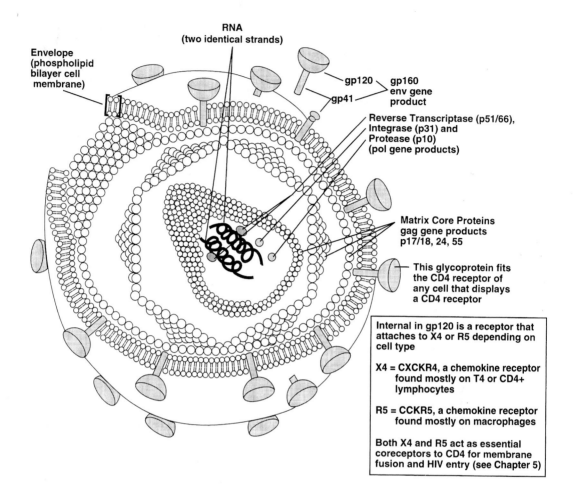

RNA
(two identical strands)

Envelope
(phospholipid
bilayer cell
membrane)

gp120
gp41
gp160
env gene
product

Reverse Transcriptase (p51/66),
Integrase (p31) and
Protease (p10)
(pol gene products)

Matrix Core Proteins
gag gene products
p17/18, 24, 55

This glycoprotein fits
the CD4 receptor of
any cell that displays
a CD4 receptor

Internal in gp120 is a receptor that
attaches to X4 or R5 depending on
cell type

X4 = CXCKR4, a chemokine receptor
found mostly on T4 or CD4+
lymphocytes

R5 = CCKR5, a chemokine receptor
found mostly on macrophages

Both X4 and R5 act as essential
coreceptors to CD4 for membrane
fusion and HIV entry (see Chapter 5)

Some members of the family have proven to be valuable tools in molecular biology research; their ability to import foreign genes into cells has been explored as a possible vehicle for gene therapy. Retroviruses also are potent disease agents, causing, among other illnesses, a form of leukemia in adult humans. Members of this family also infect chimpanzees and other simian species (simian immunodeficiency viruses or SIVs), and they infect and cause a deadly immunodeficiency syndrome in humans: AIDS.

Data that researchers have gathered during years of work comparing the genetic make-up of SIVs and HIV have shown that while primate species infected with SIVs are the long-time natural hosts to those viruses, humans are not the natural hosts of HIV.

There are three subfamilies of retroviruses, two of which are associated with human disease: **oncoviruses** (cancer-causing) and **lentiviruses** or slow viruses of which HIV-1 and HIV-2 are members. **Spumavirus** is the third group but is not known to be associated with human disease. As a lentivirus, HIV has genetic and morphologic similarities to other animal lentiviruses such as those infecting cats (feline immunodeficiency virus), sheep (visna virus), goats (caprine arthritis-encephalitis virus), and nonhuman primates (simian immunodeficiency virus or SIV).

The retroviruses and in particular the lentiviruses have presumably been present for thousands of years. Modern sociodemographic changes and other human factors have allowed rapid mutating (changing) lentiviruses, such as HIV, to find

FIGURE 3-1 Human Immunodeficiency Virus. It infects cells by a process of membrane fusion that is mediated by its envelope glycoproteins (gp120-gp41, or Env) and is generally triggered by the interaction of gp120 with two cellular components: CD4 and a coreceptor belonging to the chemokine receptor family (CXCKR4 or X4 and CCKR5 or R5). The virus is a sphere measuring 1000 Å or 1/10,000 mm in diameter. The cone-shaped core in a spherical envelope is the dominant feature. In this diagram the virus has been sectioned to better visualize its internal structure. The membrane of HIV is derived from the host cell. HIV gains the membrane while "budding" out or exiting the cell. Each free HIV leaves a hole in the cell membrane. The membrane, acquired from its host cell, consists of two lipid (fat) layers impregnated with some human proteins, for example Class I and Class II human lymphocyte antigen complexes important for controlling the immune response. The external viral membrane also contains molecules of viral glycoproteins **(gp)**—a sugar chain attached to protein. Each glycoprotein appears as a spike in the membrane. Each spike consists of two parts: **gp41,** which contains a **coiled up protein** and extends through the membrane. On interaction between HIV envelope and T4 cell coreceptors (CD4/chemokine receptors X4 and R5—depending on cell type) the gp41 coiled protein is **unsprung** and like a harpoon, pierces the cell membrane initiating the **first step** in HIV replication. **gp120** extends from the end of gp41 to the outside and beyond the membrane (the numbers 41 and 120 represent the mass of the individual gps in thousands of daltons). As a complete unit, gp41 plus gp120 is called gp160. These two membrane or **envelope** proteins play a crucial role in binding HIV to CD4 protein molecules found in the membranes of several types of immune system cells. The gp160 precursor is cleaved into envelope (gp120) and transmembrane (gp41) proteins in the cell's Golgi compartment. The HIV envelope complex is transported via vesicles to patches in the outer cell membrane. Full-length HIV RNA is complexed with capsid proteins and the nucleocapsid is transferred to the cell surface membrane at envelope-containing sites. The binding of gp to CD4 receptors makes such immune system cells vulnerable to infection. Other HIV proteins are located and described in this figure.

Within the cone-shaped core there are two identical strands of viral genomic RNA, each coupled to a molecule of transfer RNA (tRNA) that serves as a primer for reverse transcription of viral RNA into viral DNA. Also present with the RNA are an **integrase,** a **protease,** and a **ribonuclease enzyme**. The released virus is processed internally by HIV protease to form the characteristic dense lentivirus core. Most HIV appear to have initiated DNA synthesis prior to completion of budding and maturation. Actual maturation of HIV takes place after it buds out of the cell (see Figure 4-11).

new niches and host populations in which to reproduce. Now let us review some of the characteristics of HIV, the virus that causes AIDS.

HUMAN IMMUNODEFICIENCY VIRUS (HIV)

HIV is a retrovirus (Figure 3-1). Retroviruses are so named because they **REVERSE** the usual flow of genetic information within the host cell in order to reproduce themselves. In all living cells, normal gene expression results from the genetic information of DNA being copied into RNA (Figure 3-2). The RNA is translated into a specific cellular protein. In all living cell types, the directions for protein synthesis come from the species' genetic information contained in its DNA:

$$DNA \rightarrow RNA \rightarrow \text{Protein Synthesis}$$

But retroviruses have RNA as their genetic material—**NOT** DNA! In brief, retrovirus RNA is copied, using its reverse transcriptase enzyme, into a complementary single strand of DNA (Figure 3-3). The single-strand retroviral DNA is then copied into double-stranded retroviral DNA (this replication occurs in the cell's cytoplasm). At this point the viral DNA has been made according to the instructions in the retroviral RNA. This retroviral DNA migrates into the host cell nucleus and becomes integrated (inserted) into the host cell DNA. It is now a **provirus** (Figure 3-4). From this point on, the infection is irreversible—**the viral genes are now a part of the cell's genetic information.** In this respect, HIV can be considered as an acquired dominant genetic disease! A provirus, like the "mole" in a John LeCarre spy novel, may hide for years before doing its specific job. But for HIV, there is evidence that in some human cells the provirus begins to produce new copies of HIV RNA immediately after becoming a provirus or shortly thereafter.

Before the HIV provirus's genes can be expressed, RNA copies of them that can be read by the

Central Dogma

Prior to 1970, cell biologists thought that genetic information flowed only in one direction:

DNA $\xrightarrow{\text{(transcription)}}$ RNA $\xrightarrow{\text{(translation)}}$ PROTEIN SYNTHESIS

Reverse of Central Dogma

In 1970 the reverse transcriptase enzyme (RT) was found in a virus. These viruses became known as retroviruses.

Single + (plus) strand Retroviral RNA $\xrightarrow[\text{RT enzyme}]{\text{reverse transcription}}$ ds viral [1] DNA $\xrightarrow[\text{integrase enzyme}]{\text{integration into}}$ host cell Proviral DNA

transcription of Proviral DNA into

RNA Viruses to infect other cells ← Retroviral [2] RNA

[1] ds = Double stranded DNA

[2] If the RNA transcribed is spliced, RNA base sequences are rearranged. This RNA = messenger RNA and is used to make retroviral protein. If RNA transcribed is not spliced, it becomes the RNA genome of the new virus.

FIGURE 3-2 Retroviral Flow of Genetic Information. The general directional flow of genetic information in all living species is from DNA, where the information is stored, into RNA, which serves as a messenger for the construction of proteins that are the cells' functional molecules. This unidirectional flow of genetic information has been referred to as the **"central dogma"** of molecular biology. In the 1960s, Howard Temin and colleagues discovered an enzyme that copied RNA into DNA, a reverse of what was normally expected, thus the name *reverse transcriptase*.

host cell's protein-making machinery must be produced. This is done by **transcription**. Transcription is accomplished by the cell's own enzymes. But the process cannot start until the cell's RNA polymerase is activated by various molecular switches located in two DNA regions near the ends of the provirus: the **long terminal repeats**. This requirement is reminiscent of the need of many genes in multicellular organisms to be "turned on" or "off" by proteins that bind specifically to controlling sequences.

Production of Viral RNA Strands or RNA Transcripts

Within the host cell nucleus, proviral DNA, when activated, produces new strands of HIV RNA. Some of the RNA strands behave like messenger RNA (mRNA), producing proteins essential for the production of HIV. Other RNA strands become encased within the viral core proteins to become the new viruses. Whether the transcribed RNA strands become mRNA or RNA strands for new viruses depends on whether or not the newly synthesized RNA strands undergo complex processing. RNA processing means that after the RNA is produced, some of it is cut into segments by cellular enzymes and then reassociated or **spliced** into a length of RNA suitable for protein synthesis. The RNA strands that are spliced become the mRNA used in protein synthesis. The unspliced RNA strands serve as new viral strands that are encased in their protein coats (capsids) to become new viruses that bud out of the cell (Figure 3-4).

Two distinct phases of transcription follow the infection of an individual cell by HIV. In the first or early phase, RNA strands or transcripts produced in the cell's nucleus are snipped into multiple copies of shorter sequences by cellular splicing

The three actions of the Reverse Transcriptase Enzyme:

1. The polymerase portion makes a DNA strand that complements the viral RNA

   [diagram: Polymerase Region, RNase H Region, Direction of Movement, DNA, RNA]

2. The RNase H region removes the RNA

   [diagram: DNA, RNA, Direction of Movement]

3. The polymerase creates a second DNA strand

   [diagram: DNA, DNA, Direction of Movement]

Example

1. Single Stranded Retroviral RNA

   $5'$CAP - RU_5 UCCCUCUUCGCGU_3R - AAA_n $3'$ (+ single strand RNA)

2. Single Stranded DNA Synthesis (RT first function)

   Reverse Transcriptase →

   $5'RU_5$ UCCCUCUUCGCGU_3R$3'$

   LTR RU_5 AGGGAGAAGCGCU_3R LTR (– strand DNA)

3. Retroviral RNA Hydrolyzed (RT second function) Leaving Single Stranded DNA

   CC U CUU C
   U   C   CG G

   degraded RNA

4. Second or + Strand DNA Synthesized From First Strand Template (RT third function)

   RU_5 AGGGAGAAGCGCU_3R

   RU_5 TCCCTCTTCGCGU_3R (+ single strand DNA)

5. HIV DNA Integration Using Viral Integrase Enzyme Into Host Cell DNA

   [diagram 5' 3']

   AGGGAGAAGCGC
   TCCCTCTTCGCG

   } double stranded DNA now a provirus

$5'$CAP - RU_5 UCCCUCUUCGCGU_3R - AAA_n $3'$ (+ strand RNA)

If integration of provirus occurs in a T helper cell or certain other T cell subsets and those cells are immunogenically stimulated, the provirus begins making RNA that acts like messenger RNA essential for making virion proteins and copies of the RNA to be incorporated into the complete virion.

FIGURE 3-3 Proposed Production and Function of Retroviral Provirus. Note the reverse transcriptase enzyme has three functions: (1) to act as an RNA-dependent DNA polymerase transcribing single-strand DNA from viral RNA; (2) to demonstrate RNase H activity (RNase H is a subunit of the RT enzyme) by hydrolyzing the retroviral RNA off the RNA-DNA complex; and (3) to act as a DNA-dependent polymerase and transcribe the second DNA strand complementary to the first DNA strand. The process of viral RNA transcription is complex. When completed, the viral RNA gives rise to the formation of either linear or circular molecules of proviral DNA. Each end of the provirus contains an identical long series of terminal-repeating nucleotides or LTRs. LTRs are not a part of the viral genome. Although retroviral DNA integration is considered to be the normal route for RNA virus reproduction, retroviral reproduction may occur without proviral integration (see Figure 3-4).

Steps in viral replication

1. Attachment to CD4
2. Attachment to co-receptor CXCKR4 or CCKR5.
3. Uncoating
4. Reverse transcription of single strand RNA
5. DNA synthesis of second strand
6. Migration to nucleus
7. Integration
8. Viral transcription
9. RNA nuclear transport
10. Protein synthesis
11. RNA packaging and virion assembly
12. Viral proteins move into cell membrane
13. Release of virus
14. Maturation completed

FIGURE 3-4   Life Cycle of HIV in a T4 or CD4+ Lymphocyte. On average, the life cycle of HIV in an infected T4 cell is about 2 days. This means that one HIV, in one person in one year can produce about 180 generations of HIV. The lifetime of HIV in the blood is about six hours. An average HIV generation time is two to six days (generation time as the time it takes to infect a new cell and for that cell to release new HIV). After fusion of viral and cellular membranes, the inner part of HIV, called the **core,** is delivered into the cell cytoplasm. Uncoating of the core occurs, releasing two identical RNA strands, accompanying structural proteins and enzymes necessary for HIV replication. HIV RNA is then copied into HIV DNA, which is then transported into the cell's nucleus for insertion into the host cell's DNA. **This feature of the virus life cycle is essential for the spread of HIV in vivo, because it allows infection of nondividing cells such as monocytes and terminally differentiated macrophages and dendritic cells.** There is still some confusion as to whether HIV becomes a latent infection once HIV DNA becomes inserted or integrated into the host DNA. Evidence indicates that whether HIV is latent depends on the tissue that one is investigating. For example, in the T4 lymphocytes within the lymph nodes HIV is constantly being replicated, while some T4 lymphocytes in the blood carry HIV in the latent state. Depending on cell type, T4 or macrophage, chemokine coreceptors CXCR4 (FUSIN) and/or CC-CKR-5 are used by HIV to enter T4 and macrophage cells respectively. (See Chapter 5 for details on chemokine receptors and HIV cell entry.)

enzymes. When they reach the cytoplasm, they are only about 2000 nucleotides in length. These early-phase short transcripts encode only the virus's **regulatory proteins;** the structural genes that constitute the rest of the genome are among the parts that are left behind. In the second or late phase, two new size classes of RNA—long (unspliced) transcripts of 9749 nucleotides making up the new viral genome and medium-length (singly spliced) transcripts of some 4500 nucleotides—move out of the nucleus and into the cytoplasm. The 4500 nucleotide transcripts encode HIV's structural and enzymatic proteins (Greene, 1993).

Experimental results reported by Somasundaran et al. (1988) showed that when lymphoid cell lines or peripheral blood lymphocytes were infected with a laboratory strain of HIV, up to 2.5 million copies of the viral RNA were produced by cells; and within three days of infection, up to 40% of the total protein synthesized by the cells was viral protein. This is an unprecedented takeover for a retrovirus that typically makes only modest amounts of RNA and protein.

Much of what HIV does after entering the host cell or while integrated as a retroprovirus depends on the activity of its genes.

BASIC GENETIC STRUCTURE OF RETROVIRAL GENOMES

The first retrovirus was isolated from a sarcoma (a cancer) in chickens by Peyton Rous in 1911 and named the Rous sarcoma virus. The basic genetic structure of the Rous sarcoma virus and all animal retroviruses is the same. They all contain retroviral RNA sequences that code for the **same three genes** abbreviated GAG, POL, and ENV (defined here). Flanking each end of the retroviral genome is a sequence of similar nucleotides called long terminal repeats or redundancies (LTRs).

Some of the animal retroviruses such as the Rous sarcoma virus contain an additional

$$5' = \underset{\text{LTR}}{\underline{\qquad}} \overline{\text{GAG POL ENV}} \underset{\text{LTR}}{\underline{\qquad}} = 3'$$

oncogene (ONC) that, along with its LTRs, causes a rapid form of cancer in chickens that kills them in one to two weeks after infection. Without the *onc* gene the virus causes a *slow progressive cancer.*

Retroviral Genome of HIV

What sets the HIV genome apart from all other known retroviruses is the number of genes in HIV and the apparent complexity of their interactions in regulating the expression of the GAG-POL-ENV genes (Figure 3-5).

The Nine Genes of HIV— The HIV genome contains at least nine recognizable genes that produce at least nine individual proteins. These proteins are divided into three classes: (1) GAG, POL and ENV, the three major **structural** proteins; (2) Tat and Rev, the two **regulatory** proteins; and (3) Nef, Vif, Vpu, and Vpr, the four **accessory** proteins. As can be seen in Table 3-1, five of the nine genes are involved in regulating the expression of the GAG-POL-ENV genes.

The letters **GAG** stand for group-specific antigens (proteins) that make up the viral nucleocapsid. The GAG gene codes for internal structural proteins, the production of the dense cylindrical core proteins (**p24,** a nucleoid shell protein with a molecular weight of 24,000), and several internal proteins, which have been visualized by electron microscopy. The GAG gene has the ability to direct the formation of virus-like particles when all other major genes (POL and ENV) are absent. It is only when the GAG gene is nonfunctional that retroviruses (HIV) lose their capacity to bud out of a host cell. Because of these observations, the GAG protein has been designated the virus particle-making machine (Wills et al., 1991).

The **POL** gene codes for HIV enzymes, protease (p10), the virus-associated polymerase (reverse transcriptase) that is active in two forms, and endonuclease (integrase) enzymes. The integrase enzyme cuts the cell's DNA and inserts the HIV DNA. Evidence from retroviral deletion studies shows that the loss of LTRs on the 3' side of the POL gene stops viral DNA integration into the host genome. However, non-integrated DNA, without its LTRs and integrase enzyme, can still produce new viruses. This clearly demonstrates that viral DNA integration is not essential for viral multiplication even though integration is the normal course of events (Dimmrock et al., 1987).

The regulation of HIV transcription appears to be intimately related to the onset of HIV disease and AIDS. Thus interruption or inactivation of the POL gene would appear to have therapeutic effects (Kato et al., 1991).

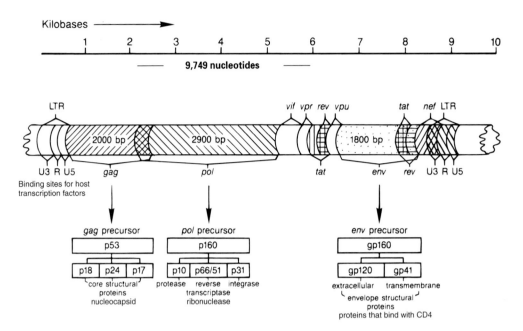

FIGURE 3-5 Genome of HIV. Nine of the genes making up the HIV genome have been identified. They are positioned as shown. Six of these genes are involved in a complex set of interactions that modify the regulation of the GAG-POL-ENV genes. Five are essential for HIV replication and six control reproduction (see text for details). The maxtrix protein, p17, forms the outer shell of the core of HIV, lining the inner surface of the viral membrane. Key functions of p17 protein are: orchestrates HIV assembly, directs gag p55 protein to host cell membrane, interacts with transmembrane protein, gp41, to retain envelope-coded proteins within HIV, and contains a nuclear localization signal that directs HIV RNA integration complex to the nucleus of infected cells. **This feature permits HIV to infect nondividing cells, a distinguishing feature of HIV** (Matthews et al., 1994).

Table 3-1 Genes of the HIV-1

Name(s)	Molecular Mass (kDa)	Function
GAG (group antigen)	p17	Matrix (protection)
	p24	Capsid (protection)
	p9, p6	Nucleocapsid (protection)
POL (polymerase)	p10	Protease (enzyme)
	p31	Endonuclease (enzyme)
	p50	Reverse transcriptase (enzyme)
ENV (envelope)	gp120	Surface envelope
	gp41	Transmembrane envelope
tat (regulator transactivator protein)[a]	p14	Transactivation of all HIV proteins
rev (differential regulator of expression of virus protein)	p13	Increase production of structural HIV protein; Transport of spliced/unspliced RNA from nucleus to cytoplasm
vif (virus infectivity factor)	p23	Required for ineffectivity as cell-free virus
nef (auxiliary protein)	p27	Retards HIV replication
vpr (virus protein R)	?	Triggers cells steroid production to produce HIV
vpu (virus protein U)	p16	Required for efficient viral replication and release-budding

[a]Transactivator gene—the product of their genes influences the function of genes some distance away.

The **ENV** gene codes for HIV surface proteins, two major envelope glycoproteins (gp120, located on the external "spikes" of HIV and gp41, the transmembrane protein that attaches gp120 to the surface of HIV) that become embedded throughout the host cell membrane, which ultimately becomes the **envelope** that surrounds the virus as it "buds" out (Figure 3-6). Studies on how HIV kills cells have revealed at least one way that the envelope glycoproteins enhance T helper cell death. The envelope glycoproteins cause the formation of **syncytia; that is, healthy T cells fuse to each other forming a group around a single HIV-infected T4 or CD4+ cell**. Individual T cells within these syncytia lose their immune function (Figure 3-7). Starting with a single HIV-infected T4 helper cell, as many as 500 *uninfected* T4 helper cells can fuse into a single syncytium. Continued creation of these syncytia could deplete a T4 cell population.

Several studies have demonstrated that the appearance of syncytium-inducing (SI) HIV strains during the chronic phase of HIV disease heralds an abrupt loss of T4 or CD4+ lymphocytes and a clinical progression of the disease. Although the SI phenotype is detected in many patients with AIDS, it has also been isolated from individuals who have not gone on to an early development of AIDS. However, the marked decrease in the T4 lymphocyte counts after shifting from non-SI (NSI) to SI strains as well as the negative effect SI strains have on primary HIV infection suggests that their appearance may not be just a consequence, but the actual cause of immune system alterations (Torres et al., 1996).

The Six Genes of HIV That Control HIV Reproduction— Collectively, the six additional HIV genes tat and rev (regulatory genes), and nef, vif, vpu, vpr (auxiliary genes) working together with the host cell's machinery actually control the reproductive retroviral cycle: adhesion of HIV to a cell, penetration of the cell, uncoating of HIV genome, reverse transcription of the RNA genome producing proviral DNA and immediate production of new viral RNA, or the integration of the provirus and later viral multiplication. The six genes allow for the entire reproductive scenario— from infection to new HIV—to occur in 8 to 16 hours in dividing cells.

Gene Sequence— The HIV proviral genome has been well characterized with regard to gene location and sequence (Figure 3-5), but the function of each gene is not completely understood. The genes for producing regulatory proteins can be grouped into two classes: genes that produce proteins essential for HIV replication (*tat* and *rev*), and genes that produce proteins that perform accessory functions that enhance replication and/or infectivity (**nef, vif, vpu**, and **vpr**) (Rosen, 1991).

FIGURE 3-6 Budding and Mature Retroviruses. HIV buds from infected cells only at special points on the cellular membrane known as "lipid rafts." The rafts are rich in cholesterol. Without the cholesterol HIV cannot fuse with new CD4+ or T4 cells (Hildreth, 2001). This is a photograph of HIV taken by electron microscopy. Note the difference between the free or mature HIV and those that are just budding out through the membrane of a T4 helper cell. This cell came from an HIV-infected hemophiliac. Closely observing the mature HIV, one can make out the core protein area surrounded by the cell's membrane (virus envelope). *(Courtesy CDC, Atlanta)*

FIGURE 3-7 Formation of T4 Helper Cell Syncytia. A single infected T4 helper cell can fuse with as many as 500 uninfected T4 helper cells. The formation of syncytia lead to a loss or depletion of T4 helper cells from the immune system. *(Courtesy of Tom Folks, National Institute of Allergy and Infectious Diseases)*

Gene Function— Each end of the proviral genome contains an identical long sequence of nucleotides, the long terminal repeats. Although these LTRs are not considered to be genes of the HIV genome, they do contain regulatory nucleotide sequences that help the six regulatory/auxiliary genes control GAG-POL-ENV gene expression (Figure 3-5). For example, the **vif** gene is associated with the infectious activity of the virus. Currently, the predominant view is that vif acts at the late stages of infection to promote HIV processing or assembly (Potash et al., 1998).

The **tat** gene is essential for HIV infection of T4 cells and HIV replication (Parada et al., 1996; Li, 1997; Stevenson, 1998). It is one of the first viral genes to be transcribed. The tat gene produces a transactivator protein, meaning that the gene produces a protein that exerts its effect on viral replication from a distance rather than interacting with genes adjacent to *tat* or their gene product. *Tat* contains two coding regions or exons—areas that contain genetic information for producing a diffusible protein—which, through the help of the LTR sequences, increases the expression of HIV genes thereby increasing the production of new virus particles. The tat protein interacts with a short nucleotide sequence called TAR located within the 5′ LTR region of HIV messenger RNA (mRNA) transcripts (Matsuya et al., 1990). Once that tat protein binds to the TAR

sequence, transcription of the provirus by cellular RNA polymerase II accelerates at least 1000-fold.

The **rev** gene (**r**egulator of **e**xpression of **v**iral protein) selectively increases the synthesis of HIV structural proteins in the latter stages of HIV disease, thereby maximizing the production of new viruses. It does this by regulating splicing of the HIV RNA transcript (cutting out nucleotide sequences that exist between exons and bringing the exons together) and transporting spliced and unspliced RNAs from the nucleus to the cytoplasm (Patrusky, 1992; Fritz et al., 1995).

The **nef** gene produces a protein that is maintained in the cell cytoplasm next to the nuclear membrane. It is believed **nef** functions by protecting the cell from dying, allowing the cell to continue producing HIV. Several antigenic forms of nef protein have been found, which suggest multiple activities of nef within HIV-infected cells (Kohleisen et al., 1992; Sagg et al., 1995). Olivier Schwartz and coworkers (Cohen, 1997) showed that **nef** can prompt cells to yank down from their surfaces a molecule known as the major histocompatibility complex (MHC), which displays viral peptides to the immune system. The group predicted that this "down-regulation" of MHC would make HIV-infected cells resistant to cytotoxic T cell killing. (Collins et al., 1998) (See Chapter 5.)

In August 2001, Yuntao Wu and colleague reported that after HIV RNA manufactures a DNA copy, but prior to its integration into the cell's DNA, the HIV DNA stimulates the production of **tat** and **nef** viral proteins. These proteins awaken T4 cells out of their dormant state. Once the T4 cells are activated, they become vulnerable to nuclear invasion by HIV DNA, allowing the virus to integrate into the T4 cell DNA structure. Not only will the activated T4 cell allow HIV DNA to enter the nucleus and insert itself into human DNA, an activated T4 cell produces a higher rate of HIV RNA replication (Wu et al., 2001).

The functions of the **vpr** gene, which codes for a **v**iral **p**rotein **R**, is associated with the transport of cytoplasmic viral DNA into the nucleus. Vpr is also involved in steroid production that in turn helps produce HIV, is required for the efficient assembly or release of new HIV viruses, and stops T4 cell division. **Vif** is necessary for complete reverse transcriptions of viral RNA into viral DNA. **Vpu** codes for a viral protein U that destroys the CD4 protein within the T4 lymphocyte, thus helping HIV to bud out of the cell. Vif, Vpr, and Vpu appear to be necessary for HIV to cause disease.

Of the HIV proteins, tat, rev, and nef are termed **early** proteins because their production results from the cutting and splicing of full-length HIV mRNA; vif, vpu, and vpr are termed **late** proteins, since their production results from unspliced or single-spliced mRNA.

UPDATE 2002, XIV INTERNATIONAL AIDS CONFERENCE Michael Malim and colleagues reported on a new aspect of the relationship between the HIV gene vif and human DNA. Their findings involve a poorly understood gene in human DNA called CEM-15 and how it can suppress the production of HIV and HIV's ability to infect cells when the vif gene is absent. Their studies indicate that if vif is absent from HIV, the CEM-15 gene slows the replication of HIV and prevents HIV from exiting the cell thereby preventing the infection of other uninfected cells. In short, HIV without its vif gene is essentially harmless. Scientists at the conference feel that this is one of the most important new findings in recent years. These data offer new hope to drug manufacturers and to those working on an anti-HIV vaccine.

How Genes Store Genetic Information and the Importance of Mutations or Change Within Genes— Genes store the information necessary for creating living organisms and viruses. In sexually reproducing organisms, the information is stored in the form of DNA organized into structures called chromosomes. Apart from sex cells (eggs and sperm) and mature blood cells, every cell in the human body contains 23 pairs of chromosomes. One of each pair is inherited from the mother, the other from the father. Each chromosome is a packet of compressed and twisted DNA. Genes are sections of DNA containing the blueprint for the whole body, including such specific details as what kind of receptors cells will have, for example, CD4, CD8, X4, R5, and so on.

DNA is made up of a double-stranded helix held together by hydrogen bonds **between specific pairs of bases. The four bases A, T, G, and C** (**adenine, thymine, guanine**, and **cytosine**) bond to each other in fixed and complimentary patterns that give humans and other species their individuality. If a gene is thought of as a sentence, and the nucleotides in DNA as letters, a change or mutation of only one letter can affect the entire sentence or the information the DNA gives the cell. To get an idea of how many mutations can occur in a cell, consider that humans have about 3.2 billion base pairs which make up about 35,000 genes or sentences that contain the information that makes a human. There are about a million differences between your 3.2 billion-letter DNA alphabet and that of another person. The kind, number, and sequence of nucleotides (bases) in human DNA and that of other species is much greater. Another way of saying this is that the closer a species resembles a human or vice-versa, the closer will be the DNA base sequences.

For example, the DNA base sequence in a chimpanzee is about 98% identical to humans. That means the difference between human DNA and chimpanzee DNA is only a base sequence difference for about 60 million base pairs out of 3.2 billion human base pairs.

Importance of Genetic Stability to a Species— The individual or collective characteristics (phenotypes) of any virus, cell, or multicelled organism depend on the expression of their genes and the interaction of gene products within a given environment. From a biological point of view, changes in phenotype (observable characteristics) that are inheritable are by definition genetic changes. Such changes occur due to changes in the kind, number, and sequence of bases in DNA. Base changes may occur by addition, substitution, and deletion. These changes are referred to as

genetic mutations. Genetic mutations provide biological heterogeneity and genetic diversity (similarity as a species but dissimilarity with regard to certain characteristics). Investigations on the rate at which genetic mutations occur in living species indicate that DNA is a stable molecule with relatively low mutation rates for any given gene. Because of low mutation rates within the DNA of a species' gene pool (all the genes that can be found in the DNA of a species) and selection pressures by a slowly changing environment, species evolution is constant but very slow.

Genetic mutations in the strain of an organism or virus produce genetic and phenotype **variants** (different members) of that strain. Regardless of the rate at which mutations occur, **they are genetic mistakes**—they are not intentional, they just happen by chance. Most mutations or genetic mistakes either make no difference to an organism or virus (silent mutations) or they cause a change. **Few genetic mistakes within a stable environment improve the species. After all, the species arrived at this point in time via genetic and environmental selection pressures—those with the best constellation of genes survived to reproduce those genes.** In species that produce large numbers of offspring, genetic mistakes that are lethal or lead to an early death are of little consequence to the species. A genetic mistake that improves the chance of survival and reproduction is retained.

Genetic Instability of HIV— A virus like HIV can produce hundreds of replicas within a single cell. Genetic mistakes during viral replication produce variant HIVs. In biological economic terms, HIV replicas are inexpensive to make. Even if most of these mutant HIV replicas are inactive or throwaway copies, it makes little if any difference to the HIV per se. However, if a few HIV replicas received environmentally advantageous mutant genes, these HIV mutants would survive as well as or better than the parent HIVs. **Both parent HIV and mutant HIV can reproduce in the same cell and exchange genes.** Over time, only the most fit mutant or variant HIVs are transmitted among people and undergo still further genetic changes. These variant HIVs could, with sufficient accumulative genetic changes, become a new type of HIV—for example, an HIV-type 3.

Investigations of some of the *RNA* viruses revealed relatively high mutation rates. Thus some of the RNA viruses are our best examples of evolution in **"real"** time. Because of their high error rate during replication they show, as expected, both high genetic diversity and biological heterogeneity in their host, and a rate of evolution about a million times faster than DNA-based organisms (Nowak, 1990). HIV, in particular, fits this category. Heterogeneity of HIV is reflected by: (**1**) the difference in the kinds of cells variant HIV infects; (**2**) the way different HIV mutants replicate; and (**3**) the way different variants of HIV harm infected cells.

It is now known that HIV is capable of enormous genetic flexibility, which allows it to become resistant to drugs, to escape from immune responses, and to avoid potential HIV vaccines. What is not known are all the factors contributing to viral diversity in individual infections. Clearly the high error rate of the reverse transcriptase (because this enzyme lacks a $3'$ to $5'$ exonuclease proofreading ability, that is, it cannot correct mistakes once made) and the high turnover rate in infected cells generate vast numbers of different virus mutants. The diversity of newly produced variants, however, is shaped by a combination of mutation, recombinations of HIV RNA, and selection forces. The main selective forces that have been proposed to drive HIV diversity are the immune response, cell tropism (cell types most likely to attract HIV), and random activation of infected cells. At the time of seroconversion a person may carry a homogeneous virus population, but then diversification occurs as HIV infects many different cell types and tissues in the body (Bonhoeffer et al., 1995).

For further information on HIV evolution, diversity, and HIV disease progression, see Chapter 7, Box 7.2.

GENETIC REVOLUTION

Genetic revolution is when an organism or virus such as, say, SIV leaves one host (chimpanzee), enters a new host (humans), and rapidly diversifies its genes in an attempt to interpret and adapt to its new environment, as when SIVcpz became HIV in humans. As HIV continued to replicate or reproduce it became more fit to survive in humans. That fitness occurs in two ways, through mutation or change in individual nucleotides making up the genes, and through recombination, a process in which there are large exchanges of sections of HIV diploid RNA.

BOX 3.1

IMPACT OF HIV ON HUMAN EVOLUTION?

Scientists are looking at the course of infections among wild animals and wondering what the history of their viral infections say about the future of HIV as it evolves in humans. Why, they ask, are wild cats, African monkeys, and, it seems, chimpanzees so impervious to illness from many of their viruses? For example, Mark Feinberg of Emory University asked why HIV-1 and HIV-2 behave so differently in the human population. It is believed that the precursor virus, HIV-1 (SIVcpz), crossed over into humans from chimpanzees and that the precursor virus to HIV-2 (SIVsm) crossed over into humans from the sooty mangabey monkeys. Both precursor SIVs evolved in humans to cause AIDS, but HIV-2 has not caused a worldwide pandemic—why? This scientists cannot answer. These primates have, over time, learned to live with their precursor HIV viruses. With respect to HIV-2, it was found that the sooty mangabeys infected with SIV-2, and African green monkeys infected with SIV-1, carried billions of SIV per drop of blood when tested, and that these virus are constantly killing large numbers of their cells, but the monkeys just replace them. It appears that to a lesser extent this is already happening with HIV-2 in humans. The virus is there and kills human cells, but infected humans appear to be far less clinically affected by HIV-2 than by HIV-1. When HIV-1 is injected into chimpanzees—human beings' closest genetic cousins—the animals become infected but usually remain unharmed, showing no sign of disease. Only one research group in the world, the Yerkes Primate Center outside Atlanta, has caused AIDS in chimpanzees using an HIV/SIV hybrid laboratory strain about 15 years ago. In 1996, only one of the chimps developed symptoms similar to human AIDS.

Stephen O'Brien of the National Cancer Institute said that the heavily viral infected monkeys who remain healthy present a picture similar to that found in wild cats. The animals have enormous numbers of viruses in their blood and tolerate the viruses' constant killing of their white blood cells. O'Brien feels this is a predictable adaptation with a clear implication for the human AIDS epidemic. O'Brien believes that when a virus gets into a population, like HIV that crossed into humans, it can kill, be 100% lethal, or just partially lethal, leaving survivors to reproduce. Over time, O'Brien said, either the virus becomes weakened or the **species changes** in order to live with that virus. Many scientists now believe that it is inevitable that HIV will alter humanity, that is, our species will change! For example, so many people are infected in some parts of Africa that future generations will have a disproportionate number of people with genetic predispositions to live with the virus. And that is how evolutionary changes occur. In short, the severity of the epidemic in some parts of the world is so profound that it will clearly impact human evolution. This is occurring in our lifetime. In the past, we've been left to infer what the impact of infection was on human evolution. But now we have the opportunity to observe it (Levin, et al., 2001). At the moment, there is no evidence that HIV is weakening.

FORMATION OF GENETIC MUTATIONS IN HIV

One mechanism for producing HIV variants or HIV mutants results from a **highly error-prone reverse transcriptase** (RT) enzyme of HIV. Preston and colleagues (1988) found that HIV transcriptase makes at least one replication error (mutation) in each HIV genome per round of replication in a cell! Other investigators say that reverse transcriptase, on average, introduces a replication mutation once in every 2000 nucleotides or about five mutations per round of replication! This unusually high rate of nucleotide misincorporation (substitution, addition, and deletion of nucleotides) as proviral DNA is being made by RT is responsible for generating the genetic diversity and heterogeneity found among the isolates of HIV. In short, the high error rate in producing proviral DNA means that each HIV-infected cell will carry variant or mutant HIV, most of which will be genetically unique (Vartanian et al., 1992). **This high rate of mutation underlies HIV's remarkable ability to become resistant to drug therapies and to hamper the production of an HIV vaccine!**

FORMATION OF GENETIC RECOMBINATION IN HIV

Subtypes are a result of the selective accumulation of mutations produced during the process of reverse transcription. Like other retroviruses, HIV produces mutations as a natural part of its replication process. However, HIV produces mutations more frequently than most retroviruses. If you drop the same virus, say in Alaska and Africa and come back 20 years later, the separate viruses will have developed their own different particularities, depending upon the environmental factors or constraints they have confronted. With HIV, there is considerable mixing of the viruses because of the large movement of infected people worldwide. If there are enough people being infected and exposed to viruses, this process will lead to the generation of intersubtype recombinants. Both mutation and recombination by RNA strand switching during transcription may contribute, equally.

When HIV replicates, each of the new virus particles being constructed incorporates two strands of viral RNA. Because two RNA molecules are packaged in each virion, reverse transcriptase (RT) may switch from one template to another during reverse transcription. If two RNAs with sequence differences are copackaged in one virion, a mosaic HIV genome containing genetic information from both RNAs could be generated, yielding novel viral genomes. Recombination can also salvage genome damage or detrimental mutations in one RNA molecule by adopting genetic information from the intact template. Thus, recombination may not only introduce genetic diversity, it may also serve as a repair mechanism for the HIV genome (Jetzt et al., 2002). Also, if two or more subtypes or genetically different HIV infect and replicate in the same cell, there is no internal organization to keep their newly forming RNA strands separate from one another. Regions of the RNA of one HIV can be spliced with those from a second HIV. These recombined, or chimeric, RNA can be packaged into new HIV and released. Andreas Jung and colleagues (2002) reported that on average, 75% to 80% of individual HIV-infected splenocytes carried three to four genetically different HIV proviruses in their DNA, evidence for large numbers of HIV recombinants.

Mutations create the changes in the genetic material of HIV, but it is recombination that quickly reshuffles these changes.

Forming a recombinant HIV is the same concept as a plant or animal hybrid. The hybrid or new species has picked up genetic information from two distinctly unrelated parents. For example, each of us is a recombinant. Each parent has its own genetic information, and the children are their recombinants. So recombination is a natural process. For us, the process doesn't usually produce large genetic changes. For HIV, the recombination process can produce tremendous change in a single replication cycle. In the case of HIV intersubtype recombinants, each parent is a different subtype, the recombinant picks up part of its genetic information from one parent, part from the other. They are also genetic hybrids.

Coinfection Produces Recombinant Subtypes

HIV infection and replication takes place in certain cells of the human immune system, T4 or CD4+ cells. In most cases, an individual's CD4+ cells are only infected with a single subtype of HIV-1 or HIV-2. But as the epidemic expands, scientists are increasingly finding evidence of individuals infected with multiple viral subtypes. This type of infection is called coinfection. That is, when a virus replicates, each of the new virus particles being constructed incorporates two strands of viral RNA. If, however, two or more viruses infect and replicate in the same cell, there is no internal organization to keep their newly forming RNA strands separate from one another. Regions of the RNA of one virus can be spliced with those from a second virus. Many rounds of recombination can go on within a coinfected individual, generating many different recombinant forms. Such recombinant subtypes give HIV a chance to survive. These recombined, or chimeric, RNA can be packaged into new viruses and released. In fact, the large proportion of recombinant strains in populations where multiple subtypes are circulating suggests that coinfection is not uncommon. Essentially, recombination is an opportunity for HIV to improve its chances of survival.

Completing the Picture on Producing HIV Genetic Variability: HIV Clades or Subtypes

Subtypes or clades are a result of the selective accumulation of mutations and recombinations that occur during the process of reverse transcription.

Recombination is probably facilitated by geographic intermixing of subtypes, coinfection of an individual with different subtypes, and coinfection of cells with different susceptibilities for different subtypes (Laurence, 1997).

Michael Saag and colleagues (1988) examined the generation of molecular variation of HIV by sequential HIV isolates from two chronically infected people. They found 39 distinguishable but highly related genomes (HIV variants). **These results indicate that HIV heterogeneity occurs rapidly in infected individuals and that a large number of genetically distinguishable but related HIVs rapidly evolve in parallel and coexist during chronic infection.** That is, whenever a drug or the immune response successfully attacks one variant, another arises in its place. Pools of genetic distinct variants that evolve from the initial HIV that begin the infection are often referred to as **quasispecies** (Delwart et al., 1993; Diaz et al., 1997).

Additional evidence indicates that some HIV genetic variants demonstrate a preference (tropism) as to the cell type they infect. This means that one genetic change may allow the virus to enter cells that were once immune to the virus. Also, a report by Helen Devereux and colleagues (2002) states that a wide variety of quasi-species circulate in each individual and that there may be HIV evolving independently in different body compartments. The rapid genetic change, which results in altered viral products, makes it very difficult to design a vaccine or drug that will be effective against all HIV variants. To date, HIV drug-resistant mutants have been found for all FDA-approved nucleoside and nonnucleoside analogs and protease inhibitors used in the treatment of HIV-infected people and AIDS patients! (Chapter 4 presents a discussion of currently used drug therapies for HIV/AIDS.)

HIV Antigenic Variation— This refers to differences in a protein that occur as a result of changes in the DNA. Each variation of protein produced elicits the production of a different antibody. Such protein changes occur, for example, as a result of DNA changes in the GAG-POL-ENV genes. Antibodies are made against the different GAG-POL-ENV gene proteins, but the antibodies made against the ENV gene protein that appear to be the most important. These antibodies neutralize the envelope glycoproteins that seem to be an essential part of HIV's infecting process. **The ENV gene is subject to the most frequent mutations, producing HIV with different envelope glycoproteins with-in a given individual.**

It now appears that **HIV can constantly change its surface antigenic composition, thereby allowing it to escape antibody neutralization.**

Thus, HIV mutations allow the virus to persist in the presence of an immune response. This immune selection viral phenomenon is not new. It is what the influenza virus does yearly so that last year's vaccine will not protect people from this year's variation. However, HIV differs from viruses such as influenza. Influenza and many other viruses do not have an RNA to DNA replication step so they are not as mutable as the retroviruses. Because of the error-prone reverse transcriptase enzyme used by the retroviruses, the possibility of genetic change far exceeds that for any other known nonretroviral human pathological virus.

DISTINCT GENOTYPES (SUBTYPES/CLADES) OF HIV-1 WORLDWIDE BASED ON ENV AND GAG PROTEINS

HIV is actually an umbrella term for two genetically distinct types of virus: HIV-1 and HIV-2. HIV-1 embraces three genetically distinct groups: M, N, and O. Of these, group M viruses, the ones that are perhaps most studied and are known to be most responsible for infections worldwide, have been subdivided into 11 genetically distinct subtypes, identified by letters A through K. Genetic analyses of HIV-2, the less virulent form of HIV, have yielded six subtypes, identified as A through F.

As stated previously, this book is about HIV-1 or HIV. In order to better understand globally circulating strains of HIV, HIV investigators have placed, based on the genetic diversity, the various HIV strains into three major groups, **M,** for the **main** HIV genotypes or **clades** found in different populations, and groups **O** and **N** for HIV genotypes or clades that are significantly different from those in the **M** group.

Group M HIV causes over 99% of the world's HIV/AIDS. **Group O** and the more recently discovered **Group N** (discussed on page 68), cause less than 1%.

Group M Subtypes

There are 11 subtypes or clades of group M: A, B, C, D, E, F, G, H, I, J, and K. The M subtypes have been analyzed with respect to the differences between them based on the variations found in their GAG and ENV proteins (Robertson et al., 1995).

Within a subtype, envelope gene sequences vary from 7% to 12%. Between subtypes the genetic

---

SIDEBAR 3.2

CROSSING FROM PRIMATES INTO HUMANS

The three major groups of HIV-1, Groups M, N, and O genetically differ from each other as much as they differ genetically from SIVcpz. These data strongly suggest that individual groups M, N, and O entered humans as separate events. HIV-2, which is very closely related to the SIV of sooty mangabeys, may have crossed over into humans on at least six occasions (Gao 1999; Gao 1992).

Although it may appear odd that distinct strains of HIV should have colonized humans from different animal species on different occasions, natural cross-species transfer has occurred frequently for other retroviruses, not just HIV. There is also a precedent with the flaviviruses, yellow fever and dengue, and with malaria. *Plasmodium falciparum* malaria, arising in Africa, is closely related to the parasite of chimpanzees, whereas *P. vivax* came from Asian monkeys.

**Why Has HIV Shown Up Now—
Is This a New Virus?**

Based on scientific evidence, different SIV strains apparently crossed into humans several times during the 20th century. There may have been many earlier introductions or precursor HIV into humans but, like Ebola or Lassa fever viral outbreaks, they may only have occurred locally, temporarily, and soon vanished. What helped HIV to become endemic, and Group M to become epidemic, might have been the huge expansion of needle and syringe use in the mid-20th century during periods of mass vaccination and injecting antibiotic use, as suggested by Preston Marx and colleagues (2001). In other words, it is not the cross-species transfer event that is new or different but the social conditions and medical practices that allowed the evolving HIV eventually to adapt to sexual transmission which allowed for its survival in humans. As described in Chapter 2, strains of SIV most likely crossed into humans around 1931, plus or minus 15 years. So, yes, this is, according to scientists, a new virus!

---

variation is up to 30%. There is the belief that a vaccine against one subtype won't offer protection against the rest. (For discussion of HIV vaccines see Chapter 9 on prevention). Subtypes B and E together make up about 14% of HIV infections worldwide. Subtypes A, C, and D make up about 84% of HIV infections.

The **11** different M subtypes or clades and O have been globally mapped (geographically located) in Figure 3-8 (Brix et al., 1996; Workshop Report 1997). This figure demonstrates the dissemination of the different subtypes from 1990 through 2002. Clearly, subtype B, closely related to subtype D, predominates in the Americas although in Brazil, Argentina, and Uruguay, substantial proportions of infections are caused by F subtype or BF recombinant viruses. Apart from these three countries, infections with non-B genetic forms are unusual; however, recently, it was reported that env subtypes A, C, and H had been identified in 5 of 11 samples in Cuba. The identification of diverse non-B subtypes in Cuba is not unexpected, considering that large numbers of Cuban military and civilian personnel had been stationed in the 1970s and 1980s in Angola, a country neighbouring the Democratic Republic of Congo (DRC), where the highest group M diversity is found, and that many of the early cases of HIV infection in Cuba were detected among these individuals. The explosive epidemic in Southeast Asia is chiefly attributable to subtype E. There are ample documented introductions of subtypes C, E, and F from endemic areas into the United States and the Western Hemisphere. Subtype C now accounts for about 40% of **new** HIV infections worldwide—particularly in China and India. **There is no one subtype that is representative of this global pandemic.**

International Genetic Subtypes

Numerous groups have shown an increase in intermixing of HIV genetic subtypes in multiple international locales. HIV subtypes A, B, C, D, F, G, and H have appeared throughout Europe; B, F, C, and D have been found in Brazil; one-third of new infections in Germany are non-B; 15% of infections in a New York City hospital are non-B; increasingly, E is found among injecting drug users in Thailand, from 24% subtype E in 1991 to 44% in 1995, and among heterosexual risk groups, a change from 86% subtype E in 1991 to

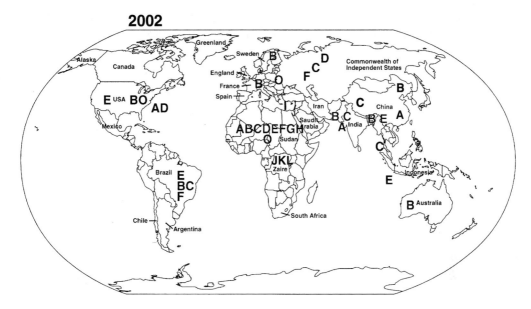

FIGURE 3-8 Global Distribution of the 11 **M** Subtypes and **O** in 2002 in areas of highest prevalence. Clearly this global map shows that HIV subtypes are **no longer** continent based—all subtypes are now present on all continents. No satisfactory explanation exists for the skewed worldwide distribution of HIV-1 subtypes. The worldwide spread of viral subtypes makes it clear that a **world vaccine** will be required, that is, one that is not subtype specific. None appears to be on the horizon, although large-scale trials with existing envelope vaccines are underway in some developing countries *(Brodine et al., 1997 updated)*.

98% in 1995; and group O has been detected in at least 12 African countries, France, Spain, and in the United States, as well as M/O dual infections. In South Africa, there is spreading of subtypes B and D throughout the homosexual population and C/E throughout the heterosexuals studied. The impact of this is an increasing spread of non-B subtypes into previous "B" areas, which has significant implications for vaccine development.

Subtypes Related to Transmission Route

While the current geographic distribution of subtypes is generally acknowledged to have arisen from accidents in viral trafficking, the perpetuation of these patterns may be due to the affinity of certain subtypes for certain targets. Max Essex of Harvard has studied Langerhans cells as a target of viral entry for subtypes E and C. He has proposed that Langerhans cells, prevalent in the female genital tract, are less hospitable to subtype B. He concluded that non-B subtypes are dominant in countries where the major mode of HIV transmission is through heterosexual contact and that this is due to the greater accessibility of subtypes E and C through

the Langerhans cells. In China, in a large group of injection drug users, a recombinant subtype AB was found to the exclusion of other subtypes. It is estimated that over half of all HIV infections worldwide are from subtype C. It is the most common subtype found in Southern Africa, China, and India.

HIV RNA Recombination

Robertson and colleagues (1995) reported that eight of the group M subtypes appear to have been involved in recombination with each other, giving rise to genetic hybrids. **These studies raise questions of whether a vaccine that works against one of the subtypes will work against a subtype hybrid.**

Group O Subtypes

Group O contains at least 30 genetically different subtypes of HIV. Group O subtypes are referred to as **"outlier"** because their RNA base sequence is only 50% similar to the known genotypes of the M group. The O variants have been known since 1987 but have been found mainly in Cameroon, Gabon, and surrounding west African countries that, to date, have only been marginally affected by AIDS. Group O viruses were of concern primarily because their divergence from group M was sufficient to miss their detection by ELISA HIV testing. (The ELISA test is discussed in Chapter 12.) Seven people in France were identified with Group O HIV in 1994. The **first** documented case of Group O HIV infection in the United States was found in April of 1996 in Los Angeles. Beginning year 2002, only two cases of HIV subtype O infection have been reported in the United States. This subtype was found in a Los Angeles county woman and a Maryland woman; both came into the United States from Africa. HIV subtype O is not routinely tested for in the United States.

New Group N Subtype?

In August 1998, Francois Simon and colleagues reported the discovery of a **new** HIV-1 isolate that **cannot** be placed in the **M** or **O** subtype category.

The authors suggest that the new isolate be classified as group **N** for **"new"** or **"non-M non-O."** The new isolate, designated **YBF30**, was found in a small number of people in the West African nation of Cameroon. The first isolate was from a 40-year-old woman who died of AIDS. This virus is similar to SIV (cpz-gab) and it either branched with the SIV strain or between it and HIV-1 group M. The authors state that future strains of SIV (cpz) could be found and strains that are closely related to YBF30 might circulate among Cameroonian chimpanzees.

SIV retroviruses are endemic in many species of primates but usually don't cause disease, which makes them natural hosts for what are known as lentiviruses or slow-acting viruses. But when they cross the species barrier into a new host like humans, these viruses may become pathogenic, causing illness. Based on evolutionary studies, researchers think SIV has existed in sub-Saharan Africa for thousands of years, adapting to several species including the African green monkey and

---

POINT OF INFORMATION 3.2

MYSTERIES OF HIV SUBTYPES

Two epidemiologic mysteries have eluded HIV/AIDS researchers for years. The **first** is why heterosexual intercourse has accounted for approximately 10% of HIV transmission in the United States and Western Europe to date, but more than 90% of HIV transmission in Asia and Africa.

The **second** mystery has centered around a subtype B HIV epidemic among injection drug users in Thailand. This epidemic began in the mid-1980s, and plateaued with less than 100,000 people infected. Several years later, however, a subtype E HIV epidemic took hold in Thailand. This epidemic has exploded among heterosexuals, with over a million people already infected. Most surprising, perhaps, is that subtype B—while present in Thailand, India, and several African countries—has not caused heterosexual epidemics in those places.

Although differences in the rate of heterosexual transmission may also be due to factors such as sexual behavior and the presence of other sexually transmitted diseases, none of these considerations has yet adequately accounted for the widespread heterosexual epidemics in Asia and Africa. Investigators have begun to focus on how biological characteristics of the individual sub-

types might also play a role. These findings about subtype cellular affinities do not suggest that subtype B cannot be transmitted heterosexually—it is throughout the United States and elsewhere. The point is that subtype B seems to be transmitted through vaginal intercourse far less efficiently than the subtypes that predominate in Asia and Africa. It has been shown that Langerhans' cells are located in specific areas, such as the vagina, cervix, and penile foreskin. They do not appear to localize in the rectal or colon mucus membranes. Experiments with HIV-infected Langerhans' cells and uninfected T4 cells showed that HIV-infected Langerhans' cells readily formed clusters and syncytia with T4 cells, resulting in efficient cell-to-cell transmission. It was also demonstrated that during the cell-to-cell interaction, Langerhans' cells not only effectively infect T4 cells but also activate them, resulting in enhanced virus replication (UNAIDS, 1997). Thus, the enhanced efficiency of subtype E to attach to Langerhans' cells may help account for the explosive heterosexual spread of the epidemic in countries such as Thailand, while the heterosexual epidemic in the industrialized world has thus far remained at a comparatively low rate (Essex, 1996).

FIRST CONFIRMED CASES OF HIV GROUP O-CAUSED AIDS

A Norwegian sailor died of AIDS in 1976 at the age of 29. So did his wife and youngest daughter, born in 1967. The members of this Norwegian family represent the **earliest confirmed cases of AIDS and the first case of HIV type O infection.** The first symptoms appeared in 1966 in the sailor, in 1967 in his wife, and in 1969 in their daughter. Between 1961 and 1965 he traveled the world's oceans, calling at ports in all six inhabited continents. On his first voyage, which began in August 1961 just after his 15th birthday, he worked as a kitchen hand on a Norwegian vessel that sailed down the west African coastline, calling at ports in Senegal, Liberia, Cote d'Ivoire, Ghana, Nigeria, and Cameroon. A gonorrheal infection during this trip shows that he was sexually active. He returned home in May 1962, and he never returned to Africa. No known evidence suggests that the sailor was bisexual, which means that sexual contact with a woman is the most straightforward explanation for his infection. This would suggest that HIV group O has been circulating in that part of Africa for at least 35 years.

SECOND CONFIRMED CASES OF HIV GROUP O-CAUSED AIDS?

The second case of Group O infection found in the literature is the second child of a French barmaid from Reims, who died in 1981. The child's clinical history is highly suggestive of neonatal AIDS. In 1992 a group O virus was isolated from the mother, who by then had AIDS.

---

sooty mangabey. There are six closely linked strains of SIV. Chimpanzees carry at least three different viral predecessors of HIV-1 that gave rise to groups M, O, and N. Sooty mangabeys carry an ancestor of HIV-2.

Simon's discovery of group N also raises other critical questions and challenges. Looking ahead, how many other SIV strains may have crossed the species barrier? Should we be mass screening for this new virus N or increasing surveillance of the other SIV strains? What about the human recombinant viruses? How well are we tracking them?

SUMMARY

HIV is a retrovirus. It has RNA for its genetic material and carries reverse transcriptase enzyme for making DNA from its RNA. HIV, using its enzyme, copies its genetic information from RNA into DNA, which becomes integrated into host cell DNA and may remain silent for years, or until such time as it is activated into producing new HIV. HIV contains at least nine genes; three of them, GAG-POL-ENV, are basic to all animal retroviruses. The six additional genes are involved in the infection process and regulate the production of products from the three genes. HIV, because of its error-prone reverse transcriptase enzyme, mutates at an unusually high rate. With time, many mutant HIV variants can be found within a single HIV-infected person. A vaccine against one mutant HIV may not work against a second—like the vaccines made yearly against different mutant influenza viruses.

A new group of HIV has been identified, Group N.

REVIEW QUESTIONS

(Answers to the Review Questions are on page 489.)

1. Why is HIV called a retrovirus?

2. What are the three major genes common to all retroviruses? How many additional genes does HIV have?

3. Why are retroviruses, and HIV in particular, believed to be genetically unstable? Give two reasons for your answer.

4. What is believed to be the major reason for the high rate of genetic mutations in HIV production?

Anti-HIV Therapy

We are constantly humbled by the devastation that something so small, HIV, can cast upon something so large, a human (Figure 4-1). This chapter provides no final answers; there is no curative therapy, no truly outstanding therapies (drugs that benefit all HIV infected without major side effects) against HIV, and, with the number of **expensive** anti-HIV drugs that are available, debate continues about the details on which drugs offer the best combination therapy and on the **standard of care** for HIV/AIDS patients. Because some 90% to 95% of HIV-infected people develop AIDS, and because 90% of all **new** HIV infections are occurring in developing nations, an **inexpensive, easily taken,** non-toxic, effective HIV-directed therapy is essential. Physicians need a drug that works against HIV as an-

tibiotics once worked against a large variety of disease-causing bacteria.

ANTI-HIV THERAPY

The ideal solution would be to prevent HIV from causing an infection. Then anti-HIV therapies would not be necessary. However, there are no means available to stop HIV from entering the body and infecting a limited number of cell types—primarily those cells displaying CD4 antigen receptor sites. Following HIV infection, there is a depletion of cells carrying CD4, especially the **T lymphocyte (T4) cells of the human immune system.** (See Chapter 5 for an explanation of cell types in the human immune system and their

William "Skip" Bluette (continued from page 23) three weeks before he died. Treatment to maintain Skip was failing—the multiple opportunistic infections were defeating the best medicine had to offer.

FIGURE 4-1 Drug Therapy for William "Skip" Bluette. Skip's treatment included amphotericin B, an antifungal drug, to combat meningitis. Starting in July 1986, he had to visit one of the hospital's clinics at least once a week to receive his treatments, which were given over several hours. Skip started taking zidovudine, a drug known to slow the progress of the disease, during the summer of 1987. Unfortunately, zidovudine also made it difficult for his body to produce blood cells. Skip stopped taking zidovudine when this occurred. In June of 1988, Skip started cleaning out his closets. He said it was part of the dying process to give belongings away "so you know where they're going." Partly, in jest, he said he wanted his ashes scattered on 42nd Street in New York—he thought that's where he "got AIDS."

He was hospitalized July 5, 1988. It was presumed that he had *Pneumocystis carinii* pneumonia, which Skip called "the killer." His breathing and speaking were labored. He had inflammation of the pancreas, for which he received morphine, and his kidneys began to fail. *(By permission of Mara Lavitt and* The New Haven Register*)*

function.) With T4 or CD4+ cell loss, over time immunological response is lost. Loss of immunological response leads to a variety of opportunistic infections (OIs). The suppression of the immune system and increasing susceptibility to OIs and cancers give HIV/AIDS a multidimensional pathology. Because HIV/AIDS is a multidimensional syndrome, it is unlikely that a single drug will provide adequate treatment or a cure (Figure 4-2).

An ideal goal for HIV drug investigators would be to find a drug that excises all HIV proviruses from the cell's DNA. It is very unlikely that this kind of drug will soon, if ever, be available. Alternatively, the **elimination** of all HIV-infected cells might be of comparable benefit, as long as irreplaceable cells are not totally lost through the process. In essence, this is the goal that the human immune system sets for itself, yet falls short of reaching, in the vast majority of HIV-infected individuals.

In the absence of a curative weapon (Figure 4-3), therapies must be designed to prevent the spread of the virus in the body. Some of these anti-HIV therapies are presented in this chapter.

Can HIV Infection Be Cured?

An effective cure means cleansing the body of the HIV. To find a cure, HIV incorporation into human DNA and subsequent reproduction of new virus must be understood. Without interference, the **HIV provirus** will remain in host-cell DNA for life. The provirus can, at any time, become activated to mass produce HIV, which leads to cell death and eventually to the individual's death. As of this writing, there is no way to prevent either the proviral state or proviral activation.

President George W. Bush's Goal: An AIDS Cure

In March of 2001, President Bush, making his first public comments on the global AIDS pandemic said his administration's primary goal is to find a cure for AIDS, a feat thought by scientists today to be all but impossible within the boundaries of contemporary biological science. The president's comments were echoed in April by Secretary of State Colin Powell in testimony before Congress in which he said the aim of the administration is to ultimately find a cure of AIDS. Health and Human Services Secretary Tommy Thompson, in his first staff briefing at the agency said, "The best thing that this department can do is find a cure for HIV and that is the best solution to a lot of our health problems." In mid-May at a luncheon speech at the World Health Assembly annual meeting in Geneva, Thompson reiterated his call for a cure. What is striking about these comments is that few, if any, AIDS researchers speak today of searching for a cure—that word hasn't been part of the epidemic language for the last 10 years.

To cure HIV infection would require one of two options: Kill every single infected cell in the body and destroy all viruses floating outside of those cells in the human bloodstream, or spare the infected cells but destroy the viruses hidden inside human DNA without damaging human genes in the process. So daunting are these tasks, so far beyond the current intellectual level of biological sciences, that the search for a cure effectively ended on the day in 1983 when French scientist Luc Montagnier announced his discovery that AIDS was caused by a retrovirus. Science has yet to discover a genuine cure for any viral disease, though it is possible to restrain some infections through vaccination.

ANTI-HIV DRUGS WITH FDA APPROVAL

Most Americans have no direct contact with the U.S. Food and Drug Administration (FDA), but their lives literally depend on the effectiveness of the agency. Charged with assuring the safety of specific foods and all medicines, the FDA has oversight over 25% of the U.S. economy. One of the FDA's key functions is approving and monitoring prescription drugs—a job that is particularly crucial for people with HIV infection or other life-threatening diseases.

POINT OF VIEW 4.1

MEDICAL BENEFIT: A CURE?

Many diseases cause death. "We can cure those diseases," people say, "but we can't cure AIDS." Tell me, how many diseases can we cure? We cannot cure very many viral diseases, nor can we cure many of the diseases that kill people, like heart disease and forms of cancer. The concept of curing people is relatively new. The strength of physicians used to come from their capacity to accompany. Accompanying a person through an illness towards health or towards death was central to the practice of medicine, but it disappeared when the issue became one of curing.

—*Jonathan Mann,* in Thomas A. Bass, *Reinventing the Future: Conversations with the World's Leading Scientists* (Addison-Wesley, 1994)

The vigil for William "Skip" Bluette (continued from page 73) 48 hours before he died. Time and therapy were running out on Skip. His last wish was to have his sisters Arlene and Nancy near when he died and they were there. On July 15, 1988, the doctors told Nancy and her mother that Skip's kidneys had failed—this time Skip would not recover. He died on July 17. He was 42 years old.

FIGURE 4-2 The Vigil for William "Skip" Bluette. The Bluette family rallied around Skip from the moment they found out he had AIDS. In April 1988, his mother had a heart attack but she survived it. Skip celebrated his 42nd birthday on May 18; it was his second birthday since his diagnosis. *(By permission of Mara Lavitt and The New Haven Register)*

The **gold standard** for determining the efficacy (effectiveness) of a new treatment is that it alters the disease in a way that is beneficial to the patient. Therefore, the end points most often used in clinical trials of therapies for a chronic disease such as HIV include prolongation of life or the extension of time to a significant disease complication.

But studies using these end points require large numbers of patients and/or the passage of considerable amounts of time. **Surrogate markers** (that is, physiological measurements that serve as substitutes for these major clinical events) can eliminate this problem if their validity and correlation with clinical outcome can be confirmed. The use

of surrogates has the potential to shorten the duration of clinical trials and expedite the development of new therapies.

Major Surrogate Markers Used Evaluating Anti-HIV Drug Therapy

The **T4 or CD4+ immune cell number** and **viral load** are the two most studied and commonly used surrogates (alternates) for clinical efficacy of anti-HIV therapies. They are imperfect measurements, however, because changes in T4 cell number per microliter of blood (a very small drop) and RNA strands per milliliter of blood are only partially explained by the therapy. T4 or CD4+ cell counts

FIGURE 4-3 Free of Pain—One with the Universe—William "Skip" Bluette. On July 20, 1988, Skip's body was cremated. There was a memorial service. On July 21, Skip's ashes were buried in Evergreen Cemetery in Connecticut. *(By permission of Mara Lavitt and* The New Haven Register*)*

exhibit a high degree of day-to-day variation in individuals, and methods used to count these cells are difficult to standardize. Recent investigations have shown that there is a T4 cell level and viral load level **disconnect.** This means that viral suppression by itself does not always predict immunological and clinical benefit. T4 cell counts and viral load can be clearly dissociated during treatment: T4 cells can increase in the presence of a high viral load, remain stable, or drop. **Clinical benefit** is more closely associated with the level of T4 cells rather than viral load. Recent data support the hypothesis that T4 cell depletion during HIV infection occurs largely as a result of the immune system's inability to generate new mature cells, and that the main effect of antiretroviral therapy is to help restore the immune system's ability to produce new T4 cells. (Perrin et al., 1998; Telenti et al., 1998; Deeks et al., 1999; Clark et al., 1999; Hellerstein et al., 1999.)

HIV/AIDS DRUGS RECEIVING FDA APPROVAL

From March of 1987 through early 2003, 17 anti-HIV drugs have received U.S. FDA approval for use in persons infected with HIV. There are more than 20 FDA approved drugs when combination pills and reformulations are included. Two other drugs have been FDA approved for **expanded access use** where standard regimes have failed. (Table 4-1).

Six of the 17 FDA-approved anti-HIV drugs are nucleoside (nuk-lee-o-side) analogs (each drug resembles one of the four nucleosides that are used in making DNA), one is a nucleotide analog and three are non-nucleosides. All ten are **reverse transcriptase inhibitors**. The other seven drugs are HIV-**protease** (pro-tee-ace) inhibitors. Cellular targets of these drugs can be seen in Figure 4-4.

THE DRUG DEVELOPMENT, APPROVAL PROCESS, AND CLINICAL TRIALS

In the United States, the drug discovery and FDA approval currently takes an average of 12 to 15 years and costs about $400 million (from the laboratory to the drugstore). In 1996, Merck & Co. claims to have spent **$1 billion** over 10 years to bring the protease inhibitor **Crixivan** to market! The odds against a new drug making it to the market are about 10,000 to 1. The clinical trial process for a drug usually includes 3 1/2 years of preclinical testing using laboratory and animal studies and 6 years of studies (clinical trials) in humans. **Phase I** includes 20 to 80 healthy volunteers and takes about a year to **test the drug's safety. Phase II** takes about two years and involves 100 to 300 persons with the disease to **assess the drug's effectiveness** and to look for side effects. **Phase III** of clinical trials lasts about three years and includes 1,000 to 3,000 patients to **verify effectiveness** and **identify adverse reactions of a drug**. Since 1989 the FDA has allowed phases I and II to be combined to shorten the approval process on new medicines for serious and life-threatening diseases. It now takes about 18 months for a drug to go through the review process for approval by the FDA. About **one in five medicines** that begin a clinical trial is **approved** for consumer use.

Global annual drug research and development spending is about $70 billion, but only 10% of that money goes to research on diseases that account for 90% of the world's infections.

THE HIV/AIDS DRUG MARKET

The anti-HIV drug therapy market is estimated to be about $8 billion a year. The $350 billion American pharmaceutical industry has been investing over $1 billion a year since the late 1980s to bring new and improved HIV drugs to market. Since 1987, a new FDA-approved antiviral drug has entered the market on average of every 9.4 months.

Beginning year 2003, 84 companies had 126 medicines and vaccines for AIDS and AIDS-related conditions in testing. This is in addition to 64 HIV and HIV-related FDA-approved medicines already on the market.

The most difficult part of presenting anti-HIV therapies to the public is the analysis of the incredible amount of new information continuously coming out in the scientific literature and attempting to make sense out of some very contradictory findings (*The Drug Development and Approval Process*, Pharmaceutical Manufacturers Association, December 1998)!

In December 1997, the U.S. House of Representatives passed into law the FDA Regulatory Modernization Act of 1997. The force of the law is to make the FDA more responsive to therapies for life-threatening diseases. The bill:

- Enabled people suffering from such afflictions to authorize their doctors to use experimental drugs or devices, not yet approved by the FDA for general use, to treat their ailments.
- Set up a registry of clinical trials to give patients and their doctors ready access to experimental treatments and drugs that might help in ministering to their illness.
- Streamlined the FDA's drug and device-reviewing process to hasten approval of new therapies for treating the severe diseases.

Clinical Trials

A clinical drug trial is a government funded and organized study of an experimental or unproven drug to determine the drug's safety and efficacy (whether or not it works). Drug trials for HIV/AIDS, sponsored by the Food and Drug Administration (FDA), are organized into the AIDS Clinical Trial Group (ACTG). Guidelines are set to determine how the ACTGs may be run and who is eligible to participate. Taking part in a trial may entitle persons to receive medical examinations and checkups and to have their overall health monitored. For many people with AIDS, the ACTGs are the only means of access to certain potentially life-saving drugs, and the only form of health care they may ever receive. Historically, FDA policy on admitting women into clinical trials has been confusing and discriminatory at best. Until recently, the FDA has had an outright ban on all women of child-bearing potential from participation in early stages of drug trials. In March of 1994, FDA took two important steps to ensure that new drugs are properly evaluated in women. **First,** it provided formal guidance to drug developers to emphasize its expectations that women would be appropriately represented in clinical studies and that new drug applications would include analyses capable of identifying potential differences in drug actions and value between the sexes. **Second,** the agency altered its 1977 policy to include most women with child-bearing potential in the earliest phases of clinical trials.

Table 4-1 Anti-HIV Therapy: Nucleoside Analogs, Non-nucleosides, and Protease Inhibitors

Name	FDA Approved	Cost/Day[a]
Nucleoside analog (reverse transcriptase inhibitor)		
Tenofovir (Viread)	October 2001	$11.33[b]
Zidovudine, AZT/ZDV (Retrovir)	March 1987	$7.96
Didanosine, ddI (Videx)	October 1991	$6.12
Zalcitabine, ddC (Hivid)	June 1994	$6.87
Stavudine, d4T (Zerit)	June 1994	$7.76
Lamivudine, 3TC (Epivir)	November 1995	$7.68
Abacavir (Ziagen)	December 1998	$9.30

Nucleoside analog reverse transcriptase inhibitors are potent in combination with other drugs; used alone, they lead to HIV resistance. *AZT, d4T, 3TC,* and *abacavir* penetrate the blood-brain barrier. Common side effect: lactic acidosis. **Four** new nucleoside analogues are in some phase of testing in the United States.[c]

Non-nucleoside compounds; (non-nucleoside reverse transcriptase inhibitors)		
Nevirapine (Viramune)	June 1996	$8.26
Delavirdine (Rescriptor)	April 1997	$6.36
Efavirenz (Sustiva)	September 1998	$13.14

Non-nucleoside analog reverse transcriptase inhibitors (NNRTIs, or non-nukes) may interact with other cytochrome *p450-processed drugs:* protease inhibitors, oral contraceptives, etc. NNRTIs have a mixed ability to penetrate the blood-brain barrier. Common side effect: mild rash. Some doctors build up drug doses slowly to avoid rash; the other worry is that dose building increases risk of drug resistance. **Six** new non-nucleoside analogs are in some phase of testing in the United States.

Protease inhibitor drugs		
Saquinavir mesylate (Invirase)[d]	December 1995 (Hoffman-La Roche)	$21.60
Saquinavir (Fortovase)	November 1997	$22.00
Ritonavir (Norvir)	March 1996 (Abbott)	$22.20
Indinavir (Crixivan)	March 1996 (Merck)	$15.00
Nelfinavir (Viracept)	March 1997 (Aguoron)	$15.75
Amprenavir (Agenerase)	April 1999 (Glaxo Wellcome)	$16.80
ABT-378 (Kaletra)[e]	September 2000 (Abbott)	$22.60
YX-478	? (Glaxo Wellcome/Vertex)	Phase III testing

Protease inhibitors (PIS) are very potent and may interact with other drugs using *cytochrome p450 metabolic pathways.* Potentially life-threatening if taken with Seldane, Hismanal, Propulsid, Halcion, or Versed. Avoid rifabutin, Nizoral, rifampin. Poor absorption may affect potency. Common side effects: liver toxicity, hypoglycemia, flatulence, bloating, lipodystrophy (fat distribution). **Six** new protease inhibitors are now in some phase of testing in the United States.

NEW DRUG CLASSES

Fusion Inhibitors—prevents HIV entry   Phase III trials, early 2001
     Pentafuside (T-20)

Integrase Inhibitors—prevents HIV DNA from entering human DNA
     Zintevir(AR-177)

Zinc Finger Inhibitors—disrupts polyprotein formation essential for HIV replication
     Benzamide-disulfide

[a]Cost is based on wholesale price of 100-pill bottle or largest size available as listed in 2001 Red Book or based on information from the manufacturer, or Hospital Formulatory Pricing Guide, 2000.

[b]Tenofovir is the first **nucleotide** analog approved for HIV treatment. It blocks HIV replication similar to the **nucleoside** analogs.

[c]Expanded Access drugs are for patients failing standard regimes. Beginning year 2003 there are at least 2 new nucleoside and 4 non-nucleoside RTI and 2 PI drugs in early anti-HIV drug trials in the United States. Telephone numbers for information concerning the use of the individual protease inhibitors are:

Saquinavir/Invirase	Hoffman-La Roche In./800-526-6367
Ritonavir/Norvir/Lopinavir	Abbot Labs/800-633-9110
Indinavir/Crixivan	Merck & Co./800-672-6372
Nelfinavir/Viracept	Agouron/888-874-2237
Amprenavir/Agenerase	Glaxo Wellcome Inc./800-722-9292
VX-478/–	Glaxo Wellcome Inc./800-722-9292

[d]Saquinavir mesylate was the first nucleotide RTI in Phase III trials. Saquinavir mesylate, ritonavir, and indinavir were approved in 97, 72, and 42 days, respectively. Abacavir is the first 2-deoxyguanosine analog reverse transcriptase inhibitor.

[e]**FDA approved Kaletra, a combination of Lopinavir and Norvir.** Lopinavir is only available in Kaletra.

Targets of Anti-HIV Drugs: Generalized Scheme

reverse transcriptase — **ssRNA**

gp120

CC-CKR-5
CXCKR-4 (fusin)

CD4 receptor

The CD4 receptor on the cell membrane binds HIV. The newly discovered **chemokine receptors (fusin & CC-CKR-5** also fuse with the virus coat an facilitate passage of the virus into the cell.

Viral RNA is released into the T4 or CD4+ cell as the virus sheds its protein coat. Reverse transcriptase **(RT)** enzyme catalyzes transcription of viral RNA to viral DNA.

RNA **RT** **ss DNA**
ds DNA
DNA

**Nucleoside Analogs'
(ZDV, ddI, ddC, d4T, 3TC, abacavir) Nonnucleoside compounds (nevirapine, delaviradine, efavirenz) Tenofovir is a nucleotide analog. All stop RT Replication of HIV-DNA**

Viral DNA is transported into the nucleus of the T4 cell. Here, it inserts itself into the T4 cell's DNA.

Viral RNA

genome RNA **messenger RNA**

Viral RNA triggers manufacture of viral proteins appropriating the cell's own machinery to do so.

Viral proteins

Immature HIV bud from the cell.

**Protease Inhibitors'
Site of Action -
Stops Protein Processing into Proper Lengths (saquinavir—two types, ritonavir, indinavir, nelfinavir, amprenavir, kaletra)**

HIV stays immature if protease is inhibited. If protease **not** inhibited, protein is processed into shorter lengths.

Mature HIV

FIGURE 4-4 Diagram of Anti-HIV Therapy. The seven FDA-approved nucleoside/nucleotide analogs, three non-nucleoside compounds, and seven protease inhibitors are represented with respect to their anti-HIV activity. The nucleoside analogs act early after infection, while the protease inhibitors act later in the HIV life cycle, after viral proteins have been synthesized into long strands. Those strands of amino acids contain the individual HIV proteins that become functional after they are cut into their appropriate amino acid sequence lengths. **NOTE: The enzyme integrase is required for HIV DNA to enter human DNA. Drugs called INTEGRASE INHIBITORS are in development.**

FDA-APPROVED NUCLEOSIDE/NON-NUCLEOSIDE ANALOG REVERSE TRANSCRIPTASE INHIBITORS AND PROTEASE INHIBITORS

All the known mechanisms by which HIV impairs the human immune system depend on HIV reproduction. Therefore, the development of anti-HIV replication drugs would appear to be a positive **first step** in controlling HIV reproduction.

Each of the seven nucleoside/nucleotide analogs, sometimes referred to as **nukes** (Figure 4-5), on entering an HIV-infected cell interferes with the virus' ability to replicate itself (Figure 4-6). That is, **when any of the seven nucleoside/nucleotide analogs are incorporated into a strand of HIV DNA being**

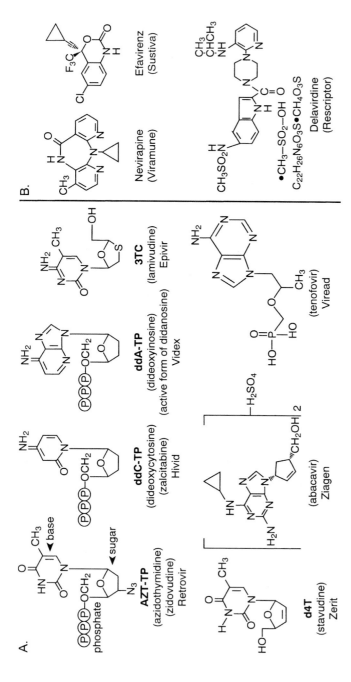

FIGURE 4-5 **A.** Structure of seven FDA-Approved Nucleoside/Nucleotide Analog Drugs Which Inhibit HIV Replication. The nucleoside analog agents competitively inhibit deoxynucleoside triphosphates (part of the HIV proviral DNA chain) when incorporated by HIV reverse transcriptase, causing DNA chain termination. Azidothymidine triphosphate (AZT-TP) competes with deoxythymidine triphosphate (dTTP), dideoxycytidine triphosphate (ddC-TP) competes with deoxycytidine triphosphate (dCTP), and dideoxyinosine (ddI) is converted to dideoxyadenosine triphosphate (ddA-TP), which competes with deoxyadenosine triphosphate (dATP). Stavudine (d4T) competes with deoxythymidine triphosphate (dTTP). Lamivudine (3TC) competes with deoxycytidine triphosphate (dCTP) and Abacavir competes with deoxyguanosine-5'triphosphate (dGTP). **B.** Structure of the Three FDA Approved non-Nucleoside Reverse Transcriptase Inhibitors. Unlike nucleoside RTI's, these drugs **do not** have a specific chemical structure that includes a base, sugar, and phosphate group. **These drugs bind directly to the reverse transcriptase.** This blocks DNA polymerase activity and stops HIV DNA replication. The introduction of these drugs brought great promise but that promise did not last long as HIV showed high levels of resistance to the drugs at a very rapid rate. **Cross Resistance:** Note the similarity in base structures among these drugs. Because of such similarities, when HIV becomes resistant to one of these drugs it also, in many cases, becomes cross-resistant to one or more of the other drugs in the nucleoside and non-nucleoside reverse transcriptase inhibitors.

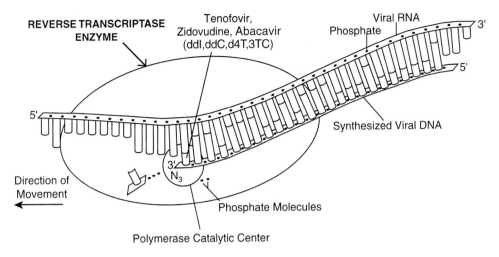

Direction of Movement ←

FIGURE 4-6 Incorporation of FDA-Approved Nucleoside/Nucleotide Analogs Preventing HIV Replication. Zidovudine (ZDV) is a synthetic thymidine analog that is widely used in the treatment of HIV disease and AIDS. HIV-RT is 100 times more sensitive to ZDV inhibition than is the **human transcriptase.** The incorporation of zidovudine-triphosphate into HIV DNA by the action of HIV reverse transcriptase terminates DNA chain extension because polymerization or the incorporation of the next nucleotide adjacent to the azide N_3 group cannot occur. Similar blockage of DNA replication occurs when FDA-approved ddl, ddC, d4T, or 3TC are used. Abacavir is the first 2'deoxyguanosine analog to be used.

newly synthesized, it stops further synthesis of that DNA strand. The nucleoside analog stops the HIV enzyme, reverse transcriptase, from joining the next nucleoside into position. The six FDA-approved nucleoside analogs are all members of the family of 2',3'-dideoxynucleoside analogs. By name they are **zidovudine** (ZDV), often **mistakenly called AZT (3'-azido-2',3'-deoxythymidine),** trade name **Retrovir; didanosine** or **ddI (2',3'-dideoxyinosine),** trade name **VIDEX; dideoxycytosine, zalcitabine** or **ddC (2',3'-dideoxycytosine),** trade name **HIVID; stavudine** or **d4T,** trade name **Zerit; lamivudine** or **3TC,** trade name **Epivir; Abacavir,** trade name **Ziagen;** and the single nucleotide analogue **Tenofovir,** trade name **Viread** (Table 4-1).

**Focus on the Seven Nucleoside/
Nucleotide Analogs**

Each of the seven drugs has limited effectiveness as a **monotherapy.** The principal limitations are: **(1)** they are not 100% effective in stopping HIV reverse transcriptase from making HIV DNA; **(2)** positive clinical effects are short term, they are not sustained; **(3)** each drug has its own set of toxic side effects; **(4)** individually they do not

delay the onset of AIDS; and **(5)** HIV rapidly becomes resistant to each of them.

Side Effects: "First Do No Harm"

Each of the seven reverse transcriptase inhibitors (RTIs) is associated with severe to moderate side effects. For example, zidovudine causes anemia (lowered blood cell count), nausea, headache, and lethargy and inhibits mitochondrial DNA replication in humans (de Martino et al., 1995); didanosine causes peripheral neuropathy (PN) (a burning pain or pins and needles-like sensation in hands and feet) and pancreatitis (a dangerous swelling of the pancreas) and is very hard for people with poor appetites to take; zalcitabine causes PN and mouth ulcers; stavudine causes PN; and lamivudine causes hair loss and PN.

In year 2000 both **Zevit** and **Videx** were associated with the lactic acidosis—a large increase in acid buildup in the body damaging the liver and/or pancreas—this can be deadly! Pregnant women are at highest risk according to the FDA. These two drugs are to be used in pregnant women **only** when benefits outweigh risks.

With respect to the non-nucleoside analogs ending 2000 and beginning 2001, the FDA has posted warnings on the use of **Nevirapine** (viramune) because of reported serious and sometimes fatal liver toxicity. Most of the cases associated with liver failure occurred in people who took the drug on first exposure to HIV—health-care workers who stuck themselves with an HIV contaminated needle.

Collectively, some 15% of HIV infected people **cannot** tolerate the **nucleoside/non-nucleoside antiretroviral drugs.** Even those who can tolerate the drugs are time-limited and right now according to Anthony Fauci, director of the National Institute of Allergy and Infectious Diseases, about 80% of those on drug therapy are rapidly running out of time.

USE OF NON-NUCLEOSIDE ANALOG REVERSE TRANSCRIPTASE INHIBITORS

Non-nucleoside reverse transcriptase inhibitors (NNRTIs), sometimes referred to as **nonnukes, are a structurally and chemically dissimilar group of antiretrovirals that can be used effectively in triple-therapy regimes.** The mechanism of action of NNRTIs is distinct from that of nucleoside analogs, even though both **prevent** the conversion of HIV RNA into HIV DNA. Nucleoside RT inhibitors constrain, or stop, HIV replication by their incorporation into the elongating strand of viral DNA, causing chain termination. In contrast, NNRTIs **are not incorporated** into viral DNA but inhibit HIV replication directly by binding noncompetitively to RT. NNRTIs at first appear to offer hope. All four tested did inhibit the RT-HIV enzyme (atevirdine, delvaridine, loviridine, and nevirapine). But this inhibition was **short-lived** because HIV-resistant mutants for each of the non-nucleoside RTI were found within weeks of their use. Combination therapies using, for example, zidovudine and nevirapine, have shown some success but it turned out that various drug combinations do not extend survival time. But they do extend the asymptomatic period! The FDA approved nevirapine (Viramune) for market in June of 1996. **The primary advantage of using NNRTIs in therapy is to delay use of protease inhibitors.**

The key to future success in using the reverse transcriptase inhibitors (RTIs) is finding RTIs that work in cells that are not undergoing division. Most RTIs currently in use work only in cells that are dividing.

FDA-APPROVED PROTEASE INHIBITORS

Recall from Chapter 3 that some HIV genes code for **reverse transcriptase** (RT) **integrase** and **protease** enzymes. Later on in the reproductive cycle of HIV a specific **protease** is required to process the precursor GAG and POL polyproteins into mature HIV components, GAG proteins, and the enzymes integrase and protease (Erickson et al., 1990). **If protease is missing or inactive, noninfectious HIV are produced.** Therefore, inhibitors of protease enzyme function represents an **alternative** strategy to the inhibition of reverse transcriptase in the treatment of HIV infection.

As research progressed, scientists found that HIV protease is distinctly different from human protease enzymes, so a drug that blocks HIV protease should not affect human normal cell function. This means that HIV protease blockers are specific to HIV protease and that reduces dangerous side effects of protease-inhibiting drugs. Beginning 2003, some 20 HIV protease-inhibiting drugs were under study, six are in clinical trials, and seven have received FDA drug approval (Figure 4-7). **PROBLEM: AT LEAST 15% OF PEOPLE MUST GIVE UP PROTEASE INHIBITORS BECAUSE OF SEVERE SIDE EFFECTS. ABOUT 15% OF PEOPLE DO *NOT* RESPOND TO PROTEASE INHIBITORS AND NEW REPORTS INDICATE THAT PROTEASE INHIBITORS ARE FAILING TO SUPPRESS HIV REPLICATION IN OVER HALF THOSE PEOPLE IN TREATMENT FROM ONE TO THREE YEARS. (Valdez et al., 1999; Clough et al., 1999) HIV IS AN IMPRESSIVE ENEMY.**

Structure and Function of HIV Protease

Following production of the HIV proteins, the core structure of HIV assembles at the cell membrane. A matrix protein, p17, appears to specify the site of assembly by associating with the cytoplasmic portion of the transmembrane envelope protein gp41. A packaging signal identifies which viral RNA transcripts (messages for making HIV proteins) are to be included into HIV. The assembled HIV core buds through the cell membrane,

Saquinavir mesylate

Saquinavir

Indinavir

Ritonavir

Nelfinavir

Amprenavir*

* FDA approved for expanded access only

FIGURE 4-7 Chemical Structures of six of the seven FDA approved Protease Inhibitors. Kaletra not shown, is a combination of two PI.

thus acquiring a human lipid envelope complete with HIV envelope proteins. Maturation of the new HIV requires cleavage by HIV protease of the long Gag and Gag-Pol proteins, which occurs during or shortly after HIV budding.

HIV protease is made up of two units, each unit consisting of 99 amino acids, with two aspartyl residues at the base of the active site serving as the target for most of the protease inhibitors under investigation. Protease has two important functions. **First,** it cuts itself loose from other components of the virus by a process known as autocatalysis (self-releasing). **Second,** the aspartyl protease of HIV cleaves the Gag (p55) and Gag-Pol (p160) polyproteins into structural Gag protein subunits and the three viral enzymes—**reverse transcriptase, integrase,** and **protease** itself (Figure 4-8). Without protease activity, only immature virions are produced that are incapable of completing a replicative cycle (Laurence, 1996). Thus, protease is absolutely essential for viral replication. HIV protease is also distinct from human proteases, making it an ideal target for antiretroviral therapy. For example, any drug inhibiting protease will also indirectly inhibit the production of Reverse Transcriptase (**RT**).

Other protease-released proteins help organize various HIV components (proteins and nucleic acid) into a mature, infectious HIV (Figure 4-9).

PROTEASE INHIBITORS

In 1988, protease inhibitors with potent and selective antiretroviral activity in cell culture were identified, but the insolubility, poor oral absorption, and rapid liver metabolism of candidate drugs delayed the identification of suitable therapeutic agents until 1992. The **protease inhibitors** made up of a small number of amino acids (up to 15) bind to the protease active site and inhibit the activity of the enzyme. This inhibition prevents cleavage of the long HIV proteins, resulting in the formation of immature **noninfectious** viral particles.

The Seven Protease Inhibitors in Use

1. Saquinavir mesylate (Invirase)— Saquinavir mesylate was the first protease inhibitor (PI) that FDA approved for use in combination with nucleoside analog drugs in persons with advanced HIV disease. At the time of approval, there were no clinical trial data on survival or progression of HIV disease using saquinavir (Nightingale, 1996).

Although HIV mutants to saquinavir have been identified, saquinavir mutants appear to develop more slowly and at a lower frequency than formation of HIV mutants to other anti-HIV drugs (Jacobsen et al., 1995). The available oral formulation of saquinavir has **poor absorption (limited bioavailability).**

A. Why HIV Protease is Essential for HIV Replication

Long Lengths of Inactive Viral Polyprotein

Units of Protease that Cut the Polyprotein into Individual Active Proteins

A Different Active Protein From Each Separate Length of Polyprotein

(1)　(2)　(3)　(4)

FIGURE 4-8
Representation of Protease and Protease Inhibitors. **A.** The function of HIV protease is to release the individual replication enzymes, core proteins, and envelope proteins so that HIV can develop into mature, infective HIV. **B.** Blocking the production of these essential HIV proteins using protease inhibitors produces immature, noninfective HIV. The action (cutting of protein lengths into active HIV components) of HIV protease occurs during and just after HIV buds out of the cell!

B. How HIV Protease Inhibitors Inhibit Viral Protease Function

A Protease Inhibitor Binds to the Cutting Site of the Protease. The Inactivited or Blocked Protease Cannot Cut the Polyprotein.

It is also the least potent of the six FDA-approved protease inhibitors. **The cost is about $648/month.**

2. Saquinavir (Fortovase)— It is a formulation of saquinivar mesylate. It is sold in a softgel capsule and is more easily absorbed by the body, making it much more effective than S. mesylate. Fortovase was FDA approved in November of 1997 and is now, according to the latest April 1998 **NIH Guidelines for the Use of Antiretroviral Agents,** recommended for use over S. mesylate. **The cost is about $660/month.**

3. Ritonavir (Norvir)— Ritonavir is the second PI to be FDA approved. **The cost is about $666/month.**

4. Indinavir (Crixivan)— This PI is perhaps the most often used of the six FDA-approved protease inhibitors. **The cost is about $450/month.**

5. Nelfinavir (Viracept)— Nelfinavir has been evaluated at doses similar to the previous four protease inhibitors. **The cost is about $473/month.**

FIGURE 4-9 Representation of HIV Assembly. During the budding process, the viral Gag and Gag-Pol polyproteins assemble at the cell membrane together with viral RNA to form immature HIV. These polyproteins are then cleaved by the HIV-coded protease enzyme to provide the structural and functional (enzyme) proteins essential to form the **mature,** infectious viral core. *(Adapted from Vella, 1995)*

6. Amprenavir (Agenerase)— It is approved for use in adults and children. It is also the **first** anti-HIV drug to appear as a result of computer imaging—a structure-based drug design. **The cost is about $504/month.**

7. ABT-378 (Kaletra)— is FDA approved and is a combination of Lopinavir and Novir—both are protease inhibitors. The cost is about $678 per month.

FDA Approved Combination Therapy— Year 2000

Two drug combinations were approved near year's end 2000. Kaletra is a protease inhibitor combination containing Lopinavir/Novir. Trizivir is the first to contain three nucleoside analogs—Ziagen (abacavir), Retrovir (Zidovudine or AZT), and Epivir (3TC); the cost of Trizivir is over $600 per month.

DEVELOPMENT AND SELECTION OF HIV DRUG-RESISTANT MUTANTS

Development of Drug-Resistant Nucleoside Analog Mutants

HIV reverse transcriptase, the enzyme that copies (transcribes) HIV RNA into HIV DNA, **is unable to edit or eliminate transcription errors during nucleic acid replication** (Roberts et al., 1988). Because there is no repair or correction of mis-

takes (as occurs in human cells), there are about one to five mutations in each new replicated HIV DNA HIV RNA strand (Coffin, 1995). This means that **each new virus** is different from all other HIV that is being produced because new virus is being produced at a rate of 1 billion to 10 billion per day! There will be 1 billion to 10 billion new HIV mutants produced each day in one person. Thus, virtually all possible mutations, and perhaps many combinations of mutations, are generated in each patient daily (Ho et al., 1995; Wain-Hobson, 1995; Wei et al., 1995; Hu et al., 1996; Mayers, 1996).

DEVELOPMENT OF DRUG RESISTANT PROTEASE INHIBITORS

HIV resistance to all seven PIs has been found in clinical trials. The development of HIV resistance to PIs is a major concern. For example, recent studies (Schmit et al., 1996) found that long-term (one year) use of **ritonavir** is associated with the production of at least nine different mutations that make HIV resistant to ritonavir. These ritonavir-resistant mutants also demonstrated cross-resistance to both **indinavir** and **saquinavir.** John Mellors (1996) reported that within 12 to 24 weeks after **indinavir** therapy, at least 10 different HIV-resistant indinavir mutations occurred and five HIV saquinavir-resistant mutations occurred with the use of the individual drugs. **Cross-resistance to ritonavir occurred in at**

BOX 4.1

PROTEASE INHIBITORS: EXTENDING LIFE; THE DOWNSIDE OF THIS GIFT—RECOVERY?

THE LAZARUS EFFECT: A RETURN TO FUNCTIONAL STATUS!

In November of 1995, one man in his late forties wrote his obituary—he had been fighting off HIV disease, then AIDS, for over 13 years. In another case, the man's T cell count was zero. He was on oxygen and morphine. Funeral arrangements were made, and his friends and family were on a death vigil. They are but two examples of several thousand men, beginning 1999, all under the age of 50, who had given up hope—they believed they were a short step away from death. Some ran up huge debts—maxed out all their credit cards and gave lavish gifts. Some regretted the way they had lived or not lived to this point, some became very angry, some made peace with themselves and others, but **all** felt death was imminent. **Then it happened**—the first results of combination therapies using nucleoside and non-nucleoside reverse transcriptase inhibitors **dropped viral load counts.** Then, a few months later, the protease inhibitors used alone or in combination with two or three of the nucleoside or non-nucleoside reverse transcriptase drugs dropped viral load counts to **unmeasurable** or **undetectable** levels in people with HIV disease and AIDS patients. **And,** those with significantly lowered viral loads demonstrated **surprising recovery—their T4 cells rebounded, in some cases from below 200 back up to, or approaching, normal!** These **"AIDS cocktails,"** as the combination therapies were soon called, gave people with AIDS a new chance at a productive life for the first time since the beginning of the pandemic in the United States in 1981.

About 50% of people diagnosed with AIDS in 1995 are still alive, meaning the median survival rate is now at least seven years—we don't know how long it will stretch out to, but that is progress.

CAN THERE BE A DOWNSIDE TO SUCH A MIRACLE?

Of course the most tragic downside is the fact that not all who would benefit from the **drug cocktail** can afford it—But that is not the issue that is relevant to the question per se. No, this question pertains to a downside, if any, for people who have access to these drugs.

WHAT KIND OF PROBLEMS EXIST?

Guilt

Many who now feel "new" again feel **guilty** because these drugs are not available to all who need them—the poor and the uninsured in the United States and those in underdeveloped nations.

Reestablishing Relationships

Depending on how long and how severe the illness, the affected became more or less isolated—even "best" friends stopped calling or dropping by. Some who also had AIDS died, while some were too sick to care or mourn them; but now that they have recovered? **WHAT NOW? Beginning year 2003, about 475,000 people in the United States were on anti-HIV therapy, which includes protease inhibitors. These drugs are not as readily available to the other 500,000 HIV infected in the United States. To date they are mostly unavailable in developing nations.**

Ability To Work Again—Loss of Disability Pay

Disability insurance has been a **cocoon of safety** for many now experiencing "new" life. Traditionally, people with AIDS received disability checks until death. But suddenly it is not so certain that that is going to be the case. People who were expected to die are going to be coming back. Nobody is prepared for this. Now that drug cocktails have extended life expectancies, it is expected that these people will be reevaluated and lose their disability payments. **They will have to go back to work.**

Across the United States, AIDS groups are deluged with calls from patients who are excited, confused, or frightened about the prospect of ending disability status and returning to work. In Miami, a psychologist has begun weekly seminars on resumé writing and job interviews for AIDS patients who have not worked in years. At AIDS Project Los Angeles, counselors field 100 calls each week on return-to-work issues.

AIDS patients face a barrage of challenges as they think about rejoining the workforce. Job

BOX 4.1 *(continued)*

skills sometimes have atrophied. Old careers do not seem fulfilling anymore after a brush with death. Potential employers may not want to hire someone with a costly disease, even though federal law bars discrimination against people with AIDS. Without clear knowledge of the new drugs' staying power, some patients fear that a return to work could be premature, leaving them in dire shape if protease inhibitors fail and they lose their jobs once again.

Dilemmas of Returning to Work: Two Examples

1. A 38-year-old software engineer shudders to think about the myriad new technologies he must master if he is to resume work. He used to be a star computer programmer, deluged with consulting assignments. Then AIDS forced him to go on long-term disability.

   "I'm going to need new software, new tools, new products" to be a success once more. He estimates that retraining courses will cost $10,000. Where will the money come from?

2. He considered taking a part-time job at a friend's hat-embroidery shop but decided against it, in part for fear of jeopardizing his government benefits, and also because he isn't sure how long his health will hold up. **"The biggest downside of this disease is that you stop being a dependable person,"** he said. "I couldn't be sure that I would be there every day. That's very hard to acknowledge."

TREATMENT DOWNSIDE

From mid-1996 into year 2003, optimism remains high on the medical advances using AIDS cocktail therapy. Though researchers applaud recent drug and immunology findings, many worry about the implications. **Treatment successes may create a false sense of security, and lead to complacency in prevention efforts. If we are close to a cure, people may say, why bother with politically sensitive issues like needle exchange programs, distribution of free condoms, sex education programs in our schools, and so on.** But the therapy is not available to the majority of HIV-infected, even in the developed countries like the United States. What of the other 42 million living HIV infected worldwide? If too many glowing promises are made too soon—before treatment is available

for all, or most of the world—people may revert back to unsafe sex and other behaviors that will increase their risk of becoming HIV-infected. **No, it is not yet time to stop teaching and providing preventive measures!**

POLITICAL DOWNSIDE

As scientists dare ask whether HIV eradication may be possible in some people in the near future (two to five years), the press may be promising more than the scientists can deliver, but press can and does influence political will. If the political will to fight this disease **weakens** due to the **premature declaration of victory,** this may be the greatest downside of all!

HIV is not yet a chronic disease and has not yet been eradicated from anyone, despite reductions in viral load to **undetectable** levels for over three years in some cases.

The Continuous Debate on the Use of Protease Inhibitors

Protease inhibitors have been hailed as life-saving antiretroviral drugs since their debut in 1996. But there is a major rift in the HIV/AIDS community concerning their use as new information about them emerges. The new drugs have saved people's lives, that's true. But the new drugs have also killed people. That's also true! They have damaged and deformed some people so badly that although they are alive, they say they wish they were dead. Drug cocktails comprised of protease inhibitors—now considered to be the standard treatment for infected patients who are both sick and healthy—have caused many to suffer liver damage, kidney failure, strokes, heart attacks, and other devastating side effects that are deemed inevitable by advocates of the new retroviral treatments, but called horrific and unnecessary by opponents. According to Joseph Sonnabend, an HIV/AIDS physician at St. Lukes–Roosevelt Hospital Center, "There is absolutely no question whatsoever that protease inhibitors have helped people. But they've probably hurt more people than they've helped. The people for whom benefit has been proven beyond a doubt are really sick people who would have died without them. But the target population for the drug therapy are those that are still healthy, and these people will almost certainly have their lives shortened by these drugs."

least 19 isolates of HIV-indinavir resistant mutants.

Rapid Production of HIV Protease Inhibitor Mutations

The high rate of viral replication found throughout the course of HIV infection and the high frequency of virus mutations occurring during each replication cycle, due to the lack of RNA proofreading or correction mechanisms, are the basis for the emergence of drug-resistant variants under the selective pressure of antiretroviral drugs. In fact, a **Darwinian** model can be applied to HIV dynamics, with the continuous production of genetically different HIV (variants) and the continuous selection of the **fittest** virus.

Unfortunately, with daily production of billions of HIV and a mutation rate that produces billions of new mutants each day, **it is likely that any single mutation already exists before any drug is introduced.**

Because resistant variants may exist before treatment is initiated and may evolve (become greater in number) under selective pressure, anti-HIV therapy can address viral resistance in three ways: (**1**) maximize the suppression of viral replication, the fewer rounds of HIV replication, the fewer HIV mutations possible; (**2**) use combination drugs requiring HIV to create multiple drug mutations for resistance; and (**3**) force the emergence of HIV variants with slower replication or decreased virulence.

Protease Inhibitor HIV Resistance Lessons Learned

Data obtained from saquinavir mesylate, saquinavir (Fortovase), indinavir, and nelfinavir studies show a dose-dependent delay in the emergence of resistance. This is the most important property of protease inhibitors that distinguishes them from nucleoside reverse transcriptase inhibitors. Higher doses of nucleosides do not delay resistance or provide a greater effect, but rather increase toxicity. **With increased dose of the protease inhibitors, a more durable reduction in viral RNA response and a delay in resistance are achieved without greater toxicity** (Mellors, 1996).

It appears, based on clinical trial data, that the best way to avoid resistance is to take the drug on time, and to not skip doses. Taking PIs in combination with other anti-HIV drugs has been shown to slow down the development of HIV PI resistance.

Selection of Drug-Resistant Mutants

Based on the large number of mutant HIV produced in any one person, **it is not surprising that HIV emerges with resistance to drugs used in antiretroviral therapy.** Such strains are referred to as **drug-resistant** mutants. HIV drug-resistant mutants are selected to reproduce most effectively under conditions of selective pressure exerted by the presence of the drugs. Those HIV able to resist the drugs continue to multiply; those that are sensitive to the drugs are destroyed—**selection!** (Figure 4-10)

The Demise of Monotherapy

Sixteen years ago (1987) the first antiretroviral drug, Zidovudine (AZT as it is often referred to) entered the fight against HIV replication. The infected person took 12 pills per day—two pills every four hours around the clock. It is a very toxic drug, but for some it meant a short extension of life. The use of Zidovudine and newer antiretrovirals as single agents had to stop.

The use of **one** anti-HIV RTI drug at a time (monotherapy) leads to HIV drug-resistant mutants. But, it took seven years before David Cooper, an AIDS-drug therapy researcher declared 1995 the year of the **"demise of monotherapy for HIV and the rise of combination drug therapy"** (Simberkoff, 1996; Stephenson, 1996). The **standard of therapy** now is that **all** anti-HIV drugs must be used in combination and that each combination include two reverse transcriptase inhibitors and a protease inhibitor. The use of three or more drugs in combination is referred to as HAART or **Highly Active Anti-retroviral Therapy** (Merry et al., 1998 updated).

The Function of HARRT: Suppression of HIV Replication and Restoration of Immune Competence

Suppression

The function of HAART is to suppress HIV replication regardless of the number of drugs used. The reasoning is to keep the viral load low so that sexual transmission of HIV becomes unlikely, and to prevent HIV mutation by reducing its

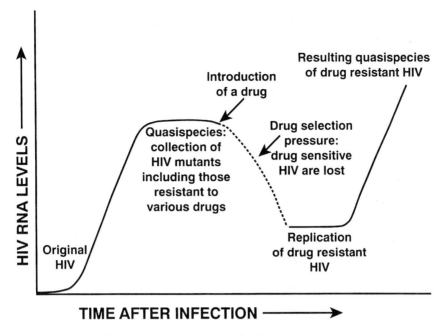

FIGURE 4-10   Enrichment of Drug Resistant HIV. The development of drug-resistant HIV variants in an individual limits available treatment. This drug-resistant HIV is transmitted such that the recipient becomes infected with one or more drug-resistant HIV variants.

ability to replicate. A number of clinical trials have demonstrated that only about half the patients placed on HAART, for the first time, are able to achieve maximal suppression—undetectable or less than 50 copies of HIV RNA per milliliter of blood. Where HAART works, most people reduce their viral load to 50 copies within 24 to 32 weeks. Less is known about the long-term durability of this suppression. Few existing clinical trials are sufficiently long lasting to provide this information. One recent report from the Frankfurt Clinic Cohort found low rates of viral breakthrough or viral rebounds in some patients continuing to take therapy for up to 3.3 years. Of those who achieve this undetectable viral load, the majority will experience a viral rebound during the first year of therapy and most everyone will experience the rebound if they stop taking the drugs (Back 2001). Currently, about 30% or 300,000 Americans living with HIV infection are untreated. Worldwide, beginning 2003, of the 42 million people living with HIV, between 6% to 10% or about 3.4 million people in developing nations need antiretroviral drugs now. But the World Health Organization (WHO) estimates that less than 3% of these people are receiving the therapy. The WHO hopes to have up to 3 million people in Africa and Asia on therapy by year 2005.

Restoration

Although antiretroviral drugs, for those who can tolerate them, have suppressed HIV replication, they have not restored the immune system such that victims can resume their previous lifestyles or even prevent their earlier-than-expected death.

Questions That Need Answers: For those who can tolerate antiretroviral drug therapy, which triple drug therapy should be used? Which three drugs can sustain the most favorable benefit/risk ratio over the longest time? Should triple-class, triple-drug therapy be used immediately, or should some be reserved for later? Many studies are underway to answer these questions, but as many experienced HIV caregivers already know, the answers may not necessarily be the same for all patients.

HOW COMBINATION DRUG THERAPY CAN REDUCE THE CHANCE OF HIV DRUG RESISTANCE

Combination drug therapy works because a single strand of RNA, the genetic material of HIV, must be multiple mutant, that is, it must carry a genetic change to become resistant to **each** new drug used. So, the greater number of drugs used, each capable of stopping HIV replication by interfering with the function of reverse transcriptase, the greater the number of genetic changes that must occur in a single RNA strand of the virus. For reasons of explanation, say that the **chance of change** in one nucleotide of HIV for resistance to a single drug occurs in **ONE** RNA strand during the production of 10,000 (10 thousand) or 1×10^4 such strands. This is a reasonable figure! Then to have a second nucleotide mutation occur in that **same** single strand for resistance to a second drug, again at 1×10^4 means that only one RNA strand in 100 million or 1×10^8 would carry both genetic changes. For three separate nucleotide mutations occurring in one RNA strand then, it would be $(1 \times 10^4) \times (1 \times 10^4) \times (1 \times 10^4)$ or **only one RNA strand out of 1,000,000,000,000 (1 trillion) would carry a resistance to all three drugs at the same time. But as small as this number is, recall that 1 billion to 10 billion genetically different RNA strands are produced each day in one individual. Also, individual RNA strands can exchange nucleotides in a process called recombination. This increases the chance of multiple resistant RNA strands.** This is why it is so important to **slow** the replication of HIV—fewer rounds of replication mean fewer RNA strands, thus fewer possibilities of producing HIV that are resistant to AIDS drug cocktails! Current AIDS drug cocktails, especially those using one or more protease inhibitors, quickly and significantly reduce HIV replication—this is why people on these combination therapies must take them **on schedule,** in prescribed doses, and maybe for the rest of their lives!

Problem—Multidrug Cocktails

Multidrug cocktails work well initially because they are attacking the strains of the HIV that are the least resistant to the drugs. But the result of that success is to encourage the rapid spread of HIV strains that are highly resistant to the drugs, which could give rise to a new and even more dangerous AIDS epidemic among people most at risk for the disease.

Several separate research investigations, using two new types of sensitive diagnostic tests, found evidence suggesting that about 30% of individuals newly infected with the HIV are carrying forms of the virus that are already resistant to one of the 17 drugs, and 14% are resistant to two of the drugs used in American combination therapy. Mutations that confer resistance to nucleoside analog reverse transcriptase inhibitors, non-nucleoside reverse transcriptase inhibitors, and protease inhibitors have all been identified in HIV-infected persons who have never been treated with antiretroviral drugs. The **first** zidovudine-resistant HIV was reported in 1989. Thus, with the wider use of antiretrovirals, pretreatment HIV resistant strains will occur in the population with increasing frequency.

It is clear that the appearance of drug-resistant HIV is a function of the number of HIV replication cycles that take place during infection, and that combination therapy that suppresses HIV replication to undetectable levels can delay or prevent the emergence of resistant strains (Figure 4-11). Abundant evidence has linked the presence of HIV drug resistance to therapy failure (Moyle, 1995).

During 10 to 20 years of a person's infection, HIV can undergo as **much genetic change (mutations)** as humans might experience in the course of millions of years, which makes it extremely **difficult to develop treatments** that have **long-term effectiveness** (*Scientific American,* August 1995).

In summary, the frequency of genetically variant HIV within an HIV population is influenced by the mutation rate, fitness of the mutant to survive, the size of the available HIV pool for genetic recombination, and the number of HIV replication cycles.

Transmission of Drug-Resistant HIV

A report at the 1998 12th International AIDS Conference stated that for the first time strains of HIV resistant to all protease inhibitors and other widely used anti-HIV drugs were being transmitted from one person to another! Prior to this announcement, scientists did not believe that such highly mutant forms of HIV could be transmitted. The transmission of a multidrug-resistant

FIGURE 4-11 Production of HIV. Each dark hole in the T4 cell membrane represents the emergence of one new HIV that came off the membrane and is loose in the body. Each HIV-infected T4 cell is producing about 3000 to 4000 viruses at any point in time. Each HIV in this photograph is genetically different from any other HIV being released from this T4 cell and most likely genetically different from any other HIV in the body. T4 or CD4+ cells live for about 80 days in a healthy person and about 25 days in an AIDS patient. *(Source: CDC, Atlanta)*

virus is now well documented. For example, a drug-resistant analysis of HIV derived from a group of 141 people from five U.S. cities with primary HIV infection drawn showed that HIV with a given drug resistance, within donors, was found in their sexual partners (Little et al., 1999; Wong et al., 2000). In addition, in February 2000, the **first** documented case of **HIV reinfection** was reported at the 7th Conference on Retroviruses and Opportunistic Infections. An HIV-infected male became reinfected with a **second** strain of HIV, one more aggressive than the HIV he carried. He acquired the second strain from a different sexual partner who harbored the variant HIV. Prior to his **reinfection** he demonstrated good health. His health declined markedly after he acquired the second infection.

Drug-Resistant HIV: A Growing Problem

At the 8th Annual Retrovirus Conference, 2001, Susan Little and colleagues reported on 394 HIV-negative people located in seven major cities. These people were followed from 1995 into midyear 2000. During that time period, those who were infected had their HIV strains checked for drug resistance. Between 1995 and 1998, 3.5% of those newly infected received a drug resistant virus. Between 1999 and mid-2000, 14% received a drug-resistant virus and 6% of these people were infected with HIV that were resistant to two drugs. This means that of the 40,000 to 50,000 new HIV infections in 2001, between 6,000 and

7,000 people received drug-resistant HIV. Little reported that patients who acquired a resistant virus were less likely to fully suppress the virus. These patients more frequently failed the drug regimens. The data also showed a more rapid disease progression for these people.

In December 2001, the RAND Corporation reported on a national survey to determine the number of HIV people on HAART that carried HIV drug-resistant mutants. In the survey of 2000, HIV infected patients revealed: 64% were getting less benefit from their HAART than they were two years ago—based on higher levels of HIV in their blood. Among those who have higher HIV blood levels, 65% have drug-resistant HIV. Even newly infected individuals, who have not taken the treatment cocktails, are showing high levels of drug resistance—one out of five infected people carry resistant viruses, acquired from their sexual or drug-use partners. This means that even by conservative use of the data, half of the people under HAART in the United States right now have drug resistant HIV. A demographic breakdown of the data on drug resistance shows that it is not the poor and IV drug users who have the highest rates of drug resistant HIV because of failure to properly take the drugs. Rather, it is the white, gay, fully insured, highly educated men who carry the most highly drug-resistant viruses. The evolution of drug resistant HIV is very similar to the way antibiotic resistant bacteria evolved after the introduction of penicillin and other antibiotics along the way until now—a time where there are few, if any, effective bacterial antibiotics!

Question: How long will it take for HAART to reach the same scenario as that which exists for the use of antibiotics against bacteria?

Most important is the fact that receiving HIV resistant to one drug limits the use of all drugs in that class of antiretroviral drugs. This resistance limits treatment options.

Drug Failure and Third Line Regimens: Salvage, Mega, or Giga HAART Therapy

Under current definition, a treatment-experienced, or so-called salvage HIV-infected patient, is one who has failed at least two HIV regimens that include at least one drug from each approved drug class. Although the HIV salvage population is on the rise as the life expectancy of patients with HIV increases, they are still underrepresented in new clinical trials because sponsors of new drugs do not expect the drugs to be effective in salvage patients. The reasons that HIV drug regimens lose their effectiveness are as varied as the patients who are undergoing treatment with them. Treatment failures, which can occur in up to 60% of patients, can develop in those with a prolonged history of sequential HIV monotherapy and in those who have built up resistance. They also can occur in patients who fail to comply with their prescribed therapy or who are given a poorly suited regimen at the outset.

Drug-resistant HIV strains are a major cause of **treatment failure** (drugs that fail to suppress HIV replication) in the management of HIV disease. Resistant viral strains can evolve whenever the virus is not fully suppressed by a particular drug treatment regimen or via long-term therapy with suboptimal drug regimens, poor drug absorption, or noncompliance with existing regimens. Drug testing is underway to design third line regimens or **salvage therapies** for patients harboring resistant HIV. Salvage therapy is the use of substitute drugs that will continue to suppress viral replication when standard therapy fails.

The Kitchen Sink— By early 2003 some patients had used all of the 17 FDA-approved, anti-HIV drugs in order to suppress HIV replication! Clearly some of the drugs were being recycled in a variety of new combinations. The try anything approach—the kitchen sink!

The number of HIV-infected persons in America and Europe requiring third line regimens or salvage therapy is increasing rapidly. In America, between 30% and 50% of those in therapy are now in salvage therapy. Because, to date, such therapies are not proving effective, deaths due to AIDS are increasing.

Throughout the developed world, one in 10 AIDS patients now requires third line or salvage therapy because they carry HIV resistant to the drugs. About one in 50 of these patients are resistant to all 17 FDA-approved antiretroviral drugs. (Kenyon 2001). In 2002, French scientists began to use mega HAART or giga HAART therapy for those with limited treatment options. The theory behind using a larger number of drugs is that not all of the virus in a person's body is going to be resistant to all of the drugs. By using many drugs with different mechanisms of blocking HIV from reproducing, it may still be possible to achieve a potent anti-HIV effect. This salvage or rescue regime consists of the following drugs: three to four nucleoside reverse transcription inhibitors (NRTIs), hydroxyurea, one or two non-NRTI, and three to four protease inhibitors! Continued studies will determine safety and effectiveness of mega/giga HAART therapies. In May 2002, the CDC published its most recent "Guidelines for Using Antiretroviral Agents Among HIV-Infected Adults and Adolescents" (MMWR 51:1–57).

Genotypic and Phenotypic Drug Resistant/Susceptibility Profiles

Assays or tests analyze the virus circulating in the patient's body the day the blood sample was drawn. Genotypic assays are faster than phenotypic assays, but the interpretation of the genotype results is not always easy.

Determining the specific drug resistant and drug susceptibility profiles for a patient strain of HIV can be very useful in order to establish when a change in therapy will best suit the patient and, if necessary, to begin a plausible salvage therapy.

Establishing a list of genetic mutations related to drug resistance is called **genotypic analysis** and indicates a given HIV isolates genetic resistance to a given drug. Note that when HIV becomes resistant to one drug, it can at the same time become resistant to others that function in the same manner (cross-resistance). The suspected degree of drug resistance, as suggested from genotypic analysis, can

Table 4-2 Understanding HIV Drug Resistance: Defining the Terms

Term	Meaning
Resistance (Drug)	A change in HIV that improves its ability to replicate in the **presence** of the drug.
Genotype	The arrangement of four nucleotides in making up HIV-DNA (RNA). A change in genotype means a nucleotide has been gained, lost or switched. For example, HIV mutant M184V is a change in genotype at codon 184 of reverse transcriptase from ATG to GTG. This alters the amino acid from methionine to valine abbreviated (M184V), resulting in resistance to lamivudine.
Phenotype	The trait or behavior that results from changes in genotype, for example, the ability of the virus to replicate in presence of drug compared with drug-sensitive control virus or wild-type-nonmutant HIV.
Cross-resistance	This occurs when **one** mutation occurs that affects HIV's susceptibility to other drugs (generally the drugs are structurally related).

be measured directly by adding the drug in question to an HIV-cell culture and determining the HIV's ability to reproduce. A virus-culture-drug assay is called **phenotypic analysis.** (Table 4-2) A check is made to see if HIV's resistance to a given drug correlates to a given genetic mutation and if other mutations offer a cross-resistance to that drug. In this way, drugs that work against the different HIV mutants can be used in **salvage therapy.**

Thus, phenotypic assays are more straightforward to interpret than genotyping results because they do not require the expert interpretation of complex mutation patterns. The drug susceptibility data provides information for the clinician to select a treatment regimen effective against the predominant viral population circulating in the patient's blood. The main use of phenotypic assays at present is to identify those antiretroviral drugs that still retain activity against the patient's virus. Phenotypic assays are useful to provide guidance after treatment failure and to select a proper combination of drugs prior to initiation of therapy. They are also useful to detect transmission of drug resistant virus and to monitor HIV patients during early viral rebound. In essence, phenotypic testing provides information to target antiretroviral therapy against the predominant HIV variant in the patient for a prolonged suppression of viral replication, decreased mortality, and lower health-care costs.

However, phenotype testing is very expensive at $800 to $1,000 per test. Because of the time element (about two to five weeks) and cost, such testing is not readily available to the patient. Thus, patients rely on the cheaper (about $400 to $500) and faster (one week) genotypic testing. Most third-party payers do not cover these tests. Geno-

type analysis is now available through five commercial laboratories and phenotype testing in two.

In general, resistance tests can't predict which drugs will work—only the ones that don't—which is why they're mostly recommended to help people whose regimens are failing. As with viral load tests, it's critical to be consistent about which tests you use. For now, experts say, the decision to change the regimens should be based primarily on increases in viral load.

UPDATE 2002 September 2001, The FDA approved Visible Genetics, Inc.'s TRUGENE HIV-1 Genotyping Kit and OpenGene DNA Sequencing System. The use of this system is intended for use in detecting HIV gene mutations in the protease and part of the reverse transcriptase regions of HIV, the region that confers resistance to specific types of antiretroviral drugs. It is intended for use as an aid to qualified clinicians in the therapeutic management of HIV-infected patients in conjunction with all relevant clinical and laboratory findings. TRUGENE offers physicians the opportunity to prescribe drugs which will enable them to reestablish control of their patients' HIV, thereby improving their quality of life.

In June of 2002, ViroLogic, Inc. announced the launch of the first-ever commercial laboratory test to evaluate the **replication capacity or viral fitness** of HIV. ViroLogic's new Replication Capacity (RC) assay measures the ability of a patient's virus to make copies of itself and is designed to provide useful additional information to physicians to select optimal antiretroviral therapy cocktails for their patients. Research studies suggest that replication capacity data, in combination with drug resistance information, viral load and CD4+ count, may allow for a more informed prediction of HIV disease progression. For example, using an RC assay, physicians can identify situations in which the replication capacity of a patient's virus is impaired, which often occurs when the virus has extensively mutated to become resistant to an antiretroviral drug regimen. In these cases, even though the antiretroviral drugs are no longer fully controlling replication of the virus, a physician may choose to maintain the regimen in order to keep the mutated, less fit strain of HIV in the patient's body, especially if the patient has few or no other treatment options.

HIV THERAPY CUT-OFF POINTS

In November 2000, the first ever "clinically relevant cut-off points" for different antiretroviral drugs were announced. A clinical cut-off point defines the highest level of a drug that can be given whereby the patient can still be helped by that drug. At resistance levels above the cutoff, patients are unlikely to respond to treatment. These cut-offs, developed by ViroLogic, were determined by using clinical trial data to evaluate the impact of changes in drug susceptibility on treatment outcomes. The new cut-off data should improve a physician's ability to guide patient drug therapy.

VIRAL LOAD: ITS RELATIONSHIP TO HIV DISEASE AND AIDS

Viral load refers to the number of HIV RNA strands in the plasma or serum of HIV-infected persons (a discussion of HIV RNA production is provided in Chapter 3; also see referenced material, Jurriaans et al., 1994; Henrard et al., 1995; Goldschmidt et al., 1998). In general, two to six weeks after HIV exposure, infected individuals develop a high level of blood plasma HIV RNA. Methods now exist to quantitate the amount of HIV RNA in the blood plasma or serum of HIV-infected people. (**Plasma** is a transparent yellow fluid that makes up about 55% of blood volume. **Removing** fibrinogen and blood clotting factors from plasma results in **serum**.)

The Purpose of HIV Viral Load Testing

People with high viral loads are much more likely to get sick or die of AIDS than people with low viral loads.

Physicians recommend viral load testing for the following reasons:

♦ to help you make decisions about starting or changing drug treatment for HIV;
♦ to find out your risk for disease progression;
♦ to show how well your drug regimen is working;
♦ to help determine your HIV disease stage.

Laboratories report HIV viral load test results as the number of copies of HIV per milliliter of blood plasma (copies/ml). Until recently, HIV viral load tests could only accurately measure HIV levels down to 400 copies. The new AMPLICOR HIV-1 MONITOR UltraSensitive viral load test can measure HIV levels down to 50 copies. **CAUTION: An "undetectable" viral load, however, is not enough. The goal is for people with HIV to live out their normal life span, free of opportunistic infections and with the fewest possible drug-related side effects.**

Pitfalls of Viral Load (HIV-RNA) Testing

Despite the potential advantage of HIV-RNA testing over that of conventional HIV-antibody testing—particularly in a high-risk population with symptoms of acute HIV—**the specificity of all commercially available HIV-RNA technologies is less than 100% and, as a result, likely to yield a significant number of false positives.** According to Chiron Diagnostics, the manufacturer of one such assay, the specificity of Qantiplex-branched DNA technology versions 2.0 and 3.0 is approximately 95% to 97% at a copy number of <3000 and <150 copies/ml, respectively. More conservative published data suggest that the specificity of the three commercially available viral load assays (**bDNA, PCR, and NASBA**) may be similar, with a false-positive rate of approximately 5% to 10%. The emotional impact of a **false-positive** screening HIV-RNA test in recently exposed persons can be extraordinarily damaging.

When Is Viral RNA Found in the Plasma?

HIV RNA strands are present during **all stages** of the disease, and the viral load increases with more advanced disease (Piatak et al., 1993; Saksela et al., 1994). Following infection with HIV, there is usually a rapid, transient increase of HIV proteins and RNA followed by a lengthy period of viral RNA replication at lower but measurable amounts (Figure 4-12). In well-characterized groups with known dates of HIV seroconversion, a high viral load immediately after seroconversion (Mellors et al., 1995) and at three years after seroconversion (Jurriaans et al., 1994) appear to be strong predictors of HIV disease progression. However, for most patients with asymptomatic HIV infection, the time of the primary infection is unknown. The levels of viral load prior to the diagnosis are also unknown. In order to determine the predictive value of an isolated viral load measurement under these circumstances, John and colleagues (1996) developed a mathematical model to predict the time to symptomatic disease based on viral load measurements in **untreated patients** with asymptomatic HIV infection and T4 cell counts greater than 500/μL of blood.

Their analysis, based on their mathematical model, shows that in the absence of antiretroviral treatment, persons with a viral load of 10^5 (100,000) copies/mL serum may begin **progression to AIDS** (PTA) in less than three years and people with a viral load half a log higher (at 500,000) may begin PTA in less than one year. [A **log** just means a 10-fold difference. For example, an increase in viral load, say from 1,000 to 10,000 (1×10^3 to 1×10^4), is one log. A decrease from 100,000 to 1,000 is a **two-log reduction.** Thus, a **one-log** increase or reduction in viral load means that the viral load has increased or decreased by 90%; a **two-log** increase or reduction is a 99% change; a **three-log** increase or reduction is a 99.9% increase or reduction, and so on. See

FIGURE 4-12   Clinical Course of HIV Disease as Related to T4 Cell Count and Level (number) of HIV RNA Copies (viral load) in Plasma. During primary infection (the time period between infection and development of HIV antibody), HIV RNA levels spike *(triangles)* and HIV disseminates *(spreads)* throughout the body. This is followed by an abrupt drop in measurable HIV RNA in the blood (probably due to the production of HIV antibody), followed by a steady rise in HIV RNA until death. Over these same time periods, there is a continuous loss of T4 cells *(squares)*. Note that the asymptomatic stage can be quite long—on average about 10 to 12 years, at which time T4 cell counts drop and HIV RNA copies increase to levels where there is high risk of opportunistic infections.

Table 4-3.] **In contrast,** people with a viral load of $10^{4.5}$ (31,600) have about two years and may have up to eight years before beginning PTA. People with a viral load of 10^4 (10,000) RNA copies/mL have about 3 years and may have up to 19 years before beginning PTA. The rate of change of the viral load was also an important predictor of HIV disease progression.

MEDICAL COMPLICATIONS ASSOCIATED WITH ANTI-HIV DRUG THERAPIES

The term medical complications is used herein to describe clinical problems in the management of HIV infection. Most doctors now agree that not everyone infected with HIV needs to take antiretroviral drugs. But everyone with HIV does need medical monitoring and care, and access to treatment when and if appropriate. Because those taking antiretroviral treatment had a fraction of the

Table 4-3   Decimal, Exponent, and Logarithms

Decimal Number	Exponential Form	Log$_{10}$ Value
100,000,000	10^8	8
10,000,000	10^7	7
1,000,000	10^6	6
100,000	10^5	5
10,000	10^4	4
1,000	10^3	3
100	10^2	2

Each number is a 10-fold change from the previous one.

death rate of those without treatment does not necessarily mean that one's chance of survival will be correspondingly increased by antiretrovirals. The reduced death rates reflect the benefit of treatment for those who needed it most, would show a positive response, and had access to the medication (Bozette et al., 2001; Freedberg et al., 2001).

For those who think AIDS is over—it is **NOT**.

For those who think the drugs are working well—they're **NOT.**

Drugs Extend Lives, But at a Cost

Over the past several years, those who take or have taken antiretroviral drugs know it is a hard life—for many there is no alternative! But the longer one uses these drugs, the greater the chance of suffering from the toxic side effects of the drugs. It has been reported that some people are taking eight or more of the antiretroviral drugs in their cocktail. They are running out of options. One **CANNOT** say how long an HIV-infected person on antiretroviral drugs can expect to live—or how well. Because each person's lifestyle, healthcare, ability not to become depressed, and genetic immune response varies, there is no way to predict how well or long one can expect to stay alive with current anti-HIV treatments. The 5- or 10-year death sentence has been reprieved for many on treatment. But how long before their drug toxicities kill, or force them off treatments? When People With AIDS (PWAs) started experimenting with going off drugs in order to avoid toxic buildup, healthcare experts coined the phrase **"drug holidays"** to describe such behavior. Pressure to remain compliant was so severe that when patients stopped taking the drugs (because they were often being hurt by them), doctors became angry and patients were accused of laziness or lack of fortitude. Only later did activists and doctors coin a new phrase **"strategic drug interruption,"** stopping HIV drugs in order to function or survive. It is now common practice. However, one cannot stay off the drugs too long because HIV will ravage their immune system. **AIDS really is not yet manageable if it is not survivable!** Rounding out what has been learned about anti-HIV drug toxicity is that HIV drugs are implicated in lipodystrophy, heart problems, bone loss (hip replacement), intercellular malfunctions called mitochondriosis, lactic acidosis, and liver and kidney dysfunction and failure. (Mitochondriosis is mitochondrial dysfunction—some side effects include fat redistribution syndrome, commonly referred to as lipodystrophy. Lipodystrophy includes increased fat in the neck or stomach; loss of subcutaneous fat from the face, arms, or legs; or enlarged breasts. Additional side effects associated with mitochondrial toxicity that interrupts cellular energy production that leads to fatigue, shortness of breath, weight loss, and rapid heart beat are hair loss; numbness and pain in the hands, arms, feet, and legs; muscle disease; heart disease; inflammation of the pancreas; increased blood acidity; and kidney irregularities.) Add in the various opportunistic infections and the drug toxicities required to treat them, and one finds many surviving AIDS patients have become antiviral and antibiotic multidrug resistant. These AIDS patients require stronger and more toxic remedies month after month and year after year. Ultimately one eventually dies, either from infection or from complications from treatments.

Management of HIV/AIDS: Treat Early, Treat Late?

Building the Ship as It Sails

There are at least three major decisions that have to be made early on in the management of HIV/AIDS patients. The **first** is when to begin antiretroviral therapy, the **second** is which drugs to use to initiate treatment, and the **third** is how long to administer the therapy.

Clinicians face a dilemma of choice when advising asymptomatic patients with established HIV infection on when to begin highly active antiretroviral therapy (HAART) and what drugs to use. **Begin early,** some researchers advise, because later there will be a higher virologic hurdle to overcome. **Begin later,** others recommend, and save potent drugs until the patient's immune system begins to fail. If therapy is started too early, cumulative side effects of the drugs used and the development of multi-drug resistance may outweigh the net benefits of the lengthening of life. If therapy is started too late, increases in disease progression and mortality outweigh the risk of adverse events.

In order to access the very best time to initiate antiretroviral therapy one needs to know the goal of antiviral therapy! Most HIV/AIDS physicians would agree that the goal is multidimensional: to prolong life while improving the quality of life; to suppress HIV replication to the limits of detection for as long as possible; to select the best possible therapy for the individual; and to minimize costs and all side effects to drug therapy. With these goals in mind, and the drugs available to suppress HIV replication and extend life with quality, the question becomes **"When should one begin antiretroviral therapy?"**

DETERMINATION OF VIRAL LOAD AND QUESTIONS PEOPLE ASK

Viral load blood tests have been developed to show how much HIV is in the blood. Through 2001 only two have been licensed by the FDA. Not all doctors order viral load tests because not all insurance companies pay for them. However, as viral load tests become more widely available, insurance coverage will be there.

The amount of HIV in a patient's blood is important, especially since only about 2% of HIV is in circulating blood. The other 98% is in the lymph system and other body tissue. A low level indicates the disease is stable and a high level may mean treatment should begin or be changed.

AVAILABLE VIRAL LOAD TESTS

Three types have been developed: through 2001 only two have received FDA approval, Amplicors Q-PCR (quantitative polymerase chain reaction, Figure 12-5) and Amplicor's HIV Monitor Ultra Sensitive test that measures viral load down to 50 copies. The other two tests are the bDNA (branch-chain DNA, Figure 12-7) and NASBA (nucleic acid sequence-based amplification). All three measure the amount of HIV RNA present in the blood of HIV-infected patients. Test results are usually given per milliliter (mL) of blood. Because each HIV carries two copies of RNA, if there are 100,000 copies of HIV RNA it means there are 50,000 copies of the virus present.

RESULTS OF VIRAL LOAD TESTS

Results of viral load tests can range from almost zero to over a million; low numbers mean fewer viruses in the blood and less active disease; high numbers mean more active disease.

The three tests usually give similar results. However, if the patient's viral load is very low, the bDNA may not detect the HIV RNA. Newer versions of all tests may be more accurate and more sensitive. In general, it is best to stay with one type of test for consistency.

RELEVANCE OF VIRAL LOAD TESTING

The test is new and researchers are still trying to decide on the important values for viral load. In general, though, results can be interpreted as follows:

HIV Viral Load Result	Interpretation
	Death within 6 years
5000 or fewer	6%
10,000 or fewer	18%
10,000 to 30,000	35%
Over 30,000 copies	70%

Viral load numbers will depend on the viral load test used. For example, a 25,000 RNA strand number determined using a branched DNA (bDNA) test might be read as 50,000 RNA strands using Amplicors' FDA-approved PCR-RT (polymerase chain reaction-reverse transcriptase) test and higher or lower numbers using other HIV RNA testing procedures. Overall however, the lower the viral load, the better. But no single test of any type gives a complete picture of health. Trends over time are important, as are nutrition, physical condition, psychological outlook, and other factors. Current viral load tests can now detect as few as 5 to 20 RNA strands/mm^3.

DETECTABLE VS. UNDETECTABLE LEVELS OF HIV RNA

What does an **undetectable** level of HIV RNA mean? Many individuals now have an undetectable level of HIV-RNA in their blood after taking combination therapy. But undetectable RNA levels do not mean that the person is cured or no longer infectious. **An undetectable RNA level means that too few RNA strands are present to measure. The number of RNA strands is below the level of tests of sensitivity.** Currently, tests measure between 50 and 400 copies/ml. There are experimental assays used in research that are more sensitive and can detect levels of RNA as low as five copies/ml.

Achieving **undetectable** viral loads is now the **gold standard** for successful HIV treatment. The more rapidly one's viral load becomes **undetectable** and the longer it remains suppressed, the better the drug and chance for long-term survival. A measurable viral load after it was once undetectable is regarded as a sign of drug failure. Never reaching undetectability is also considered a drug failure for that person.

TYPICAL QUESTIONS ABOUT VIRAL LOAD

1. What is the viral **set point?** The viral set point represents an equilibrium between the virus, which wants to replicate, and the host, which tries to control or contain the replication (viral reproduction is about equal to viral clearance). It appears that each patient establishes his or her own set point within two to six months after initial infection with HIV. HIV drugs appear to alter the set point for HIV by reducing its ability to replicate. This helps lower the body viral load and gives the body a chance to restore some of the lost immune function.

2. **What is the cost of a viral load test? Does insurance pay for it?** Beginning 2003, a viral load test cost between $100 and $200. Some insurance policies pay for the test.

3. **If a viral load test result was 12,000 and six months later it is 18,000, is the change im-** portant? Viral load may rise and fall without any change in health. The rule of thumb is that viral load change is not significant unless it more than doubles.

4. **How often should viral load be measured?** Measuring viral load every four months, at the same time T4 cells are measured, has been suggested.

5. **Can viral load be associated with determining anti-HIV therapy?** Measuring viral load about four weeks after changing antiretroviral medications can be useful for finding out whether the new treatment is working.

6. **A person's T4 cells had been between 400 and 600 for several years, and suddenly his viral load rose to 50,000 and his physician recommended drug therapy. Why?** Research suggests that people with viral loads over 10,000 are at higher risk for the progression of HIV disease, regardless of T4 cell counts.

2001 U.S. Department of Health and Human Services Guidelines for the Use of Antiretroviral Therapy

In general, the U.S. Department of Health and Human Services guidelines are the most aggressive on when to start therapy, followed by French guidelines. The Brazilians are the least aggressive, recommending dual nucleoside therapy for those with earlier disease and lower viral loads. Overall, the various guidelines involve expensive strategies that can only be used in more developed countries, or in the wealthier sectors of less developed countries.

The 2001 Guidelines for people with **symptomatic** disease or T4 (CD4+) cell counts of less than 200/µL are the same as in the year 2000 Guidelines. However, there are two major changes for treatment of the **asymptomatic.** Year 2000 guidelines suggested drug therapy be implemented either when the T4 or CD4+ cell count dropped below 500/µL or a viral load of 10,000/ml. The new guidelines delay therapy until values of T4 cells drop to less than 350/µL and viral load is greater than 30,000/ml by bDNA assay or 55,000/ml by RT-PCR assay. These changes were made in order to delay side effects and drug resistance associated with antiretroviral therapy. These changes suggest that the virus should be **Hit Later-Hit Carefully** rather than **Hit Early-Hit Hard.** These changes suggest that relatively healthy, HIV-infected people should not receive early HAART therapy. The new British guidelines delay the start of therapy even longer. They recommend therapy when the T4 or CD4+ cell count drops below 200, regardless of viral load.

Early Treat, Early Stop: Timing Is Everything

In early 2002, the implementation of Early Treat-Early Stop (ET-ES) began on a limited basis. The ET-ES or pulse regimen is to provide the drugs as early as possible after infection and then as soon as the patient experiences a reduction in viral load to about 50 copies of HIV/milliliter of blood—stop treatment. The idea is that immediate drug treatment protects the capabilities of their immune system, leaving them basically intact. At the same time, their short, pre-therapy exposure to HIV is analogous to a vaccine. The immune defenses of early-treated patients are a step ahead of the virus, and these people may, over time, be able to stop therapy completely at some point. Problems with this concept is the same as for the other regimens of Hit Early-Hit Hard or Hit Later-Hit Carefully—how is a population of the early-infected identified and after placed on therapy, how to individually monitor them over prolonged time periods, how to eliminate the toxic side effects of the drugs, how to stop viral resurgence, and how to control the mutant virus that are in the rebound viral population. And, of course, there is the question of how late is too late to obtain the expected impact of HAART that occurs with early treatment?

The Future For HAART=SMART?

The National Institute of Allergies and Infectious Disease (NIAID) is funding a study to resolve which is the better HAART strategy—Hit Early-Hit Hard or Hit Later-Hit Carefully or Hit and Run, that is, Interrupted Therapy. The major reasons for the study are the growing concerns about the drugs' toxic side effects and the increase in resistance to them. This critical long-term study to determine which of the common HIV treatment strategies ultimately is better began in January 2002, at 21 national locations in 14 states and the District of Columbia, and several sites in Australia. The study called SMART, or Strategies for Management of Anti-Retroviral Therapies, will eventually enroll 6000 people who will be monitored for up to nine years. The study is being conducted by the Community Programs for Clinical Research on AIDS (CPCRA), a network of community-based researchers.

SMART differs from previous AIDS treatment clinical trials in several ways. For example, although the effectiveness and toxicity of various anti-HIV therapies have been studied, this is the first study to do so over a prolonged period. SMART will compare two distinct treatment approaches and will follow enrollees for an average of seven years. In addition, while most AIDS treatment trials measure indirect indicators of AIDS development, such as the amount of virus or number of CD4+ T cells in the blood, SMART will measure clinical events such as progression to AIDS or to death, which take longer to occur. The study's length is a major reason for great emphasis on patient and physician education both prior to enrollment and the study. SMART's enrollment criteria are broad—teenagers as well as adults are eligible—so the findings will be applicable to as many people as possible.

During the first year, 2002, study investigators enrolled 1000 HIV-infected people and randomly assigned them to either a "go-slow" or a "hit-hard-early" treatment strategy. The hit-hard-early strategy (in which drugs are used to suppress HIV levels to low or undetectable levels) is recommended in guidelines employed by many physicians in the United States. Study participants in the go-slow arm of the study will agree not to take antiviral drugs unless their T4 or CD4+ T cell count crops below 250 per cubic milliliter (mm^3) of blood, and then they will take the drugs only until their CD4+ T cell counts rebound above 350. The long-term feasibility of the study will be evaluated after the first year. Based on a favorable outcome, an additional 5000 people will be enrolled over the next three years. To take advantage of the wealth of information predicted to come from such a large and lengthy trial, the SMART study will incorporate several substudies. One, which examines treatment effects on the heart, is the first of its kind. Another will examine whether and how treatment changes body fat distribution and bone density—significant side effects of HAART. The successful completion of this study should provide groundbreaking information on how to approach treatment of HIV disease.

Reality of the 2001 Guideline Suggestions

First, it must be recognized that HIV can persist without ever replicating. So, if it does not copy itself, current antiretroviral drugs will not work! No amount of current HIV drug therapy will ever eliminate this reservoir—this disease is virtually incurable using current antiretroviral drug therapy.

The combination of the release of many anti-HIV medications and a lack of long-term research on their effects has resulted in confusion concerning the best course of treatment using the drugs. Some physicians and researchers subscribe to an aggressive regimen, while others adhere to a reactive regimen that initiates medication in response to condition. There is still debate over which strategy provides the best chances for survival.

Concerns are greatest about the toxicity of the regimens and adherence problems. Some studies have shown that HIV quickly eliminates the T4

RATION OF HIV/AIDS PHYSICIANS TO THE POPULATION AND THE HIV-INFECTED

In America there are an estimated **5,000** HIV/AIDS-**experienced** physicians. This represents one physician per 57,000 people. **Given that an estimated 900,000 HIV-infected need the care of these physicians, the ratio drops to one experienced physician for every 180 HIV-infected people!** (Data from the CDC.) In contrast, in Northern India within a land mass of the size and population of the United States, there are an estimated **seven** experienced HIV/AIDS physicians, or one physician per 40 million people (Katz, 2000). **Given that an estimated 2 million HIV-infected need the care of these seven physicians, the ration drops to one experienced HIV physician for every 286,000 HIV infected people!**

In South Africa with 42 million people there are an estimated **25** HIV/AIDS-experienced physicians or 1/1.7 million people. Given that an estimated 4 million HIV-infected need the care of these 25 physicians, the ratio drops to one experienced HIV physician for every 160,000 HIV-infected people! (Data from the World Health Organization.) These data indicate that even if the **antiretroviral drugs** were available and affordable, in countries with poor medical and distribution infrastructure, the presence of these drugs may not in itself be of great significance.

Class Discussion: Offer pro/con information of significance that would alter or eliminate the infrastructure problems in getting the antiretroviral drugs to those who need them. How best can we produce HIV-experienced physicians rapidly?

cells that coordinate the immune attack against the virus and that these cells do not appear to regrow, even after the reduction of viral load through treatment. This evidence indicates that it may be best to try to reduce viral levels as soon as possible to save these cells so the body can mount an effective attack against the virus. In short, there are about as many physicians for early therapy as physicians and their reasons for the use of therapy later in the disease.

The information coming out of the February 2000 and 2001 Retrovirus and Opportunistic Infection meetings indicates that HIV enters inactivated T4 cells **within three days** after infection and that HAART therapy does not affect such cells. That is, the viruses aren't really gone, they've simply been sequestered in cells and tissues that HAART cannot reach (for example, HIV in macrophages and dendritic cells). In most patients who have spent months or years on HAART, either the virus levels rise again or the drug toxicities become intolerable. HAART, in and of itself, is neither a cure nor a safe enough medication to realistically be taken for a decade or more. Many patients are now approaching their seventh year on HAART and strange ailments are turning up, including diabetes, bone loss, cholesterol-associated heart and liver diseases, body fat distribution, and a host of cancers. All this adds to already existing confusion on when to start therapy. Keep in mind that **without antiretroviral drugs,** an HIV-infected person on average will live 10 or 11 years without serious discomfort—they are for the most part asymptomatic. The drugs are **toxic.** They have seriously damaged people who were put on the drugs after receiving falsely positive tests. Taken off the drugs because of their severe illness from the drugs, they recovered, but not completely.

CLASS QUESTION: TREAT EARLY-TREAT LATE, YOUR DECISION IS?

TWO MOST SOBERING REPORTS ON AIDS-RELATED DEATHS

James Witek and colleagues reported that "among an urban population representative of today's pandemic, mortality continues to be significant even with early access to HIV care and HAART," and that "patients who died in 1999 had lower viral loads on presentation to care, longer time in care, and higher final T4 counts. Those who died in 1999 had taken more antiretroviral regimens (3 vs 2), had better adherence and appeared more likely to have had a virologic response to HAART (59% vs 16%). Eleven out of

MONETARY REASONS FOR PRODUCING ANTIRETROVIRAL DRUGS

From a drug developer's standpoint, AIDS must be the most attractive disease on Earth. There are four obvious reasons: **(1)** the drugs are very expensive, **(2)** many patients are privately insured because they are healthy and working, **(3)** thanks to advocacy groups the government pays for drugs for many people who can't afford them, and **(4)** the drugs don't cure anybody—they appear to be necessary for a lifetime! Where else in American medicine is there a population of **uninsured** patients of whom 79% have access to HIV/AIDS antiretroviral drug therapy that costs between $12,000 and $20,000 a year? Is there anywhere else in American medicine where such expensive health care has been made available to the poor and disenfranchised populations? According to the U.S. **De**partment of **H**ealth and **H**uman **S**ervices, 60% of those needing HAART therapy receive it.

Economics of Producing Antiretroviral Drugs

In 1998, the markets for HIV/AIDS therapeutics totaled more than $2 billion in U.S. revenues and according to Frost & Sullivan (http://www.frost.com), these markets are projected to reach nearly $13 billion by 2005. These figures represent revenues derived from the following HIV drug product classes: protease inhibitors (PIs), nucleoside reverse transcriptase inhibitors (NRTIs), and non-nucleoside reverse transcriptase inhibitors (NNRTIs). Frost & Sullivan is an international marketing, consulting, and training company that monitors the health care industry for market trends, market measurements, and strategies.

Death Prevention Profits

In 1995 there were 51,000 AIDS-related deaths. Using the new antiretroviral drugs, in 1996 the number of deaths fell to 38,000. By 1998 deaths dropped to 18,000, and by 2002 to 14,000. Using year 1995 as a baseline for number of deaths, each year thereafter the fewer that died, the greater the number that must continue to take the drugs for the rest of their lives. Until there are preventative and therapeutic vaccines, or some form of cure available, the number of drug consumers continues to grow. Just in the United States there were an estimated 50,000 new HIV infections in 2001 and in 2002. Why wouldn't a company commit itself to producing HIV/AIDS drugs? Toby Casper (2000), reported that the profits on antiretroviral drugs is enormous. He gave the following examples: In 1999, Glaxo Wellcome made $589 million on $4.1 billion of Combivir (AZT + 3TC) sales. Profits between 1997 through 2001 for AZT, about $800 million; for 3TC about $1.6 billion; for ddI about $400 million and for d4T $1.4 billion. Cost to develop each new drug from idea to the drug store is between $250 million and $400 million.

---

40 patients died with viral loads less than 5,000 copies, seven of whom had viral loads less than 400 copies." Tanvir Chowdhry and colleagues reported that "though mortality has fallen progressively from 1995 to 1998, there is a recent trend to an increase in death rates in our large HIV clinic," and "deaths are occurring in persons with greater levels of immune capacity as reflected in T4 cell counts and also in persons under good virologic control. These observations underscore the need both to monitor the etiologies of HIV-associated mortality and to better understand the relationship between immune defenses, treatment related toxicities and end organ failure in HIV disease." Such data along with other information presented in this chapter do not bode well for the clinical course of this disease in the year 2003 and beyond.

Readers may further wish to confuse themselves by reading the **Pro and Con** on this issue as presented by Bruce Walker and colleagues **"Treat HIV Infection Like Other Infections—Treat It"** (1998—Pro) and William Burman and colleagues, **"The Case For Conservative Management of Early HIV Disease"** (1998—Con).

Structured Therapy Interruptions (STI): HIT and RUN

There are two main justifications for STI. The **first** is simply to provide patients with a break from the rigors of HAART. While a rebound in plasma HIV is almost always observed, the STI does allow patients a break from the demands and toxicities of HAART regimens. The **second** justification is that rebound HIV that occurs during an

CURRENT PROBLEMS USING COMBINATION THERAPY

First, DURATION: Many patients ask how long they will have to continue combination therapy. But why would they ask this—it's keeping them alive. The combinations often involve taking 20 to 70 or more antiretroviral and opportunistic disease pills a day that must be swallowed according to a rigid schedule that would tax even the most compulsive individual. The timing centers around an empty stomach, and the drugs often cause severe stomach irritation. In one case, a patient had to discontinue therapy after 26 weeks because of gastrointestinal intolerance. The viral load went from **undetectable to 98,600 copies/mL** and the T4 cell count fell from 307 to 227/mm^3 within two weeks! **Pills rule life!** (See Figure 4-13.)

Second, ADHERENCE or COMPLIANCE: Health care providers have been dealing with the issue of client **adherence** or **compliance** for centuries. The medical literature shows that it is difficult for patients to adhere to even the simplest treatment regimens. In the hypertension literature, one-third of patients take medications as directed, one-third take little or no medication, and one-third are intermittently adherent. Age, race, sex, educational level, socioeconomic status, and a past history of alcoholism or drug use are not reliable predictors of poor adherence. Regimen simplicity, however, does affect adherence. For example, in hypertension; once-daily therapy is associated with rates of 90% adherence, twice-daily with 80%, and three or more times daily with 65%. Other factors shown to be associated with better adherence to medications include a severe illness and belief in the efficacy of treatment. Factors associated with poor adherence include unstable housing, mental illness, and major life crises. **Adherence** to a drug regimen means taking all the prescribed anti-HIV drugs at the scheduled times and not missing any doses. Anytime people are asked to change and/or maintain new behaviors to treat an existing condition or to prevent a threatened one, there is a good chance that they will not comply, consistently and correctly, to the prescribed activities. Combination drug therapy for HIV infection does not cause new compliance issues; it just highlights the known difficulties of an existing problem. **The Achilles Heel of Anti-HIV Therapy:** Skipping only a few pills can trigger the emergence of drug-resistant

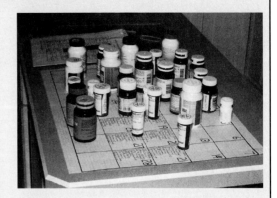

FIGURE 4-13 Patient Compliance. People with HIV disease and AIDS take many different drugs daily, depending on their prescribed medications for the various opportunistic infections and combinations of drugs necessary for anti-HIV therapy. The patient's drug intake, when this photograph was taken, numbered 28 different pills daily. If this patient took 27 pills each day for 10 years, this person would ingest **98,550 pills. Is it any wonder that people fail to take all of their medications?** *(Photograph courtesy of the author)*

strains of HIV. Such a development could create a worse problem than the initial infection because the resistant virus could overwhelm the individual taking the drugs and anyone else to whom the individual transmitted the virus.

There is a present danger that the behavior of underdosing (not taking enough) or partial compliance (taking the protease inhibitor when they feel like it) or patients who modify their dosage regimens—**to extend their prescription**—may create HIV strains resistant to all currently available drugs. This would lead to an even more devastating AIDS pandemic! The major reason given by 202 HIV-positive people on combination anti-HIV therapy was, **I FORGOT!** (33%). Clearly, the degree of compliance to therapy affects treatment outcome. Andrea Barthwell (1997) reported that from 12 years of research, the clearest finding is that nonadherence is the norm in medical care.

Stephen Becker and colleagues (2002) report a mean overall adherence rate of only 53% among a population of over 3700 Medicaid receipients. Barely one quarter of subjects achieved an adherence rate of 80% or higher, and adherence was worst among those aged 18–24 years. Clearly much more needs to be done to improve these rates of adherence, or many patients will be embarking on a rapid route to resistance and treatment failure.

Third, COSTS: AIDS is a disease of poverty. The majority of HIV-infected in the United States and worldwide will **never** get a first dose of a protease inhibitor or an AIDS cocktail. The cost of **just** protease inhibitors is between $12,000 and $20,000 per year! The cost to treat the 475,000 Americans, beginning year 2003, who are receiving HIV treatment (about 80% receive the three-drug cocktail) is about $7.6 billion a year. To treat the estimated 900,000 HIV-infected at the same rate would cost about $18 billion per year. Over **half the costs** are for antiretroviral medication—the pills can cost between $5 and $16 each. At 10 to 30 pills a day the cost per person can run up to about $500 a day or over $180,000 a year. Worldwide, **if** people received equal treatment, the bill for all people living with HIV/AIDS outside the United States beginning year 2003 would be about $21 billion per day ($500/day×41 million infected people).

Currently (2003) less than 3% of the 40 million people in developing nations who need HAART are receiving the drugs. According to Peter Piot, Executive Director of UNAIDS, in Africa about 30,000 HIV-infected people are receiving HAART and 2.2 million died of AIDS in 2002. In North America, over 500,000 are on HAART with 25,000 deaths. Under new pricing arrangements, HAART drugs can be purchased in Africa for as little as 67 cents a day. But for most, this sum can be too costly. In Uganda, for example, gross national income per capita is about $300 a year, or 83 cents a day.

Antiretroviral Drugs as a Viable Option in Africa

In addition to the cost of drugs, other major obstacles that have to be considered are food or the lack of it. Hundreds of thousands get to eat, at most, every other day! Many of the drugs have to be taken with food and clean water, another problem. But what if suddenly the drugs were available to all. Who will monitor those on drugs as to their timely adherence? Most do not own a watch. Who will diagnose the disease and prescribe the drugs? As found in developed nations, drug regimes are based on the individuals'

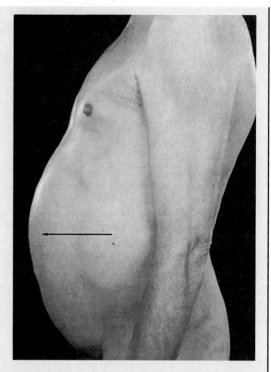

FIGURE 4-14 Protease Paunch—Also Referred to as Crix Belly. This lipid disorder (lipodystrophy) occurs in many patients using protease inhibitors for anti-HIV therapy. In addition to the visual effects of antiretroviral therapy, there are a number of dangerous side effects—see text for details. *(Photograph courtesy of Dr. David Cooper)*

needs. Yet, as seen in Point of Information 4.1, HIV/AIDS physicians are in extremely short supply in Africa. Who will monitor the change in drug regimens as drug resistance emerges? Medical problems in addition to AIDS abound in Africa, tuberculosis, malaria, measles, and a large list of other adult and childhood diseases that currently kill millions each year. The problem of health and heath care in Africa has been out of control for centuries. HIV/AIDS appears to have awakened the continent but Western style medicine and care is a long way off.

Larry Kramer, a cofounder of Gay Men's Health Crises, states that the cost of his drugs to combat AIDS, **which do not include a protease,** amounts to about $19,000 a year; this does not include visits to his doctor or the batteries of blood tests that he routinely requires. And he is asympto-

FIGURE 4-15 Buffalo Hump. The enlargement of a cervicodorsal fat pad. Buffalo hump develops after use of protease inhibitors for anti-HIV therapy. In addition to the visual effects of antiretroviral therapy, there are a number of other dangerous side effects—see text for details. *(Photograph courtesy of Dr. David Cooper)*

matic. *A New York Times* article in 1997 estimated that drugs for someone with symptomatic AIDS cost about $70,000 a year; in response, a New York University adjunct law professor and gay-rights advocate wrote a letter to the editor saying that his drugs cost $84,000 a year using protease inhibitors; the annual drug cost can exceed $150,000. At these prices, how many of the nation's 900,000 HIV-infected will be able to afford proper HIV therapy? **AT THESE PRICES PEOPLE HAVE TO CHOOSE WHETHER TO PAY RENT, BUY FOOD, OR PAY FOR THEIR MEDICINE— SOME CHOICE!**

Fourth, SIDE EFFECTS: The paradox of HIV treatment is that sometimes the cure feels worse than the disease, especially when treatment begins before symptoms arise. Sometimes the cure also looks worse than the disease. For example, fat redistribution, a side effect of antiviral treatment, can appear at a time when a person's HIV disease might otherwise be invisible—both to others and to him or herself. To date, all FDA-approved protease inhibitors (PIs) have important side effects in a large number of PI users (25% to 65% in different surveys). To name a few, PIs have been associated with: dry skin, cracked lips, loss of body hair, sexual dysfunction in men, oral warts, loss of bone mineral density, gastrointestinal problems (diarrhea etc.), high triglycerides and cholesterol levels associated with coronary artery disease, increased blood sugar levels and diabetes, and abnormal body fat metabolism and distribution or **lipodystrophy.** This occurs particular on the abdomen, central obesity, referred to as the **protease paunch** (Figure 4-14), and on the back between the shoulder blades, called **"buffalo hump"** (Figure 4-15) and may include a loss of fatty tissue in the arms, legs, and face. Women may experience narrowing of the hips and breast enlargement (Lo et al., 1998; Miller et al., 1998; Lipsky, 1998; Carr et al., 1998; A-E and Gervasoni, et al., 1999). Although abnormal fat distribution may not be considered serious in life and death situations, it probably does matter to the asymptomatic person who cares about body image and who cares about cardiovascular problems in the future.

Some of the newer, not yet FDA-approved PIs may cause kidney failure and liver problems. PIs also appear to increase blood levels of **VIAGRA,** the new male impotence drug by inhibiting liver enzymes that would normally eliminate Viagra.

Fifth, WEIGHING THE UNKNOWN: Without taking any drugs, about 50% of the HIV-infected will be well some 10 years after they have become infected!

Help: for those experiencing drug side effects or who want to know more about the drugs call:

AIDS Treatment News: 800-341-2437

Project Inform: 800-822-7422

Women Alive: 800-554-4876

World: 510-658-6930

TESTIMONY ON SIDE EFFECTS: ONE WOMAN'S EXPERIENCE

(This anecdotal account was sent to the author from Ms. Colleen Perez and is used with her permission and the author's appreciation.)

I am a single parent with three children—they are the medicine that lights my heart afire and keeps me going! The side effects I lived with from taking Saquinavir/Fortovase (not simultaneously), 3TC, and AZT were a nightmare. Firstly, I suffered from a severe peripheral neuropathy in my arms. I'd awaken drenched with sweat, unable to feel my arms, that is until the shooting pains hit! Then came severe edema, I went from 145 lbs. to 180 and still climbing in less than one year. I looked full term 9 months pregnant. In fact, not a day went by that someone didn't ask me when the baby was due? You may initially think me vain, but let me tell you that I labored to breathe, and had great difficulty making the smallest movement. I also suffered from acid reflux disease that was so bad I was nauseous, burping, and farting uncontrollably, and constantly! Having always been fairly fit and athletic in the past, those drugs made my life little more than a living hell. The cost of the drugs is around $1,200 a month. The tab is picked up by our local MIP (Medically indigenous person) and somewhat federally funded health insurance plan. The pharmacist here in Guam tells me health care is going to collapse.

It was at the 12th World AIDS Conference in Geneva that I became incensed over the unfairness of North/South, bridging the gap! The gap is just getting wider. Thanks to the giant pharmaceutical companies and their medical marketers. I had never seen such bullshit, it made me ashamed to be human. The drug companies all had their stuff strutting displays, talking to me because I'm kind of white, and ignoring my Asian companions. It made me sick and I flushed all my Fortovase down a Swiss toilet. Why the organizers chose to hold a global conference in one of the world's most expensive cities is beyond me. By the way, I had a breakdown there, right at the Geneva airport, I read my ticket wrong and missed my flight by 12 hours. I spent the night in a Swiss hospital, well at least that was free! I have stopped taking the drugs and started vitamins and mineral supplements, lost the "baby" (fat belly induced from the drugs) and at last I feel OK. My viral load is high at 532,000, my T cells low at 193, my doctor is a bitch and our ONLY HIV/AIDS specialist here. But the worst thing that has happened to me is a whopping coat of white esophagal thrush! I would like to try something that will bring my viral load down. I really don't want to take protease again. Please don't ask me to consult my doctor because she told me to find my own treatment. I'm tough and ornery and you'll continue to come across me and my philosophies like, "no pain, no pain!", far into the next millennium.

STI may actually boost the immune response to HIV in the same way that a booster immunization would. This enhancement in HIV-specific immunity might allow better control of viral replication in the future. This sounds good in theory, but in reality it does not appear to work for the majority of patients placed on STI. After reviewing many controlled studies on STI the conclusion is that there are **NO** significant lasting beneficial changes in T4 or CD4+ cell counts in patients placed on STI. And there are no consistent data to suggest that STI will lead to durable control of viremia when HAART is discontinued (Blankson et al., 2001)! In HIV infection, a dynamic equilibrium exists between viral replication and the HIV-specific immune response. In the vast majority of cases, the immune system is eventually overwhelmed by the extraordinary rates of viral replication. While HAART dramatically inhibits HIV

replication, it also dulls or deadens the HIV-specific immune response. So, when HAART is discontinued, HIV replication occurs in the presence of diminished immunity, which may explain the tendency of viral loads to exceed retreatment levels during STIs. The overall dynamics of STI is not understood. Clearly some patients are helped but it appears, at the moment, most are not. The theoretical advantages of enhancing HIV-specific immunity must therefore be weighed against the real risk of losing T4 cells and the potential risk of drug resistance.

UPDATE 2002: 9TH RETROVIRUS CONFERENCE, SEATTLE, WA, FEBRUARY 24–28 Three thousand six hundred specialists from 59 countries met at the 9th Conference on Retrovirus and Opportunistic Infections. The mantra to date has been if there are drugs that work, use them and refine them while searching for newer and better

COMMENTS FROM AN ASYMPTOMATIC HIV-INFECTED MALE

He asks about the image the drug companies producing the anti-HIV drugs are presenting to help those who are infected. And he quickly answers his own question: "Open any gay magazine and see the major drug company ads depicting sexy people living, thriving, partying, and having sex with AIDS. They climb mountains (without nearby toilets) and sail across oceans while popping handfuls of happy AIDS pills. Surely AIDS is no longer a bad disease. And check out those young handsome 'come love me' AIDS drug models. If I take the drugs will I have sex, too? Of course you will, unless you become disfigured by lipodystrophy or find yourself on dialysis. You can always date in between IV therapy and emergency room visits. Pardon the sarcasm but the point is this: The image presented in the media depicting AIDS patients is a lie invented to sell AIDS drugs. Living with HIV sucks. It starts out sort of OK but it goes downhill much too quickly."

CONCLUSION

For many thousands of people living in America with HIV, successful treatment has raised the bar of expectations, and this can be unsettling for clinicians. Over the past six years (1996–2002), people with HIV were relieved not to be dying or hospitalized; medication side effects were a welcome exchange for longer lives. Now, as their lives have been extended over the long term, side effects have become less tolerable. Many people with HIV have unexpectedly sensed the possibility of normal lives and are reacting to the limitations of a progressively distorted figure, diarrhea, peripheral neuropathy, and constant fatigue. Some clinicians have responded to this with impatience, and some disdain; their belief is that the side effects are a small price to pay for being alive. In some cases, this response stems from clinicians' feelings of not being able to be of more help, in others, from a fear that altering a successful regimen might compromise an individual's HIV status and cause their progression toward AIDS.

BOX 4.2

CAN COMBINATION THERAPY USING NUCLEOSIDE ANALOGS WITH PROTEASE INHIBITORS CURE HIV DISEASE? AN ALTERNATIVE—REMISSION?

MISSION IMPOSSIBLE

Beginning 2002, studies showed the HIV-infected people have **compartments or sanctuaries** of replication-competent HIV residing in resting (nondividing) T4 and T4 memory cells, macrophage, and other cell types and tissues (for example, brain, nervous system, kidney, and testes). HIV recovered from the pool of cells/tissues, although they did not show resistance to anti-HIV drugs, were still present. That is, after three years on combination drug therapy, HIV were still present in persons that had **no** measurable HIV RNA in their blood. Such data clearly indicates that the body's reservoir of HIV has a very slow rate of cleansing itself of HIV. The worst case scenario: it may take between 5 and 20 years of uninterrupted aggressive anti-HIV therapy before the pool of latent HIV is cleared from the body. (AIDS Clinical Care 1998; Schrager et al., 1998; Balter, 1997; Wong et al., 1997 Chun et al., 2000) Anthony Fauci (Figure 5-10) and other HIV/AIDS scientists told those at the 12th International AIDS Conference (June–July 1998) that every patient, even those in successful therapy for three or more years, have latent HIV pool that is formed early in infection and remains despite the most effective treatment.

People attending the conference were also told that

♦ HIV/AIDS vaccines are at least 10 years away,

♦ drug resistance and often unbearable side effects from the most powerful of the new drugs are causing many patients to discard them,

♦ although prevention campaigns are succeeding in a few countries, those successes are spotty even in the developed nations, and

♦ cases of HIV resistant to all **protease inhibitors** and **reverse transcriptase inhibitors** are being transmitted from one person to another.

BOX 4.2 *(continued)*

In mid-1999, Diana Finzi and colleagues reported that HIV can remain dormant in resting T4 cells. They described the decay rate of the inactive reservoir of HIV in 34 adults who are taking combination therapy and whose plasma levels had fallen to below-detectable level. On average, the half-life of the latent HIV was 43.9 months, which could mean **eradication could take as long as 60 years, a lifetime if the source of the latent virus holds only 1×10^5 or 100,000 cells.** As a result, the researchers say, latent infection of dormant T4 cells provides an opportunity for HIV to remain in all patients, including those who consistently take antiretroviral therapy. This work implies that most HIV-infected people will not be able to stop their anti-HIV medications. Yet, **current drug therapy** most likely **cannot** be tolerated for a lifetime. To date, most people taking anti-HIV drugs have been on them for two to four years. The longest experience, for relatively few who participated in the early clinical trials for testing of drug cocktails has been about six years.

AN ALTERNATIVE—REMISSION

HIV/AIDS investigators remain reluctant to use the word "cure," but they are beginning, in increasing numbers, to believe in **long-term remission** for most HIV-infected people. Cecil Fox, one of the first HIV/AIDS investigators to search for HIV in human lymphoid tissue, believes that the HIV/AIDS scientific community should be relating the treatment and results of treating HIV/AIDS patients much the same as people undergoing cancer therapy with the goal of getting the patient into remission.

To this point HIV/AIDS therapists have been treating HIV/AIDS patients for an **infectious disease.** They are looking for a cure: Get rid of every last microbe—in this case HIV. But remission, keeping HIV under control is much more reasonable. Make HIV/AIDS into a long-term, manageable disease with medications that are tolerable—fewer side effects. The model for this alternative outlook on anti-HIV therapy can be seen in long term, nonprogressors. These people make up a small percent of the HIV/AIDS population, **but they are infected and remain healthy.**

THE HAART OF THE MATTER

Robert Siliciano of John Hopkins Medical Institute calculated that it would take up to 12 years to eradicate from the body those latent HIV-infected cells that are somehow protected from the drugs. Other scientists estimate that it would take 60 years on Highly Active Antiretroviral Therapy (HAART) for the last of the HIV-infected cells to die off! How does one adhere to the demanding drug regimens for all that time? And adherence is a must because any failure could be enough to restock the body with newly protected HIV infected cells and then the whole drug treatment process would have to begin again!

The AIDS cocktail may not provide the light at the end of the tunnel, but for now, at least, it has lengthened the tunnel for those with AIDS. **THE AIDS COCKTAIL IS NOT A CURE AND THERE IS NO EFFECTIVE MORNING-AFTER-A-CARELESS-NIGHT PILL. THERE IS NO REASON TO ABANDON SAFER SEX PRACTICES!**

therapies. But, by what was presented at the 9th Retrovirus Conference (9th RC), no new drugs are ready for use and many HIV/AIDS patients are running out of time. They are on last-hope, salvage therapies that don't work because of viral drug resistance. A Tibotec-Virco study has shown that one in four of the 12,000 U.S. patients it surveyed were resistant to all three classes of drugs: nucleoside/non-nucleoside, and protease inhibitors. All of these drugs, now on the market, block one of the two enzymes the virus uses to incorporate its genes into T4 or CD4+ cells and uses them to reproduce itself. These HIV enzymes are called reverse transcriptase and protease. Currently,

researchers know of at least 250 different mutations in the HIV genetic code that can make it drug-resistant.

The most pressing needs for those in HIV/AIDS treatment are new therapies for the thousands of patients having to go on salvage therapy. The now-overturned "hit early, hit hard" guidelines, which some say precipitated the influx of drug-resistant strains, have made researchers and HIV/AIDS patients more attuned to what is coming down the drug pipeline. The problem is, however, what is in the drug pipeline, based on the reports at the 9th RC, is more of the same. There have been no major breakthroughs in HIV/AIDS drug

BOX 4.3

TESTING OF ANTI-HIV DRUGS FOR POST-EXPOSURE PREVENTION (PEP)

The Forum— A woman has sex with her HIV-positive husband and the condom breaks. A woman is raped by a man who is HIV-positive. A child is sodomized by an HIV-positive male. A prison guard is bitten by an HIV-positive inmate. A couple has unprotected sex—a one-night stand. These were some of the cases brought up by experts as they debated whether doctors should be prescribing AIDS drugs as a **morning-after or post exposure prophylaxis or prevention (PEP) treatment for those exposed to HIV.**

In mid-October 1997, San Francisco became the first city in the United States to offer new PEP drugs to individuals trying to prevent HIV infection.

72-Hour Window— The **standard of practice** for about three years at most medical centers is to offer antiviral drugs promptly when health care workers of AIDS patients are stuck with needles or come into contact with body fluids from infected patients. Many researchers believe the drugs must be given within 72 hours of exposure—the time it takes for HIV to integrate into human cells' DNA after infection. The treatments are given for four weeks.

Beginning year 2003 over 1000 American health-care workers have received PEP care—nine have become HIV positive, but they admitted to continuing to practice high-risk behavior. Regardless, over the past 10 years, PEP has become the standard of care for occupational exposure to HIV. Over this time period, much has been learned about the safety and efficacy of the drugs used and optimal patient management (Henderson et al., 2001).

Of interest is the fact that—like sexual behavior and injection drug use—not all potential exposures are equal. When thinking about sex and drug exposures, every sexual exposure is not associated with the same risk of becoming infected; neither is every type of injection drug use exposure.

Risk of Infection by Route of Exposure

Sexual Activity— HIV exposure takes many forms and needs to be assessed to determine risk. Exposure to body fluids through kissing and through oral sex poses a risk that is considered to be very small. Oral sex is not, however, risk-free. Efforts to quantify the risk-per-episode of various sexual activities have yielded results that are misleadingly low. For example, receptive anal intercourse has the highest risk, 0.8% to 3.2%. This risk appears low; a gambler might feel very safe with such odds. But—as too many HIV-positive individuals can attest—all it takes is once. Receptive vaginal intercourse (female risk) carries a per-episode risk estimated at 0.05% to 0.15%. Insertive vaginal sex (male risk) is estimated to cause HIV infection 0.03% to 0.09% of the time. With these numbers in mind, when one considers PEP following sexual exposure, it becomes obvious that efforts to provide prophylaxis after every sexual exposure would be neither feasible nor sensible. Other factors need to be addressed.

Needle Stick Injury— The average risk of infection after any exposure through any needle stick is 0.3%.

Treatment Guidelines— There are guidelines published by the CDC for prophylaxis following needle stick or occupational exposures to HIV in the health-care setting. Currently, there are no published guidelines for the initiation of PEP after sexual exposure to HIV. This does not mean that PEP does not exist in these cases. But to date, recommendations come through inference, judgment, and thoughtful intention. There is a wide spectrum of situations to consider, but there are no absolutes when it comes to the right choices regarding PEP. PEP after sexual exposure is recommended because of the knowledge that in some cases it works. The guidelines established by the CDC came about after studying the effectiveness of PEP following exposure to HIV through needle sticks or splashes of infectious material in the health-care setting. The use of zidovudine (ZDV) for PEP reduced the transmission of HIV by 79%. Similarly, it is well recognized that the use of ZDV in pregnant women dramatically reduced vertical transmission of HIV to newborns. It is therefore conceivable that the use of antiretroviral medication following sexual exposure to HIV will also be effective. However, to date, there are no studies supporting this.

For those who think PEP is or will be a magic bullet like some of our antibiotics were—**no way**—better to focus on practicing medical procedures correctly or being safe the night before.

UPDATE 2002— The findings of a two-year study conducted at the Sunninghill Clinic in Sandton, Johannesburg, South Africa on the use

BOX 4.3 *(continued)*

of drugs to prevent HIV infection in raped women provide hard evidence that they work. Adrienne Wulfsohn, who conducted the study, said that she monitored over 1000 raped women who were put on anti-HIV drugs within 72 hours of exposure and none became HIV infected! Her findings will form a part of the world's first guidelines for PEP after sexual assault to be issued by the CDC sometime in 2002. In South Africa, the risk of HIV infection after rape is 40%. The South African Law Commission Report of 1999 says that South Africa has about 1.6 million rape attacks a year! PEP is now being offered to raped women in 20 European countries, Botswana, Thailand, and in several American states and in Canada.

Conclusion— At this point in our knowledge and understanding of HIV, there are no absolutes or final answers. This problem is not one that will go away. Indeed, with 30% of gay black men in their 20s in America now estimated to be HIV infected, the demand for PEP after sexual

exposure will increase. It cannot be overstated, however, that the key to reducing sexual transmission of HIV is not PEP, but safer sex practices. Public health officials, physicians, and patients must continue working toward reducing the need for PEP by advocating and encouraging safer sex practices for everyone.

More information on PEP research is available by calling (800) 367-2437 [(800)-FOR-AIDS]. Information is also available on the **internet** at hivinsite.ucsf.edu by clicking on "Key Topics." As yet, there is no national list of PEP programs. Your local AIDS service organization may be able to help. The CDC published the "**Updated U.S. Public Health Service Guidelines for the Management of Occupational Exposures to HBV, HCV and HIV and Recommendations for Post Exposure Prophylaxis**" in June 2001, a must-read for those with questions on PEP.

Class Discussion: With your current knowledge about HIV/AIDS, if you knew that you had just been exposed to HIV would you ask for immediate therapy? Why?

---

development since the introduction of protease inhibitors in 1996. Lee Klosinski, director of programs for AIDS Project Los Angeles, said that progress in the field of AIDS research has been absolutely glacial for the past three years. Ideas on some novel drug therapies discussed at the 9th RC are years away from the marketplace. With AIDS drug research in a slump and the rate of HIV infection increasing, better control of the AIDS epidemic is going to take a lot longer than scientists had expected or predicted even a few years ago. The number of new HIV infections in the United States has increased from approximately 40,000 infections per year since 1988 to 50,000 infections in years 2000 through 2002. Although antiretroviral treatment has dropped the annual number of AIDS-related deaths from 40,000 to about 15,000, many people have stopped therapy because of the side effects of the drugs or because they are experiencing resistance to treatment.

Novel Drugs in the Pipeline but Years Away From Clinical Prescription

Entry Inhibitors (See Figure 5-5)— HIV enters cells in a complex, three-part series. HIV first anchors itself to a receptor on T4 lymphocytes, called CD4, then to a co-receptor, CCR5. Once

hooked, it fuses its membrane to a cell membrane, easing itself inside. Several different compounds under investigation are able to make it more difficult for the virus to enter the cell. One such drug that attempts to block this first step is Bristol-Myers Squibb's experimental medicine, code named BMS805. The drug works by blocking gp120 on the surface of HIV that attaches to the CD4 receptor of the cell. In the test tube, it appears to work against strains of HIV that can resist all the other anti-HIV drugs. However, it has not yet been tried on people. It is an orally ingested drug.

Another drug, SCH-C, developed by Schering Plough, an orally ingested drug, blocks the next step in viral entry, the attachment of HIV to CCR5. In a pilot study of 12 people, the drug used alone for one week dropped viral levels dramatically. Furthest along in testing is Roche's and Trimeris' T20 or Pentafuside (enfuvirtide or fuzeon), which blocks the third step of viral entry. T20 binds to the gp41 protein on the surface of HIV, stopping HIV from binding to the CD4 receptor on the cell membrane. Large-scale studies are underway, and the company is seeking Food and Drug Administration approval. T20 must be kept refrigerated and injected twice daily, and will cost up to $16,000 a year. Initially, T20 will be used as a third line or salvage therapy. To date, fuzeon is in short supply. Roche pharmaceuticals say there is only enough of the drug to treat 25,000 people through year 2003.

UPDATE 2002   In June 2002, Xiping Wei and colleagues (2002) reported that T20 HIV-resistant mutants rapidly emerged during the first 10 days of a clinical trial in which 16 HIV-infected people took part. Other studies are in progress.

Robert Gallo, Director of the Institute of Human Virology said at the 2002 14th International AIDS Conference that "in two or three years, the protease inhibitors will go away, replaced by viral entry inhibitors and more intelligent use of reverse transcriptase inhibitors. The entry inhibitors that are being tried now—five, six, seven of them—will cause the next wave of excitement by the next conference in Bangkok, Thailand in 2004."

Laurie Garrett, writing in *Esquire* in March 1999, "The Virus at the End of the World," quotes Spencer Cox, New York AIDS activist involved in Treatment Action Group (TAG), who said our worst case scenario now is that it's 1987 all over again for an ever-increasing number of HIV-infected people—for them there are no effective treatments! Clinical studies now suggest that 60% of patients experience

---

SIDEBAR 4.3

CURRENT STATE OF HIV DRUG THERAPY

The Present— Nothing better describes the current state of this epidemic and the treatment of it than to say a job half done. While so much has been accomplished, still there is the lack of ability to truly save lives. At best, today's treatment and care programs offer a respite in the fight against AIDS—a time in which the virus is not gone but at least subdued into temporary submission. But the price for this, in both dollars and quality of life, is much too high. It is still too early to know how long people will be able to live with the current drugs. For some, it is but a matter of a few years before drug side effects and viral resistance begin to outweigh the benefits. For others it has been nearly seven years since potent triple-drug therapy became available (1996) and shifted the balance in the battle between virus and the immune system. Some are still doing well on drug therapy and experiencing only minor side effects, others are dying. With time it has become very clear that most people will not be able to stay on treatment for the rest of their lives. Between cumulative drug resistance, long-term side effects and simple weariness with the demands of the various regimens, it is almost naïve to expect people to be able to succeed for periods of 20 to 50 years or more. But that's what it will take to allow people to live a normal life span despite HIV.

The Future— In theory, better drugs are coming, but their reality seldom meets expectations. Even more worrisome is that a variety of economic and social factors are rapidly making HIV/AIDS a less than attractive target for the

pharmaceutical industry. AIDS activists may debate the extent of this problem, or its possible causes, but not its reality. Two companies, Pharmacia & Upjohn and Dupont Pharmaceuticals, have already sold off their HIV product lines. Several others quietly ended their HIV research projects after protease inhibitors were first approved. Another major firm has narrowed its HIV research program and will only continue with one or two drug candidates already in development, forgoing any investment in new approaches or viral targets. Still others have shifted their interest to vaccine work. More worrisome, from the companies' point of view, is that few of the recently approved drugs have been successful in the market place. Some argue that, despite their improvements over current therapy, new drugs will have a rough time facing off against the 17 better-known drugs already available unless they offer clear-cut advantages. It is more advantageous at the moment to reformulate currently FDA approved drugs into combination pills lowering the number that have to be taken daily.

NEW DRUGS

The pipeline of new drugs beyond the next few years does not look promising. The economic trend is for more of the available drugs to become concentrated within fewer companies. This places the power over production and pricing in the hands of the remaining companies and greater dependence upon them for future drug development.

HIV suppression **failure** during first line antiviral drug treatment. About 70% to 80% experience salvage or second line drug treatment failure.

PEDIATRIC ANTI-HIV THERAPY

Most of the questions in the 1998 AIDS Update concerning **when** and **what** should be used in treating pediatric patients have been somewhat resolved in that the CDC issued new pediatric guidelines that advise aggressive antiretroviral therapy for all HIV-infected children younger than 12 months of age "regardless of clinical, immunologic, or virologic status" (Guidelines, Pediatric, 2000; also see Chapter 11). In 1999, Sylvia Lee-Huang and colleagues of New York University, Harvard Medical School, and the National Institutes of Health reported on the discovery of three enzymes in urine of pregnant women with anti-HIV activity. The enzymes are **lysozyme** and two separate **ribonucleases.** Lysome is believed to break down the outer membrane of HIV while the ribonucleases degrade HIV's genetic material. Because these are proteins already present in the body, their use as antiviral agents should be well tolerated. Investigations continue.

PROTEASE INHIBITORS AND PREGNANCY

The use of zidovudine (ZDV) during pregnancy has cut the transmission rate of HIV into children to 8%. In mid-1997, researchers began putting HIV-infected mothers on combination therapy with protease inhibitors to see if they could cut the rate to lower levels. But protease inhibitors are more powerful and potentially more toxic than zidovudine and no one knows what harm it might do to the developing fetus.

For additional considerations for antiretroviral therapy in the HIV-infected pregnant woman, see "Guidelines for the Use of Antiretroviral Agents in Adults: Updated Recommendations." (2000).

DISCLAIMER

The author does not accept any responsibility for the accuracy of the information or the consequences arising from the application, use, or misuse of any of the information contained herein, including any injury and/or damage to any person or property as a matter of product liability, negligence, or otherwise. No warranty, expressed or implied, is made in regard to the contents of this material. This material is not intended as a guide to self-medication. The reader is advised to discuss the information provided here with a doctor, pharmacist, nurse, or other authorized healthcare practitioner and to check product information (including package inserts) regarding dosage, precautions, warnings, interactions, and contraindications before administering any drug, herb, or supplement discussed herein.

SUMMARY

New results in the field of HIV therapy have given HIV-infected persons new hope in their battle against HIV disease and AIDS. First, combinations of nucleoside analogs were shown to have a clinical benefit (prolonged survival and fewer AIDS-defining events) when given to symptomatic individuals. Next came the demonstration of the extraordinary capability of protease inhibitors. The introduction of the protease inhibitors is the most powerful intervention against HIV to date. Marked reductions in viral load, striking clinical improvement, and reduction in mortality have been observed among patients able to take these medications **properly.** Whether to initiate protease inhibitor therapy in the very early stages of HIV disease is controversial.

Neither protease inhibitors, nucleoside, or non-nucleoside inhibitors work for all HIV-infected persons; the reasons for this lack of efficacy are not completely understood. Long-term adverse effects of protease inhibitors are beginning to show.

Antiviral drugs have certainly shown tremendous success in reversing the trend of HIV infection that leads to disease. But with up to 40% of treated individuals now showing HIV strains that are strongly resistant to anti-HIV drugs, the reality of the dangerous cellular reservoirs of HIV must be better appreciated.

Looking at the problem of resistance, it's now known that unless the virus is virtually eliminated from the blood—again, an unlikely prospect—it's only a matter of time before a viral mutant emerges that is resistant to therapy. Current estimates are that the virus mutates once each time it copies itself—up to 1 billion times a day. It's like going to Las Vegas. HIV just keeps spinning its bases (its genetic building blocks), looking for a jackpot.

Over the past year, progress in HIV has continued to resemble an electrocardiogram. The sharp dips represent difficult roadblocks that have blunted our hopes for a cure. The peaks mark scientific breakthroughs and new approaches used to bring HIV under control. As we closed year 2002 and move within the new millennium, the overall picture remains mixed and varies greatly among individuals battling the virus. But there are many reasons to be optimistic and even excited about the state of research, at least from a scientific point of view, without losing sight of the real battles we face. The brief three-year honeymoon that began with the arrival of protease inhibitors has now experienced significant setbacks. Concerns about serious drug side effects and drug resistance linked to long-term use of HIV combination therapies have replaced optimism, causing

a growing number of people on therapy to reconsider the benefits versus the risk of potent antiviral therapies and to seek alternative approaches. In response, pharmaceutical manufacturers have worked to simplify drug regimens and create more potent, less toxic products. It appears now that HIV/AIDS scientists and clinicians may have been a bit too optimistic about what the drugs could do. Today the treatment community is unanimous about one thing: The next generation of drugs must be more powerful and easier to take. They should also improve the problems associated with the present generation of drugs, such as resistance, dosing, absorption, and bioavailability (the active part of a drug that's available to fight the virus).

At the moment, current treatments are inadequate because they do not lead to a cure; at best, they slow disease progression. They are complicated to administer, require close medical monitoring, and can cause significant side effects. They are also very costly and, as a result, are inaccessible to the majority of people living with HIV/AIDS.

SOME AIDS THERAPY INFORMATION HOTLINES

For HIV/AIDS treatment information, call:
The American Foundation for AIDS Research: 800-39AMFAR (392-6237)

AIDS Treatment Data Network: 212-268-4196

AIDS Treatment News: 800-TREAT 1-2 (873-2812)

For information about AIDS/HIV clinical trials conducted by National Institutes of Health and Food and Drug Administration-approved efficacy trials, call:
AIDS Clinical Trials Information Service (ACTIS): 800-TRIALS-A (874-2572)

For more information about HIV infection, call:
Drug Abuse Hotline: 800-662-HELP (4357)

Pediatric and Pregnancy AIDS Hotline: 212-430-3333

National Hemophilia Foundation: 212-219-8180

Hemophilia and AIDS/HIV Network for Dissemination of Information (HANDI): 800-42-HANDI (424-2634)

National Pediatric HIV Resource Center: 800-362-0071

National Association of People with AIDS: 202-898-0414

Teens Teaching AIDS Prevention Program (TTAPP) National Hotline: 800-234-TEEN (8336)

General information:
English: 800-342-AIDS (2437)

Spanish: 800-344-7432

TDD Service for the Deaf: 800-243-7889

General information for health care providers:
National Clinician's Post Exposure Treatment: 800-448-4911

HIV Telephone Consultation Service: 800-933-3413

OTHER ORGANIZATIONS AND WEBSITES

AIDS Action Council
This organization provides advocacy and information on public policy and access to treatment. 1875 Connecticut Avenue NW, Suite. 700, Washington, DC 20009; 202-986-1300

AIDS Clinical Trials Information Service (ACTIS)
Info in Spanish and English on federal and other clinical drug trials. 800-TRIALS-A; TTY/TDD 800-243-7012; www.actis.org

In February 2000, the National Institutes of Health announced the launch of the first phase of a consumer-friendly database with information on more than 4,000 federal and private medical studies involving patients and others at more than 47,000 locations nationwide. The new database may be reached at http://clinicaltrials.gov/.

AIDS Education Global Information System (AEGIS)
Daily news updates, newsletters, trials, search engines; run by Sister Mary Elizabeth, www.aegis.com.

aidsinfonyc.org
Cooperative site run by ATDN, PWA Health Group, Treatment Action Group (TAG), and other organizations. www.aidsinfonyc.org

AIDS Project Los Angeles (APLA)
1313 North Vine St., L.A., CA 90028; 213-993-1600; 204.179.124.76/apla/; Nutrition and Protease Inhibitors

AIDS Treatment Data Network (ATDN)
Clinical trials listing, many glossaries, ADAP, alternative treatments; also in Spanish. 611 Broadway, Ste. 613, NYC, NY 10012; 800-734-7104; aidsin-fonyc.org/network

Critical Path AIDS Project
Treatment info, clinical trials, newsletter library. www.critpath.org

Gay Men's Health Crisis (GMHC)
Legal issues, prevention, treatment, counseling and support groups. 129 W. 20th St., NYC, NY 10011; 212-367-1000; Hotline 212-807-6655; www.gmhc.org

Gay and Lesbian Medical Association
459 Fulton St., Ste. 107, San Francisco, CA 94102; 415-255-4547

Health Care Communications
A commercial website with updates on conferences and physicians' and activist reports; www.healthcg.com

HIV/AIDS Treatment Information Services (ATIS)
Info in English and Spanish on FDA-approved treatments. www.hivatis.org

HIV Law Project
Legal advocacy; 212-674-7590

HIV Insite
A top-notch website run by UCSF; hivinsite.ucsf.edu

HIVNet-Information Server. www.hivnet.org

HIV/AIDS Treatment Information Service—http://www.hivatis.org

Good source for federally approved treatment guidelines.

Housing Works
Info, advocacy for HIV-positive homeless. 594 Broadway, NYC, NY 10012; 212-966-0466

International Association of Physicians in AIDS—http://www.iapac.org current information on drug therapies and treatment guidelines.

International AIDS Society-USA—http://www. iasusa.org Focus on medical education for physicians to improve treatment.

JAMA HIV/AIDS Information Center—http://www. ama-assn.org
Compilation of drug and treatment updates. "Best of Net" internet links.

John Hopkins AIDS Service—http://www.hopkins-aids.edu
Monthly case rounds—medical management of HIV infection.

Lambda Legal Defense and Education Fund
120 Wall St., 15th Fl., NYC, NY 10005; 212-809-8585

National Association of People with AIDS
Info, advocacy, referrals. 1413 K St. NW, 7th Fl., Washington, DC 20005; 202-898-0414

Project Inform
1965 Market St., Ste. 220, San Francisco, CA 94103; Treatment hot line 800-822-7422; 415-558-8669; www.projinf.org

PWA Health Group
Buyers' club that provides treatment info. 150 W. 26th St., Ste. 201, NYC, NY 10001; 212-255-0520; aidsin-fonyc.org/pwahg

San Francisco AIDS Foundation
HIV info. treatment, newsletter, referrals. P.O. Box 426182, San Francisco, CA 94142; 415-487-3000; www.sfaf.org

Internet Addresses
1998 NIH Guideline—Anti-HIV Therapy for Adults/Adolescents or for Pediatrics: http://www.hivatis.org

To locate a physician, call your local or state Medical Society.

Note: This is not an all-inclusive list. For other sources of information, contact your state HIV hotline. State HIV hotline numbers are located at the end of the "Introduction."

REVIEW QUESTIONS

(Answers to the Review Questions are on page 489.)

1. Can HIV infection be cured?

2. What is a surrogate marker?

3. From _____ of 1987 through _____ of 2002 _____ anti-HIV drugs were FDA approved.

4. How many FDA-approved anti-HIV drugs are nucleoside or nucleotide analogs?

5. What is the proper drug name for the following drug acronyms: ZDV, ddI, ddC, d4T, and 3TC?

6. How do nucleoside analogs inhibit HIV replication?

7. What are the two major problems in the use of nucleoside and non-nucleoside analogs in HIV therapy?

8. What is HIV viral load? What can its quantitative measurement reveal?

9. Name the seven protease inhibitors that have FDA approval for use in the United States.

10. Which of the seven FDA-approved protease inhibitors appears to be the most effective and why?

11. How do non-nucleoside drugs inhibit HIV replication?

12. Briefly describe the focus of HIV combination drug therapy.

13. After starting antiretroviral therapy, what is an acceptable target for viral load that indicates the therapy is effective?

    A. 5,000 copies/mL

    B. 5,000–10,000 copies/mL

    C. 10,000–15,000 copies/mL

    D. No acceptable target level has been set.

14. Which of the following statements is correct regarding HIV pathogenesis?

    A. HIV contains two copies of the viral DNA genome.

    B. Viral polyproteins are cleaved by protease.

    C. The RNA copy is integrated in the host-cell chromosome.

    D. gp120 envelope glycoprotein facilitates entry of HIV core particle into the cell's cytoplasm.

15. Some medical centers are offering drug therapy that may be able to:

    A. Cure AIDS

    B. Help prevent HIV infection shortly after exposure

    C. Effectively treat HIV/AIDS without side effects

    D. Prevent HIV infection

    E. Prevent AIDS

16. Go to the library/internet and write a report on the most recent advance in antiretroviral therapy.

17. Compared with the money the federal government spends on research and treatment to combat other health and medical problems such as heart disease and cancer, **do you think federal spending on AIDS research and treatment is too high, too low, or about right? Support your choice with credible evidence.**

The Immunology of HIV Disease/AIDS

THE IMMUNE SYSTEM

All living organisms are continually exposed to substances that are capable of causing harm. Most organisms protect themselves against such substances in more than one way—with physical barriers, for example, or with chemicals that repel or kill invaders. Animals with backbones, **vertebrates,** have these types of general protective mechanisms, but they also have a more advanced protective system called an **immune system.** The immune system is a complex network of organs containing cells that recognize foreign substances in the body and destroy them. It protects vertebrates against pathogens, or infectious agents, such as viruses, bacteria, fungi, and other parasites.

Although there are many potentially harmful pathogens (agents that cause diseases), no pathogen can invade or attack all organisms because a pathogen's ability to cause harm requires a susceptible victim, and not all organisms are susceptible to the same pathogens. For instance, the virus that causes AIDS is strictly a human pathogen; it does not cause a disease in animals such as dogs, cats, and mice. Similarly, humans are not susceptible to the viruses that cause canine distemper or feline (cat) leukemia.

DEVELOPMENT OF HUMAN IMMUNE SYSTEM CELLS

The immune system begins to develop during the **first month** of fetal development with occurrence of blood stem cells in the yolk sac. By the third month of development, blood cell development occurs predominantly in the liver until the skeletal elements of the fetus are formed. Thereafter, bone marrow is the major site of blood cell formation. Blood stem cells differentiate into granulocytes, monocytes, and lymphocytes, as well as megakaryocytes and erythrocytes. Beginning two months into development, lymphocytes destined to become T cells move from the bone marrow into the developing thymus to complete their maturation. The maturation of B lymphocytes occurs in bone marrow under the influence of the stromal reticular cells. By birth, the immune system has developed into a sophisticated network, connecting central locations of immune cell production with peripheral tissues for immune surveillance. These peripheral components of the immune system include the blood, thymus, lymphatic system, spleen, skin, and mucosa. **Host defense is the culmination of a carefully orchestrated cellular and molecular interaction within the immune system and between the immune system and the rest of the body.**

Function of the Immune System

A man dies because his body rejected a heart transplant; a woman is crippled by rheumatoid arthritis; a child goes into a coma that is brought on by cerebral malaria; another child dies of an infection because of an immunodeficiency; an elderly man has advanced hepatic cirrhosis caused by iron overload. These five clinical situations are as diverse as can be, yet all have one thing in common: **a malfunction of the human immune system!**

The immune system filters out foreign substances, removes damaged and dead cells, and acts as a security system to destroy mutant and cancer cells. It is composed of a number of specialized cells, several organs, and a group of biologically active chemicals. The human immune system is like a jigsaw puzzle—many parts come together to form an overall defense against disease-causing agents. If parts of the immune system are missing or damaged, illness may occur due to an immune deficiency.

Separating Friend from Foe: How the Immune System Decides

Skin prevents disease-causing agents from entering the body. But they can enter through body openings, cuts, or wounds. Whether the invader is a life-threatening bacterium or a relatively harmless cold virus, your immune system must control it. A single infectious microorganism that survives and multiplies causes illness. Some infectious agents resemble the body's own cells. **How do immune cells know which to attack and which to ignore?** The answer is, once an agent enters the body, it triggers an **immune response** if the body does not recognize the substance or agent as a part of itself or **"self."** All body cells have special molecules, called **class I proteins,** on their membranes that are like flags or barcodes with the word **"self"** on them.(Figure 5-1) The cells of the immune system try to destroy anything present in the body that is not carrying the self molecules—anything

that is **"nonself."** Nonself is any substance or object that triggers the creation of antibodies. Such nonself substances are called **antigens.** Antigens may be whole virus or organisms or parts of virus, organisms, or their products.

In general, most cellular organisms that damage cells do so from the outside by producing toxic chemicals or in some way externally interfering with the cell's metabolism. But viruses generally invade or **enter** different cell types, forcing them to produce viral replicas at the expense of the cells' own essential metabolic functions. Gradually, like a machine wearing out, host cells start to malfunction and die. The best thing a

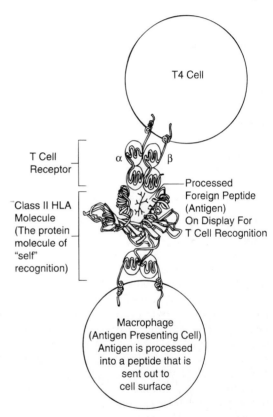

FIGURE 5-1 Interaction Between a Human Leucocyte Antigen **"Self"** Protein (HLA), a Foreign Peptide (Antigen), and a T Cell Receptor. The diagram represents the trimolecular interaction of a processed antigen into a peptide that is being presented on the surface of the antigen-presenting cell to a T4 cell. The presence of the class II HLA self identity marker and the presence of the foreign peptide stimulate the T4 cell into action. *(Adapted from Sinha, 1990)*

CLASS I AND CLASS II PROTEINS

There is a series of genes located on human chromosome 6 that is referred to as the *Human Leucocyte Antigen (HLA)* or as the **major histocompatibility** (tissue type) **complex (MHC).** The genes in this region produce a series of proteins that are **almost** unique to the individual. Because these proteins belong to the individual, they would be recognized as foreign or as an **antigen** when placed in another human, for example, as in a transplanted heart **(transplantation antigens). Almost** all cells in an individual have a sample of their own HLA proteins or transplantation antigens located on the surface of each cell's membrane. Thus, a person's transplantation antigens are recognized as **self-proteins** by their immune system. Such HLA proteins are referred to as **class I** (type 1) tissue compatibility proteins. Every individual has their own set of class I proteins on their cell membranes. It is these proteins that cause **transplant graft rejections.** With minor exceptions, there is not much of your body tissue that would not be rejected if placed in another human body because your class I proteins would be recognized as foreign by the recipient body's immune system. **But how does the recipient's immune system recognize these class I proteins as foreign? ANSWER:** By using a second class of HLA proteins, **class II.** Relatively few human cell types carry this **protein on their cell membranes.** All such cells carrying the class II protein are derived from a monocyte-macrophage cell series, which includes macrophages located in the lung, liver and spleen, dendritic cells of the gut, skin, spleen and lymph nodes, Langerhans' cells of the skin, and microglial cells of the nervous system.

The class II protein, located on the membrane of these cell types, allows these cell types to act as the body's police force. These cells **digest** foreign protein into smaller products. Some of these products, a small series of amino acids or **peptides,** are then escorted to the cell surface alongside a molecule of the class II protein. In this way, the cells carrying a class II protein **serve up** or **present** the foreign substance or antigen alongside or adjacent to the class II protein or "self molecule" so that immune system cells, **notably** the T4 cells and B cells, can sense the presence of the foreign protein and initiate an immune response against it—the activation of a variety of immune system attack cells (cytotoxic T cells, killer T cells) and the production of very specific antibodies.

In medically important viral infections, neutralizing antibodies are generated within 6 to 14 days. In contrast, such protective antibodies generally appear 50 to 150 days after infection with HIV and the hepatitis B virus (HBV) in humans (Pianz et al., 1996).

PROCESSING "FOREIGN" PROTEIN AND LOADING OF THEIR PEPTIDES ONTO CLASS I AND CLASS II MOLECULES

Protein processing and loading of peptides onto class I molecules that are carried out to the cell membrane is taking place all the time in most body cells. There is always plenty of material to feed the processing machinery, because worn-out, damaged, and misfolded internal proteins are continuously being degraded and replaced by new ones.

By contrast, the processing of proteins from outside the cell and the loading of peptides onto class II molecules are normally restricted to B cells, macrophages, and dendritic cells, which are very efficient at taking in material. Although most class I and class II molecules form complexes with peptides derived from proteins inside and outside the cell, this demarcation is by no means absolute.

As a consequence of protein processing, the surfaces of a body cell becomes adorned with peptide-laden HLA molecules, amounting to about 100,000 to 300,000 class I or class II products of each of the HLA genes. Because each HLA molecule has one peptide bound to it, **uninfected** cell displays hundreds of thousands of self peptides on its surface. Some of these peptides are present in the thousands, whereas others are represented by a few copies; most peptide species have 100 or so copies on the surface of each cell. Each cell thus displays a heterogeneous collection of peptides, and the surface of a cell resembles rows of well-stocked stalls at a bazaar, with bargain hunters looking over the stock. But if, in this metaphor, the vendors are the HLA molecules and the peptides the goods, who are the potential buyers? They are a group of lymphocytes reared in the thymus and then turned loose to roam the body—**the T cells** (Klein et al., 2000a; Klein et al., 2000b).

virus can do is find a host cell that does not die and that can produce replicas indefinitely. In a biological time frame, new disease-causing viruses are often very deadly to new hosts. If a new virus strain is too deadly, it kills its host before other hosts are infected, and the ensuing epidemic dies out. For example, the **Ebola virus,** which makes its victims very weak shortly after infection and kills them in 7 to 14 days, has had eight brief outbreaks since its first appearance in 1976, the latest in October 2000. This virus kills quickly and vanishes. Its origin is still unknown. Over biological time, successful viruses and their new hosts learn to accommodate each other. This will most likely

---

BOX 5.1

HOW LARGE IS A TRILLION?

The human body is made up of many trillions of cells. For example, the human immune system contains at least a trillion lymphocytes dedicated to destroying foreign substances that endanger health. But, a trillion of anything is a very large number. Can we **really appreciate just how large a trillion of something is?** Perhaps the following will help.

1. A stack of 1 trillion one-dollar bills would reach a height of 69,000 miles.

2. It would take a person 11.5 days to count to 1 million and 31,688 years to count to 1 trillion—1, 2, 3, 4, 5 . . . !

3. A stack of 1 trillion HIV (Figure 5-2) would be **over** 62 miles high (diameter of HIV=1,000 angstroms: $(1\times10^{12})(1000)$ $(1\times10^{-10})=1\times10^{5}$ meters$=62.15$ miles)

FIGURE 5-2   Dimensions of HIV in Angstroms. HIV has a diameter of 1000 angstroms (Å). It would take 254,000 HIV laid side by side to equal 1 inch in length. *(Illustration courtesy of the author)*

happen with human-HIV associations, but how many people over how many years will have to die before human cells learn to accommodate HIV is unknown. Perhaps it will never happen. Smallpox virus has been infecting humans for thousands of years and has never been accommodated by humans.

HUMAN LYMPHOCYTES: T CELLS AND B CELLS

The hallmark of the human immune system is its ability to mount a highly specific response against virtually any foreign entity, even those never seen before in the course of evolution. It is able to do this because of the number of different kinds of cells called lymphocytes. The human immune system contains about 2 trillion (2×10^{12}) lymphocytes, a relatively small number when compared to the 100 trillion cells in the body (see Box 5.1, Figure 5-2). Most mature lymphocytes recirculate continuously, going from blood to tissue and back to blood again as often as one to two times per day. They travel among most other cells and are present in large numbers in the thymus, bone marrow, lymph nodes, spleen, and appendix (Figure 5-3). By 1968, lymphocytes had

been divided into two classes: **lymphocytes called B cells** that are derived from and mature in bone marrow, and **lymphocytes called T cells** that are derived from bone marrow but travel to and mature in the thymus gland (Figure 5-4). T cells make up 70% to 80% of the lymphocytes **circulating** in the body. Circulating T cells are a heterogeneous group of cells with a wide range of different functions. When a T cell encounters another cell, it uses various probes on its surface—known as receptors and CD4 coreceptors—to examine protein fragments arrayed on the cell's surface. The fragments tell the T cell whether the cell being scanned is normal, and to be left unharmed, or infected, and to be destroyed. The protein fragments are cupped inside tiny holders called class II major histocompatibility complexes (class II MHCs). To be more specific, each individual T cell expresses a receptor (**T cell antigen receptor, TCR**), which recognizes a ligand (a compound that fits a particular receptor) composed of an antigenic peptide, 8–15 amino acids long, bound to a **self-major-histocompatibility-complex (MHC) molecule** (also **referred to as HLA-human leukocyte antigen system**) (see Point of Information 5.1). Thus, a T cell does not directly recognize a soluble antigen, but rather recognizes an antigen displayed on the surface of an **antigen-presenting**

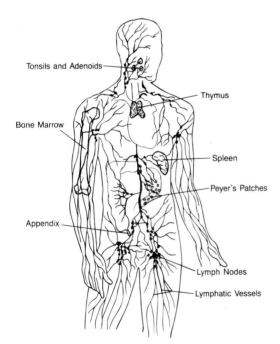

FIGURE 5-3 Organs of the Human Immune System. The organs of the immune system are positioned throughout the body. They are generally referred to as lymphoid organs because they are concerned with the development, growth, and dissemination of lymphocytes, or white cells, that populate the immune system. Lymphoid organs include the bone marrow, thymus, lymph nodes, spleen, tonsils, adenoids, appendix, and the clumps of lymphoid tissue in the small intestine called Peyer's patches. The blood and lymphatic fluids transport lymphocytes to and from all the immune system organs. Gut-associated lymphoid tissue contains 50% to 60% of the body's lymphocytes, and those lymphocytes, according to Peter Anton at UCLA, contain six times more CD4 receptors than do CD4+ or T4 cells circulating in the blood. These data may mean that the gut is the preferred site of HIV replication in untreated patients.

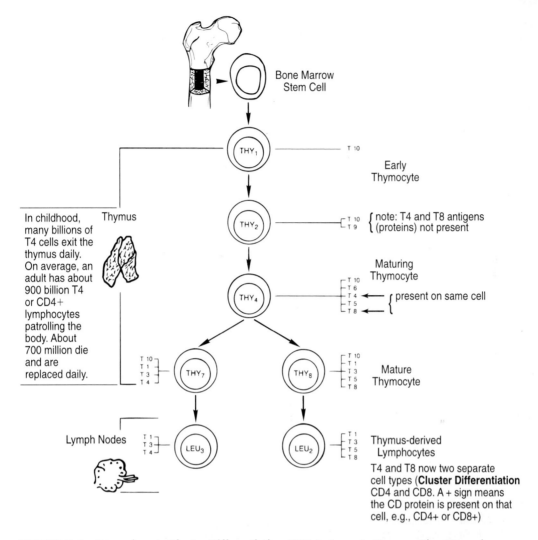

FIGURE 5-4 T Lymphocyte **Cluster Differentiation (CD)** Antigens in Humans. The CD marker or antigen on a T cell tells something about what the cell does. For example the CD4 and CD8 T cells have different Jobs to do. Stages of thymic differentiation (that is, the presence of the different antigens or proteins on their membrane surfaces) are defined on the basis of reactivity to monoclonal antibodies. Schematic pictures of cells represent thymocytes within specific stages of a defined phenotype: T1-T10.

cell (APC) like a B cell or macrophage (Table 5-1). There are about 10 billion APCs located in the lymphoid organs. The receptors of T cells are different from those of B cells because they are "trained" to recognize fragments of antigens that have been combined or complexed with HLA class II molecules. As T cells circulate through the body, they scan the surfaces of body cells for the presence of foreign antigens that have become associated with the HLA molecules. The antigen present on the APC signals the T cell on whether the APC should be left unharmed or that the APC is infected and should be destroyed. This function is sometimes called **immune surveillance.**

Two of the important kinds of T cells are **cytotoxic or killer T** lymphocytes, (CTL) and

Table 5-1   Cells of the Human Immune System

Cell Type	Function
Stem cells	Self-perpetuating cells that give rise to lymphocytes, macrophages, and other hematological cells
T helper cells (T_H), also called T4 or CD4+ cells	Cells that interact with an antigen before the B cell interacts with the antigen
Cytotoxic T cells (Tc)	Recruited by T helper cells to destroy antigens
Suppressor T cells (Ts)	Cells that dampen the activity of T and B cells; they somehow inhibit the immune response
B cells	Bone marrow stem cells that differentiate into plasma cells that secrete antibodies
Plasma cells	Cells devoted to the production of antibody directed against a particular foreign antigen
Monocytes	Precursors of macrophages
Macrophages	Differentiated monocytes that serve as antigen-presenting cells to T cells; they can also engulf a variety of antigens and antibody-covered cells
Killer cells (K)	Lymphocytes that recognize and kill any cell that is coated with antibody
Natural killer cells (NK or null cells)	Lymphocyte cells that detect and kill tumor cells and a broad range of foreign cells

helper T lymphocytes. Killer T cells carry the **CD8 antigen.** Helper T cells carry the **CD4 antigen** and are called **T4 or CD4+ cells** (for an explanation of CD8 and CD4 antigens, see Box 5.2, T lymphocytes). The CD4 and CD8 proteins (antigens) located on their respective T lymphocytes act as a bar code or number on a football jersey; the antigens identify the cell type. Killer or CTL T cells bind to cells carrying a foreign antigen and destroy them. **T4 cells do not kill cells; they interact with B cells and CTL cells and help them respond to foreign antigens.** The T4 cell has the role of a quarterback in football, it calls the plays for the rest of the lymphocyte team.

It is believed that T4 cells recognize only those antigens of viruses, fungi, and other parasites; and trigger only those parts of the immune system necessary to act against these agents. Indeed, it is the viruses, fungi, and other parasites that produce the majority of opportunistic infections when the T4 cells have been depleted by HIV.

It was unknown if B cells begin to malfunction soon after HIV infection. In late 2001, investigators at the National Institute of Allergy and Infection Diseases (NIAID) reported that the presence of HIV in infected patients causes B cells (a) to produce excessive amounts of nonessential antibodies, (b) to fail to respond to physiological signals, and (c) are at risk of becoming cancerous.

Some of these changes can be reversed with the use of antiretroviral drugs (Moir et al., 2001).

In Summary

The two types of **lymphocytes, B cells and T cells,** play different roles in the immune response, though they may act together and influence one another's functions. The part of the immune response that involves B cells is often called **humoral immunity because it takes place in the body fluids.** The part involving T cells is called cellular immunity because it takes place directly between the T cells, other cells, and the antigens. This distinction is misleading, however, because strictly speaking, all adaptive immune responses are cellular—that is, they are all initiated by cells (the lymphocytes) reacting to antigens. **B cells** may initiate an immune response, but the triggering antigens are actually eliminated by soluble products that the B cells release into the blood and other body fluids. **These products are called antibodies and belong to a special group of blood proteins called immunoglobins.** When a B cell is stimulated by an antigen that it encounters in the body fluids, it transforms, with the aid of a type of T cell called a helper T cell, into a larger cell, a blast cell. The blast cell begins to divide rapidly, forming a clone of identical cells. Some of these transform further into plasma cells—in essence,

— BOX 5.2 —

TO UNDERSTAND THE DIFFERENCE BETWEEN HEALTH AND DISEASE, PEOPLE NEED TO UNDERSTAND THE IMMUNE SYSTEM!

BASIC IMMUNE SYSTEM TERMINOLOGY

Of the many mysteries of modern science, the mechanism of **self** versus **nonself recognition** in the immune system must rank near the top. The immune system is designed to recognize foreign invaders. To do so it generates on the order of 10^{12} or 1 trillion different kinds of immunological receptors so that no matter what the shape or form of the foreign invader there will be some complementary receptor to recognize it and effect its elimination. Understanding how the immune system responds to any foreign substance is puzzling enough, but the added mystery is that the immune system can distinguish foreign carbohydrates, nucleic acids, and proteins from those that exist within us, often in shapes barely distinguishable from the invaders. When the immune system is working well it never gets activated by self substances, but unerringly responds to the nonself substances. When the system is not working well this distinction gets blurred and **diseases of autoimmunity occur—our immune cells attack our own tissue!**

To understand the human immune system certain basic terminology is reviewed:

Antibody—an immunoglobulin (a protein) that is produced and secreted by B lymphocytes in response to an antigen. Antibodies are able to bind to and destroy specific antigens. Antibodies contribute to the destruction of antigen by their interaction with other components of the immune system.

Antigen—a substance that is recognized as foreign by the immune system when introduced into the body. An antigen can be a whole microorganism (such as a bacterium or whole virus) or a portion or a product of an organism or virus.

Leukocytes—all white blood cells (WBCs) including neutrophils, lymphocytes, and monocytes (phagocytes).

Lymphocytes—mononuclear WBCs that are critical in immune defense because they provide the specificity and memory needed for immune function and long-term or even life-long immunity. The two major classes of lymphocytes are B cells and T cells; both recognize specific antigens. (For an excellent review of lymphocyte life span and memory, see Sprent et al., 1994.)

Lymphocyte Surface Receptors—Proteins are located on cell surfaces to serve a physiologic function. Some are enzymes, some are transport proteins, and many are **receptors**. All cells use specific receptors to communicate with their environment or with other cells. The receptors found on lymphocytes may be loosely classified according to their function. Thus lymphocytes require receptors that recognize antigen. They need receptors for antigen-presenting cells and receptors for the many factors that regulate lymphocyte responses.

Chemokines—also called cytokines, activate and **DIRECT** the migration of leukocytes. There are 28 known chemokines separated into two subfamilies, those whose protein amino acid structure begins with cytosine–amino acid–cytosine, called the CXC chemokines, and those whose protein amino acid structure begins with cytosine–cytosine, called the CC chemokines.

Cytokines—soluble factors secreted by T cells, B cells, and monocytes that mediate complex immune interactions by acting as messengers. Subcategories of cytokines include: (1) lymphokines (secreted by lymphocytes), and (2) monokines (secreted by monocytes and macrophages). Specific cytokines include interleukin-1 (IL-1), interleukin-2 (IL-2), gamma interferons (γINF), B cell stimulating factor (BCSF), and B cell differentiating factor (BCDF).

Two Branches of the Immune System—The two branches of the human immune system are: Cellular Immunity and Humoral Immunity. Basic terms for each are provided, but as the terms will show, the two branches overlap to provide our immunity. (Adapted from *Mountain-Plains Regional HIV/AIDS Curriculum*, 1992.)

I. *Cellular Immunity*—immune protection resulting from direct action of cells of the immune system. Key cell types offering cellular immunity are:

A. *Phagocytes*

1. Phagocytes are leukocytes that are specialized for ingesting particles and molecules.

2. The most active phagocytic cells are monocytes and macrophages. Monocytes circulate in the blood but eventually

BOX 5.2 *(continued)*

move into body tissues (brain, muscle, etc.) where they mature into macrophages.

3. Phagocytes initiate the cellular immune response. When an invader (a virus or bacteria) enters the body, it will be trapped and digested by a phagocyte. This attack against invaders occurs in various places in the body: the lining of the gut, throat, skin, bloodstream, or in organized lymphoid tissue such as the tonsils, other lymph nodes, or the spleen.

4. The phagocyte ingests the foreign invader and partially digests it. Pieces of the invader (antigens) can then be displayed on the phagocyte's surface, making the phagocyte an **antigen-presenting cell.** This process alerts other cells in the immune system that a foreign substance is present.

B. *Lymphocytes*

1. Ninety-eight percent of lymphocytes reside in lymphoid tissue (Pantaleo et al., 1993). Lymphocytes are uniquely specialized. Each lymphocyte has receptors on its surface for one, and only one, of the many millions of possible antigens that can invade the body. When the receptors lock with their matched antigen, the process of neutralizing, inactivating, or destroying the foreign particle begins.

2. This requires that the body have an immense variety of receptors for an immense number of antigens.

3. Humans usually have about 2 trillion lymphocytes. Several types of these lymphocytes play major roles in the immune response.

   a. *T Lymphocytes* mature in the thymus and play a central role in the immune response by destroying infected cells, controlling inflammatory responses, and helping B cells make antibodies. There are several subsets of T lymphocytes *(Subsets of T cells display different proteins in groups (antigens) on their cell membranes. For this reason they are referred to as cluster differentiation (CD) antigens.* At least 180 different cluster differentiating antigens are known to reside on different human cell types. The different CD antigens lo-

cated on T lymphocyte subsets allow investigators to distinguish between the different T cell lines. For example, in physical appearance it is nearly impossible to distinguish T cells from B cells. But each carries a different CD antigen. T lymphocytes attached by HIV carry type 4 antigen and are referred to as CD4+ T lymphocytes or T4 cells, likewise for T8 cells. B lymphocytes do not carry the T4 or T8 antigen.)

4. *Helper T cells* (T_H) alert the immune system to the presence of an antigen and activate other cells in the system. Helper T cells carry about 10,000 copies of the CD4 protein molecule on the surface of each helper T cell so these **CD4+** cells are often referred to as **T4** cells.

   a. T4 cells have receptors (TCR) on their surface that are specialized for the recognition of antigens found on the surface of antigen-presenting cells. It has been estimated that 10^{11} to 10^{15} different TCRs can be generated in humans. The total of the different TCR specificities of a given individual constitutes their "T-cell repertoire." This is a rough measure of the capacity of a given individual to respond to the myriad of foreign microbes, antigens, and so forth, that he or she will be confronted within his or her lifetime.

   b. When the T4 cell randomly contacts the surface of a phagocyte, its receptor binds to antigen on the phagocyte and the T4 cell becomes activated.

   c. The T4 cell then begins to secrete a variety of stimulatory factors *(lymphokines) into the space around it.*

   d. The T4 cell will eventually divide into two cells of exactly the same specificity. If the foreign substance persists, the two daughter cells will divide, and so on. Thus, the number of cells specific for that foreign antigen is greatly expanded.

   e. The T4 cell probably does little to repel the intruding substance on its own, but it is vital for activating the other main classes of lymphocytes

BOX 5.2 *(continued)*

(for example, B cells, natural killer cells and phagocytes). It does this by means of the lymphokines it secretes when activated. The most familiar of these are interleukin-2 (IL-2) and gamma interferon (γIFN).

  f. As a result of activation by T4 cells, B lymphocytes multiply and produce specific antibodies. The antibodies attach to the antigens on free organisms and infected cells, leading to inactivation and destruction of organisms and cells.

5. ***Inducer T cells*** (T_i) were previously known as the delayed sensitivity T cells. Inducer T cells also carry the CD4 molecule.

  a. When an inducer T cell recognizes antigen on the surface of a phagocyte and is helped by factors from a T4 cell, it also becomes activated and secretes its own family of lymphokines, IL4, IL5, and IL10. These factors attract many more phagocytes from around the body that accumulate in the area where antigen is being recognized.

  b. Phagocytes are specialized for ingesting and destroying the foreign invader.

6. ***Cytotoxic T*** lymphocytes (CTL) are also known as killer T cells. CTLs express the CD8 molecule and are most often referred to as **T8** cells. They are crucial for the immune response to viral infections. Although they cannot neutralize free virus, by eliminating virus infected-cells they are largely responsible for recovery from a viral infection.

  a. The recognition of invading microbes by CTLs is a complex business. An infected cell must first chemically chop up the microbe's protein into small fragments, or peptides. These peptides are transported to the cell surface, where they become bound to specialized molecules called human leukocyte antigens (HLAs). Special receptors on the CTL recognize the HLA-peptide complex, and the CTL then kills the infected cell by unloading a cocktail of cytotoxic chemicals into it. But even a small mutation can change the microbes peptide's structure enough that it

will no longer bind to HLA—or, alternatively, so that the peptide is no longer transported to the cell surface—and the infected cell then becomes "invisible" to the CTL.

  b. As the infected cell breaks apart, infectious particles can be released from the cell. The released infectious particles may be phagocytized, neutralized by antibody, or may infect new cells.

  c. Cytotoxic T8 cells have antigen specificity; this specificity is determined when the cytotoxic T8 cell is exposed to the antigen.

C. ***B Lymphocytes*** or ***B cells*** arise principally in the bone marrow and are responsible for making antibodies. The B cell response is referred to as humoral immunity.

1. B lymphocytes have receptors for antigen and also require help from T4 cells to become activated.

2. When activated, they release large amounts of immunoglobulins, called *antibodies,* (about 2000 per second) into the bloodstream and mucosal surfaces.

3. Antibodies circulate in body fluids. When they encounter the specific antigen with which they can interact, they bind to it.

4. Antigen–antibody interactions block the antigen's harmful potential in a variety of ways. For example, if the antigen is a toxin it may be neutralized or if it is a virus, it may lose its ability to bind to its target tissue.

5. In addition, the complex of antigen and antibody activates a group of proteins in the blood called *complement,* which then facilitates the removal of the antigen by calling in a large number of phagocytes.

D. ***Memory cells*** recall their history, quickly

1. Two groups of T and B lymphocytes become separate T and B memory cells for when the same antigen invades the body again.

2. Memory cells initiate immune response upon reexposure to an antigen.

3. Memory cells remember, recognize, and induce a more rapid immune response against the antigen.

BOX 5.2 *(continued)*

4. Memory cells are responsible for disease resistance after immunization and are also responsible for natural immunity.

E. **Suppressor T cells**

1. The function of suppressor lymphocytes in the immune system is not well understood, nor has a single kind of lymphocyte been identified that acts as a suppressor cell!

2. Suppressor cells turn off antibody production and other immune responses after an invader has been destroyed or eliminated from the body. This provides a balance in the immune system and allows it to rest when its functions are not required.

F. **Natural killer (NK) cells**

1. NK cells are antigen nonspecific lymphocytes that recognize foreign cells of many different antigenic types. That is, one NK cell can recognize many different types of invaders. Therefore, NK cells can attack without first having to recognize specific antigens.

2. NK cells are important in fighting viral infections.

II. **Humoral Immunity**—immune protection by the circulating antibodies that are produced by B cells. (See preceding section on **B Lymphocytes.**)

---

antibody-producing factories. These **plasma cells produce a single type of antigen-specific antibody of about 2000 antibodies per second.** The antibodies then circulate through the body fluids, attacking the triggering antigen.

What Happens to the Immune System after HIV Infection

HIV enters the body via infected body fluids: blood, semen, and vaginal secretions. Once inside, HIV specifically infects a type of white blood cell called the T4 cell. These cells direct the body's immune response against infection. As HIV takes over the T4 cells, it alters their growth and reproduction through a complicated process that leads to the T4 cells' destruction. The ratio of T4 cells to T8 cells then changes. In healthy people, the number of T4 cells is greater than the number of T8 cells. In HIV-infected individuals, a decline in the T4 count signals the progress of immune system deterioration. The results are debilitating: The T4 cells are not as responsive to antigen identification, macrophages become less responsive, and B cells produce fewer specific antibodies and lose their normal responsiveness. At this point, the immune system becomes dysfunctional and the host becomes vulnerable to attack from opportunistic infections.

ANTIBODIES AND VIRUSES

Twenty-four hours a day, 365 days a year, the body's lymphocytes must be on the lookout for harmful bacteria, viruses, and other pathogens. These agents of disease don't look very different, biochemically, from most of the regular molecules lymphocytes normally encounter in the blood. Yet a mistake by these immune cells can leave the body open to infection.

The immune system has evolved antibodies for distinguishing the body's own molecular debris from potentially harmful material.

The Antibody

Antibodies are Y-shaped molecules that bind to specific foreign proteins, or pieces of protein, called antigens.

When antibodies on the surface of a B cell snag an undesirable or foreign protein, **both disappear inside the cell.** Eventually, a bit of the foreign protein may reemerge, attached to a "self" recognizable protein molecule called a **class II protein** (Figure 5-4). The pair, the small piece of foreign protein attached to a "self" **class II protein,** acts as a red flag to T4 cells, which set off an aggressive immune response.

The self or class II protein molecules play a critical part in the immune defensive response because they determine which viral peptides will be displayed on the antigen-presenting cells (APC), and how effectively they are showcased. Any two individuals are likely to differ in the precise structure of these class II molecules they possess. Thus, they will also differ in the peptides their cells exhibit and in the ability of the class II-peptide units to attract the attention of the immune system.

HIV AND THE IMMUNE SYSTEM IN PERSPECTIVE

Signs and symptoms of an illness is often an indicator that your body is responding to one or more of a variety of invaders from the outside—virus, bacteria, fungus, protozoa, etc. The pus around the splinter in the finger that got infected is a sign of immunological effort—white blood cells are building up as they do battle against the foreign object. The same is true when the body responds to HIV. A biological war begins inside; it's the immune system vs. the virus, and even without medicinal help, it usually takes years for HIV to conquer the immune system. Deciding whether to go on drugs or not is a tough decision. For 95% of people the virus will eventually win regardless, but it appears that the current anti-HIV drugs can improve the quality and length of life for many of the HIV infected.

Having HIV means having to learn some of the names of different cells that play a part in the immune system. The human immune system is a complex network of cells and organs that work together to defend your body from viruses and other microorganisms. There are two types of immune response: innate (inherited, present at birth) and acquired (not inherited, resulting from the effects of the environment). The innate part starts very quickly after infection and does not depend on recognizing a specific type of foreign substance that is present in the body. Natural killer cells and macrophages are components of innate immunity.

Acquired immune response starts more slowly, but is longer-lived. In addition, the acquired part of the response is specific to certain foreign substances and it contains cells that record the history of past infections. This memory allows the immune system to react quickly if there is a re-infection with the same virus or microorganism. Two important components of acquired immunity are antigens and antigen-presenting cells. An antigen is a foreign substance, usually protein from one of the invading agents. The foreign antigen causes an immune response from the body. Certain cells called antigen-presenting cells digest these agents and display a part of the antigen on their cell surface. Antigen-presenting cells then seek out other immune cells that will respond to the specific antigen they are displaying on their surface. One type of cell that antigen-presenting cells look for is called a B cell, a specific type of lymphocyte of the immune system. Each B cell recognizes one and only one

type of antigen. When the antigen-presenting cells find B cells that recognize that antigen, those B cells become active and begin to reproduce. Most of the new B cells release a specific antibody to that antigen. Antibodies play several roles, including marking foreign agents and infected cells for destruction by other parts of the immune system. Once the infection is under control, these antibody-creating B cells are no longer needed and they die. However, when B cells reproduce, they also produce memory B cells, cells that have recorded the history of what just happened. These memory cells can live for years. If the same antigen is encountered again, the memory B cells activate and reproduce more quickly than the first time, in a day or so, rather than two weeks to a month.

Antigen-presenting cells can also look for T lymphocyte cells. Like B cells, T cells are specific to exactly one type of antigen. Again, once the right T cells are found, they become active and reproduce. But instead of producing antibodies, T cells release special chemicals called cytokines. Once produced, cytokines direct immune cells to attack a specific antigen. There are two types of T cells: CD4+T or T4 cells and CD8+T or T8 cells. CD4+T cells are also called helper T cells because they help other parts of the immune system respond to infection. Specifically, CD4+T cells stimulate B cells to respond and increase the production of CD8+T cells. Although CD8+T cells have many roles, one of the most important is to kill the cells that have become infected by an antigen. In this case the antigen is HIV. These CD8 cells are also called killer cells or cytotoxic T lymphocytes (CTLs). As with B cells, once the infection is under control, many of these T cells are no longer needed and they die. However, some of these T cells also become memory cells, which can respond quickly if the antigen is encountered again. HIV, though, is a formidable enemy to the immune system. It reproduces by installing itself in the CD4+ cells that coordinate the immune response. Once HIV is inside them, these T cells become virus factories, producing thousands of viral particles before dying. A person infected with HIV produces millions to billions of new viral particles everyday. The more CD4+ cells HIV kills off, the more powerless the immune system becomes to fight off other disease-causing viruses and microorganisms. Most often it is these agents, some of which may have been inside the body and controlled by the immune system since child-hood, that cause the infections during the course of HIV disease. Because they take advantage of the opportunity provided by your weakened im-mune system, these illnesses are known as oppor-tunistic infections, or OIs. There are drugs to combat OIs, but over the long term, the viruses and microorganisms like HIV become resistant to the drugs, and the HIV infected progresses to death.

Immune Based Therapies

The discovery of HIV in 1983 led to an intensive search for therapies that might inhibit the virus' life cycle—a search that eventually produced the 17 antiretroviral drugs that are on the market today. Finding treatments that might work by improving the function of the immune system—immune-based therapies (IBTs)—has been a dif-ficult task, mainly because the mechanisms by which HIV impairs immunity are still not fully understood. Without that understanding, IBTs have largely been shots in the dark, with some attempting to improve overall immune function (and thus prevent or delay opportunistic infec-tions), and others attempting to specifically improve the immune response to HIV. Over the years, many approaches have been pro-posed and studied, sometimes with great fan-fare, but all have so far failed to demonstrate any measurable health benefit. As yet, there are no IBTs approved for the treatment of HIV infection or AIDS.

Most people infected with HIV seem to recognize just a few of the many potential small peptide units generated from the virus's proteins, usually be-tween one and 10.

At the time, scientists did not know where the cell degraded this undesirable protein and at-tached it to a **"self"** recognizable protein.

In mid-1994, four research teams announced the discovery of a special compartment, or or-ganelle, inside cells where this processing occurs. Using sophisticated biochemical and immunolog-ical techniques, they independently determined that both the **"self"** recognizable protein and the antibody-antigen complex wind up in this com-partment called an **endosome** (Amigorena et al., 1994; Pennisi, 1994; Schmid et al., 1994; Tulp et al., 1994).

The characterization of this specialized vesicle is an important step. It permits an understanding of the trafficking events and defines the intracellular event of antigen processing. (For an excellent re-view of the concept of antigen processing and pre-sentation, see Unanue, 1995; for class I and class II proteins, Strominger et al., 1995; for the concept of self, Zinkernagel, 1995; for cell-mediated immuni-ty, Doherty, 1995).

B Cells Make Antibodies and Release Them into the Bloodstream

After an antibody and virus join, they are digested by macrophages or cleared from the blood by the liver and spleen. **Some B cells and T cells become memory cells, which are stored by the immune system.** Memory cells appear to recall their histo-ry and remember the antigen they have previous-ly encountered. If the same antigen ever gets into the bloodstream again, these cells rapidly begin antibody production. However, if the antigen, say a virus, has mutated (changed), as the flu virus does yearly, previous antibodies will not affect it. New antibodies must be created to neutralize the new mutant virus. While this antibody produc-tion is taking place, the viral invader has time to multiply and infect new cells, and the infected person suffers the symptoms of the flu.

Can the Immune System Remember HIV Exposure?

The immune system works because it produces antibody against an antigen and in addition cre-ates immune memory cells—special cells that have instant recall of a past exposure to that anti-gen. But this does not appear to occur when the immune system is exposed to HIV. Yes, antibody is made, but when HIV disappears (is reduced to below measurable levels using HAART), so does the immune defense against it. There are few if any memory cells to protect us should HIV re-bound or break through drug suppression repli-cation. In the mid-1990s, Francis Plummer and colleagues at the University of Nairobi stunned scientists when they announced discovery of a group of Kenyan female prostitutes who appeared resistant to HIV infection, surviving infection for years despite more than six customers a week **without condom protection** in a society where upward of one in five (20%) of their customers were likely to be HIV positive. Vaccine researchers were ecstatic because the discovery offered evidence that people could successfully become immune to HIV—something cynics had argued might be impossible. But at the 7th Conference on Retroviral and Opportunistic Infections (Febru-

ary 2000) Plummer's group had distressing news: 10% of the apparently resistant prostitutes became HIV positive from 1996 to 1999. Their infections coincided with the women's decisions to **decrease their exposure to HIV by having fewer customers or insisting that the men wear condoms.** Kevin De Crock, an HIV investigator, said, "It suggests that HIV antigen stimulation is required for the maintenance of resistance." **De Crock said it may be that the immune system is not capable of remembering without a constant presence of**

SIDEBAR 5.2

MEASURES AND COUNTERMEASURES: THE HUMAN IMMUNE SYSTEM VS. VIRUSES

A war has existed between humans and viruses that invade human cells and cause disease. Probably from the first encounter, prehuman to first humans, viruses became able to **hide** inside human cells. The immune system in turn adapted by developing a means of surveying and identifying cells containing hidden virus. Virus then adapted by deceiving the immune surveillance system; the immune system then evolved a better means to **mark** cells carrying the virus. This game of hide-and-seek between the virus and the immune system continues. Learning the means by which the virus attempts to trick the immune system carries over into the study of **tumor cells.** They must also escape the immune system's surveillance system and do so by using several of the same ploys used by the virus. From what microbiologists have learned so far, different viruses have evolved different ways of getting rid of expression of class 1 proteins, the flagpole of self proteins. But the mechanisms are amazingly different in different viruses. Examples are:

Cytomegalovirus (CMV)—A virus that may cause birth defects in the fetus and the rapid onset of blindness in people with AIDS. On entering a cell, CMV stops self identity proteins from reaching the cell membrane. If the class 1 proteins can't reach the membrane neither will pieces of CMV. The immune system is blinded to the fact the CMV is inside the cells. The immune system counters with a natural killer cell that destroys all cells that do not contain a self protein on their surface! But CMV over time evolved a means to produce a **fake** self protein that passes for the real one. The natural killer cells are successfully fooled.

Adenovirus—The virus causing common colds. This virus can also stop self proteins from reaching the membrane carrying identifying pieces of virus. Further, this virus is able to make the **cell divide** so it can replicate itself. The cell then becomes cancerous (replication out of control), begins to destroy itself—but the virus has evolved a way to stop the cell's self-destruction, so the cell continues to divide. The process is similar to what happens in tumor cells.

HIV—This virus has the most deadly scheme of all. This virus infects cells of the immune system—most often the T4 cells that is essential to the initiation of the immune response. Similar to other viruses, HIV has to disable the self alerting system. One of HIV's genes, call **nef,** makes a protein that attaches to the **self proteins,** just inside the cell's membrane. The other end of the nef protein carries an address label, readable by the cell's internal sorting system that directs proteins to their proper place. The message carried by the nef protein says, in the cell's sorting code, "Haul to garbage dump and recycle," tricking the infected cell into pulling down its self proteins and destroying them. The nef protein also tags the CD4 proteins for destruction in the same way. Like the self proteins, the CD4's stick up through the cell membrane. What does HIV gain from having the cell destroy CD4 proteins? That's the million dollar question investigators are working on. The reason may be to prevent other viruses from entering the cell or because in latching onto the CD4 proteins, the nef protein dislodges and energizes another protein that is known to activate the T cells. The cell's activation to make more HIV may be the answer.

HIV (too few memory cells made?). This would appear to be an HIV catch 22—to control HIV it must be present, but the control will over the long run be insufficient to stop the progression to AIDS.

ANTIBODIES AND HIV DISEASE

Resistance to HIV does not seem to be the same as the more common examples of immunity. The body's protective countermeasures against measles and mumps are absolute. Years after exposure, there is no hint within the body of the foreign agents that cause those diseases. After children become immune to mumps, they can no longer infect other people. Immunity to these diseases occur because the immune system makes **neutralizing** antibody that destroys the infecting agent. Memory immune cells are able to produce neutralizing antibody whenever these infecting agents enter the body. In contrast, it has been shown that although the immune system of most people initially produce neutralizing HIV antibodies, the continued evolution of HIV in their bodies results in a series of mutant HIV that are not efficiently neutralized via antibody response. Thus over time, the ratio of effective neutralizing antibody production to new virus production becomes disproportionate, that is, more virus than effective neutralizing antibody is made and at this time the level of T4 or CD4+ cells begin to drop. T4 cells drop because antibodies to HIV reduce circulating HIV in the plasma (viral load) without affecting HIV replication or cell-to-cell spread of HIV. This means that the production of mutant HIV to existing antibody never ceases, resulting in continued T4 cell infection and loss. Eventually there are too few T4 cells to ward off opportunistic infections (see Chapter 7 for additional information on T4 cell replacement and HIV production).

The rapid production of HIV mutants without the same rapid production of a neutralizing antibody against each mutant means that sometime after infection, much if not most of the antibody in some people may be nothing more than useless antibody copy (antibody to the initial strain or strains of HIV). In these people, HIV disease would most likely progress more swiftly than in persons whose immune system can keep up with the production of new antibody to match the formation of HIV mutants. This may be one important reason why some people progress to AIDS and death so rapidly when compared to other HIV-infected people.

HIV Protected from Human Antibodies

Humans create antibodies against a number of HIV proteins, namely the envelope proteins (gp120), the transmembrane protein (gp41), and the proteins of HIV's core (gp24). **But, antibodies cannot enter cells.** The antibody can only attack HIV in the plasma. Plasma is the fluid part of the blood and does not include the blood cells. **Once inside a host cell, HIV is protected from antibody.** Such cells, monocytes, and macrophage and dendritic cells carry HIV internally. All these cell types serve as **HIV**

POINT OF INFORMATION 5.2

THE BIG QUESTIONS:

♦ How does HIV, which at first glance does not appear to be a highly formidable foe, persist in the body for such long periods of time and continue multiplying and progressively causing more and more damage until a fatal outcome is reached?

♦ Why does the immensely powerful immune system of the body, an organ system that has evolved over millennia of challenges from a wide variety of infectious and noninfectious invaders to become an exceedingly effective defender of the body against agents far more virulent than HIV, now appear to be powerless against it?

THE ANSWER:

Because HIV, unlike other agents that enter the human body, (virus, bacteria, fungus, and protozoa) infects immune system cells, in particular **the T4 or CD4+ cell that governs the response of the entire immune system!** Without T4 cells the immune system cannot function—like a car without gas, all the parts are there but nothing happens when called on to operate.

reservoirs in the body. In addition, these cells travel to all distant points within the body and deliver HIV. The self-antiretroviral chemicals that these cells generate appear to be ineffective against their hidden traveling companion, HIV (Moir et al., 2000; Olinger et al., 2000). Perhaps the most disturbing discovery concerning HIV reservoirs in 2001 is the work of Robert Siliciano at Johns Hopkins University. This discovery is disturbing because little is known about memory cells' lifespan and whether they can be eradicated. Memory cells are programmed to do nothing but sit and wait for viruses to attack; their job is to keep a record of the germs that the body has previously encountered so that the immune system will be ready the next time it is confronted with the antigens. What HIV has done is tap into the most fundamental aspect of the immune system, and that is a person's immunological memory. It's the perfect mechanism for the virus to ensure its survival. Because the cells are the immune system's memory, they must survive for a long time, creating a latently infected reservoir of HIV in the body. This reservoir is the single biggest obstacle to getting rid of HIV. Anthony Fauci, director of the National Institute of Allergy and Infectious Diseases said, "We are not going to be eliminating this reservoir. Whether you can measure it or not doesn't seem to have a significant im-

pact on the clinically relevant phenomenon of what happens when you stop taking the drug."

Once HIV gets inside these cell reservoirs as a **provirus,** it is likely to remain there for the rest of the cell's life (person's life) unless some other antiviral mechanism within the body or some chemical agent is able to destroy the provirus. To date, no such drug has been found to be effective against the HIV **provirus.**

IMMUNE SYSTEM DYSFUNCTION

When HIV first arrives in the body, there are no immune memory T cells that know how to deal with it. The body has never experienced HIV. As with any other first exposure to an infection, it is the job of **naïve or unexposed** T cells to respond. Returning to the scene in the lymph nodes, naïve or unexposed T4 or CD4+ cells get recruited to fight HIV and in turn they become infected. As these infected T cells begin to divide, HIV is able to replicate and release new viruses from each infected cell. Viral load counts in the blood will usually rise rapidly during this period called **primary or acute infection.** It is during the acute phase that HIV also seeds latent HIV reservoirs in lymphoid tissue. During this period, a small fraction of the T cells that are activated to fight HIV revert

---

POINT OF INFORMATION 5.3

WHAT ARE CELL RECEPTORS?

In the study of cells, the term **receptor** is used to describe any molecule that interacts with and subsequently holds onto some other molecule. The receptor is like the **hand** and the object held by the hand is commonly called the **ligand.** The interaction between the receptor and ligand implies specificity; a receptor known to bind with substance X would not normally bind with a different substance. For example, a two-slotted electrical wall outlet is a receptacle (receptor) for a two-pronged plug (ligand). A three-pronged plug will not fit into this receptacle. Depending on the type of two-slotted receptacle, even some two-pronged plugs may not fit.

Where Are Cell Receptors Located?

Receptors can be found inside a cell, and especially embedded within all the membranes that

a given cell may have. In humans there are organ systems present, and a given receptor may be found associated only with a particular type of cell that comprises a particular type of tissue that makes up a particular organ.

What Do Receptors Do?

Receptors are critical to the life of all cells, whether or not the cells represent an animal, a plant, a fungus, or a bacterium. Every function, response, interaction, pathway, process, and any other term you might think of that concerns the moment-to-moment existence of a cell, is controlled by various receptor/ligand-induced systems. Essentially, you are what your genetically coded receptors allow you to become.

back to a resting, or **memory,** state. As the cells rest, so do the viruses they harbor. **In effect, HIV causes two infections: an active infection that spreads via infected T4 cells to other parts of the body, including the brain; and a dormant, or latent infection that persists in lymphoid tissue cell reservoirs.**

If this process is allowed to continue unchecked, the large pool of naïve T cells become slowly drained. To understand why, think of the lake metaphor. The water still flows out of the lake at the same rate, so if the siphoning isn't stopped, the lake eventually empties. Studies have shown that the naïve T cell pool does indeed dwindle in HIV infection. In fact, recent study shows that the loss of newly produced naïve T4 cells is strongly linked to disease progression.

HIV also affects the **memory T4 or CD4+ cell pool.** Studies have shown that people with HIV lose their ability to respond to a variety of infections. When a person progresses to AIDS, he or she often gets sick from old infections that were previously controlled by memory T cells. A critical fact is that the body only has a certain amount of room for memory T cells. Immunologists have proposed that when a new memory T cell matures in response to a new infection, an existing memory cell has to die off to make room. This sounds like a recipe for disaster, but an average person has enough room in their memory T4 cell pool to accommodate all the memory T cell squads they need to stay healthy (for example, the herpes zoster squad, the Pneumocystis carinii pneumonia squad, the cytomegalovirus squad). If a particular memory T cell squad gets low on members, when new memory T cells show up, other T cells can always be recruited if the infection reappears.

HIV infection, however, appears to lead to the continual addition of defective HIV-specific memory T cells to the pool. This accumulation causes a reduction in the number of functional memory squads needed to control other infections. This may explain the occurrence of different infections,

---

POINT OF INFORMATION 5.4

THE FIRST LOOK AT HOW HIV's gp120 ENVELOPE GLYCOPROTEIN CHANGES SHAPE TO ATTACH TO CD4 AND CHEMOKINE RECEPTORS

In three **landmark** studies, published in two scientific journals, Carlo Rizzuto and colleagues (1998), Richard Wyatt and colleagues (1998), and Peter Kwong and colleagues (1998) revealed and discussed the crystal structures of gp120, HIV's surface (envelope) glycoprotein. These reports have **very important** implications for the virology, immunology and vaccine development against HIV and most other viruses that infect humans. These papers came after 10 years of frustrating efforts to crystallize gp120—a prerequisite to determining its structure by x-ray crystallography. David Baltimore, noted laureate and head of a U.S. government advisory panel on AIDS vaccines said, "This is a big deal." Other notable HIV researchers believe these findings are a major advance in the collective knowledge of the virology and immunology of HIV infections. Revealing the structure of gp120 was to reveal the **passkey** on how HIV escapes antibody attack and invades T lymphocytes. First, **gp120** attaches to the T cell receptor, CD4; then gp120 changes shape, unveiling a binding site that allows HIV to attach to a second T cell receptor, one of the chemokines, with both attachments secured, HIV enters the cell. A computer-generated snapshot of the HIV infection process is very informative (Figure 5-5). The picture shows, for example, that some of the virus' most stable—and therefore vulnerable—structures are either located at the bottom of crevices, where the relatively bulky antibodies of the immune system can't reach them, or obscured by great forests of sugar molecules. It appears that the immune vulnerable structures are covered by a top similar to a moveable roof on a stadium. One possible antibody target comes out of hiding but only in that brief moment after gp120 latches onto the CD4 receptor and before it attaches to the chemokine receptor—much too briefly for the immune system to react. Because HIV keeps its immune-vulnerable structures hidden until the last possible moment, HIV is now called the **"Houdini of viruses."** However, most drugs are very small molecules—much smaller than antibodies. Properly designed drugs might be able to infiltrate some of those crevices in HIV's outer walls.

FIGURE 5-5 UNRAVELING THE SECRET TO HIV CELL INFECTION: ATTACHMENT, FUSION AND ENTRY. A. The process begins with interactions between a cluster of proteins on HIV's outer coat, sometimes referred to as the gp160 spike—and CD4 and one of the chemokine receptors (either CCR5 or CCR4) on the cell surface. This interactive complex is made up of three transmembrane glycoproteins (gp41), which anchor the cluster to the virus, and three extracellular glycoproteins (gp120), which contain the binding domains for both CD4 and the chemokine receptors. **B.** The first step in fusion involves the attachment of the CD4 binding domains of gp120 to CD4. CD4 attachment inhibitors (e.g., PRO 542) act here. **C.** One gp120 is bound with CD4 protein, the envelope complex undergoes a structural change, bringing gp120 close to the chemokine receptor, allowing for a more stable two-pronged attachment. Antagonists or co-receptor blockades of CCR5 (SCH-C) and CXCR4 (AMD-3100) act here. If the virus attaches to both CD4 and the chemokine receptor, additional conformational changes allow gp41 to enter CD4+ cell membrane. **D.** The collapse of the extracellular portion of gp41 to form a hairpin, which is sometimes referred to as a coiled-coil bundle. The fusion inhibitors T-20 and T-1249 act here resulting in a poorly formed hairpin. In the absence of an inhibitor, the hairpin structure brings the virus and cell membrane close together, allowing fusion of the membranes and subsequent entry of viral RNA. *(Illustration adapted from The PRN Notebook, Vol. 7, March 2002, www.prn.org).*

including opportunistic microorganisms, during the more advanced stages of HIV infection. It also explains why some people on HIV therapy remain vulnerable to opportunistic infections. They may have lost their "memory" to these infections.

How Invading HIV Gets to the T4 Cell

Based on the recent investigations of American and Dutch scientists, it appears that HIV hijacks immune cells to enter the body's immune system.

Dendritic cells are the watchdogs of the immune system. They are located just below the skin surface and under moist mucosal tissue on surfaces like those of the vagina, urethra, and penis. When dendritic cells see a foreign invader such as a microorganism, or virus, they capture it, shred it, and display pieces of proteins from the invading pathogen on their surfaces. These displayed proteins serve to alert other immune system cells such as T4 cells that the body is under attack. What recent investigations now show is that HIV attaches to dendritic cells and hitches a ride into the lymphoid tissues where it then infects T4 cells. The dendritic cell has finger-like projections that carry a protein receptor called **DC-SIGN** (dendritic cell specific ICAM-3-grabbing nonintegrin). HIV adheres to DC-SIGN and is carried from the mucosal lining of the cervix or rectum to the lymph nodes where it transfers HIV to the T4 cells through their coreceptors R4 and R5 (Steinman, 2000; Geijtenbeck, et al., 2000). Thus, another puzzle piece is in place toward the complete understanding of how HIV successfully attacks the human immune system.

How HIV Enters T4 or CD4+ Cells and Macrophage

HIV researchers have known since 1984 that human CD4 cell membrane receptors alone are sufficient for **binding** HIV to the T4 lymphocyte membrane but CD4 receptors are not sufficient for **HIV envelope fusion** with the T4 cell membrane or for **HIV penetration** or entry into the cell's interior. This knowledge has enticed many groups of AIDS researchers to search for additional receptors, **coreceptors** to CD4, that HIV uses to enter a cell after binding to it. Various candidate receptor molecules were put forward, sometimes with more fanfare than fact, but have not stood the test of critical examination.

FUSIN O3R CXCKR-4 (R4)

In May of 1996, Ed Berger (Figure 5-6) and colleagues reported finding a receptor that allowed

---

SIDEBAR 5.3

THE DENTRITIC CELL AND NEW-FOUND FUNCTION

Dendritic cells—among the first cells in the body to encounter infectious organisms—are key players in initiating an immune response. These cells arise in the bone marrow but migrate to tissues throughout the body. Before dendritic cells encounter an infectious agent, they are immature and act as roving sentinels of the immune system. Upon an encounter with an infectious agent, the dendritic cell reaches maturity—capturing the infectious agent and processing it for presentation to the T-cell, thus initiating a cascade of immune events that fight infection.

Researchers at the Whitehead Institute for Biomedical Research have discovered that a dendritic cell initiates an immune response that is tailor-made for specific infectious organisms. The researchers found that dendritic cells turn on different sets of genes, or a signature pattern of gene response, depending on whether the organism is a bacteria, virus, or fungus. This study shows that even at the earliest stages of infection, the human body knows the nature of the infectious organism, or pathogen, and responds with a specific type of immune response to eliminate the pathogen.

Dendritic cell maturation—as a result of its recognition of a pathogen—is highly specialized. The dendritic cell fine tunes its response based upon the nature of the pathogen. For every pathogen, there is a specific set of genetic programs that are activated or not activated, which then impacts how the immune system as a whole reacts to the infectious agent. The knowledge that dendritic cells are able to sense and respond specifically to each pathogen could ultimately help clinical scientists detect the presence of particular pathogens and measure the nature of the immune response by looking for the signatures of pathogen-specific genes.

FIGURE 5-6 Edward A. Berger, chief of the molecular structure section, Laboratory of Viral Diseases at the National Institutes of Allergy and Infectious Diseases. In the spring of 1996, he and colleagues discovered the **first** coreceptor **CXCKR4** or **FUSIN** that HIV needs to complete its attachment and entry into T4 lymphocytes. *(Photograph courtesy of Edward A. Berger)*

syncytium-inducing (SI) strains of HIV (HIV that causes T4 cells to form clusters—they attach to each other) to enter T4 cells. Strains of HIV that do not induce T4 cell syncytium formation (NSI) could not enter T4 cells. Berger and colleagues named this T4 cell receptor **FUSIN.** In August of 1996 Conrad Bleul and colleagues identified a chemokine, **CXC stromal cell-derived factor-1 (SDF-1)** that binds to the **FUSIN** receptor and blocks HIV entry. They named this chemokine **CXCKR-4.** This coreceptor functions preferentially for T cell line-tropic HIV strains.

What Are β-Chemokine Receptors and β-Chemokines— β-Chemokine receptors are cell-surface proteins that bind small peptides (a short chain of amino acids) called β-chemokines to their surface. Chemokines are classified into three groups depending on the location of the amino acid cysteine (**C**) in the peptide. These are C_ _, C-C_ _ _ _, and CXC_ _ _chemokines. The X in CXC represents any other amino acid. The chemokine receptors are identified by the individual chemokine(s) that binds to them. In that sense, **a reference to a specific chemokine(s) also identifies its receptor.**

CC-CKR-5 (R-5) RECEPTOR

Within two months after the FUSIN receptor data was reported, **five separate research teams** reported on an additional coreceptor called **CC-CKR-5** (R-5). R-5 is the fifth of seven known human chemokine receptors that respond to β-chemokines. The function of β-chemokines is to attract macrophages and other immune cells to sites of inflammation. R-5 is known to be a receptor for three β-chemokine proteins called RANTES, MIP–1α, and MIP–1β. The β-chemokine RANTES (**r**egulated-upon-**a**ctivation **n**ormal **T** **e**xpressed and **s**ecreted), chemokine MIP-1α and 1β (**m**acrophage **i**nflammatory **p**roteins) are all produced by T8 cells and are known to inhibit HIV replication, particularly in **macrophage-tropic HIV strains** (HIV strains that infect macrophage over T4 cells) (Deng et al., 1996; Dragic et al., 1996) **and are powerful suppressors of HIV infection, especially HIV infection of macrophages!** That is, these three chemokine proteins suppress HIV entry into macrophage by somehow blocking the coreceptor R-5. Members of the research teams who have contributed to the discovery of the R-5 receptor believe that **macrophage-tropic or M-tropic HIV strains occur in greatest number early on after HIV infection and then, sometime later during HIV disease the predominant HIV strain shifts to HIV strains that use the FUSIN receptor (R-4) on T4 cells.** HIV, by shifting receptors, may be avoiding the suppressive activity of the chemokines that block the R-5 receptor. Figure 5-7 shows a diagram of this suggested **receptor swap** that occurs sometime during HIV disease progression. One of the great unsolved puzzles of HIV disease is **why**, during disease progression, does HIV lose its ability to infect macrophage and become T-cell tropic? **Why does HIV switch to other cell receptors?**

Macrophage-tropic HIV

T cell-tropic HIV

R-5 — CD4

R-5 fusin

CD4 fusin(X4)

Macrophage

T4 cell circulating in the blood

T cell line

FIGURE 5-7 Coreceptors Required for HIV To Enter Human Cells. HIV can broadly be divided into two classes: those more suitable (tropic) to infecting macrophage, a major reservoir of HIV, and those that infect T4 cells in the lymph nodes or other tissues. Macrophage-tropic nonsyncytium-inducing (NSI) HIV isolates infect macrophages but fail to infect HIV T cells lines, while T4 HIV syncytium-inducing (SI) strains fail to infect macrophage. But HIV of both classes efficiently infect T4 cells isolated from peripheral blood mononuclear cells (PBMC). **Macrophage-tropic NSI HIV appear to be preferentially transmitted by sexual contact and constitute the vast majority of HIV present in newly infected individuals (Zhu, 1993). The T-tropic SI viruses generally appear late in the course of infection during the so-called "phenotypic switch" that often precedes the onset of AIDS symptoms (Conner, et al., 1994).** The molecular basis of HIV-1 tropism appears to lie in the ability of envelopes of macrophage-tropic and T-tropic viruses to interact with different coreceptors located on macrophage or T4 cells. Macrophage-tropic viruses primarily use R-5 and less often R-3 and R-2, newly described seven-transmembrane domain chemokine receptors, while T-tropic HIV tend to use FUSIN (R-4), a previously identified seven-transmembrane protein (Hill et al., 1996; Moore, 1997).

CCKR-2 (R-2) AND CCKR-3 (R-3) RECEPTORS

Recent studies have shown that at least two additional chemokine receptors participate in allowing HIV cell entry. HIV can use both CCKR-2 (R-2) and CCKR-3 (R-3) to help its invasion of cells. For example, dual tropic HIVs use R-2 and R-3 to enter cells and studies with microglial cells (**non-CD4 type cells**) show that both R-5 and R-3 permit HIV to enter these **brain** cells (McNicholl et al., 1997). Current research involves finding ways to block or fill the chemokine receptors with a harmless molecule, thus blocking HIV's binding site on the cell (Chen et al., 1997).

GENETIC RESISTANCE TO HIV INFECTION

At this point in the HIV/AIDS pandemic it is believed that about 95% of HIV-exposed people are susceptible to HIV infection and HIV disease progression. This statement is made because it has long been known that persons who have deliberately avoided safer sex practice and who have had unprotected sex with HIV-infected persons failed to become HIV-infected! The question that has continued to puzzle HIV investigators is, how can multiple HIV-exposed persons remain uninfected? Pieces of that puzzle began to fall into place when two gay males who, despite repeated unprotected sex with companions who died from the

RANTES: A DOUBLE-EDGED MOLECULE

DOES IT HELP OR HARM?

Confusion reigns as to why some people do not become HIV-infected regardless of exposure; why some people are more easily infected than others and why some people progress to AIDS more quickly than others. **NOW** there is genetic evidence that the gene for **Rantes increases the risk of HIV infection and at the same time delays the progression to AIDS** (McDermott et al., 2000)!

David McDermott and colleagues at the National Institute of Allergy and Infectious Diseases looked at variations in a gene called RANTES in HIV-infected and HIV-resistant people. Specifically they looked for tiny changes in a single base pair, also known as single nucleotide polymorphism (SNP). They found that one such SNP appears significantly more often in HIV-positive than HIV-resistant individuals, and this particular alteration increases the activity of the RANTES

gene and is associated with up to twice the risk of HIV infection. However, individuals with this SNP who become infected with HIV take about 40% longer to develop AIDS!

The reason for this paradoxical effect is not clear. This specific SNP may cause overproduction of the RANTES immune system molecule. This molecule then creates an inflammatory response that widens the space between cells, which permits HIV to enter more easily. At the same time, an overabundance of this molecule, which attaches to T cell receptors, may slow HIV by blocking viral attachment—because RANTES gets there first.

Several companies are trying to develop RANTES-based therapies to slow HIV progression, but researchers must remember that higher RANTES levels may increase the likelihood of acquiring HIV.

---

disease, remained HIV negative. Neither quite understood why he was spared but they were public-spirited enough to press scientists to come up with the answer. HIV investigators Rong Liu and coworkers (1996) and Michel Samson and coworkers (1996) reported that repeated HIV-exposed but uninfected people have a **32-nucleotide deletion in the gene that produces the R-5 receptors on macrophage**. The protein produced by this gene is severely damaged and does **not** reach the cell surface to act as a chemokine receptor. Without these receptors, the envelope of HIV cannot fuse with the envelope of macrophage to gain entrance into the cell. Thus, people who carry both defective R-5 genes' **homozygotes** (they received one defective gene from each parent) are resistant to HIV infection. If one is **heterozygous** (that is, one carries one defective gene and one normal gene), one will produce the R-5 receptor that HIV needs to penetrate macrophage, but they may be fewer in number. Thus, chemokines (the chemicals that the receptors were made for) would have fewer receptors to fill so there is a greater chance that fewer R-5 receptors are open or available for HIV attachment. As a result, heterozygous people may be **less** resistant to HIV infection than the homozygous mutant (receptorless) people, but may

be **more** resistant than people who have two normal genes (homozygous normal) who are the most susceptible to HIV infection. (O'Brien 1998)

Michael Dean and colleagues (1996) presented evidence that the frequency of R-5 deletion heterozygotes (those with one copy of the gene) was significantly elevated in groups of individuals who had survived HIV infection for more than 10 years, and, in some risk groups, twice as frequent as their occurrence in **rapid progressors to AIDS**. Michael Marmor and colleagues (2001) reported that white gay males who are heterogeneous (have one copy of the mutant gene) were 70% less likely to become HIV infected than those without the mutation. Survival analysis also shows that disease progression is slower in R-5 deletion heterozygotes than in individuals with the normal R-5 gene. Jesper Eugene-Olsen and colleagues (1997) reported that individuals who are heterozygous for the 32-base-pair deletion in the R-5 gene have a slower decrease in their T4-cell count and a longer AIDS-free survival than individuals with the wild-type gene for up to 11 years of follow-up.

Sean Philpott and colleagues reported in 1999 that children who inherit the R5 mutation are protected from vertical HIV infection (mother to newborn via breast milk).

Will the Mutant R-5 Gene Protect People from All Subtypes of HIV?

This genetic defect, the 32-nucleotide deletion, prevents infection only with the strain of HIV (Subtype B) that is transmitted sexually and is prevalent in the United States and Europe. It does not necessarily protect against other strains of HIV transmitted through intravenous drug use or blood transfusions, or strains prevalent in Africa.

Should I Be Tested for the Presence of the R-5 Gene?

Researchers agree that getting tested for the gene would not be difficult, but it would not be of great value because the tested person could still be infected by other strains of HIV. It must be assumed that most people do not carry a pair of defective R-5 genes because 95% or more of HIV-exposed people become HIV-infected!

Who Carries the Defective R-5 Gene?

Perhaps most surprising, HIV investigators found that the homozygous genetic defect (a person having two defective genes) is common: **It is present in 1% of whites of European descent**. But it appears to be absent in people from Japan and Central Africa; about 20% of whites are heterozygous for this gene.

UPDATE 2002 Recent studies conducted at Stellenbosch University show that this particular mutation, the R5 gene deletion, is virtually absent in the South African black population. The investigators believe that this is but one factor that affects a black person's susceptibility to HIV infection. Most likely there are other genes involved in the complexity of susceptibility to infection. Aside from the issue of susceptibility to infection, there is no consensus on whether blacks or Hispanics, after infection, progress more quickly than whites towards AIDS.

Why Does This Gene Exist?

Scientists speculate that the mutant form of R-5 protected against some disease that afflicted Europeans but not Africans. The obvious candidate would be the Black Death of 1346, the plague. If the mutant R-5 blocked plague bacteria, the survivors would be more likely to carry the trait and pass it to the next generations. Stephen O'Brien said that the

chance of this gene randomly reaching its current frequency in the white population is about **zero**. The idea that a mutant gene can confer protection against a specific infection is not new. The mutation that causes sickle cell anemia provides people carrying one copy of it with resistance (but not immunity) to malaria. There is some evidence that the cystic fibrosis mutation may protect against typhoid fever.

How HIV Kills the T4 or CD4+ Immune Cells

In July 2001, Jacques Corbeil and colleagues at the University of California at San Diego reported for the first time on how HIV assaults the human immune T4 or CD4+ cell. Using sophisticated technology, the team of researchers looked within the body's immune cells and recorded the molecular events triggered by invasion of HIV. They created a detailed account of the devastating progression of cellular injury following HIV infection. For this study, an HIV-infected CD4+ T-cell line was monitored following infection at eight time intervals, from 30 minutes to 72 hours after exposure. They monitored some 7,000 genes over this time period in an attempt to discover what effect HIV's genes would have on the cell's genes. For each interval, 10 million infected cells were applied to a microarray gene chip. A control sample of healthy cells was analyzed at the same intervals for comparison. According to the researchers, HIV invades and swiftly overpowers the DNA of the immune cells and inserts its own genes. HIV interrupts the cells genes and alters the cellular mitochondrial energy source. In addition, it suppresses the immune cells' DNA repair mechanisms while inducing other genes to initiate their own death. The first observation by the researchers came 30 minutes after infection. At that time HIV had already suppressed more than 500 genes in the infected cells and had activated 200 other genes that included suicide genes, or those activated as part of the normal cycle of cell death, known as apoptosis. Three days after infection of 1,400 genes expected to be active, based on healthy cell measurements, half were suppressed—not functioning. The research has moved the study of HIV from observing clinical signs and symptoms of HIV to studying the molecular changes HIV forces on a living cell. Such research may lead to new drug therapies and the next step in finding an effective vaccine.

T4 CELL DEPLETION AND IMMUNE SUPPRESSION

In addition to the new insight as to how HIV kills T4 or CD4+ cells, there are other ways in which these immune cells are depleted.

Recent research using the **polymerase chain reaction** (a method of amplifying present but unmeasurable quantities of HIV DNA in T4 cells into measurable quantities) has revealed that about *one in every 10 to 100* **T4 cells is HIV-infected in an AIDS patient**. Thus T4 cells serve as reservoirs of HIV in the body (Schnittman et al., 1989; Cohen, 1993). Collectively, T4 cell depletion leads to cumulative and devastating effects on the cell-mediated and humoral parts of the immune system.

Means by Which T4 Cells May Be Lost

1. *Filling CD4 Receptor Sites*— There is evidence from in vitro studies that HIV can attack CD4 receptor sites in at least two ways. First, HIV can attach, via its gp160 "spikes," to CD4 receptor sites. Second, HIV is capable of releasing or freeing its exterior gp120 envelope glycoprotein, thereby generating a molecule that can actively bind to CD4-bearing cells (Gelderblom et al., 1985). As a result of filling the receptor sites on the T4 cells, the T4 cells lose their immune functions; that is, the T4 cell does not have to be infected with HIV to lose immune function. In addition, CD4-bearing cells that attach the free gp120 molecule then become targets for immune attack by antibody-mediated antibody-dependent cell cytotoxicity (ADCC) and non-antibody-mediated cytotoxic T cells. Both events can result in the destruction of uninfected CD4 bearing cells. The extent to which this occurs in vivo depends on the level of gp120 synthesis, secretion, and shedding. Free gp120 has not yet been measured in the circulation, but this is not surprising given its powerful affinity for CD4 (Bolognesi, 1989).

2. *Syncytia Formation*— The formation of syncytia involves fusion of the cell membrane of an infected cell with the cell membranes of uninfected CD4 cells, which results in giant multi-nucleated cells (Figure 3-7). A direct relation between the presence of syncytia and the degree of the cytopathic effect of the virus in individual cells has been demonstrated in vitro, and HIV isolated during the

accelerated phase of infection in vivo has a greater capacity to induce syncytia in vitro. Syncytia have rarely been seen in vivo.

In the asymptomatic phase of HIV infection, predominantly nonsyncytium inducing (NSI), HIV variants can be detected. In about 50% of the cases SI HIV variants emerge in the course of infection, preceding rapid T4 cell depletion and progression to AIDS (Groenink et al., 1993).

3. *Superantigens*— Superantigens are bacterial or viral antigens that are capable of interacting with a very large number of T4 cells. Unlike a conventional antigen, which usually evokes a response from less than one in a million (0.01%) T4 cells, a superantigen can interact with 5% to 30% of T4 cells. They directly bind to the exposed surfaces of MHC class II molecules on **antigen-presenting cells (APCs)** and to the variable region of the T cell receptors (TCR) β chain ($V_β$) on the responding T cells. Therefore, superantigens can interact with a large fraction of T cells, resulting in cellular activation, proliferation, anergy (absence of reaction to an antigen), or deletion of specific T cell subsets. Bacterial superantigens include staphylococcal enterotoxins and the toxic shock syndrome toxin-1, which are the causative agents for several human diseases such as food poisoning and toxic shock syndrome (Phillips et al., 1995). The superantigen hypothesis regarding HIV infection stems from the observations that endogenous or exogenous retroviral-encoded super-antigens stimulate murine T4 cells in vivo, leading to the anergy or deletion of a substantial percentage of T4 cells that have the specific variable β regions (Pantaleo et al., 1993).

4. *Apoptosis*— Programmed cell death, or apoptosis (a-po-toe-sis), is a normal mechanism of cell death that was originally described in the context of the response of immature thymocytes to cellular activation. It is a mechanism whereby the body eliminates autoreactive clones of T cells.

In a typical day, 60 billion or 70 billion cells perish in your body. Much of this normal cellular turnover involves **apoptosis**. When apoptotic pathways are defective, insufficient cell death can lead to cancers and autoimmune diseases, and excessive cell death can result in neurodegeneration or stroke. Accordingly, much work is being done to define key players in apoptosis.

It has recently been suggested that both qualitative and quantitative defects in T4 cells in patients with HIV infection may be the result of activation-induced cell death or apoptosis. Because apoptosis can be induced in mature mouse T4 cells after cross-linking CD4 molecules to one another and triggering the T4 cell antigen receptor, there has been speculation that cross-linking of the CD4 molecule by HIV gp120 or gp120-anti-gp120 immune complexes prepares the human cell for the programmed death that occurs when a MHC class II molecule in complex with an antigen binds to the T4 cell antigen receptor. Thus activation of a prepared cell by a specific

antigen or superantigen could lead to the death of the cell, without direct infection by HIV (Pantaleo et al., 1993). For an excellent review of apoptosis and its role in human disease, see Barr et al., 1994; Hengartner, 1995; and Yeh, 1998.

5. *Cellular Transfer of HIV*— Infected macrophages, or antigen-presenting cells, which normally interact with the T4 cells to stimulate the immune function, can transfer HIV into uninfected T4 lymphocytes. **In any case, immediate viral or proviral replication, kills the T4 cell**.

6. *Autoimmune Mechanisms*— One of the older theories, namely that HIV tricks the immune system into attacking itself is back because of the recent work of Tracy Kion and Geoffrey Hoffmann (1991). Their work showed that mice immunized with lymphocytes from another mouse strain make antibodies to the HIV envelope protein gp120, as do autoimmune strains of mice, even though **none of the animals had ever been exposed to the AIDS virus**. One implication of these results is that some component on the lymphocytes resembles gp120 closely enough so that antibodies directed against it can recognize gp120 as well. The converse is that antibodies to gp120 should also recognize the lymphocyte component so that an immune response directed against HIV might also interfere with normal lymphocyte function. The autoimmune theory is consistent with results that show there is a selective loss of particular subsets of T cells in AIDS patients.

7. *Cofactors May Help Deplete T4 Cells*— HIV-infected people who are asymptomatic show a wide variation in HIV disease time and progression to AIDS. It is believed that cofactors may be responsible for some of the time variation with regard to disease progression.

Many agents may act as cofactors to activate or increase HIV production. Although, in general, it is not believed that any cofactor is necessary for HIV infection, cofactors such as nutrition, stress, and infectious organisms have been considered as agents that might accelerate HIV expression after infection. Three new human herpes viruses (HHV-6, 7, and 8) may be cofactors and play a role in causing immune deficiency. They have been shown to infect HIV-infected T4 cells and activate the HIV provirus to increase HIV replication (Laurence, 1996). Cytomegalovirus and the Epstein-Barr virus have also been associated with increased HIV expression. Over time, investigators expect to find other sexually transmitted diseases that behave as cofactors associated with HIV infection and expression.

Drugs may also be cofactors in infection. Used by injection drug users (IDUs), heroin and other morphine-based derivatives are known to reduce human resistance to infection and produce immunological suppression. *Pneumocystis carinii* pneumonia is about twice as frequent in heroin users as in homosexuals. It is believed that the heroin has an immunosuppressive effect within the lungs (Brown, 1987).

Blood and blood products may also act as cofactors in infection because they are immunosuppressive. Because blood transfusions save lives, their long-range effects are generally overlooked. Transfusions in hemophiliacs, for example, result in lowered resistance to viruses such as cytomegalovirus (CMV), Epstein-Barr (Berkman, 1984; Blumberg et al., 1985; Foster et al., 1985), and perhaps HIV. Seminal fluid (fluid bathing the sperm) may also act as a cofactor in infection because it also causes immunosuppression. One of its physiological functions is to immunosuppress the female genital tract so that the sperm is not immunologically rejected (Witkin et al., 1983; Baxena et al., 1985).

Epidemiologically, homosexuals at greatest risk of AIDS are those who practice passive anal sex, that is, **anal recipients** (Kingsley et al., 1987). It is generally considered that this sexual behavior is a cofactor that enables the AIDS virus to enter the bloodstream by means of traumatic lacerations of the rectal mucosa.

Last but not least of the agents that can suppress the immune system and thereby act as a cofactor in HIV infection is **stress**. Stress can be mental or physical; but it is easier to measure the effects of physical stress.

Although moderate exercise appears to stimulate the immune system, there is good evidence that intensive exercise can suppress the immune system. We still do not really know why (Fitzgerald, 1988; LaPierre et al., 1992). The effect of stress on the immune system is one of the reasons why physicians did not want Earvin "Magic" Johnson to play basketball (see Box 8.5 in Chapter 8).

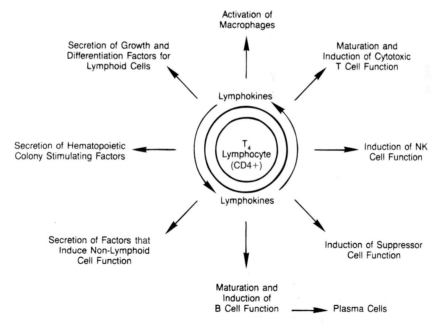

FIGURE 5-8 The T4 Cell Role in the Immune Response. T4 lymphocytes are responsible directly or indirectly for inducing a wide array of functions in cells that produce the immune response. They also induce nonlymphoid cell functions. T cell involvement is effected for the most part by the secretion of soluble factors or **lymphokines** that have trophic or inductive effects on the cells presented in the figure. Lymphokines serve to transfer control of the immune response from the external environmental proteins to the internal regulatory system consisting of ligands and receptors. *(Adapted from Fauci, 1991)*

IMPACT OF T4 CELL DEPLETION

The overall impact of T4 cell depletion is multi-faceted. HIV-induced T4 cell abnormalities alter the T4 cells' ability to produce a variety of inducer chemical stimulants such as the **interleukins** that are necessary for the proper maturation of B cells into plasma cells and the maturation of a subset of T cells into cytotoxic cells (Figure 5-8). Thus the critical basis for the immunopathogenesis of HIV infection is the depletion of the *T4 lymphocytes*, which results in profound immunosuppression.

Presumably, with time, the number of HIV-infected T4 cells increases to a point where, in terminal AIDS patients, **few normal T4 cells exist**.

Saha Kunal and colleagues reported on the isolation of CD8+ lymphocytes from HIV-infected patients who produced new HIV. The HIV produced by the CD8+ cells were able to infect both the CD4+ (T4) and CD8+ (T8) cells. CD4+ produced HIV infected CD8+ cells without using the R4 or R5 coreceptors that HIV use to infect CD4+ cells. These data are additional evidence of HIV's ability to adapt to existing biology and to continue to replicate itself.

ROLE OF MONOCYTES AND MACROPHAGES IN HIV INFECTION

Some scientists now believe that T4 cell infection alone does not cause AIDS because not enough T4 cells are destroyed. They believe that equally important to T4 cell infection is **monocyte** and **macrophage** infection (Bakker et. al., 1992). Monocytes change into various types of macrophages (given different names) in order to search and destroy foreign agents within tissues of the lungs, brain, and interstitial tissues, tissues that connect organs. Despite the name changes, all forms of macrophages basically work the same way: They ingest things. Some macrophages travel around within the body, others become attached to one spot, ingesting.

Macrophages are often the first cells of the immune system to encounter invaders, particularly in the area of a cut or wound. After engulfing the invader, the macrophage makes copies of the invader's antigens and **displays** them on its own cell membrane. These **copies of the invader antigens sit next to the self molecules. In effect, the macrophage makes a "wanted poster" of this new**

invader. The macrophage then travels about showing the wanted poster to T4 or CD4+ cells, which triggers the T4 cells into action. Macrophages also release chemicals which stimulate both T4 cell and macrophage production and draw macrophages and lymphocytes to the site of infection.

Macrophages may play an important role in spreading HIV infection in the body, both to other cells and to HIV's target organs. First, HIV enters macrophage and spreads from macrophage to macrophage before the immune system is alerted. **Second,** macrophages, in their different forms, travel to the brain, the lungs, the bone marrow, and to various immune organs, carrying HIV to these organs.

HIV's ability to infect brain tissue is particularly important. The brain and cerebral spinal fluid (CSF) are specially protected sites. CSF cushions the brain and the spinal cord from sudden and jarring movements. The brainblood barrier, a chemical phenomenon, normally stops foreign substances from entering the brain and the CSF. But HIV-infected monocytes can pass through this barrier. **For HIV, monocyte-macrophages are Trojan horses, enabling HIV to enter the immune-protected domain of the central nervous system—the brain, the spine, the rest of the nervous system.**

HIV isolates taken from macrophages appear to grow better in macrophages than in lymphocytes. In human cell culture experiments, HIV isolates taken from lymphocytes appear to grow better in lymphocytes than in macrophages. These peculiarities of replication rates may be evidence of separate tissue-oriented HIV strains.

HIV-infected macrophages have proven to be a major problem in efforts to control and stop HIV infection.

Clinical Latency: Where Have All the Viruses Been Hiding?

The immunodeficiency syndrome caused by HIV is characterized by **profound T4 or CD4+ cell depletion.** Prior to the progressive decline of T4 cells and the development of AIDS, there is a symptom-free period that may last for 10 or more years, during which the infection is thought to be clinically latent. Scientists thought little if any viral replication occurred during this period. In recent years, a number of studies have offered an alternative view. Some investigations suggest that there is no real la-

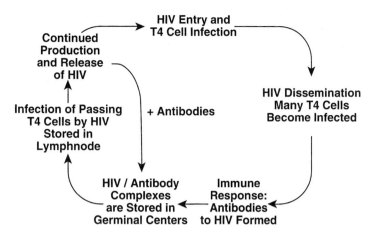

FIGURE 5-9 The Role of HIV Antibody in HIV Seeding of the Lymph Glands and Infection of New T4 Cells. To rid the body of HIV requires a way to cleanse the lymph nodes of HIV. *(Adapted from Fox, 1996)*

tency period in HIV infection. Instead, **starting from the moment of infection, there appears to be a continuous struggle between HIV and the immune system, the balance of which slowly shifts in favor of the virus.** Cecil H. Fox of the Yale School of Medicine reported in December 1991 that HIV is not lying dormant at all but is continually infecting immune cells in the **lymph nodes** (Figure 5-9).

The **lymph nodes,** which are pea-sized capsules that trap foreign invaders and produce immune cells, are all over the body and are connected by vessels much like those that transport blood. Deep within the lymph nodes of 18 HIV-infected patients, researchers found millions of viruses. Based on those data, Fox suggested that HIV uses the lymph nodes as places to meet up with most immune cells. Fox believes that HIV begins replication in T4 cells in the lymph nodes soon after it enters the body. Infected T4 cells leave the lymph nodes and new uninfected cells arrive to become infected. Years later, when enough immune cells have been killed, the patient's defenses become so impaired that he or she is vulnerable to any one of a wide array of opportunistic infections—AIDS has arrived.

Anthony Fauci (Figure 5-10), the head of the National Institute of Allergy and Infectious Diseases (NIAID), and Sonya Heath and colleagues (1995) agree that there are many more HIVs in the lymph nodes than in the blood. Studies in his

FIGURE 5-10 Anthony S. Fauci, M.D. Director, National Institute of Allergy and Infectious Diseases, National Institutes of Health; Associate Director of NIH for AIDS Research. In 2001, he received the Annunzio Humanitarian Award for his impact on the understanding and treatment of infectious diseases/AIDS. *(Photograph courtesy of National Institute of Allergy and Infectious Diseases)*

laboratory have shown there are many millions of HIV particles stuck to what are known as **follicular dendritic cells** in the lymph nodes of an infected individual.

The follicular dendritic cells, which have thousands of feathery processes emanating from them and whose **normal function is to filter and trap antigens for presentation to antibody-producing B lymphocytes, serve as highly effective trapping centers for extracellular HIV particles.** Virtually every lymphocyte in a lymph node is enmeshed in the processes of these cells. Follicular dendritic cells themselves are susceptible to HIV infection, and appear to place huge numbers of virus particles into intimate contact with other cells that are susceptible to HIV infection (Haase et al., 1996; Knight, 1996).

During the clinically latent phase, the lymph nodes of an infected individual are slowly destroyed.

In the final phase of an infection, the follicular dendritic network completely dissolves and the architecture of the lymph node collapses to produce what Fauci called a **"burnt-out lymph node."** With this collapse, large amounts of HIV are released into the circulatory system and an ever-increasing number of peripheral cells are infected with HIV (Baum, 1992; Edgington, 1993).

In 1995, David Ho and colleagues, Xiping Wei and colleagues, and Martin Nowak and colleagues published separate reports on the rapid production of HIV that begins soon after initial HIV infection.

Rapid viral replication countered by a strong immune response is not unknown; on the contrary, it is characteristic of acute, short-lived viral infections, such as measles or the flu. But in those infections, the immune system most often wins: It rids the body of the virus and builds resistance to future infection. The question is why can't the immune system do the same against HIV? Perhaps it's the length and intensity of the struggle that ultimately does in the immune system by encouraging the emergence of mutant viruses that outstrip the immune system's ability to continue making new types of antibody. During the time when the immune system is functioning well and producing new antibody against each new HIV variant, the struggle between HIV production and immune suppression of the viral load must move repeatedly from the virus to the immune system and back until the immune system is, with time, over-

whelmed with the number of different types of antibody it must rapidly produce in large quantity.

Implications of a High HIV Replication Rate

Based on Ho and colleagues kinetic studies of viral replication, it can be estimated that the population of HIV undergoes between 3000 and 5000 replication cycles (**generations**) over the course of 10 years, producing a **minimum of 10^{12} (1 trillion) HIV** in an HIV-infected person. This creates a lot of opportunity for HIV RNA evolution because genetic mutations occur most commonly during replication. Some mutations will weaken HIV in such a way as to expose it to attack by the immune system. But other mutations will aid the virus, speeding its replication and increasing the chances it can evade the immune system. Because HIV gets so many chances to replicate, it evolves and mutates, and those strains with the greatest replication efficiency gradually win out. **This is Darwinian evolution going on in one patient.**

HIV has been shown to have a random (any base has an equal chance of changing) mutation rate of approximately 1 mutation per 10,000 nucleotides **AND** one mutation caused by reverse transcriptase copy error (**transcription error**) per round of replication. The **combination** of events results in too many variants for the immune system to handle. For example, a single HIV-infected person, by the time he or she is diagnosed with AIDS, may have billions of HIV variants in his or her body. With so many variants present, some will be resistant to most if not all drugs currently used in therapy and to drugs that have **not yet been created!** The constant production of variant HIVs produce the drug-resistant mutants and not the action of the drug.

In 1996 the hope was that HAART could wipe out HIV. This hope was based on two ideas, both later proved to be wrong: that the drugs would completely stop the virus from reproducing, and that there were **no reservoirs where the HIV could hide.** But HIV has the uncanny ability to reestablish itself in a variety of cell types. Even the most rigorous attempts to reduce or eliminate HIV from these reservoirs have failed. Scientists had vastly **underestimated** the extent of virus activity in an HIV-infected person, particularly during the asymptomatic or clinically latent phase. These and other recent studies should satisfy the major unanswered question concerning HIV disease/AIDS, which was, **"Where is the virus?"** During the 1980s, it was difficult to find medium to high levels of HIV in persons with HIV disease or even in those persons in the later stages of AIDS.

We now know that there are large amounts of HIV present early on in the lymph nodes of HIV-diseased people and in viral reservoirs. Perhaps the most troubled group of researchers now may be those currently developing AIDS vaccines.(See Chapter 9 for a discussion about possible HIV vaccines.)

SUMMARY

After a healthy person is HIV-infected, he or she makes antibodies against those viruses that are in the bloodstream, but not against those that have become integrated as HIV proviruses in the host immune cell DNA. Over time the immune system cells that are involved in antibody production are destroyed. Evidence is accumulating that cofactors such as nutrition, stress, and previous exposure to other sexually transmitted diseases that increase HIV expression are associated with HIV infection and HIV disease. Agents that suppress the immune system may also play a significant role in establishing HIV infection. In short, HIV infection is permanent. HIV attaches to CD4-bearing cells and enters those cells using one or more of at least four chemokine receptors—**CC-CKR-2, CC-CKR-3, CXCKR-4 (FUSIN), and CC-CKR-5.** These coreceptors allow HIV to fuse with the cell membrane, and enter the cell, after HIV attachment to the CD4 receptor. And, as seen in Chapter 3, HIV undergoes rapid genetic change, and, as far as is known, **attacks only human cells—mostly of the human immune system.** It has recently become quite clear that large amounts of the virus are produced within weeks after HIV infection. The virus remains, for the most part, in the lymph nodes until very late in the disease process.

REVIEW QUESTIONS

(Answers to the Review Questions are on page 489.)

1. Which cell type is believed to be the main target for HIV infection? Explain the biological impact of this particular infection.

2. What is CD4, where is it found, and what is its role in the HIV infection process?

3. Is there a period of latency after HIV infection—a time when few or no new HIV are being produced?

4. True or False: HIV is the cause of AIDS.

5. True or False: HIV primarily affects red blood cells.

6. True or False: Lymphocytes have a major role in the immune response to antigens.

7. True or False: All T and B lymphocytes inhibit or destroy foreign antigens.

8. True or False: CD4 and CD8 molecules are antibodies.

9. True or False: HIV belongs to the family of retroviruses.

10. True or False: Cytotoxic and suppressor T lymphocytes are the main targets of HIV.

11. True or False: The latent period is that time between initial infection with HIV and the onset of AIDS.

12. True or False: HIV can spread to infect new cells after it buds out of infected cells.

13. True or False: HIV causes the gradual destruction of cells bearing the CD4 molecule.

14. The most effective use of T4 cell counts in the clinical management of patients with HIV infection is for:

    A. Determining when to initiate therapy.

    B. Assessing risk of disease progression.

    C. Deciding on prophylaxis for opportunistic infections.

    D. Measuring the antiretroviral effect of initial therapy.

6 Opportunistic Infections and Cancers Associated With HIV Disease/AIDS

CHAPTER CONCEPTS

♦ Suppression of the immune system allows **harmless** agents to become **harmful** opportunistic infections (OIs).
♦ OIs respond well to Highly Active Antiretroviral Therapy (HAART).
♦ OIs in AIDS patients are caused by viruses, bacteria, fungi, and protozoa.
♦ About 95% of the HIV infected are coinfected with herpes 1 and/or 2.
♦ Human Herpes Virus-8 may be the cause of Kaposi's sarcoma.
♦ In the United States, 14% of AIDS patients are coinfected with tuberculosis.
♦ The cost of treating OIs can be very high.
♦ There are two types of Kaposi's sarcoma (KS): classic and AIDS-associated.
♦ KS is rarely found in hemophiliacs, injection drug users, and women with AIDS.
♦ The clinical presentation of OIs has been impacted by the use of protease inhibitors.

WHAT IS AN OPPORTUNISTIC DISEASE?

Humans evolved in the presence of a wide range of parasites—viruses, bacteria, fungi, and protozoa that do not cause disease in people with an intact immune system. But these organisms can cause a disease in someone with a weakened immune system, such as an individual with HIV disease. The infections they cause are known as **opportunistic infections** (OIs). Thus, OIs occur after a disease-causing virus or microorganism, normally held in check by a functioning immune system, gets the opportunity to multiply and invade host tissue after the immune system has been compromised. For most of medical history, OIs were rare and almost always appeared in patients whose immunity was impaired by either cancer or genetic disease.

With improved medical technology, a steadily growing number of patients are severely immunosuppressed because of medications and radiation used in bone marrow or organ transplantation and cancer chemotherapy. **HIV disease also suppresses the immune system.** Perhaps as a corollary to their increased prevalence, or because of heightened physician awareness, OIs seem to be occurring more frequently in the elderly, who may

be rendered vulnerable by age-related declines in immunity. New OIs are now being diagnosed because the pool of people who can get them is so much larger, and, in addition, new techniques for identifying the causative organisms have been developed. However, most of the infections considered opportunistic are not reportable, which interferes with a clear-cut count of their growing numbers.

Although OIs are still not commonplace, they are no longer considered rare—they occur in tens of thousands of HIV/AIDS patients. But despite this increase, physicians and their patients have reasons to be optimistic about their ability to contain these infections. The reasons are: (**1**) In a massive federal effort, driven by the HIV/AIDS epidemic, researchers are finding drugs that can prevent or treat many of the OIs; and (**2**) various anti-HIV drug therapies have shown promise for warding off OIs by boosting patients' immune systems.

THE PREVALENCE OF OPPORTUNISTIC DISEASES

The prevalence of OIs in the United States is very high. There are some 250,000 HIV-seropositive individuals with T4 or CD4+ cell counts below

200/μL of blood. More than 100 microorganisms—bacteria, viruses, fungi, and protozoa—can cause disease in such individuals, even though only a fraction of these (17) are included in the current surveillance definition for clinical AIDS. In a large survey from the Centers for Disease Control and Prevention (CDC), such OIs were diagnosed in 33% of individuals at one year and in 58% at two years after documentation of a T4 cell count below 200/μL. In 1995, 1997, 1999 and in 2001 the CDC presented guidelines for prevention and treatment of OIs in HIV-infected persons (*MMWR*, 2001). The new treatments for OIs have extended the survival of AIDS patients, but they have also opened new issues. With the growing proportion of long-term AIDS survivors, new OIs have become prominent, together with concerns about cost, compliance, drug interactions, and quality of life (Laurence, 1995; *MMWR*, 1995). The six most common AIDS-related OIs are bacterial pneumonia, candidal esophagitis, pulmonary/disseminated TB, mycobacterium avium complex disease, herpes simplex reinfection, and *Pneumocystis carinii* pneumonia or PCP. **The year 1997 marked the first time, since the AIDS pandemic began in the United States, that the incidence of AIDS-defining OIs among HIV-infected persons fell in number from the previous year's total.** The number of OIs dropped 7% in 1997 compared to 1996 (HIV/AIDS Surveillance Report, 1997).

PROPHYLAXIS AGAINST OPPORTUNISTIC INFECTIONS

Drug prophylaxis against OIs has become a cornerstone of treatment for AIDS patients. For example, the prevalence of PCP dropped from about 80% in 1987 to about 20% by mid-1994 because of excellent drug therapy. The mortality of PCP without treatment is almost 100% (Dobkin, 1995). Researchers at the University of California, San Francisco, found that on average it costs $215,000 to extend by one year, the life of an HIV-infected patient with PCP who is treated in an intensive care unit (Laurence (1996)). That is more than twice the comparable care cost for 1988. Part of the reason given was that as people with AIDS survived longer, they were presenting with third, fourth, and fifth episodes of PCP, superimposed on other chronic infections. The downside to OI

prophylaxis is that it is difficult to find drugs that work without harmful side effects. In addition, viruses and organisms that cause OIs become resistant to the drugs over time. This is one of the primary reasons researchers are looking for ways in which to boost an immunosuppressed patient's immune system.

OPPORTUNISTIC INFECTIONS IN HIV-INFECTED PEOPLE

AIDS is a devastating human tragedy. It appears to be killing about everyone who demonstrates the symptoms. One well-known American surgeon said, **"I would rather die of any form of cancer rather than die of AIDS."** This statement was not made because of the social stigma attached to AIDS, or because it is a lethal condition. It was made in recognition of the slow, demoralizing, debilitating, painful, disfiguring, helpless, and unending struggle to stay alive.

Because of a suppressed and weakened immune system, viruses, bacteria, fungi, and protozoa that commonly and harmlessly inhabit the body become pathogenic (Figure 6-1). In addition, organisms and viruses from old infections that have lingered in the body reactivate. The suppression of the immune system presents an **opportunity** for the harmless to become harmful. Prior to 1998 about 90% of deaths related to HIV infection and AIDS were caused by OIs, compared with 7% due to cancer and 3% due to other causes. Now, with the use of antiretroviral drugs, OIs cause about 50% of deaths. Liver and kidney organ failure, heart disease, and various cancers are on the increase as the cause of death in AIDS patients.

HIV-Related Opportunistic Infections Vary Worldwide

The course of HIV infection tends to be similar for most patients: infection with the virus is followed by seroconversion and progressive destruction of T4 or CD4+ cells. Yet the opportunistic infections and malignancies that largely define the symptomatic or clinical history of HIV disease vary geographically. People with HIV and their physicians in different regions confront distinct problems, mainly because of differences in exposure, in access to diagnosis and care, and in general health.

Comparisons between the data about opportunistic infections in different countries must be

FIGURE 6-1 General Progression of Opportunistic Infections after HIV Infection. Normal T4 or CD4+ cell count in adolescent/adults is, on average, about 1000/μL of blood. There is a relationship between the drop in T4 lymphocytes and the onset of opportunistic infections (OIs). The first sign of an OI begins under 500 T4 cells/μL. As the T4 cell count continues to drop, the chance of OI infection increases. Note the variety of OIs found in AIDS patients with 200 or less T4 cells/μL.

THE CHANGING SPECTRUM OF OPPORTUNISTIC INFECTIONS

Only 10 years ago there was hardly any standardized use of protective agents to block the infectious complications or opportunistic infections (OIs) associated with HIV-induced immunodeficiency. Now there is an array of drugs that can be used in strategies to prevent or delay nearly all the major OIs. With this advancement has come the need to weigh the pros and cons of various strategies. Cost, antimicrobial resistance, drug interactions, and pill overload are all important considerations.

EFFECT OF ANTI-HIV THERAPY ON OPPORTUNISTIC INFECTIONS

As presented in Chapter 4, the use of anti-HIV combination drug therapy (AIDS drug cocktails) has produced a number of unexpected results in patient response to those drugs. Soon after combination therapy began, physicians witnessed a rather **confusing** or **unusual** presentation of OIs. In some cases certain OIs improved, in others the situation deteriorated! Such changes in OIs expression are occurring now, at a time when hundreds of thousands of HIV-infected people need **Highly Active Antiretroviral Therapy (HAART).**

TREATMENT IN THE HAART ERA

HAART therapy appears to scramble the human immune system. When HIV patients take retroviral medicines that control HIV replication, their immune systems begin to recuperate in ways that are puzzling and controversial. For example, patients recover immunity to some deadly opportunistic infections but appear unable to fight diseases for which they were vaccinated as children, for example, tetanus, or to target HIV itself. Collectively, such observations indicate HAART patients can only raise successful immune responses against pathogens they see **regularly.** For example, cytomegalovirus is an organism found in everybody's blood, so the immune systems of HAART patients see the pathogen constantly and generate cells and antibodies that attack it. But tetanus is something people rarely encounter, so HAART patients, unlike their HIV-negative counterparts, fail to raise immune responses against it. And the ultimate irony is that HAART, when successful, kills all but a few million HIVs that are forced into hiding. Therefore, the immune system doesn't see

HIV anymore and stops making cells and antibodies against the virus.

Recent studies suggest that the incidence of esophageal candidiasis and, by inference, other forms of *Candida* infection has fallen by 60% to 70% on patients treated with HAART. The use of HAART dramatically changed the epidemiology of opportunistic infections and is clearly associated with gradual recovery of the immune system (Powderly et al., 1998; Ledergerber et al., 1999).

This information aside, when HIV is controlled with the antiretroviral drugs, immunity to infections—**other than HIV**—usually starts to return. As a result, some opportunistic infections go away without specific treatment; and sometimes patients can stop prophylactic treatment for certain opportunistic diseases. However, entering year 2002, it is still unclear who can stop prophylaxis safely, and who cannot.

Studies from 1998 through 2001, using protease inhibitor drugs in HAART have shown that virtually no patient whose T4 level rose to and stayed over 100 per microliter of blood (μl) developed an OI. This is the strongest evidence to date that immune reconstruction is occurring with protease inhibitor therapy, and suggests that it occurs early and with quite modest improvements in T4 cell levels. The implication is that the search for immunorestorative therapy other than with the current antiretroviral is somewhat less urgent than previously believed, though still a clear priority.

Rates of Most HIV-Related Diseases No Longer Falling

A hallmark of the HAART era (1996 to present) has been the dramatic decline in the incidence of AIDS-related opportunistic illnesses (OIs). This was evident even within the first year of widespread use of HAART, and the downward trend continued for several years. A report from the CDC presented trends in the incidence of 26 OIs and malignancies during the period from 1995 to 1999. The analysis was based on data from 20,455 HIV-infected patients seen at 11 U.S. treatment centers. The population appeared to be generally representative of the overall U.S. population, but with greater representation of minority populations. Women comprised 26% of the study group and were analyzed separately from men. Overall, the annual trends in incidence showed significant decreases in 20 of the 26 OIs from 1995 to 1999. Among men, significant decreases were seen in 19 of the 25 OIs with no trend observed for the remaining 6. Among women, 11 of the 26 OIs showed decreasing trends, 14 had no trend, and cervical cancer was shown to be increasing. From 1998 into 2000, however, there was no change in the incidence of any OIs except for decreasing rates of cerebral toxoplasmosis and DMV retinitis. This leveling off is consistent with the perceptions of some clinicians with large HIV practices who have noted a resurgence of certain opportunistic diseases. While this partly comprises patients who first present with advanced HIV disease, there is also the possibility that some patients are now seeing the limits of the durability of the clinical benefit from HAART (Bartlett, 2002).

OMINOUS SHADOWS

It is now clear that sustained viral suppression is not feasible in all patients receiving HAART. **A third post-HAART era is projected, during which resurgence of opportunistic infections will be seen. This era may be marked by a higher rate of infection by antimicrobial-resistant microorganisms in patients with HIV infection than in the pre-HAART era of the late 1980s to the late-1990s.**

VIRAL LOAD RELATED TO OPPORTUNISTIC INFECTIONS

HIV-clinicians have recently looked at the predictive value of plasma HIV RNA for the development of three OIs: PCP, CMV, and MAC. Using a database of patients participating in AIDS Clinical Trial Groups (ACTG), for every 1-log increase in plasma HIV RNA, the risk of developing one of these OIs was increased 2- to 3-fold. Plasma HIV RNA level was predictive of an increased risk of an OI independent of T4 cell count, which also predicted OI risk. This information confirms that maintaining control of viral replication may be a critical component of preventing OIs in HIV-infected patients.

---

made with care. But, most developing nations lack the facilities and trained personnel to identify opportunistic infections correctly; consequently, their prevalence may be underreported. Clinicians in developed countries can order sophisticated laboratory analyses to identify pathogens. Those in developing countries must rely on signs and symptoms to make their diagnoses. Oral candidiasis and herpes zoster are easy to diagnose without laboratory backup because the lesions are visible. While some pneumonias and types of diarrhea can be specified, others, such as extrapulmonary tuberculosis, cytomegalovirus infections, cryptococcal meningitis, and systemic infections such as histoplasmosis, toxoplasmosis, microsporidiosis, and nocardiosis, go underreported due to the lack of laboratory facilities.

Socioeconomic Factors

Geography explains much about the varying patterns of opportunistic infections, but a decisive factor is often financial capacity. On the most fundamental level, **money** is needed to create an infrastructure that limits exposure to pathogens. Thus, while few people with HIV in wealthy countries develop certain bacterial or protozoal infections, they are a major cause of death in poor areas that cannot provide clean water and adequate food storage facilities.

Financial resources also affect clinicians' abilities to diagnose AIDS and, when appropriate, to provide the proper medicine. AIDS patients in Africa often die of severe bacterial infections because they don't have the antibiotics or the clinical care they need. They don't survive long enough to develop diseases such as PCP.

United States, Europe, and Africa— The United States and Europe on one end, and Africa on the other, represent the global extremes of financial resources for health care. The most common opportunistic infections each region faces reflect the overall quality of health care, sanitation, and diet. For example, Thailand and Mexico belong to the large group of nations that have intermediate incomes and correspondingly intermediate patterns of HIV complications (Harvard AIDS Institute, 1994).

AIDS patients rarely have just one infection (Table 6-1). The mix of OIs may depend on lifestyle and where the HIV/AIDS patient lives or has lived. Thus, a knowledge of the person's ori-

Table 6-1 Some Common Opportunistic Diseases Associated With HIV Infection and Possible Therapy

Organism/Virus	Clinical Manifestation	Possible Treatments
Protozoa		
Cryptosporidium muris	Gastroenteritis (inflammation of stomach-intestine membranes)	Investigational only
Isospora belli	Gastroenteritis	Trimethoprim-sulfamethoxazole (Bactrim)
Toxoplasma gondii	Encephalitis (brain abscess), retinitis, disseminated	Pyrimethamine and leucovorin, plus sulfadiazine, or Clindamycin, Bactrim
Fungi		
Candida sp.	Stomatitis (thrush), proctitis, vaginitis, esophagitis	Nystatin, clotrimazole, ketoconazole
Coccidioides immitis	Meningitis, dissemination	Amphotericin B, fluconazole, ketoconazole
Cryptococcus neoformans	Meningitis (membrane inflammation of spinal cord and brain), pneumonia, encephalitis, dissemination (widespread)	Amphotericin B, fluconazole, itraconazole
Histoplasma capsulatum	Pneumonia, dissemination	Amphotericin B, fluconazole, itraconazole
Pneumocystis carinii	Pneumonia	Trimethoprim-sulfamethoxazole (Bactrim, Septra), pentamidine, dapsone, clindamycin, trimetrexate
Bacteria		
Mycobacterium avium complex (MAC)	Dissemination, pneumonia, diarrhea, weight loss, lymphadenopathy, severe gastrointestinal disease	Rifampin + ethambutol + clofazimine + ciprofloxacin +/- amikacin; rifabutin, clarithromycin & azithromycin
Mycobacterium tuberculosis (TB)	Pneumonia (tuberculosis), meningitis, dissemination	Isoniazid (INH) + rifampin + ethambutol +/- pyrazinamide
Viruses		
Cytomegalovirus (CMV)	Fever, hepatitis, encephalitis, retinitis, pneumonia, colitis, esophagitis	Ganciclovir, Foscarnet
Epstein-Barr	Oral hairy leukoplakia, B cell lymphoma	Acyclovir
Herpes simplex	Mucocutaneous (mouth, genital, rectal) blisters and/or ulcers, pneumonia, esophagitis, encephalitis	Acyclovir Famciclovir
Papovavirus J-C	Progressive multifocal leukoencephalopathy	none
Varicella-zoster	Dermatomal skin lesions (shingles), encephalitis	Acyclovir, Foscarnet
Cancers		
Kaposi's sarcoma	Disseminated mucocutaneous lesions often involving skin, lymph nodes, visceral organs (especially lungs and GI tract)	Local injection, surgical excision or radiation to small, localized lesions; Chemotherapy with vincristine and Bleomycin
Primary lymphoma of the brain	Headache, palsies, seizures, hemiparesis, mental status, or personality changes	Radiation and/or chemotherapy
Systemic lymphomas	Fever, night sweats, weight loss, enlarged lymph nodes	Chemotherapy

Patients with compromised immune systems are at increased risk for all known cancers and infections (including bacterial, viral, and protozoal). Most infectious diseases in HIV-infected patients are the result of proliferation of organisms already present in the patient's body. Most of these opportunistic infections are not contagious to others. The notable exception to this is tuberculosis.

(Disclaimer: This table was developed to provide general information only. It is not meant to be diagnostic nor to direct treatment.)

(Adapted from Mountain-Plains Regional Education and Training Center *HIV/AIDS Curriculum*, 4th ed., 1992 updated, 1997; and from *MMWR* 2002.)

gins and travels may be diagnostically helpful. (Note: a number of the symptoms listed in the CDC definition of HIV/AIDS can be found associated with certain of the OIs presented.)

Fungal Diseases

In general, healthy people have a high degree of innate resistance to fungi. But a different situation prevails with opportunistic fungal infections, which often present themselves as acute, life-threatening diseases in a compromised host (Medoff et al., 1991).

Because treatment seldom results in the eradication of fungal infections in AIDS patients, there is a high probability of recurrence after treatment (DeWit et al., 1991).

Fungal diseases are among the more devastating of the OIs and are most often regional in association. AIDS patients from the Ohio River basin, the Midwest, or Puerto Rico have a higher-than-normal risk of histoplasmosis *(his-to-plaz-mo-sis)* infection. In the Southwest, there is increased risk for coccidioidomycosis *(kok-sid-e-o-do-mi-ko-sis).* In the southern Gulf states, the risk is for blastomycosis. Other important OI fungi such as *Pneumocystis carinii (nu-mo-sis-tis car-in-e-i), Candida albicans (kan-di-dah al-be-cans),* and *Cryptococcus neoformans (krip-to-kok-us knee-o-for-mans)* are found everywhere in equal numbers. Because of their importance as OIs in AIDS patients, a brief description of **histoplasmosis, candidiasis,** *Pneumocystis carinii* **pneumonia, and cryptococcosis are presented.**

Histoplasmosis (Histoplasma capsulatum)— Spores are inhaled and germinate in or on the body (Figure 6-2). This fungal pathogen is endemic in the Mississippi and Ohio River valleys. Signs of histoplasmosis include prolonged influenza-like symptoms, shortness of breath, and possible complaints of night sweats and shaking chills. In AIDS patients, there is a multisystem involvement: The liver, central nervous system, lymph nodes, and gastrointestinal tract are affected, while mucosal ulcers and enlarged spleen may also occur. Histoplasmosis in an HIV-positive person is considered diagnostic of AIDS. In about two-thirds of AIDS patients with histoplasmosis, it is the initial OI. Over 90% of cases have occurred in patients with T4 cell counts below 100/µL (Wheat, 1992).

In non-HIV-infected patients, amphotericin B is almost always successful in treating histoplas-

mosis (Table 6-1). Only 50% to 80% of AIDS patients respond, however, and relapse is common during maintenance therapy. Nonetheless, amphotericin B followed by weekly maintenance therapy remains the recommended strategy. Amphotericin B is a toxic drug, increases one's temperature, and may also cause uncontrollable shaking; it is sometimes referred to as the "shake and bake" treatment. Earlier reports suggested ketoconazole as a potential alternative for initial or maintenance therapy, but it had an even higher failure rate than amphotericin B and is no longer recommended in HIV-infected patients.

Itraconazole (Sporanox) is approved for treating histoplasmosis and some consider it the drug of choice for HIV-related histoplasmosis (Daar et al., 1993; *Guidelines, U.S. Public Health Service, 2001).*

Candidiasis (Candida albicans)— This fungus is usually associated with vaginal yeast infections. It is a fungus quite common to the body and in particular inhabits the alimentary tract. It is normally kept in check by the presence of bacteria that live on the linings of the alimentary tract. However, in immunocompromised patients, especially those who have received broad spectrum antibiotics, candida multiplies rapidly. Because of its location in the upper reaches of the alimentary tract, if unchecked, it may cause mucocutaneous candidiasis or thrush, an overgrowth of candida in the esophagus and in the oral cavity (Figure 6-3, A and B). Mucosal candidiasis was associated with AIDS patients from the very beginning of the AIDS pandemic (Powderly et al., 1992). In women, overgrowth of candidiasis also occur in the vaginal area.

Some people with oropharyngeal candidiasis may experience a sore mouth. This is particularly painful when acidic foods and juices are taken. In addition, the taste of food is often altered. Treatment is aimed at relieving the symptoms, as therapy is rarely successful at eliminating the fungus (Hay, 1991).

Impaired cell-mediated immunity, as occurs in people with HIV disease, may allow for a disseminated infection (distributed to other areas of the body). **Oral or esophageal candidiasis** causes thick white patches on the mucosal surface and may be the first manifestation of AIDS. Because other diseases can cause similar symptoms, candidiasis by itself is not sufficient for a diagnosis of AIDS.

Pneumocystis carinii— The life cycle and reproductive characteristics of *P. carinii* are not

FIGURE 6-2   A. Anal Histoplasmosis. Histoplasmosis is caused by *Histoplasmosis capsulatum* and causes infection in immunocompromised patients. *(Courtesy CDC, Atlanta)* **B.** AIDS patient's tongue showing multiple shiny, firm Histoplasma erythematous nodules (see arrow A) and thrush (see arrow B). *(Photograph courtesy of Marc E. Grossman, New York)*

Soft
Palate

FIGURE 6-3 Thrush. **A.** An overgrowth of *Candida albicans* on the soft palate in the oral cavity of an AIDS patient. **B.** Creamy patches of candida that can be **scraped off,** leaving a red and sometimes bleeding mucosa. *(A, Courtesy CDC, Atlanta; B, Schiodt, Greenspan, and Greenspan 1989. American Review of Respiratory Disease, 1989, 10:91–109. Official Journal of the American Thoracic Society. © American Lung Association)*

completely understood because the organism is difficult to culture for laboratory study. However, the molecular biology and molecular taxonomy are now being rapidly constructed (Walzer, 1993; Stringer et al., 1996). Virtually everyone in the United States by age 30 to 40 has been exposed to *P. carinii.* It lies dormant in the lungs, held in check by the immune system. Prior to the AIDS epidemic, *P. carinii* pneumonia was seen in children and adults who had a suppressed immune system as in leukemia or Hodgkin's disease and were receiving chemotherapy. In the AIDS patient, the onset of *P. carinii* pneumonia is insidious— patients may notice some shortness of breath and they cannot run as far. It causes extensive damage within the alveoli of the lungs.

The *P. carinii* fungus develops from a small unicellular trophozoite into a cyst containing eight sporozoites. These sporozoites are spread throughout the body, but they show a greater affinity for the lungs, where they multiply in the spaces between the lung sacs and cause pneumonia (Figure 6-4). Prior to 1981, fewer than 100 cases of *P. carinii* infection were reported annually in the United States; yet 80% of AIDS patients develop *P. carinii* pneumonia at some time during their illness. This is one of the few AIDS-related conditions for which there is a choice of relatively effective drugs. The first of these to be made available was the intravenous and aerosolized versions of pentamidine. There are frequent recurrences of this infection. With treatment, there is a 10% to

30% mortality with each PCP episode (Montgomery, 1992). PCP accounted for a diagnosis of AIDS in over 65% of AIDS cases in 1990. In 1994 it had fallen to 20% due to available therapy (Ernst, 1990; Murphy, 1994). The triad of symptoms that almost always indicates the onset of PCP during HIV disease is fever, dry cough, and shortness of breath (Grossman et al., 1989). *P. carinii* pneumonia is unlikely to develop in people with HIV disease unless their T4 cell count drops below 200 (Phair et al., 1990).

FIGURE 6-4 Scanning electron microscope image of *P. carinii* attached to embryonic chick lung cells in culture. Note the tubular extensions through which it extracts nutrients from host lung tissue. *(Propagation of Pneumocystis carinii in Vitro, © Pediatric Research, 11:305–316)*

Cryptococcosis (Cryptococcus neoformans)— Since its discovery in 1894, *C. neoformans* has been recognized as a major cause of deep-seated fungal infection in the human host. The infection can affect many sites, including skin, lung, kidney, prostate, and bone. However, symptomatic disease most often represents infection of the central nervous system. Cryptococcal meningitis is the most common form of fungal meningitis in the United States (Ennis et al., 1993). This fungus is shed in pigeon feces, the spores of which enter the lungs. If the lung does not eliminate it, it gets into the bloodstream, travels to the brain, and can cause cryptococcal meningitis.

In a healthy person, *C. neoformans* may cause pulmonary problems or meningeal infection (infection of the membranes that envelop the brain and spinal cord). It is more commonly seen in people with immunosuppression, especially in HIV/AIDS cases. *C. neoformans* is a fatal OI that occurs in about 13% of AIDS patients (Brooke et al., 1990). It is acquired through the respiratory tract and most commonly causes cryptococcal meningitis. Disseminated *C. neoformans* infection may involve bone marrow, the central nervous system (CNS), and the lungs, causing cryptococcal pneumonia. In AIDS patients, *C. neoformans* also causes infection of the skin, lymph nodes, and kidneys. *Cryptococcus* cannot be cured and it does recur. What drugs should be used is a subject of controversy.

Viral Diseases

In late 1999, **hepatitis C (HCV)** was classified as an OI because the relative risk for liver-associated death is increased 7-fold in HIV-positive patients compared to **NON**-HIV-infected individuals. It is estimated that 200 million people worldwide are infected with the hepatitis C virus. Over 4 million of the infected live in America.

Because of a depleted T4 or CD4+ cellular component of the immune system, AIDS patients are at particularly high risk for the herpes family of viral infections: cytomegalovirus, herpes simplex virus types 1 and 2, varicella-zoster virus, and Epstein-Barr virus.

Cytomegalovirus (CMV)— This virus is a member of the human herpes virus group of viruses. CMV is the perfect parasite. It infects most people asymptomatically. When illness does occur, it is mild and nonspecific. There have been no epidemics to call attention to the virus. Yet CMV is now considered the most common infectious cause of mental retardation and congenital deafness in the United States. It is also the most common viral pathogen found in immunocompromised people (Balfour, 1995).

A **latent state** follows initial infection, with CMV probably located in the white blood cells and involving many organs and organ systems. Later it is reactivated, usually by some form of immunosuppression such as organ or bone marrow transplantation, cancer chemotherapy, or HIV disease (Jacobson et al., 1992; Hardy, 1996).

The virus is very unstable and survives only a few hours outside a human host. It can be found in saliva, tears, blood, stool, cervical secretions, and in especially high levels in urine and semen. Transmission occurs primarily by intimate or close contact with infected secretions. The incidence of CMV infection varies from between 30% and 80% depending on the geographical community tested. However, over 90% of homosexual males have tested positive for CMV (Jacobson et al., 1988). CMV causes the more important viral infections in AIDS patients. This virus causes a broad spectrum of diseases in HIV-infected people, ranging from mild or severe gastrointestinal problems to infections of the brain, the liver (hepatitis), and the onset of fulminant (sudden and severe) pneumonia. Gastrointestinal infection may result in severe ulceration of the esophagus, stomach, small intestines, and colon. CMV pneumonia occurs in 10% to 20% of AIDS patients and can be lethal because therapy is unsuccessful.

CMV infection of AIDS patients usually results in prolonged fever, anemia (too few red blood cells), leukopenia (too few white blood cells), and abnormal liver function. CMV also causes severe diarrhea and HIV-associated retinitis resulting in eventual blindness (*Emergency Medicine*, 1989; Lynch, 1989; Dobkin, 1995).

Perhaps 75% of AIDS patients have an eye disease, with the retina the most common site (Russell, 1990). The retina, which is a light-sensitive membrane lining the inside of the back of the eye, is also part of the brain and is nourished by blood vessels. **AIDS-related damage to these vessels produces tiny retinal hemorrhages and small cotton wool spots**—early indicators of disease that are often detected during a routine eye examination (Figure 6-5).

FIGURE 6-5
Cytomegalovirus retinitis. The disease, as seen in this photograph, involves the posterior pole of the right eye. Fluffy white infiltrate **(cotton wool spots)** with a small amount of retinal hemorrhage can be seen in the distribution of the superior vascular arcade. *(Courtesy of Scott M. Whitcup, M.D., National Eye Institute, National Institutes of Health, Bethesda, Md.)*

Symptoms of CMV retinitis may be subtle, such as blurred vision, haze or floaters, or small dim spots in side vision. In unusual circumstances, the virus can produce dramatic symptoms, such as loss of vision within 72 hours. Without treatment, CMV can destroy the entire retina in three to six months after infection.

Herpes Viruses Types 1 & 2 (HSV 1 & 2)— Herpes infections are one of the most commonly diagnosed infections among the HIV/ AIDS population. Almost all HIV-infected individuals (95%) are coinfected with HSV 1 and/or HSV 2. Both viruses cause **severe** and progressive eruptions of the mucous membranes. HSV 1 affects the membranes of the nose and mouth. Also, when herpetic lesions involve the lips or throat, 80% to 90% of the time they either precede or occur simultaneously with **herpes-caused pneumonia** (Gottlieb et al., 1987). Bacterial or fungal superinfections occur in more than 50% of herpes-caused pneumonia cases and are a major contributory cause of death in AIDS patients.

Mortality from HSV pneumonia exceeds 80% (Lynch, 1989). Herpes may also cause blindness in AIDS patients. The following is from Paul Monette's *Borrowed Time:*

> I woke up shortly thereafter, and Roger told me— without a sense of panic, almost puzzled—that his vision seemed to be losing light and detail. I called Dell Steadman and made an emergency appointment, and

I remember driving down the freeway, grilling Roger about what he could see. It seemed to be less and less by the minute. He could barely see the cars going by in the adjacent lanes. Twenty minutes later we were in Dell's office, and with all the urgent haste to get there we didn't really reconnoiter till we were sitting in the examining room. I asked the same question—what could he see?—and now Roger was getting more and more upset the more his vision darkened. I picked up the phone to call Jamiee, and by the time she answered the phone in Chicago he was blind. *Total blackness, in just two hours!*

The retina had detached. (An operation on retinal attachment was successful and sight was restored. The cause of the retinal detachment was a herpes infection of the eyes.)

HSV 2 also affects the membranes of the anus, causing severe perianal and rectal ulcers primarily in homosexual men with AIDS. Herpes of the skin can generally be managed with oral **acyclovir** (Zovirax), Foscavir, or Famvir (Table 6-1).

Herpes Zoster Virus (HZV)— Like herpes simplex, this virus has the potential to cause a rapid onset of pneumonia in AIDS patients. Untreated HZV pneumonia has a mortality rate of 15% to 35%. HZV is now monitored as an early indicator that HIV-positive people are progressing toward AIDS.

Protozoal Diseases

An increasing number of infections **that have not been observed in immunocompromised patients**

BOX 6.1

A PHYSICIAN'S AGONIZING DILEMMA

Opportunistic infections are the primary threat to patients with AIDS; they are the main causes of illness and death. The cruel irony is that although there are 30 or more FDA-approved drugs to treat these infections, most cannot be used in patients receiving zidovudine (ZDV) *because the combination drug therapy is devastatingly toxic to bone marrow.*

EXAMPLE:

Cytomegalovirus (CMV) Retinitis

CMV retinitis is one of the *worst* of the opportunistic infections and it develops in 90% of AIDS patients (Gottlieb et al., 1987). Both the patient who contracts CMV retinitis and the treating physician confront an almost impossible dilemma: whether to continue the zidovudine and risk blindness or to treat the retinitis and risk death from another infection. A physician recently said, "In my experience, I have never yet been able to combine zidovudine with the experimental drug ganciclovir (DHPG), which is the only recognized treatment for CMV retinitis, because the combination destroys the bone marrow. I therefore face the virtually impossible task of asking a 25-year-old person: 'Which of these options do you prefer: to take zidovudine and keep on living but go blind, or to preserve your sight by having retinitis treatment but risk dying?' That is a truly terrible question to ask of any patient, especially a young one." He continued, "Recently, I treated just such a young patient. He had been taking zidovudine for AIDS when he contracted CMV retinitis. When I presented him with this agonizing choice, he told me, 'I definitely don't want to go blind. I want to be treated for this retinitis.' So he stopped taking zidovudine and was started on DHPG treatment. He started to have seizures, which were a consequence of the toxoplasmosis brain abscess that eventually ended his life. Just before he died, he told me that the worst decision he ever made was to stop taking zidovudine. 'I should have stayed on it,' he said, 'and gone blind.'" (Robert J. Awe, M.D., 1988)

Cryptococcal Meningitis

The situation for AIDS patients with cryptococcal meningitis is similarly depressing. Because of the severe bone marrow toxicity, it is virtually impossible to use amphotericin B, the effective treatment for this meningitis, at the same time as zidovudine. Besides, the use of amphotericin B has its own side effects as can be noted from this excerpt from Paul Monette's *Borrowed Time: An AIDS Memoir:*

Amphotericin B is administered with Benadryl in order to avoid convulsions, the most serious possible side effect. It was about nine or ten when they started the drug in his veins, and I sat by the bed as nurses streamed in and out. A half hour into the slow drip, the nurse monitoring the IV walked out, saying she'd be right back, and a couple of minutes later Roger began to shake. I gripped him by the shoulders as he was jolted by what felt like waves of electric shock, staring at me horror-struck. Though Cope [the physician] would tell me later, trying to ease the torture of my memory, that "mentation" [mental activity] is all blurred during convulsions, I saw that Roger knew the horror (page 336).

When the nurse returned she looked at him in dismay: "How long has this been going on?" Then she ordered an emergency shot of morphine to counteract the horror. When at last he fell into a deep sleep they all told me to go home, saying they would try another dose of the ampho in a few hours. I was so ragged I could barely walk. So I left him there with no way of knowing how near it was [Roger's death], or maybe not brave enough to know.

Whichever option is chosen, the patient is bound to suffer, and perhaps die, either of cryptococcal meningitis or of some other infection.

---

are being found in AIDS patients. Three such infections are caused by the protozoans *Toxoplasma gondii, Isospora belli,* and *Cryptosporidium muris.*

Toxoplasma gondii— *T. gondii* is a small intracellular protozoan parasite that lives in vacuoles inside host macrophages and other nucleated cells. It appears that during and after entry, *T. gondii* produces secretory products that modify vacuole membranes so that the normal *fusion* of cell vacuoles with lysosomes containing digestive enzymes is blocked. Having blocked vacuole-lysosome fusion, *T. gondii* can successfully reproduce and cause a disease called **toxoplasmosis** (Joiner et al., 1990).

It can infect any warm-blooded animal, invading and multiplying within the cytoplasm of host cells. As host immunity develops, multiplication slows and tissue cysts are formed. Sexual multiplication occurs in the intestinal cells of cats (and apparently only cats); oocysts form and are shed in the stool (Sibley, 1992). Transmission may occur transplacentally, by ingestion of raw or undercooked meat and eggs containing tissue cysts or by exposure to oocysts in cat feces (Wallace et al., 1993).

In the United States, 10% to 40% of adults are chronically infected but most are asymptomatic. *T. gondii* can enter and infect the human brain causing **encephalitis** (inflammation of the brain). Toxoplasmic encephalitis develops in over 30% of AIDS patients at some point in their illness (Figure 6-6). The signs and symptoms of cerebral toxoplasmosis in AIDS patients may include fever, headache, confusion, sleepiness, weakness or numbness in one part of the body, seizure activity, and changes in vision. These symptoms can get worse and progress to coma and death unless toxoplasmosis is promptly diagnosed and treated. Toxoplasma infection affecting other parts of the body is rare, and symptoms vary depending on which organs the disease affects. Similar to a variety of other OIs manifested in HIV-infected people, toxoplasmosis appears to represent a reactivation of an earlier infection. In the United States, 30% of the population between the ages of 10 and 19 demonstrate serological evidence (anti-body) to *T. gondii* exposure. *T. gondii* lies dormant in the reticuloendothelial system until it becomes reactivated within the immunocompromised host. Thus, for most AIDS patients, it is believed that *T. gondii* is latent within their bodies and is reactivated by the loss of immune competence. Once activated, symptoms can be as mild as chills, headaches that do not respond to common pain killers, low fevers, and delusions; or as severe as hard seizures, coma, and death. Arthur Ashe, tennis champion who died in February of 1993, was being treated for *T. gondii* infection. (Figure I-1)

***Cryptosporidium*—** *Cryptosporidium* is the cause of cryptosporidiosis, and is a member of the family of organisms that includes *Toxoplasma gondii* and *Isospora*. Its life cycle is similar to that of other organisms in the class Sporozoa. Oocysts are shed in the feces of infected animals and are immediately infectious to others. In humans, the organisms can be found throughout the GI tract, including the pharynx, esophagus, stomach, duodenum, jejenum, ileum, appendix, colon, and rectum. Various case reports of patients with AIDS describe infection in the gallbladder and pulmonary dissemination which clinically resembles *Pneumocystis carinii* pneumonia. *Cryptosporidium* **causes profuse watery diarrhea of 6 to 26 bowel movements per day with a loss of 1 to 17 liters of fluid (a liter is about 1 quart).** It is an infrequent infection in AIDS patients, usually occurring late in the course of disease as immunological deterioration progresses.

Studies of transmission patterns have shown infection within families, nursery schools, and from person to person, probably by the fecal-oral route. The infection is particularly common in homosexual men, perhaps as a consequence of anilingus (oral-anal sex).

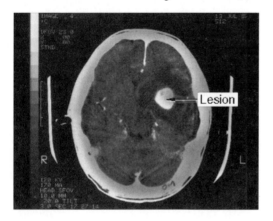

FIGURE 6-6 *Toxoplasma gondii* Lesions in the Brain. Radiographic imaging shows a deep ring-enhancing lesion located in the basal ganglia. *(By permission of Carmelita U. Tuazon, George Washington University)*

***Isospora belli*—** *Isospora belli* enters the body via feces-contaminated food and drink or is sexually transmitted (DeHovitz, 1988). This organism infects the bowels. Isosporiasis is characterized by an acute onset of profuse watery diarrhea (**8 to 10 stools per day),** fever, malaise, cramping, abdominal pain, and in some cases significant weight loss and anorexia. According to the 1987 revised definition for AIDS, isosporiasis persisting for longer than one month and a positive test for HIV is indicative of AIDS.

Bacterial Diseases

There is a long list of bacteria that cause infections in AIDS patients. These are the bacteria that normally cause infection or illness after the ingestion of contaminated food, such as species of *Salmonella*. Others, such as *Streptococci, Haemophilus,* and *Staphylococci are* common in advanced HIV disease. A number of other bacteria-caused sexually transmitted diseases such as syphilis, chancroid, gonorrhea, and chlamydial diseases are also associated with HIV disease.

One difference between AIDS and non-AIDS individuals is that bacterial diseases in AIDS patients are of greater severity and more difficult to treat. Two bacterial species, *Mycobacterium avium intracellulare* and *Mycobacterium tubercu-*

losis are of particular importance as agents of infection in AIDS patients (Table 6-2).

Mycobacterium avium intracellulare (MAI)— Over the past 40 years, MAI has gone from a rare, reportable infection to something that is common in most large American communities. Unlike tuberculosis, which is almost exclusively spread person to person, MAI is, in most instances, environmentally acquired. MAI exists in food, animals, water supplies, and soil, and enters people's lungs as an aerosol when they take showers.

When an elderly person develops MAI infection, it is invariably confined to his or her lungs. In contrast, MAI infections in AIDS patients run rampant and are clearly systemic (Zoler, 1991).

Table 6-2 Categories of Organism and Viral Involvement in Opportunistic Diseases

Symptoms	Causative Agent	Symptoms	Causative Agent
Generally Present		Proctocolitisa[a]	*Entamoeba histolytica*
Fever, weight	*Pneumocystis carinii*	(diarrhea,	Campylobacter
loss, fatigue,	Cytomegalovirus	abdominal pain,	Shigella
malaise	Epstein-Barr virus	rectal pain)	Salmonella
	Mycobacterium avium intracellulare		*Chlamydia trachomatis*
	Candida albicans		Cytomegalovirus
		Proctitisa[a]	*Neisseria gonorrhoeae*
Diffuse Pneumonia		(pain during	Herpes simplex
Dyspnea, chest	*Pneumocystis carinii*	defecation,	*Chlamydia trachomatis*
pain, hypoxemia,	Cytomegalovirus	diarrhea, itching	*Treponema pallidum*
abnormal chest	*Mycobacterium tuberculosis*	and perianal	
X-ray	*Mycobacterium avium intracellulare*	ulcerations)	
	Candida albicans		
	Cryptococcus neoformans	**Neurological Involvement**	
	Toxoplasma gondii	Meningitis,	Cytomegalovirus
		encephalitis,	Herpes simplex
		headaches,	*Toxoplasma gondii*
Gastrointestinal Involvement		seizures, dementia	*Cryptococcus neoformans*
Esophagitis	*Candida albicans*		Papovavirus
(sore throat,	Herpes simplex		*Mycobacterium tuberculosis*
dysphagia)	Cytomegalovirus (suspected)	Retinitis	Cytomegalovirus
Enteritis	*Giardia lamblia*	(diminished	*Toxoplasma gondii*
(diarrhea,	*Entamoeba histolytica*	vision)	*Candida albicans*
abdominal pain,	*Isospora belli*		
weight loss)	Cryptosporidium		
	Strongyloides stercoralis		
	Mycobacterium avium intracellulare		

[a]Especially in those persons practicing anal sex.

Adapted from Amin, 1987.

For Sexual Exposures—People should use male latex condoms during every act of sexual intercourse to reduce the risk of exposure to cytomegalovirus, herpes simplex virus, and human papillomavirus, as well as to all other sexually transmitted pathogens. Use of latex condoms will help prevent the transmission of HIV to others. Avoid sexual practices that may result in oral exposure to feces (oral-anal contact) to reduce the risk of intestinal infections such as cryptosporidiosis, shigellosis, campylobacteriosis, amebiasis, giardiasis, and hepatitis A and B (*MMWR*, 2002).

The fact that MAI produced disseminated disease in AIDS cases was recognized in 1982. The epidemiology of MAI continues to evolve. MAI occurs in 18% to 43% of people with HIV disease and has been implicated as the cause of a nonspecific **wasting syndrome.** AIDS patients demonstrate **anorexia** (inability to eat), weight loss, weakness, night sweats, diarrhea, and fever. Some patients also experience abdominal pain, enlarged liver or spleen, and malabsorption. In contrast to viral infections, this bacterium rarely causes pulmonary or lung problems in AIDS patients. Among persons with AIDS, the risk of developing disseminated MAI increases progressively with time. AIDS patients surviving for 30 months had a 50% risk of developing disseminated MAI. It appears most HIV-infected persons will develop disseminated MAI if they do not first die from other OIs (Chin, 1992).

Mycobacterium tuberculosis— Tuberculosis (TB) infects one-third of the world's population and is now the leading cause of illness and death in people infected with HIV. Tuberculosis is an infectious disease caused by the bacterium *Mycobacterium tuberculosis,* which is spread almost exclusively by airborne transmission. TB has been observed in elephants, cattle, mice, and other animal species. In 1993, TB was transmitted from an infected seal to its trainer in Australia. In the United States, monkeys are the primary source of animal-to-human transmission.

The disease can affect any site in the body, but most often affects the lungs. When persons with pulmonary TB cough, they produce tiny droplet nuclei that contain TB bacteria, which can remain suspended in the air for prolonged periods of time. (With respect to transmission, the cough to TB is similar to sex to HIV.) Anyone who breathes air that contains these droplet nuclei can become infected with TB. It has been suggested that there is a minimal chance of inhaling HIV in blood-tinged TB sputum (Harris, 1993).

A person who becomes infected with the TB bacillus remains infected for years. Usually a person with a healthy immune system does not become ill, but is usually not able to eliminate the infection without taking an antituberculosis drug. This condition is referred to as a **latent tuberculosis infection.**

About 10% of otherwise healthy persons who have latent tuberculosis infection will become ill with active TB at some time during their lives (*MMWR,* 1992). With HIV disease, the risk is 10% per year (Daar et al., 1993). It has been estimated that through year 2002, 15 million HIV-infected people worldwide are coinfected with TB.

Tuberculosis is not generally considered to be an OI because people with healthy immune systems contract TB. After infection with *M. tuberculosis* about 5% of immunocompetent individuals will develop TB (Daley, 1992). But, people with a depressed immune system are much more likely to develop the disease (Zoler, 1991). Tuberculosis in people with AIDS does not look like ordinary tuberculosis. In the usual presentation of the disease, TB is usually restricted to a given area in the chest. People with AIDS may have tuberculosis throughout the chest cavity.

TB AND HIV

There is a strong association between HIV disease and TB: HIV infection is the highest risk factor for progression from latent *M. tuberculosis* infection to TB (Bermejo et al., 1992).

HIV infection is now considered to be the single most important risk factor in the expression of TB. HIV disease is associated with the reactivation of a dormant or inactive TB infection (Stanford et al., 1993).

M. tuberculosis infection occurs in about 35% of HIV-infected individuals, usually as the result of *M. tuberculosis* reactivation from a latent prior infection (Brooke et al., 1990). The CDC defines extrapulmonary TB combined with an HIV-positive test as diagnostic of AIDS.

According to the World Health Organization, TB is, worldwide, the leading cause of death in HIV-infected people and among adults from a single, infectious organism. TB has killed at least 200 million people since 1882, the date of the discovery of the bacterium that causes TB. Millions more die from TB each year. Globally, TB was estimated to account for 30% of AIDS-related deaths in 1999, and greater than 30% in 2000 and 2001. **March 24 of each year is recognized as World TB Day.**

In the United States, 14% of AIDS patients are also coinfected with TB. Health officials state that between 40% and 60% of those developing multidrug-resistant TB will die (Ezzell, 1993).

Other Opportunistic Infections

Other opportunistic infectious organisms and viruses and the diseases they cause and possible therapies are listed in Table 6-1. Table 6-2 separates OIs into the body parts most affected by a particular organism or virus.

From diagnosis until death, the AIDS battle is not just against its cause, HIV, but against those organisms and viruses that cause OIs. Opportunistic infections are severe, tend to be disseminated (spread throughout the body), and are characterized by multiplicity. Fungal, viral, protozoal, and bacterial infections may be controlled for some time but are rarely curable.

CANCER OR MALIGNANCY IN AIDS PATIENTS

The word malignancy means a cancer. Specifically, cancer is an abnormal growth of cells that divide uncontrollably and may spread to other parts of the body. There are many kinds of cancer, which can involve just about any part of the body.

HIV infection carries with it a high susceptibility to certain cancers. Because of the severe and progressive impairment of the immune system, host defense mechanisms that normally protect against certain types of cancer are lost. Cancers develop in approximately 40% of AIDS patients. Four kinds of cancer that occur with increased frequency are: **progressive multifocal leukoencephalopathy, squamous cell carcinoma** (oral and anal), **non-Hodgkin's lymphoma**, and **HIV/AIDS-associated Kaposi's sarcoma (KS).** None of these cancers, except for KS, is considered to be an opportunistic infection because they are not infections. They are cancers arising from cells that have lost control of their division processes. Of the nine types of AIDS-associated cancers, KS occurs with the greatest frequency and is discussed in some detail. Lymphomas are briefly described (Table 6-3). (For a recent review of HIV/AIDS-related cancers read Hessol, 1998; Grulich 2000.)

Kaposi's Sarcoma (cap-o-seas sar-com-a)

No other HIV/AIDS-related opportunistic disease attacks and singles out one segment of the population as KS does with HIV-positive gay men. Men with KS outnumber women approximately 95% to 5%; HIV-positive homosexual men with KS outnumber heterosexual men almost as significantly. KS is extremely rare in hemophiliacs with HIV. In fact, in one major study of hemophiliacs with HIV, only one in 93 developed KS, and he happened to be a gay man.

HIV infection represents an overwhelming risk factor for the development of KS, which was rare in the United States (incidence less than 1/100,000/year) before the HIV epidemic. Today, KS still remains one of the most frequent diseases affecting HIV-infected individuals. It is an aggressive disease, with

Table 6-3 Malignancies Associated with HIV/AIDS

Kaposi's sarcoma (epidemic form)
Burkitt's lymphoma
Non-Hodgkin's lymphomas
Hodgkin's disease
Chronic lymphocytic leukemia
Carcinoma of the oropharaynx
Hepatocellular carcinoma
Adenosquamous carcinoma of the lung
Cervical cancer
Anal cancer
Squamous cell carcinoma
Progressive multifocal leukoencephalopathy
Vulva cancer

BOX 6.2

LIFE GOES ON!

by Wendi Alexis Modeste

What this epidemic has cost me is the complete faith I had in the medical profession. I was raised believing that doctors were second only to priests and God. They were never to be questioned. Whatever the doctor said was law. If a person didn't get well after seeing the doctor, somehow they (the patient) had done something wrong. This was pretty much standard thinking for middle-class African-Americans. For a variety of reasons (mainly no self-esteem) I became a drug addict, prostitute, convict, battered, homeless woman, in that order! With the exception of emergency room admissions (which are a joke and a whole 'nother story) I had no access to health care.

Now, as a PWA (person with AIDS) fortunately/unfortunately on SSI, Medicaid pays for my nine different AIDS medications, clinic visits, treatment, tests, etc. When I received the "exciting news" that I was eligible for "all" Medicaid benefits, I was still under the impression doctors were those super-intelligent, gifted, Christian, saint-like people. Girlfriend, I am here to tell you, AIDS has totally shot that Marcus Welby theory straight to hell!

Early in my diagnosis, I went to my physician because my tongue was almost completely covered with what looked like cottage cheese. There was also a horrible pink lesion dead center. The first time I showed it to my doctor he said, "Ugh," and made a face. He told me to wait a month. If nothing changed or got worse when I returned he'd have someone look at it. Being ignorant about the disease at that time, and still blindly believing in the medical profession, I waited a month, then returned. Again I showed the doctor my tongue. He asked me if I wanted him to write me a prescription for codeine and Valium. I totally freaked! By this time, I'd done some reading and realized I probably had thrush and some sort of herpes. This physician was aware of my serostatus. He also knew that I was a person with a 20-year history of drug abuse. I'd been in recovery less than a year and this jerk wanted to prescribe for me two of the most addictive and abused prescription drugs. I'd never mentioned being in pain or that I was experiencing any type of anxiety. I contacted the Executive Director of this health facility and asked to have a different doctor assigned to me. In an attempt to make me feel guilty about requesting a change, I was told about the problems doctors have in getting Medicaid reimbursement. I was neither intimidated nor impressed. A new doctor was assigned. My new physician was very nice. After *I* told *him* what I thought my diagnosis was, he prescribed the appropriate medications. He was not trained in AIDS/HIV. I could have dealt with his ignorance because I knew he was trying. His nurse, however, was a different story. Every time she came to do my vitals she'd say the same thing: "I always get nervous when taking the temperature of you guys." She'd then force a little chuckle and go on to say, "Oh, well, I figure we all have to die of something." (I assume this was to show me what a courageous Florence Nightingale she was.)

Let me tell you, when you are burning up with a 103 degree temp. and your bowels haven't stopped running for a week, causing your butt to feel like it's on fire, it's real hard to be the patient, understanding AIDS educator. I really get crazy when the person I'm forced to educate is someone whose been privileged to more information than myself.

But life goes on!

One day I had a toothache. I go to the dentist. After waiting half the day, I'm brought into the treatment room for an X-ray. At first I thought the dental assistant had made a mistake. Surely this room had been prepared for a paint job. Everything was draped in white towels. The entire dental unit, including where my head, arms and feet went, was completely covered. The seat of the unit was securely wrapped up, as was the metal extension arm that holds the overhead dental lamp. All surfaces of the walls were also draped. When I asked the reason for this "painter preparation," I was informed it was done because I have AIDS, and they had to protect their other patients from coming into contact with my contaminated blood. Needless to say, I saw red! I knew I had to protect myself. I mean, what kind of dentistry were they practicing if they were concerned about my blood splattering that far and wide? What was even more frightening was that they'd done all this unnecessary draping and I was only having an X-ray. I filed a complaint with the Human Rights Dept.

BOX 6.2 *(continued)*

I became a patient at the AIDS Care Center in Syracuse. My physician, a woman (need I say more?), is a caring person and well-educated about AIDS/HIV. My nurse/social worker is excellent, but as all of us living with AIDS know, shit happens. One day I awaken with enough yeast in my body to make all the baked goods in Central New York rise. My doctor isn't in. I wait a couple of days but can no longer stand the discomfort. I beg to see a doctor in the AIDS Care Unit. I'm assigned the doctor who sees the HIV-infected prisoners. (My heart and soul truly go out to those guys.) First he talks with me over the phone to find out if I can possibly wait another week when my doctor is due to return. I tell him my tongue is unrecognizable, the yeast in my esophagus is burning like a heart attack, and the Roto-Rooter service couldn't satisfy the itch caused by the yeast in my vagina. HELL NO, I can't wait another week! I go in to see him. I show him my tongue. I can't believe it, but like the first doctor, he uses that medical term, "Ugh," then says, "That does look nasty." At this point I'm ready to French kiss this idiot. But it gets worse. He won't touch me, let alone examine anything. He asks me what I think will work. I feel too badly to curse, so I tell him Mycelex, Myastatin suspension, Monistat 7. He writes the prescriptions and for good measure increases my acyclovir. For this he gets paid? He did nothing!

I'm now as educated as a lay person can be about HIV disease/AIDS. In addition to my doctor at the AIDS Care Center, I have a private primary care physician. Sometimes it's easier to get in to see this doctor. I call his office one day because there is swelling and burning on the sides of my tongue. I cannot eat. My regular doctor isn't in, but one of his associates assures me if I come in to the office he'll see me right away and give me something to ease the pain so I can at least eat. As a fat person who proudly admits a genuine fondness for food, I can tell you not being able to eat registers serious panic in my soul. Nothing stops me from eating. I was probably the only overweight homeless dope addict living on the streets of NYC. Being scared is putting it mildly. I scrape up the carfare and go to the office. After waiting an unreasonably long time, Doogie Howser's twin comes in to see me and announces he's Dr. Jones, whom I spoke to on the phone. OK, I know not to judge a book by its cover. I mean, Doogie is pretty good on TV. Dr. Jones looks at my tongue and proceeds to ask a zillion questions, all of which are an-

swered in my chart. Finally he says he's never seen an HIV-infected person or a person with AIDS, and frankly he doesn't know what to do. He then suggests I eat popsicles for a few days because the cold will soothe the pain and the sugar should help give me energy. I kid you not, this actually happened. This jerk prescribed me popsicles. I truly wished I could transmit the virus by biting at this point. He used me so he could write in his journal or resume (or somewhere) that he'd treated a person with AIDS. He could also charge Medicaid for nothing.

But this type of quackery must stop.

The last gripe I'm going to list is this patient statement I hear all the time when I get an unexplained fever or infection and no one can determine its origin. I'm told, "there hasn't been enough studies done on the paths this disease takes in women. Even less has been done on the effects of different AIDS medications on people of color." This is said to me as if it's my fault they don't know. This disease has been documented for ten years in both men and women. I know African-Americans were dying of AIDS long before the gay white community mobilized and, thank God, refused to lay down and die quietly. There is no excuse for the fact that there's no studies done on these populations.

I am thankful to Dr. Sallie Klemmens and nurse/clinician/social worker Judith Swartout at University Hospital's designated AIDS Care Center here in Syracuse. I am thankful for Dr. Barbara J. Justice who with God's help kept me alive when I lived on the streets of NYC. They are all examples of what the medical profession should be about. Dr. Justice made me feel that I counted and should be assertive about my health care. Though no longer my surgeon, she continues to be a source of inspiration and a fountain of information for me. These three are gems in a field I think is greatly overrated, overpaid, and run by capitalist male chauvinist pigs.

Though medical people wear white, that absence of color symbolizing purity and goodness, I beg you all, "Don't believe the hype!" We need a national health care system for everyone. As PWAs we must be assertive about our health care. Good health care is a right not a privilege.

As a child I cried when I learned there was no Santa Claus. When my illusion about the medical profession was shattered I got angry. I decided to fight with the only ammunition I had, education! **Knowledge gives one power**. A close friend of mine told me I shouldn't submit this

BOX 6.2 *(continued)*

article because I might offend some members of the medical profession. He also felt because I'm on Medicaid I'm not supposed to complain, I should be grateful. To his comments I respond, raised with two college-educated parents, never wanting or needing anything, I wasn't supposed to be a drug addict. Unfortunately I was. After 20 years of addiction, I wasn't supposed to be able to stop. I've been in recovery almost two years now. I'm not supposed to be living with

AIDS, but with God's help I'm happy and living large (as the kids say now).

The best things I do have always been what I'm not supposed to do!

Power to all PWAs!

Wendi Alexis Modeste, a PWA who was diagnosed in 1990, died August 25, 1994.

Source: Modeste, W.A., August 1991, Issue 68, *PWA Coalition Newsline*. Reprinted with permission.

---

involvement of the gut, lung, pleura, lymph nodes and the hard and soft palates.

In the United States, Kaposi's sarcoma is at least 20,000 times more common in people with HIV/AIDS than in the general population, and 300 times more common than in other immunosuppressed groups (Beral et al., 1990).

KS was first described by Moritz Kaposi in 1877 as a cancer of the muscle and skin. Characteristic signs of early KS were bruises and birthmark-like lesions on the skin, especially on the lower extremities. KS was described as a slow-growing tumor found primarily in elderly Mediterranean men, Ashkenazi Jews, and equatorial Africans.

Kaposi's sarcoma as described by Moritz Kaposi is called classic KS and it differs markedly from the KS that occurs in AIDS patients (Figure 6-7 A, B). Classic KS has a variable prognosis (forecast), is usually slow to develop, and causes little pain (**indolent**). Patient survival in the United States ranges from 8 to 13 years with some reported cases of survival for up to 50 years (Gross et al., 1989). Symptoms of classic KS are ulcerative skin lesions, swelling (**edema**) of the legs, and secondary infection of the skin lesions.

Kaposi's Sarcoma and AIDS

The AIDS epidemic has brought a more virulent and progressive form of KS marked by painless, flat to raised, pink to purplish plaques on the skin and mucosal surfaces that may spread to the lungs, liver, spleen, lymph nodes, digestive tract, and other internal organs. In its advanced stages it may affect any area from the skull to the feet (Figure 6-8). In the mouth, the hard palate is the most common site of KS (Figure 6-9) but it may also occur on the gum line, tongue, or tonsils.

KS in AIDS patients comes on swiftly and spreads aggressively. However, there have been **no**

reported AIDS deaths due to just KS. But, KS can have enormous psychological impact particularly if the lesions occur on exposed areas.

Some of the most inconvenient and uncomfortable KS targets include the soles of the feet, the nose, and the oral cavity. Lesions on the lower extremities or on the feet, are often associated with edema and swelling, causing not only severe pain but difficulty putting on shoes and walking. Swelling can be complicated by bacterial cellulitis, ulceration and skin breakdown, often with gram-negative bacterial infections. In addition to the obvious cosmetic damage, lesions on the face may be accompanied by swelling around the eyes that can sometimes progress to the point where patients literally cannot open their eyes. Finally, oral lesions can be painful and make eating and speaking problematic.

The prevalence of KS among gay men in 1981 was 77%; by 1987, it had fallen to 26% and by 1995 to less than 20%. This drop in KS among gay men was paralleled by a fall in CMV cases. KS continues to decline in frequency.

Proposed Kaposi's Virus— Most HIV/AIDS researchers now believe that HIV is not the primary pathological agent for Kaposi's sarcoma. Beral and colleagues (1990) at the Centers for Disease Control and Prevention concluded that the epidemiological data on Kaposi's distribution suggest that it is caused by a sexually transmitted pathogen other than HIV.

In December of 1994, Yuan Chang and colleagues reported that they found DNA sequences that appear to represent a **new human herpes virus (HHV-8)** in KS tissue. Gianluca Gaidano and colleagues (1996) report that their data confirm that HHV-8 DNA sequences are found, at high frequency, with selected types of AIDS-related KS. Evidence continues to accumulate indicating

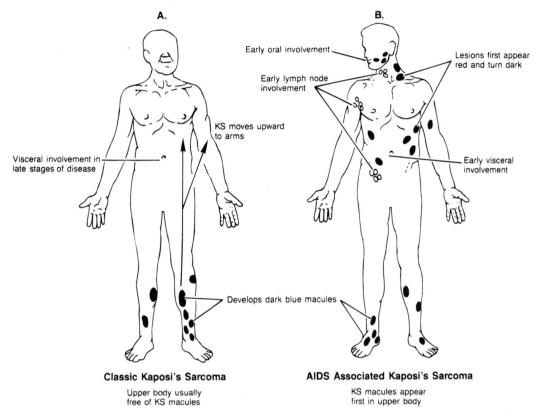

A.

Early oral involvement

Early lymph node involvement

KS moves upward to arms

Visceral involvement in late stages of disease

B.

Lesions first appear red and turn dark

Early visceral involvement

Develops dark blue macules

Classic Kaposi's Sarcoma
Upper body usually free of KS macules

AIDS Associated Kaposi's Sarcoma
KS macules appear first in upper body

FIGURE 6-7 Classic and AIDS-Associated Kaposi's Sarcoma. **A.** Patients with classic KS (non-AIDS-related) demonstrate violet to dark blue bruises, spots, or macules on their lower legs. Gradually, the lesions enlarge into tumors and begin to form ulcers. KS lesions may, with time, spread upward to the trunk and arms. The movement of KS appears to follow the veins and involves the lymph system. In the late stages of the disease, visceral organs may become involved. **B.** For AIDS patients, initial lesions appear in greater number and are smaller than in classic KS. They first appear on the upper body (head and neck) and arms. The lesions first appear as pink or red oval bruises or macules that, with time, become dark blue and spread to the oral cavity and lower body, the legs, and feet. Visceral organs may be involved early on and the disease is aggressive. However, death is not caused by KS.

that HHV-8 is the infectious agent responsible for KS (Kledal et al., 1997; Said et al., 1997).

UPDATE 2002 During the first four years many research papers on whether Herpes virus 8 causes KS were published in recognized scientific/medical journals (Figure 6-10). It appears there is a cause and effect relationship; HHV-8/KS (Martin et al., 1998; O'Brien et al., 1999; Antman et al., 2000; Rinaldo et al., 2001; Osmond et al., 2002).

The work of Charles Rinaldo and colleagues (2001) reveals that healthy non-HIV-infected people who carry HHV8 have a healthy immune response and control virus. HIV-infected persons

who carry HHV8 have a poor immune response to the virus, which then becomes a precursor for the expression of KS.

The Kaposi's virus may have entered the same population in which HIV is endemic, which would explain why the two are often transmitted together (O'Brien et al., 1999). HIV may produce the right conditions for Kaposi's development by causing growth factor production, and possibly by suppressing the body's immune defenses against cancer.

The work of Dennis Osmond and colleagues states that a KS-associated herpes virus was present in about 25% of gay males in San Francisco

FIGURE 6-9 Oral Kaposi's Sarcoma. KS can be seen on the hard palate and down the sides of the oral cavity. *(Courtesy of Nicholas J. Fiumara, M.D., Boston)*

FIGURE 6-8 Kaposi's Sarcoma on Lower Leg of an AIDS Patient. *(Courtesy of Nicholas J. Fiumara, M.D., Boston)*

in 1978, several years before the CDC reported on the immune deficiency disease later called AIDS. As evidence mounts that genital herpes plays an important role in facilitating HIV acquisition, researchers are debating whether herpes screening and treatment should be considered for an HIV prevention strategy.

Lymphoma (lim-fo-mah)

Lymphomas are the second most common cancer in HIV and are now the seventh most common cause of death for people with AIDS. A lymphoma is a neoplastic disorder (cancer) of the lymphoid tissue (Figure 6-11). *B cell* lymphoma occurs in about 1% of HIV-infected people, but makes up about 90% to 95% of all lymphomas found in people with HIV disease (Herndier et al., 1994). Although it occurs most often in those demonstrating persistent generalized lymphadenopathy (swollen lymph glands), the usual site of lymphoma growth is in the brain, the heart, or the anorectal area (Brooke et al., 1990). The most common signs and symptoms are confusion, lethargy, and memory loss. Lymphomas are increasing in incidence primarily due to the extension of the life span of AIDS patients, by medical therapy (Table 6-1).

Progressive Multifocal Leukencephalopathy

Progressive multifocal leukoencephalopathy (PML) is an opportunistic infection caused by a papovavirus [Jamestown Canyon virus (JCV)] affecting 4% of AIDS patients. It is usually fatal within an average of 3.5 months and there is no treatment. In a few patients spontaneous improvement and prolonged survival have been reported. Some observations have indicated that cytosine arabinoside, a potent antiviral, may reverse the symptoms of PML. Symptoms of PML include altered mental status, speech and visual disturbances, gait difficulty, and limb incoordination (Guarino et al., 1995).

HIV Provirus: A Cancer Connection

In early 1994 AIDS investigators reported that HIV, on entering lymph cell DNA, activated nearby cancer-causing genes (oncogenes). The evidence suggests that HIV itself may trigger cancer in an otherwise normal cell.

These findings may mean that a variety of retroviruses that infect humans may also cause cancer (McGrath et al., 1994). Such findings raise concerns for developing an HIV vaccine. Using a weakened strain of HIV to make the vaccine may, when used, increase the incidence of lymphoma and other cancers.

Kaposi's Sarcoma-Associated Herpesvirus (KSHV)

FIGURE 6-10 Kaposi's Sarcoma-associated Herpesvirus (KSHV) or Human Herpesvirus-8 (HHV-8). Saliva is a major source of many infectious herpesviruses, including Epstein Bar Virus (EBV) and Cytomegalovirus (CMV) as well as KSHV; and by analogy to other saliva-borne herpesvirus, KSHV in saliva is a likely source for transmission. *(Three-Dimensional Model of KSHV created by Louis E. Henderson, Ph.D. Reproduced with permission from the* PRN Notebook™, *March 2002. Published by Physicians' Research Network, Inc.®,NY, USA. All rights reserved. ©March 2002.)*

POINT OF INFORMATION 6.3

CLASSIFICATION OF LYMPHOMAS

Lymphomas are generally classified into two types: **Hodgkin disease (HD),** and **non-Hodgkin lymphoma (NHL),** and they originate in the lymphoid tissues. The difference between them is entirely morphological, that is, the anatomic cellular characteristics are different. Hodgkin disease tumors contain giant cells of uncertain origin. Research suggests that B cells give rise to HD. The cells of NHLs have a more conventional appearance and can be classified as having arisen from T cells, B cells, or monocytes. There is otherwise little difference between these lymphomas in terms of location and progression of disease. Hodgkin disease is more common in the overall population, while NHLs are relatively rare. Yet NHL is the second most frequent cancer among HIV-infected patients. In general, AIDS patients are not more prone to develop breast, lung, and colon cancer. Collectively, scientists do not know much more about why AIDS patients develop certain cancers and diseases than they did 21 years ago when this pandemic started.

FIGURE 6-11 HIV/AIDS Patient Demonstrating a Lymphoma of the Neck. *(Courtesy CDC, Atlanta)*

NEUROPATHIES IN HIV DISEASE/AIDS PATIENTS

Soon after it enters the body HIV colonizes in the brain and other nerve tissues. Within the compartment of the nervous system, the virus remains, often at high concentrations and with time can lead to a spectrum of problems spanning from localized disease of the brain to distal peripheral neuropathy.

Neuropathies are functional changes in the peripheral nervous system; therefore, any part of the body may be affected. Although neuropathies are not OIs, they may result from the presence of certain OIs. **Peripheral neuropathy** is caused by nerve damage and is usually characterized by a sensation of pins and needles, burning, stiffness, or numbness in the feet and toes. It is a common, sometimes painful, condition in HIV-positive patients, affecting up to 30% of people with AIDS. At autopsy, two-thirds of AIDS patients have neuropathies (Newton, 1995). Neuropathy has been a continuous problem for patients throughout the HIV/ AIDS epidemic. It is most common in people with a history of multiple opportunistic infections and low T4 or CD4+ cell counts. There is a wide range of expression among patients with neuropathy, from a minor nuisance to a disabling weakness. The kinds of neuropathies occurring in people with HIV/ AIDS are numerous and must be identified before appropriate treatment can be prescribed. The underlying cause of the most common type of peripheral neuropathy remains elusive. What was a common complaint early in HIV infection of severe neuropathy—usually, burning feet, causing patients to walk on their heels—has diminished. The decrease in such complaints may be attributable to the antiviral effects of the drug ZDV. On the other hand, new varieties of drug-induced nerve damage (neuropathies) have been recognized with the use of nucleoside, non-nucleoside reverse transcriptase inhibitors, and protease inhibitor antivirals.

DISCLAIMER

This chapter is designed to present information on opportunistic infections in HIV/AIDS patients. The author does not accept any re-

SUMMARY

One of the gravest consequences of HIV infection is the immunosuppression caused by the depletion of the T4 or CD4+ helper cell population; suppressed immune systems allow for the expression of opportunistic diseases and cancers. It is the OI, end organ failures, and cancers that kill AIDS patients, not HIV per se. It is the cumulative effect of several OIs that creates the chills, night sweats, fever, weight loss, anorexia, pain, and neurological problems.

One tragic disease that does not result from an OI is Kaposi's sarcoma (KS), characterized as a cancer that can spread to all parts of an AIDS patient's body. About 20% of AIDS patients, mostly gay men, have KS. It is not usually found in hemophiliacs, injection drug users, or female AIDS patients.

REVIEW QUESTIONS

(Answers to the Review Questions are on page 489.)

1. Define opportunistic infection (OI).

2. Which OI organism expresses itself in 80% of AIDS patients? Where is it located and what does it cause?

3. Which of the protozoal OI organisms causes weight loss, watery diarrhea, and severe abdominal pain?

4. Which of the bacterial OIs causes "wasting syndrome," night sweats, anorexia, and fever?

5. True or False: Kaposi's sarcoma (KS) is caused by HIV. Explain.

6. Name the two kinds of KS.

7. True or False: KS affects all AIDS patients equally. Explain.

8. True or False: Candidiasis and ulceration may be present in patients with HIV infection.

9. True or False: Oral candidiasis occurs frequently with HIV infection.

10. True or False: The use of combination anti-HIV drug therapy, especially those combinations containing a protease inhibitor have substantially **decreased** the **severity** and **number** of OIs in AIDS patients.

HIV/AIDS SELF-EDUCATION QUIZ

Before you begin reading Chapters 7 through 13, take this quiz to help determine your current knowledge about HIV infection and AIDS.

1. HIV infects only homosexual persons.	T	F	?
2. AIDS affects only adults.	T	F	?
3. The agent that causes AIDS is HIV.	T	F	?
4. HIV is a bacterial agent.	T	F	?
5. The risk of an HIV infection from a blood transfusion is low, but it can happen.	T	F	?
6. Patients with AIDS have reduction in T4 or CD4+ cells.	T	F	?
7. People who have antibodies to HIV always develop AIDS.	T	F	?
8. HIV has been found in vaginal secretions, saliva, blood, and other body fluids.	T	F	?
9. AIDS is not a disease, but a syndrome.	T	F	?
10. HIV is easily transmitted to people.	T	F	?
11. The period from exposure to HIV to the expression of AIDS may be at least a year.	T	F	?
12. There is no known cure for HIV disease.	T	F	?
13. There is no known cure for AIDS.	T	F	?
14. HIV carriers without signs of active disease can transmit the virus.	T	F	?
15. All HIV-infected persons progress to AIDS.	T	F	?
16. All persons with AIDS die prematurely.	T	F	?
17. An effective HIV vaccine will be developed by 2007.	T	F	?
18. A person can be diagnosed with AIDS but have no outward symptoms.	T	F	?
19. One can have a zero T4 cell count and still be alive.	T	F	?
20. AIDS is considered a new disease of the twentieth century.	T	F	?

The correct answers to these questions are: 1.F; 2.F; 3.T; 4.F; 5.T; 6.T; 7.F; 8.T; 9.T; 10.F; 11.T; 12.T; 13.T; 14.T; 15.F; 16.T; 17.?; 18.T; 19.T; 20.T.

The following chapters will help in your understanding of this new sexually transmitted disease.

A Profile of Biological Indicators for HIV Disease and Progression to AIDS

HIV DISEASE DEFINED

The diagnosis of AIDS in the 1980s was most often associated with a quick death. Mortality came quickly and was inevitable within a few months of the diagnosis.

By the mid-1980s the CDC had learned enough about HIV infection to call it a disease. That made sense, as the vast majority of those who became infected became ill. HIV infection leads to the loss of T4 or CD4+ cells, which in turn produces a variety of signs and symptoms of a **nonspecific disease** with initial acute fever associated illness or mononucleosis-like symptoms that may last up to four weeks or longer. After the initial symptoms, most individuals enter a clinically asymptomatic phase (see Case in Point 7.1). This means the infected person feels well while his or her immune system is slowly compromised. It has been shown that long-lasting symptomatic **primary** HIV infection predicts an increased risk of rapid development of HIV-related symptoms and AIDS, but it is not known whether the different responses to HIV infection are caused by viral, host factors, or both.

Virulent strains of HIV have been characterized by their rapid replication, **syncytium-inducing (SI)** capacity, and tropism (attraction) for various types of T cells. It is known that the biological properties of HIV strains in asymptomatic HIV-infected individuals with normal T4 or CD4+ cell counts may predict the subsequent development of HIV-related disease, and that patients who harbor SI isolates develop immune deficiency more rapidly. It is not clear whether the appearance of more virulent strains during the symptomatic phase of the infection is a cause or an effect of progressive immune deficiency (Nielson et al., 1993). Several studies have demonstrated that a long period of fever around the time of **seroconversion (the presence of detectable HIV antibody in the serum)** is associated with more rapid development of immune deficiency (Pedersen et al., 1989).

Spectrum of HIV Disease

Because the immune system slowly falters, HIV disease is really a spectrum of disease (Figure 7.1 A, B). At one end of the spectrum are those infected with

VARIATION OF INITIAL SYMPTOMS AFTER HIV INFECTION

Case I: Male, Age 35, Los Angeles, California

One evening, for no apparent reason, John began sweating profusely. Soon after, a red rash began on his arms, face, and legs and then covered his body. Simultaneously, breathing became difficult and he was rushed to an emergency room. By then he was shaking violently. After medication and a battery of tests his problem could not be defined. This brief illness passed, but some years later, during a blood screen for insurance purposes he came up HIV positive. He immediately reflected back on his earlier illness and its cause.

Case II: Male, Age 29, Los Angeles, California

This case is in marked contrast to Case I. Feeling the pinch of a sore throat, this male went to his physician for an antibiotic. On examination, he had a yeast infection that appeared far back in his throat. This raised suspicion and he agreed to an HIV test. It came back positive. He had no other illness, he was treated, the sore throat vanished, and he is thriving in a long asymptomatic period.

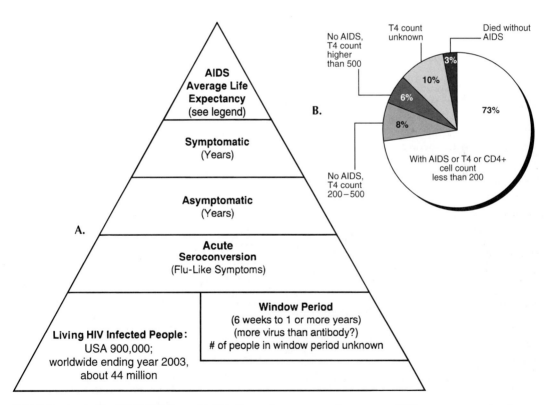

FIGURE 7-1 **A.** The HIV/AIDS Pyramid. This figure demonstrates that current AIDS cases are coming from an existing pool of HIV-infected persons. In the United States, of those infected, about 40% do not yet know they are HIV positive. Although both the asymptomatic and symptomatic periods may last for years, once diagnosed with AIDS the average life expectancy **without AIDS drug cocktails is two to three years.** Life expectancy for those now on combination drug cocktails depends on the state of the individual's immune system and response to antivetroviral therapy. **B.** Clinical outcomes 10 to 16 years after HIV infection in a population tracked by the San Francisco City Clinic from the beginning of the AIDS outbreak.

FIGURE 7-2 HIV/AIDS: The Beginning and the End. **A.,** Because he has no electricity in his office in Cite Soleil, Haiti, this physician uses a flashlight to examine an HIV-positive patient who is in the first stages of the infection. This physician sees, on average, one new HIV-infected person each day. **B.,** At age 28, Jean David looks at his X-ray, which, along with his medical history, according to his physician, indicates his impending death from AIDS. Jean David died soon after this picture was taken. He left an HIV-infected wife and HIV-infected 14-month-old daughter. *(Photos by Mike Stocker/South Florida* Sun-Sentinel)

HIV who look, feel, and are perfectly healthy. At the opposite end are those with advanced HIV disease (**symptomatic AIDS**) who are visibly sick and require significant medical and psychosocial support (Figure 7-2 A, B). Between these two extremes, HIV-infected people may develop illnesses that range from mild to serious. Symptoms can include persistent fevers, chronic fatigue, diarrhea, swollen lymph nodes, night sweats, skin rashes, significant weight loss, visual problems, chest pain, and fungal infections of the mouth, throat, and vagina. Illness from these conditions can be **severe** and **disabling**, and some people may die without ever being diagnosed with AIDS. Also, people with HIV disease may develop neurologic disorders, which can cause forgetfulness, memory loss, loss of coordination and balance, partial paralysis, leg weakness, mood changes, and dementia. These symptoms may occur in the absence of any other symptoms. The interval between initial HIV infection and the presence of signs and symptoms that characterize AIDS is variable and may range from several months to a median duration of about 11 years (Figure 7-3).

Defining Incubation and Latency

Because of the long delay in determining what happened after HIV infection and progression to AIDS, the terms **incubation** and **latency** are used,

in many cases interchangeably, causing some confusion. In this chapter, the two terms are used with respect to **clinical** observations as follows: **Clinical incubation** is that period after infection through the window period or when anti-HIV antibody production is measurable. **Clinical latency** is the time period from detectable anti-HIV antibody production (seroconversion—the person now tests HIV-antibody positive) through the asymptomatic period—a time prior to the expression of opportunistic diseases. This time period, being asymptomatic, may last from 1 to 25 years—the average being 11 years. The beginning and end of these periods will vary from person to person and their susceptibility and expression of HIV disease.

STAGES OF HIV DISEASE

The course of the disease in the infected individual varies substantially. At the extremes are individuals who show either little evidence of progression (loss in T4 cells) 10 to 25 years following infection (about 3%) or extremely rapid progression and death within less than two to three years. In general, HIV-infected adults experience a variety of conditions, categorized into four stages: **acute infection, asymptomatic, chronic symptomatic,** and **AIDS.**

Adult/Adolescent HIV Disease Continuum to AIDS

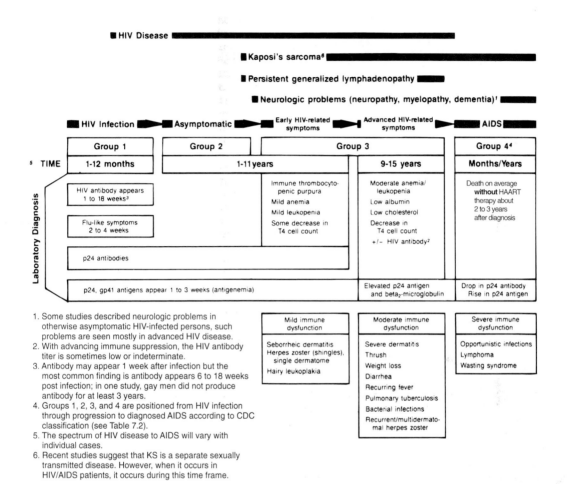

1. Some studies described neurologic problems in otherwise asymptomatic HIV-infected persons, such problems are seen mostly in advanced HIV disease.
2. With advancing immune suppression, the HIV antibody titer is sometimes low or indeterminate.
3. Antibody may appear 1 week after infection but the most common finding is antibody appears 6 to 18 weeks post infection; in one study, gay men did not produce antibody for at least 3 years.
4. Groups 1, 2, 3, and 4 are positioned from HIV infection through progression to diagnosed AIDS according to CDC classification (see Table 7.2).
5. The spectrum of HIV disease to AIDS will vary with individual cases.
6. Recent studies suggest that KS is a separate sexually transmitted disease. However, when it occurs in HIV/AIDS patients, it occurs during this time frame.

FIGURE 7-3 Spectrum of HIV Infection, Disease, and the Expression of AIDS. Seroconversion means that HIV antibodies are measurably present in the person's serum. With continued depletion of T4 or CD4+ cells, signs and symptoms appear, announcing the progression of HIV disease to AIDS. Although HIV antibodies have been found as early as 1 week after exposure, **most often seroconversion occurs between weeks 6 and 18; 95% within 3 months, 99% within 6 months** (see Figure 7-5). The early stage of HIV infection can be separated from the symptomatic stage by years of **clinical latency.** Early infection is characterized by a high number of infected cells and a high level of viral expression. AIDS is characterized by increased levels of viremia and p24 antigenemia, activation of HIV expression in infected cells, an increased number of infected cells, and progressive immune dysfunction. Stages of HIV disease blend into a continuum ranging from the asymptomatic with apparent good health, to increasingly impaired health, to the diagnosis of AIDS. Thus the spectrum of HIV disease ranges from the silent infection to unequivocal AIDS. Clinical expression moves from one condition to another, often without a clear-cut distinction. The level of an individual's infectiousness is believed to be greatest within the first months after infection and again when the T4 cell count drops below 200. **However, people who are HIV-infected can transmit HIV at any time.**

HLABISA, AN AIDS-RAVAGED TOWN IN KWAZULU NATAL PROVINCE

In 1994, 10% of adults in Hlabisa (Sha-BEE-sa) were HIV infected. Beginning 2003, over 30% or 75,000 people are HIV positive.

In the desperately crowded clinics and hospital wards, the scale of the epidemic is clear enough. This district of 250,000 people sits amid the hills of KwaZulu Natal, which has the highest adult rate of HIV infection of any province in South Africa. It is one of the few communities in South Africa in which government researchers have kept statistics on HIV infection rates for nearly a decade. Its story offers a rare and intimate look at one community ravaged by the plague. It marks the faces of young widows who trudge the road in somber capes and skirts, traditional mourning garb. It inspires the medicine makers who brew slivers of tree bark and bundles of dried leaves into elixirs sold in used Coca-Cola bottles. "Two spoons in the morning, two spoons in the afternoon," advises a herbalist who charges $1.25 a bottle. Chilled bodies that are often stacked one on top of another swamp the morgue.

Fear, Denial and Guilt

Professional men in Hlabisa boast over beers about extramarital affairs and the pleasures of unprotected sex. Some church leaders burn condoms and assail people with the virus as sinners. Prominent community members die in silence because the disease is considered so shameful. The disease is so deadly and so frightening that many hospital employees are reluctant to call it by name. They say a patient is immune, compromised, or that he suffers from "that disease." Others simply say, "You know what he's got." It is as if uttering the word might infect the tongue.

Healthcare Choice: Hospital or Healer?

Hospitals—On any given day there are more patients than available beds. In the male ward, 80% of men are HIV positive and about half the nursing positions are vacant. The first event in morning rounds is to count those who died of AIDS or a combination of HIV infection and tuberculosis. Of those who die, about half are under age 30! In the first six months of 2001, of 500 people who took HIV tests, 63% tested positive. One of the staff nurses has six children, four daughters and two sons. She leaves boxes of condoms on their bedroom dressers. The two things that give her the greatest sense of peace are taking her pills and watching those boxes empty. The children do not comment—she watches and replenishes the condom supply as needed.

Healers or Sangomas—In Southern Africa, a sangoma undergoes a long apprenticeship studying plant lore and making diagnoses that can include playing a guessing game with the patient, dancing into a trance, reading cast bones or waiting for the answer to come in a dream. In Hlabisa, physicians believe that virtually all their patients first visit a sangoma—a traditional healer. Donald McNeil describes the residence of one of the pre-eminent sangomas in Hlabisa. She is 57 years old. The walls of her home are covered with dried birds, the python skins she stabbed herself, and a crocodile her husband speared—from which, she says, she can make a lotion that renders a man's skin bulletproof. The floor is covered with hundreds of medicine containers, as humble as a Yum Yum peanut butter jar and as ornate as a set of gourds covered with beadwork. But there is also a box of latex gloves, which she wears when inspecting sores. When she injects a patient with a porcupine quill tipped with brown gunk from the Yum Yum jar, she makes a point of wiping the quill **afterward** with alcohol. Asked about those precautions, she proudly displayed the framed certificate from a 1998 workshop on "The Traditional Healer's Role in AIDS: Sexually Transmitted Diseases and Primary Health Care" offered at Hlabisa Hospital. One of the sangomas patients said that her illness was sent to her from her ancestors as a test. She also has a goat's bladder tied into her hair to remind her ancestors that she had sacrificed a goat to them.

Traditional Therapy—Because traditional Zulu medicine focuses chiefly on digestion, bile, and mucus, sangomas often give emetics or enemas. Some are simply dishwashing liquid or toothpaste. But others contain powerful herbs that can cause serious drug interactions. Enemas are used for anything from constipation to hysterical crying. However, enemas can rapidly dehydrate patients and send them into kidney or liver failure. For those who receive herbs causing them to throw up (emetics), it defeats the use of antiretroviral drugs.

Primary HIV Infection or the Acute Disease Stage

The clinical syndrome of primary HIV infection was recognized and documented in 1985, about two years after the initial identification of the causative agent of AIDS. By 1991 it was known that this symptomatic period is associated with an explosive replication of the virus, which is then partially controlled as the illness resolves spontaneously. Reports in 1993 further showed the population of HIV during this early period of infection to be quite homogeneous, in distinct contrast to the diverse quasispecies that are typically found in chronically infected persons. The course and time frame of the infection is illustrated graphically in Figure 7-3. The course of Primary HIV Infection (PHI) is limited to a few weeks or months, whereas the entire course of HIV infection can span many years. Specifically, PHI is the period after infection with HIV but before the development of detectable antibodies (see Figure 7-4).

The acute stage usually develops in two to eight weeks during PHI. Up to 70% of infected individuals develop a self-limited (brief) illness similar to influenza or mononucleosis: high spiking fever, sore throat, headaches, and swollen lymph nodes. Some may develop a rash, vomiting, diarrhea, and thrush (yeast infection in the mouth). This is referred to as the **acute retroviral syndrome**. The symptoms generally last about one to four weeks and resolve spontaneously (Table 7-1). The acute stage can be over quickly and easily missed. The acute phase is marked by high levels of HIV production, in excess of 1 million copies per milliliter of blood. During this phase, large numbers of HIV spread throughout the body, seeding themselves in various organs, particularly lymphoid tissues such as the lymph nodes, spleen, tonsils, and adenoids (Figure 7-4). During this time frame, HIV-infects monocytes, macrophage, T4 or CD4+ cells and follicular dendritic cells. Within these **safe** havens, HIV can persist for years despite **Highly Active Antiretroviral Therapy (HAART)**. This pool of latently infected cells is established very early after HIV enters the body—even if the person takes drug therapy immediately after exposure to HIV.

Table 7-1   Clinical and Laboratory Analyses of Acute HIV Infection

---

Signs

Erythematous truncal maculopapular rash
Generalized urticaria, roseola-like exantham, palm and sole desquamation
Generalized lymphadenopathy, splenomegaly
Acute meningo-encephalitis
Myelopathy, Guillain-Barre syndrome
Radiculopathy (brachial or sacral plexopathy)
Peripheral neuropathy
Myopathy
Pharyngitis
Hepatitis
Mental changes
Oral or esophageal ulcerations
Weight loss
Fever

Symptoms

Night sweats, chills, malaise, fatigue
Arthralgias, myalgias
Anorexia, nausea and vomiting, abdominal cramps, diarrhea
Headache, retro-orbital pain, photophobia, lethargy
Sore throat, dry cough

Laboratory Analysis

Mild-moderate neutropenia, relative monocytosis
Lymphopenia to lymphocytosis/atypical lymphocytes
Elevated erythrocyte sedimentation rate
Appearance of HIV antibodies
HIV in serum and/or CSF
Abnormal liver function tests
Raised levels of beta-2 microglobulin

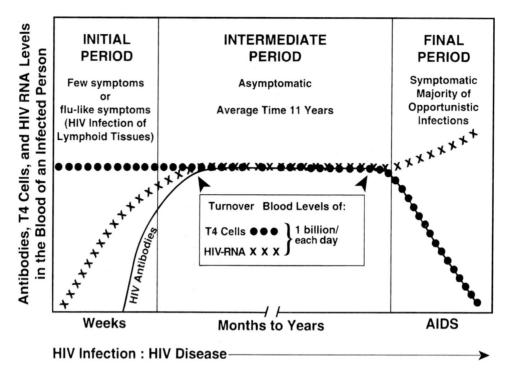

FIGURE 7-4 Relationship of T4 or CD4+ Cells, HIV Antibodies, and HIV RNA Levels (Viral Load) Beginning with HIV Infection Through AIDS. Within a week to weeks after HIV infection, HIV becomes seeded throughout the body's blood and lymph system. HIV reproduction (infection of T4 cells) begins almost immediately in the lymph system. The T4 cell population also begins rapid reproduction to replace T4 cell loss. This is why the T4 graph line stays at the same level through the **asymptomatic** period. The immune system begins to turn out HIV antibodies, in general 6 to 18 weeks later (window period, see Figure 7-5). Note that during the asymptomatic period T4 cell and HIV replication and antibody production keep pace. With time, however, T4 cells fail to replace losses, HIV continues to replicate, antibody levels drop due to loss of T4 signals to B cells to produce antibodies, and opportunistic infections begin—the **symptomatic** period. **Without** therapy this period lasts on average about two to three years. For people using HAART, the average number of years one can survive in the symptomatic period has yet to be determined.

During acute primary infection, patients have extremely high levels of viral replication **but a variable antibody immune response**. The level of cytotoxic T lymphocytes (CTLs) targeted against HIV appears to increase significantly, an attempt by the cellular part of the immune system to contain the high rate of HIV replication. Plasma HIV RNA levels may reach 10^5 (100,000) to 10^6 (1 million) copies/ml. It is now believed that the increase in the presence of CTLs and chemical factors they produce bring about a milder illness and a reduction in HIV to a **lower set point**—a steady state of viral load. The higher this set point the more rapidly HIV disease progresses to AIDS. (The presence of CTLs and long-term survival is presented in Box 7.3.) At this time in HIV infection and in some cases for weeks or months, neutralizing antibodies to HIV are not measurable—thus antibody testing, whether at clinical labs or using a home testing kit, is negative. This period of high viral replication in the absence of detectable antibody is called the **window of infectivity before seroconversion** or window period. During this period, patients may be highly infectious. The viral burden in genital secretion is particularly high during this time. Mathematical models suggest that 56% to 92% of all HIV infections may be transmitted during this period of acute infection (Quinn, 1997).

A true state of **biological latency**, according to the work of Xiping Wei and coworkers (1995) and David Ho and coworkers (1995), does not exist **in the lymph nodes** at any time during the course of HIV infection. The Wei and Ho investigations show that from the time of infection HIV replication is rapid and continuous, and within two to four weeks the infecting HIV strain is replaced by drug-resistant mutants. Each day over 1 billion HIV are produced and mostly destroyed and millions of T4 cells are infected, dying, and replaced. Over time the immune system fails to destroy HIV and replace its T4 cell losses and HIV disease progresses. Also, over time, many T4 cells in the lymphoid organs probably are **activated** by the increased secretion of certain cytokines such as tumor necrosis factor-alpha and interleukin-6. T4 or CD4+ cell **activation** allows uninfected cells to be more easily infected and causes increased replication of HIV in infected cells. Other components of the immune system are also chronically activated, with negative consequences that may include the suicide of cells by a process known as programmed cell death or apoptosis (pronounced a-po-toe-sis) and an inability of the immune system to respond to other invaders.

It is during this stage that many clinical HIV/AIDS investigators have recommended the use of **HAART** in order to stop rapid HIV reproduction and the infection of T4 lymphocyte (Vanhems et al., 1999). However, in February 2000, new antiretroviral therapy guidelines issued by the National Institutes of Health state that drug treatment should be delayed until the total T4 count falls below 350/microliter of blood and/or a viral load of 30,000/milliliter of blood. Prior recommendation was to start drug therapy at 500/microliter of blood and/or a viral load of 10,000/milliliter of blood (Centers for Disease Control and Prevention, 2001).

Asymptomatic HIV Disease Stage

Following acute illness, an infected adult can remain free of symptoms from 6 months to a median time of about 11 years. During the asymptomatic period, measurable HIV in the blood drops to a lower level but it continues to replicate and to destroy T4 cells within the lymph nodes while the body continues to produce new T4 cells and antibodies to the virus (Figure 7-5). An asymptomatic

---

POINT OF INFORMATION 7.1

ONE MISTAKE COST HIM HIS LIFE

I held my son today while he died from AIDS. There is no pain like the pain in a mother's heart. He was 28 years old, and now, he is dead.

This wonderful young man will never have a family. He will never again have a chance to do the things he enjoyed so much—water ski, snow ski, travel. He loved *Star Trek* and music. He loved working for the airlines and traveling all over the world. He was delightful and smart—a computer whiz—could take one apart and put it back together.

He wasted away from a handsome young man to a skeleton—nothing more than skin and bones. His weight dropped from 160 pounds to 80 pounds. His hair fell out. His beautiful teeth fell out. Sores broke out all over his body. He couldn't hold down any food, and eventually, he starved to death.

No, young people, he was not gay, nor was he a drug user. He just went to bed with a girl he didn't know.

His Mom

(Source: Ann Landers, syndicated columnist, 1994)

---

individual appears to be healthy and performs normal activities of daily living.

Symptomatic HIV Disease Stage

The symptomatic phase can last for months or years before a diagnosis of AIDS occurs. During this phase, as viral replication continues, T4 or CD4+ cells drop significantly. As the number of immune system cells decline, the individual develops a variety of symptoms such as fever, weight loss, malaise, pain, fatigue, loss of appetite, abdominal discomfort, diarrhea, night sweats, headaches, and swollen lymph glands. Ultimately, HIV overwhelms the lymphoid organs. The follicular dendritic cell networks break down in late-chronic stage disease and virus trapping is impaired, allowing spillover of large quantities of virus into the bloodstream. The destruction of the lymph node structure seen late in HIV disease may stop a successful immune response against HIV and other pathogens as well. Individuals at this stage, with a T4 cell count of 200 or less/μL of blood, often develop thrush, oral lesions, and

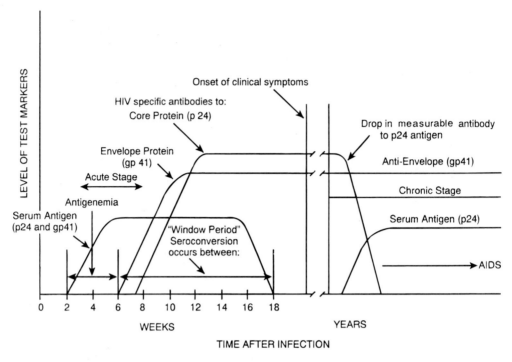

FIGURE 7-5 Profile of Serological Changes after HIV Infection. The dynamics of antibody response to HIV infection was determined by enzyme immunoassays (EIA). Note that during antigenemia, specific HIV proteins (antigens) can be detected before seroconversion occurs. Perhaps other HIV proteins will allow even earlier detection of HIV infection. Once antibodies appear, some antigens like p24 and gp41 disappear only to show up again later on. Note also that although antibody production is a sign that the immune system is working, in HIV-infected people, it is not working well enough. Although envelope and core protein antibodies are being produced as clinical illness begins, as the p24 antibody drops, the illness becomes more serious. *(Adapted from Coulis et al., 1987)*

other fungal, bacterial, and/or viral infections. The duration of these symptoms varies, but it is common for HIV-infected individuals to have them for months at a time. Of those persons in the symptomatic stage, and not using HIV drug therapy about 30% developed AIDS-associated infections within five years.

AIDS: Advanced HIV Disease Stage

The diagnosis of AIDS is a marker, not an end in itself. Currently, most people recover from their first, second, and third AIDS-defining illnesses. People with AIDS are a very heterogeneous group—some feel well and continue working for several years, others are chronically ill, and some die rather quickly.

Patients with AIDS became an even more diverse group after the 1993 expansion of the Centers for Disease Control and Prevention's (CDC's) definition of AIDS. People in excellent health are diagnosed with AIDS if their T4 or CD4+ cell count is less than 200/μl of blood.

The 26 clinical conditions used in the diagnosis of AIDS can be found in Table 7-2.

The final stage of HIV infection is called AIDS. During this time there is continued rapid viral replication that finally upsets the delicate balance of HIV production/T4 cell infection to T4 cell replacement. The virus largely depletes the cells of the immune system. It has been suggested that during the AIDS stage, serious immunodeficiency occurs when HIV diversity exceeds some threshold beyond which the immune system is

WHAT IS MEANT BY THE TERM WASTING DURING HIV DISEASE

Body wasting during HIV disease is sometimes referred to as AIDS WASTING. Wasting is not well understood, but it involves the involuntary loss of more than 10% of body weight, plus more than 30 days of either diarrhea or weakness and fever. Wasting is linked to disease progression and death. Part of the weight lost during wasting is fat. More important is the loss of muscle mass. This is also called lean body mass, or body cell mass. Lean body mass can be measured by bioelectrical impedance analysis (BIA). This is a simple, painless office procedure. AIDS wasting together with lipodystrophy can cause serious body shape changes. Wasting is the loss of muscle. Lipodystrophy is a loss of fat from one area and the accumulation of fat in another area of the body (see Figures 4-14 and 4-15).

Cause of Wasting—Several factors contribute to wasting—a) poor appetite, b) oral opportunistic infections, c) poor nutrient absorption, d) an altered food processing metabolism, e) changes in hormone levels due to the infection. There are no standard treatments for AIDS wasting.

unable to control HIV replication (Nowak et al., 1990; Wei et al., 1995; Cohen, 1995).

Finally the Question—How Long Can an HIV Infected Person Live?

The average time someone survives from the moment of HIV infection until death continues to increase. At the beginning of the epidemic, the average time was about 10 years. Many people confuse the date of diagnosis with the date of actual infection. The latter date is most often not known. Many years may separate the dates of infection and diagnosis. It currently is estimated at least 25% of persons infected with HIV today, utilizing drugs and treatments available, will survive on average for about 25 years. Average survival of persons infected 5–10 years ago is about 15 years from moment of infection until death. But averages are exactly that—averages. More precise estimates for individuals depend on current and past HIV RNA levels, current and past T4 or CD4+ cell counts, number of antiretroviral regimens used,

Table 7-2 List of 26 Conditions in the AIDS Surveillance Case Definition

- ◆ Candidiasis of bronchi, trachea, or lungs
- ◆ Candidiasis, esophageal
- ◆ Cervical cancer, invasive[a]
- ◆ Coccidioidomycosis, Disseminated or extra-pulmonary
- ◆ Cryptococcosis, extrapulmonary
- ◆ Cryptosporidiosis, chronic intestinal (>1 month duration)
- ◆ Cytomegalovirus disease (other than liver, spleen, or nodes)
- ◆ Cytomegalovirus retinitis (with loss of vision)
- ◆ HIV encephalopathy
- ◆ Herpes simplex: chronic ulcer(s) (>1 month duration); or bronchitis, pneumonitis, or esophagitis
- ◆ Histoplasmosis, disseminated or extrapulmonary
- ◆ Isosporiasis, chronic intestinal (>1 month duration)
- ◆ Kaposi's sarcoma
- ◆ Lymphoma, Burkitt's (or equivalent term)
- ◆ Lymphoma, immunoblastic (or equivalent term)
- ◆ Lymphoma, primary in brain
- ◆ *Mycobacterium avium complex* or *M. kansasii*, disseminated or extrapulmonary
- ◆ *Mycobacterium tuberculosis*, disseminated or extrapulmonary
- ◆ *Mycobacterium tuberculosis*, any site (pulmonary[a] or extrapulmonary)
- ◆ *Mycobacterium*, other species or unidentified species, disseminated or extrapulmonary
- ◆ *Pneumocystis carinii* pneumonia
- ◆ Pneumonia, recurrent[a]
- ◆ Progressive multifocal leukoencephalopathy
- ◆ Salmonella septicemia, recurrent
- ◆ Toxoplasmosis of brain
- ◆ Wasting syndrome due to HIV

[a]Added in the 1993 expansion of the AIDS surveillance case definition.

(Adapted from the CDC, Atlanta, Georgia.)

adherence to therapy, response to therapy, and current health status. At least 5% of HIV-infected persons are estimated to be long-term, non-progressors. That is, in the absence of therapy, these individuals maintain a T4 or CD4+ cell count of 450 cells per microliter of blood and typically have HIV RNA

HIV: CASE PRESENTATIONS

Case 1—A 28-year-old man visited his family physician complaining of flulike illness. The physician obtained a drug-use and sexual history, through which it was discovered that in the past year the patient had engaged in unprotected sex with several partners. HIV testing was ordered. It showed a T4 count of 550 μl and a plasma HIV RNA level of 735,000 copies/ml.

Diagnosis: Acute HIV Infection—The illness may present dramatically, with features such as painful mouth ulceration, lymphadenopathy, or a rash indistinguishable from that of mononucleosis. It may even have neurologic manifestations, such as Bell's palsy. Typically, however, the illness is hard to distinguish from influenza and an array of nonspecific viral illnesses. It may even be essentially asymptomatic. Except perhaps in retrospect, the patient usually fails to recognize the symptoms as marking acquisition of HIV infection.

Case 2—A 22-year-old woman in the first trimester of her first pregnancy reported being in fair health. She underwent routine HIV screening as part of the antepartum evaluation. The T4 count was 275/μL, and the plasma HIV RNA level was 127,000 copies/ml.

Diagnosis: Asymptomatic Chronic HIV Infection—HIV infection was detected by routine screening. Here the infection has moved from its acute phase to a latent phase during which the virus is residing in sites such as the lymph nodes, its replication still counterbalanced by host immune responses. Today detection by routine screening occurs most often in pregnant women. Indeed, as many as two-thirds of HIV cases in women are diagnosed during pregnancy.

Case 3—A 34-year-old man presented at an emergency department seeking treatment for a chest rash typical of herpes zoster. Thinking that the patient was surprisingly young to have shingles, the physician identified a history of recreational cocaine use. The patient insisted that his drug use was purely intranasal, not intravenous. He said he had never had thrush or pneumonia. The HIV antibody test was positive.

Diagnosis: Symptomatic Chronic HIV Infection Complicated by Herpes Zoster—Although zoster can occur at any time of life, it most often occurs in patients of advanced age or in those with serious conditions such as malignancy or long-term steroid therapy. In chronic HIV infection, zoster is now recognized to have an increased chance of preceding, often by a long period, other opportunistic infections. In this instance, the patient had not had thrush or Pneumocystis carinii pneumonia. Measurement of the HIV viral RNA level was deferred because of the presence of inflammation, which may cause a misleading spike in plasma HIV RNA, regardless of the underlying condition causing the inflammation. (Reproduced with permission. John Bartlett et al., Primary Care of HIV Infection. *Hospital Practice*, 1998; 33 (12:53–56, 61–64, 67–69) © 1998. The McGraw-Hill Companies, Inc.)

---

levels of less than 5000 copies/ml of blood. It is not clear what immunologic features distinguish these individuals from the other 95% of HIV-infected persons.

Symptoms and Impairment

In the symptomatic stages of HIV disease, an individual's ability to carry on the activities of daily living is impaired. The degree of impairment varies considerably from day to day and week to week. Many individuals are debilitated by the symptoms of the disease to the point that it becomes difficult to hold steady employment, shop for food, or do household chores. It is also quite common for people with AIDS to experience phases of intense life-threatening illness, followed by phases of seemingly normal functioning, all in a matter of weeks. For a good review on the mechanisms of HIV disease, read "The Immunopathogenesis of HIV Infection" by Giuseppe Pantaleo et al. (1993), Bucy (1999), and Yu (2000).

HIV Can Be Transmitted During All Four Stages

A person who is HIV-infected, even while feeling healthy, may unknowingly infect others. **The greatest risk of HIV transmission occurs within**

AIDS: A MANAGEABLE AND CHRONIC DISEASE?

It would appear, from reviewing the research and applied drug therapy literature that the holy grail of HIV therapy is to contain, control, and force HIV infection into a manageable and chronic disease. Jose Catalan and colleagues (2001) state that HIV disease has always been a chronic disease. But while it is now better managed than ever, HIV infection/disease has never been a truly manageable condition. Prior to the beginning of antiretroviral therapy (HAART) in 1996, the HIV-infected died of a variety of opportunistic infections (OI) and at varying times from their initial infection. Treatment and management of the virus and for many of the OIs was poor at best. Beginning 1996, many patients, about half, placed on HAART therapy recovered from conditions in which they were close to death. Others, using the drugs, delayed the progression of their HIV disease. But again who would respond to the therapy, for how long, and why they responded while others did not, still leaves this disease as remarkably unmanageable for at least half of the infected population. And as HIV resistance to the drugs continues to increase, the conditional management of those who once responded to therapy are once again becoming desperate for improved management of their disease. No, HIV disease has never really been manageable, rather for most, drug therapy offers a temporary reprieve for a failing immune system.

Jose Catalan and colleagues write that chronic is an umbrella term used in opposition to "acute," a time-limited, self-contained disease. The term chronic hides a wide range of diseases with few things in common: they do not go away easily, they last for a long time, and on the whole, they are never successfully eradicated. It is useful to realize that HIV infection has always been a chronic illness, in the sense that it develops over a number of years. In the early days of the epidemic, it was calculated that only about 50% of HIV-infected individuals would develop HIV-related opportunistic conditions within 10 years of infection, although once these problems appeared, decline tended to be rapid—survival after an AIDS diagnosis sometimes lasting less than two years. HIV infection is still a chronic disease, but for those with access to HAART, the time span has extended beyond these original expectations. So, is HIV infection a chronic illness? To the extent that it lasts years and, to date, cannot be cured, it is a chronic illness and has always been one. Longer survival, to date, has meant more time for more adverse consequences to develop because of HAART. And because HAART is allowing some people to live longer, they express some bizarre forms of disease never encountered before in HIV-infected patients.

the acute period, the first several months after infection, and again when the T4 cell count drops below 200.

HIV DISEASE WITHOUT SYMPTOMS, WITH SYMPTOMS, AND AIDS

Michael is a 31-year-old Hispanic male who complains of fatigue, headache, muscle aches, sore throat, and nausea. Physical assessment demonstrates a skin rash on his trunk and swollen lymph glands. His temperature is 98°F (37°C); other vital signs are within normal limits. Laboratory findings including white blood cell count, platelet count, and blood chemistry are normal. Michael states that his symptoms began one week ago. Subsequent laboratory testing will confirm that Michael has acute retroviral syndrome which accompanies primary HIV infection (PHI). But the odds are high that in almost every emergency room or physician's office in the country, Michael will be misdiagnosed. He is likely to be told that he has a viral infection, probably the flu, and sent home with instructions for supportive care.

A person may have no symptoms (**asymptomatic**) but test HIV positive. This means that the virus is present in the body. Although he or she has not developed any of the illnesses associated with HIV disease, it is possible to transmit the virus.

In time, most people with HIV disease progress to AIDS. A person has AIDS when the defect in his or her immune system caused by HIV disease has progressed to such a degree that an unusual infection or tumor is present or when the T4 or CD4+ cell count has fallen below $200/\mu l$ of blood. In AIDS patients, a number of diseases are known to take advantage of the damaged immune system. These include opportunistic infections and tumors such as Kaposi's sarcoma or lymphoma,

— BOX 7.1 —

EVOLUTION OF HIV DURING HIV DISEASE PROGRESSION

HIV is a unique retrovirus. For example, mitosis, a form of cell division, is a requirement for the nuclear entry of most retroviral nucleic acids. In contrast, mitosis does not appear to be required for nuclear entry of HIV nucleic acids, particularly in terminally differentiated cells (for example, macrophages and dendritic cells) (Freed et al., 1994). Second, HIV lacks any mechanism to correct errors that occur as its genetic material is being duplicated. This means that every time the virus makes a copy of itself there will be, on average, at least one genetic "mistake" incorporated in the new virus. A few days or weeks after initial infection, there may be a large population of closely related, but not identical, viruses replicating in an infected individual. In the **quasi**—steady-state condition, there are successive generations of viral progeny, with each generation following the next by about 2.6 days. Approximately 140 generations of virus are produced over the course of a year and 1,400 generations over the course of 10 years, allowing production of an extraordinary number of genetic variants. Some variants can provide preexisting drug-resistant forms or enable rapid development of resistance under drug pressure, and some enable the viral population to escape immune activity.

VIRAL POOL

The viral pool in an HIV-infected person is estimated to be about 10 billion viruses and each is genetically different from all other HIV in the pool. It is known from experimental data that about 1 in 1,000 particles is infectious, so the infectious viral pool may be on the order of 10 million viruses. With a genome of approximately 10^4 nucleotides, and from 1 to 10 billion HIV variants made daily, mutations most likely occur at every nucleotide position on a daily basis (Ho, 1996). This creates an enormous potential for viral evolution. On average, the HIV that is transmitted to another individual will be over 1,000 generations removed from the initial HIV infection. This extent of replication per transmitted infection (transmission cycle) is probably without equal among viral and perhaps bacterial infections (Coffin, 1995). Regardless of the underlying mechanism of immunodeficiency, it is becoming apparent that **the force that is**

driving the disease is the constant repeated cycles of HIV replication. Simon Wain-Hobson (1995) suggests that because of 24-hour-a-day HIV replication, as shown by Wei and coworkers (1995), an HIV-infected asymptomatic person can harbor at least 1 billion distinct HIV variants and an AIDS patient 10 billion HIV variants. With so many genetic variants, **some are going to be resistant to any given drug. (This would include drugs not yet used in therapy).** During the investigations of Ho and coworkers (1995) and Wei and coworkers (1995), variants of HIV, resistant to the drugs, ABT-538, **now called Ritonavir,** (a protease inhibitor), and nevirapine (a non-nucleoside agent that inhibits reverse transcriptase function), occurred within days or weeks! Alan Perelson and colleagues (1996) reported data collected from five HIV-infected people after administering Ritonavir through 7 days. Each person responded with a similar pattern of decline in plasma HIV RNA. Their results: Infected T4 cells had an average life span of 2.2 days. Plasma HIV RNA had an average life span of 0.3 days. The results also suggest that the minimum duration of the HIV life cycle in human T4 cells is 1.2 days on average and that the average HIV generation time—defined as the time from release of a virus until it infects another cell and causes the release of a new generation of HIV—is 2.6 days. The life time of HIV in resting or latent T4 cells may range from 6 months to perhaps an infinite amount of time. Such cells can produce HIV when activated.

Number	1 to 10 billion HIV produced each day.	Many million of T4 cells infected each day.
After two days	Half of HIV are destroyed and are replaced by about an equal amount of new HIV.	About half the infected T4 cells die and are replaced by new T4 cells.
After 14 days	After mutations, most new HIV are drug resistant.	T4 cell count decreases and new T4 cells are infected with the drug-resistant viruses.

BOX 7.1 *(continued)*

HIV CLEARANCE

Douglas Richman (1995) states that the HIV clearance rate can be calculated based on the rate of reduction in viral RNA load. In cases in which viral RNA load attains a constant level, it can be assumed that there is a dynamic equilibrium resulting in a steady-state level, with production rates matching clearance rates. When viral resistance emerges, as in cases of drug resistance, the production of resistant virus may double every two days. The proportion of virus with resistance mutations can also be calculated. According to Richman, in the case of the nonnucleoside reverse transcriptase inhibitors, this has been found to be approximately 1 to 2 per 1,000 RNA copies circulating in the plasma; that is, a patient with 60,000 copies/mL plasma has approximately 100 copies/mL of resistant mutants prior to the **beginning of treatment.** A similar scenario probably holds for all drug-resistant mutations. Thus it is reasonable to expect the HIV-resistant mutants will emerge to any antiretroviral compound.

TREATMENT FAILURE

Virologic Failure

Failure to reduce the viral load to an undetectable level *or*
Failure to reduce the viral load by at least 2 to 2.5 $\log_{10}$ *or*
A persistent increase in viral load following a period of adequate suppression

Immunologic Failure

Failure to restore the T4 or CD4+ cell count to more than 200 cells/mm^3 *or*
Failure to significantly increase T4 cell count *or*
A persistent decline in T4 cell count after a period of immune reconstitution

Clinical Failure

Development of new opportunistic infections (OI) *or*
Failure to resolve pretreatment OI, wasting, or dementia
(Adopted from Soloway et al., 2000)

With new techniques for quantitating plasma HIV RNA, infected individuals can be evaluated for response to antiretroviral therapy.

MUTANT HIV OVERWHELM THE IMMUNE SYSTEM

As HIV multiplies and mutant forms are produced, the immune system responds to these new forms. But ultimately the sheer number of **different** viruses to which the immune system must respond becomes overwhelming. It's a bit like the juggler who tries to keep too many balls in the air: The result is disastrous. Once the immune system is overwhelmed, the latest escape mutant—which may not necessarily be the most pathogenic one to come along—will predominate and immune deficiency will progress (Japour, 1995).

---

a malignancy of the lymph glands. The presence of one of the opportunistic diseases or a T4 cell count of less than 200, along with a positive HIV test establishes the medical diagnosis of AIDS. Thus the disease we call AIDS is actually the end stage of HIV disease. It is important to remember that AIDS itself is not transmitted—the virus is. AIDS is the most severe clinical form of HIV disease.

The term full-blown AIDS is often used on TV and in the lay press but not in this textbook. Terms such as advanced HIV disease or advanced AIDS are not only more accurate but also more meaningful.

ASPECTS OF HIV INFECTION

HIV infection depends on a variety of events, for example, the amount and strain of HIV that enters the body (some strains of HIV are known to be more pathogenic than others), perhaps where it enters the body, the number of exposures, the time interval between exposures, the immunological status of the exposed person, and the presence of other active infections. These are referred to as cofactors that contribute to successful HIV infection.

Incubation and Window Period

The time from HIV infection to the first signs and symptoms of HIV disease is called the **clinical incubation period**. Evidence suggests that the route or manner of HIV infection may influence the **incubation period**. For example, exposure through sexual intercourse has a mean incubation time of 6 months. Infection by transfusion has a mean incubation time of 2.5 years. It appears that for unknown reasons, **free viruses** (those not inside cells) present at the time of infection do not stimulate the immune system. Infected cells in the transfused blood have a **biologically latent** (inactive) proviral state and antibody will not be made until new viruses are produced which then engender HIV disease symptoms. Infected newborns have a mean incubation period of 10 months. (Newborns in general begin making their own antibody about 3 to 6 months after birth, but may not make antibody against HIV for several years.)

The time between infection and the presence of first HIV antibody or seroconversion is called the window period. Because it can be quite lengthy, HIV antibody tests performed during the window period that are negative may be **falsely negative** (Figure 7-5).

PRODUCTION OF HIV-SPECIFIC ANTIBODIES

During the 20 years (1983–2003) since the discovery of HIV, scientists have constructed a serological or antibody graph of HIV infection and HIV disease. The graph reveals how soon the body produces HIV-specific antibodies after infection and about when the virus begins its reproduction. Different parts of the graph (Figure 7-5) have been filled in by Paul Coulis and colleagues (1987), Dani Bolognesi (1989), and Susan Stramer and colleagues (1989). **The history of the HIV antibody is not yet complete, but the order of appearance and disappearance of antibodies specific for the serologically important antigens over the course of HIV disease has been described.**

The time period from seroconversion to the presentation of clinical symptoms is quite variable and may last for 11 or more years in adults and adolescents, but occurs earlier in children and older persons with HIV disease. The time period for moving from clinical symptoms of HIV disease to AIDS is also quite variable (Figure 7-3). Much depends on the individual's genetic susceptibility and his or her response to medical intervention. Note that Figure 7-5 shows that HIV plasma viremia (the presence of virus in blood plasma) and antigenemia (an-ti-je-ne-mi-ah— the persistence of antigen in the blood) can be detected as early as two weeks after infection. This

---

Table 7-3 CDC Classification of HIV-Related Diseases

HIV Disease

Group 1: Acute infection—HIV antibodies absent; asymptomatic or if symptomatic mononucleosis-like symptoms that subside in most cases

Group 2: Asymptomatic infection—HIV antibodies present; eventually moves on to

Group 3: Persistent generalized lymphadenopathy; eventually moves on to Group 4

AIDS

Group 4:

Subgroup A: Constitutional symptoms (previously called ARC, aids-related complex) and <200 T4 cells/μl of blood.

Subgroup B: Neurologic, symptoms (AIDS dementia complex, neuropathy)

Subgroup C

Category C-1: Secondary infections listed in the CDC surveillance definition for AIDS: *Pneumocystis carinii* pneumonia, recurrent pneumonia, chronic cryptosporidiosis, CNS toxoplasmosis, extraintestinal strongyloidosis, isosporiasis, esophageal candidiasis, cryptococcosis, histoplasmosis, *Mycobacterium avium intracellulare* or *Mycobacterium kansasii*, cytomegalovirus, chronic or disseminated herpes simplex, progressive multifocal leukoencephalopathy

Category C-2: Other specified secondary infections: oral cell hairy leukoplakia, multidermatomal herpes zoster, recurrent *Salmonella* bacterium, nocardiosis, pulmonary tuberculosis, oral candidiasis

Subgroup D: Secondary cancers: Kaposi's sarcoma, non-Hodgkin's lymphoma (small, noncleaved lymphoma; immunoblastic sarcoma), primary brain lymphoma

Subgroup E: Other conditions: lymphocytic interstitial pneumonitis, neoplasms, infections not previously listed

---

demonstrates that viremia and antigenemia occur prior to seroconversion. Using HIV proteins produced by recombinant DNA methods (making synthetic copies of the viral proteins), antibodies specific for gp41 (a subunit of glycoprotein 160) are detectable prior to those specific for p24 (a core protein) and persist throughout the course of infection. Levels of antibody specific for p24 rise to detectable levels between six and eight weeks after HIV infection but may disappear abruptly. The drop in p24 antibody has been shown to occur at the same time as a rise in p24 antigen in the serum. This strange phenomenon is thought to be due to the loss of available p24 antibody in immune complexes—too little p24 antibody is being made to handle the new virus being produced. It is believed that this imbalance is one of the important factors that moves the patient toward AIDS. Thus a sudden decrease in anti-p24 is considered by many scientists to be a prognostic indicator that people with HIV disease are moving toward AIDS.

Some AIDS researchers and health care professionals believe that 90% to 95% of those persons infected with HIV will eventually develop AIDS. **Without antiretroviral drugs, approximately 50% of people with HIV disease will progress to AIDS within 8 years after infection.** At 10 years 70% will have developed AIDS. After that, an additional 25% to 45% of the remainder will develop AIDS. It is **most improbable** that 100% of those infected will develop AIDS.

Classification of HIV/AIDS Progression

There are several classifications that spell out the progression of signs and symptoms from HIV infection to the diagnosis of AIDS. The classifications were developed to provide a framework for the medical management of patients from the time of infection through the expression of AIDS. All classification systems are fundamentally the same—they group patients according to their stage of infection, based on signs that indicate a failing immune system (Royce et al., 1991).

The most widely accepted classification because of its greater clinical applicability, comes from the CDC (Table 7-3). **The CDC classification uses four mutually exclusive groupings** (Figure 7-6). The groupings are based on the **presence** or **absence** of signs and symptoms of disease, and clinical and/or laboratory findings and the chronology of their occurrence. Group 1, acute infection, means the person is **viremic** (that is, many virus particles are present in his or her blood or serum). There are **no measurable antibodies;** one is HIV positive but lacks HIV antibodies and signs and symptoms of HIV disease.

The majority of people in Group 1 remain asymptomatic. Some may experience flu- or mononucleosis-like symptoms that generally disappear in a few weeks. In relatively few cases the patient moves rapidly from mild symptoms into severe opportunistic infections and is diagnosed with AIDS.

In Group 2, antibodies are present but most patients remain free of HIV disease symptoms. Regardless of the lack of outward clinical symptoms, 90% of those who are asymptomatic experience some form of immunological deterioration within five years (Fauci, 1988).

In Group 3, asymptomatic people from Groups 1 and 2 become symptomatic and demonstrate lymphadenopathy in the neck, armpit, and groin areas. Although a number of other diseases may cause the lymph nodes to swell, most swelling

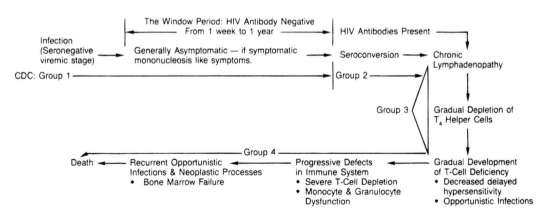

FIGURE 7-6 Clinical History of HIV Infection According to Center for Disease Control and Prevention Groupings. Seroconversion means that HIV antibodies are measurably present in the person's serum. With continued depletion of T4 cells, various signs and symptoms appear announcing the progression of HIV disease into AIDS. Although HIV antibodies have been found as early as 1 week after exposure, most often seroconversion occurs between weeks 6 and 18 but may not occur for up to 1 year or more.

——— BOX 7.2 ———

DEVELOPMENT OF AIDS OVER TIME

PROGRESSION TO AIDS WITHOUT DRUG THERAPY

A spectrum of clinical expression of disease can occur after HIV infection. Approximately 10% of HIV-infected subjects progress to AIDS within the first 2 to 3 years of HIV infection **(rapid progressors).** People with greater than 50,000 HIV RNA copies/mL at 6 months after infection are the most likely to be rapid progressors. About 60% of adults/adolescents will progress to AIDS within 12 to 13 years after HIV infection **(slow progressors).** Approximately 5% to 10% of HIV-infected subjects are clinically asymptomatic after 20 to 25 years. They have stable peripheral blood T4 cell levels of greater than 500 **(nonprogressors).** (Haynes et al., 1996; Schanning et al., 1998).

It has been estimated that from 3% to 5% will **NEVER** progress to AIDS. But, current data, on 50 known or reported cases of nonprogressors, indicate that the incidence of nonprogressors is more like 1 person in every 25,000 infected! Regardless, nonprogressors all have one thing in common, a functional squad of **memory T4 or CD4+ cells** that respond to HIV infection. Such people have an immune system that **remembers** HIV and controls it over time.

UPDATE 2001— An important chemical signal (or cytokine) used by cells in interlukin 10 (IL-10). When produced in large amounts by cells, IL-10 can weaken the immune response against viruses, bacteria, and fungi. Some researchers think HIV may trick the immune system into producing large amounts of IL-10, weakening the body's ability to fight the virus. Researchers at Mt. Sinai Hospital in Toronto reported at the 8th Conference on Retroviruses and Opportunistic Infections that T lymphocyte cells taken from nonprogressors and healthy HIV-negative people produced relatively low levels of IL-10. But such cells taken from people with AIDS produced between two to five times more IL-10. The researchers found that those who took highly active antiretroviral therapy (HAART) were able to significantly reduce their levels of IL-10.

One thing is clear from the studies of nonprogressors thus far: Not all are the same. Some show distinct features not shared by others, yet somehow all experience nonprogression. The reasons behind this phenomena may be virologic, immunologic, or both. However, no common genetic correlate has yet been identified to explain long-term nonprogression.

AIDS: LONG-TERM SURVIVORS WITHOUT THERAPY

People with AIDS with a very low T4 cell count who have survived for exceptionally long periods of time (5 years or more) are usually described as long-term survivors. Some 6% of persons diagnosed with clinical AIDS are long-term survivors (Laurence, 1996).

AIDS: LONG-TERM SURVIVORS WITH DRUG THERAPY

Current and contained use of AIDS drug cocktails containing at least one protease inhibitor has increased the number of long-term survivors! Survival after the onset of AIDS, without HAART, has been increasing in industrialized countries from an **average** of less than 1 year to over 4 years at present. With therapy, survival time has been increased by 3 to 10 years, depending on the case and therapy. Survival time with AIDS in developing countries remains short and is estimated to be, on average, less than 1 year. Longer survival appears to be directly related to routine treatment with antiretroviral drugs, the use of drugs for opportunistic infections, and a better overall quality of health care.

The majority of AIDS cases occur before age 35, and over 90% of all AIDS deaths occur in people under the age of 50 worldwide.

Philip Rosenberg and colleagues (1994) reported that the length of incubation and progression from HIV infection to AIDS varied according to the age at the time of infection. Younger ages were associated with a slower progression to AIDS. The estimated median treatment-free clinical incubation period was 12 years for those infected at age 20, 9.9 years for infection at age 30, and 8.1 years for infection at age 40.

LONG-TERM AIDS SURVIVORS

Parade Magazine, January 31, 1993, carried a review of 16 long-term survivors who date back to 1982. On April 16, 1995, the same magazine

BOX 7.2 *(continued)*

reported that 12 of the 16 had since died of AIDS. On April 6, 1997, the magazine continued its followup on the four remaining survivors seen in Figure 7-7. On July 23, 2000, the magazine reported on the **three remaining survivors.** They are Michael Leonard Marshal, 54, who is studying psychology at Santa Monica College in California; George Melton, 47, who now works as a colorist in a hair salon in San Francisco; and Niro Asistent Markoff, 55, who now works in a school of healing in East Hampton, New York.

FIGURE 7-7 Long-Term AIDS Survivors. In 1988, *Parade Magazine* began tracking 16 long-term AIDS survivors. The longest living of these survivors was diagnosed with AIDS in 1982. Only one of the 16, a woman, was HIV-infected through a heterosexual relationship. Her sexual partner was bisexual. In June 1990, 13 were alive. By January 1993, six of the original 16 were alive. In April 1997, *Parade Magazine* updated interviews—four remained. Since then, Cristofer Shihar, on the right in this photograph, died. As of July 2002, three survive. Their lives continue. *(© Blake Little)*

Marshal began taking an AIDS cocktail of anti-HIV drugs in 1996. Melton began taking the drugs in 1997. Both men have undetectable levels of HIV in their blood and "feel great." Niro Markoff said that it has been many years since she has had any trace of HIV in her blood—she has never taken HIV/AIDS drugs.

declines as the other symptoms of illness fade. However, with HIV infection, the lymph nodes remain swollen for months, with no other signs of a related infectious disease. Consequently, lymphadenopathy is sometimes called **persistent generalized lymphadenopathy** (PGL). People with PGL may experience night sweats, weight loss, fever, on-and-off diarrhea, fatigue, and the onset of oral candidiasis or thrush (a fungus or yeast infection of the oral cavity) (see Figure 6-3). Such signs and symptoms are prodromal (symptoms leading to) for AIDS. Studies have shown that people in Group 3 appear to become more infectious as the disease progresses.

People in Group 4 have been diagnosed with AIDS. They fit the 1987 CDC criteria for AIDS diagnosis. (The CDC AIDS diagnostic criteria are listed in Tables 7-3 and 1-1.) Hairy leukoplakia (Figure 7-8, Table 7-3, Category C-2) is virtually diagnostic of AIDS in Group 4 patients. Statistics show that about 30% of all the newly HIV-infected will progress to Group 4 (AIDS) every 5 years, so that about 90% will have been diagnosed with AIDS within 15 years. Not all the opportunistic diseases (OIs) or cancers

will appear in any one AIDS patient. But some OIs, like *Pneumocystis carinii* pneumonia occur in some 80% of AIDS patients prior to their deaths.

PROGNOSTIC BIOLOGICAL MARKERS RELATED TO AIDS PROGRESSION

The **ideal marker** would be able to predict HIV disease progression, be responsive to antiretroviral therapy, and explain the variance in clinical outcome due to therapy. It is, however, unlikely that any one marker will be able to fulfill all these criteria in HIV infection. Therefore, individual markers used to track HIV infection to AIDS are presented.

p24 Antigen Levels

p24 is a specific protein located in the core or inner layer of HIV. Because the immune system produces antibody against foreign protein, antibody is made against p24. A positive test for p24 antigen in the blood means that HIV production is so rapid that it overcomes the available antibody (Figure 7-5). This raised p24 antigen level condition occurs

FIGURE 7-8 Oral Hairy Leukoplakia (lu-ko-pla-ki-ah) of the Tongue. An early manifestation, it is virtually diagnostic of AIDS. The white shaggy-appearing or corrugated "hairy" patches typically occur on the lateral borders of the tongue and are caused by the Epstein-Barr virus (EBV).These white plaques cannot be removed. **A.** A milder form of the disease. **B.** A more severe manifestation of the disease. Note that the white plaques may cover the entire tongue. *(Schiodt, Greenspan, and Greenspan 1989.* American Review of Respiratory Disease, 1989, 10:91–109. *Official Journal of the American Thoracic Society.* © American Lung Association)

at least twice; once shortly after infection and again during the AIDS period when the immune system is rapidly deteriorating and unable to produce sufficient antibody to deal with newly produced HIV.

Those who, during the early stage of HIV infection, test p24 antigen positive are likely to progress to AIDS earlier **than those** who test p24 negative. Thus, a positive p24 test is an early and serious warning sign for HIV-infected people (Escaich et al., 1991; Phillips et al., 1991a).

p24 Antibody Levels

High levels of p24 antibody indicate that the immune system is functioning well and clearing the body of free HIVs. High antibody levels appear to slow the progression toward AIDS. Typically, p24 antibody levels are high during a person's asymptomatic or latent stage (Figure 7-4). However, antibody levels begin to decrease and p24 antigen levels rise, indicating a loss of immune function.

Other Markers

Beta-2 microglobulin (B-2M) is a low molecular weight protein that is present on the surface of almost all nucleated cells. As cells die, this compound is released into body fluids. Thus there is always some B-2M in the blood because of normal cell degeneration and replacement.

However, in a chronic illness with increased cell destruction, as in HIV infection, B-2M increases beyond normal levels.

To date, a B-2M level of 5 mg/L or higher is the best available indicator of progression to AIDS within three years. Levels below 2.6 are considered normal. B-2M protein increases dramatically shortly after infection occurs, then declines, and finally rises again with AIDS. B-2M can be used with T4 counts to foretell which HIV-positive individuals face the greatest immediate risk of progressing to AIDS.

T4 and T8 Lymphocyte Levels

The most extensive use of data for AIDS progression risk identification involve the number of T4 or CD4+ and T8 or CD8+ cells circulating in the blood (Anderson et al., 1991; Burcham et al., 1991; Phillips et al., 1991b).

T4 cells and the ratio of T4 cells to T8 cells found in the blood have, beginning 1997, been widely used as prognostic indicators for AIDS progression. T4 cell counts, however, are not ironclad predictors of HIV disease progression. In some cases persons with HIV disease and very low (less than 50 or 100) T4 counts remain healthy; conversely, some HIV-diseased persons have relatively high counts (over 400) and are quite ill. **T4 counts are notoriously fickle**, their counts can vary widely between labs or because

BOX 7.3

ARE THERE LONG-TERM ADULT NONPROGRESSORS OF HIV DISEASE—YES!—WHY?

Long-term nonprogressors of HIV disease in the absence of HIV drug therapy, are defined as those persons who are still alive 10 or more years after they tested HIV positive, with sero-conversion documented by history or stored serum samples, absence of symptoms, and normal and stable T4 cell counts (at least 600 T4 cells/microliter of blood). The long-term nonprogressors who are of particular interest to AIDS investigators, are those who after 8 years, in the absence of antiviral therapy, continue to maintain T4 or CD4+ cell counts of 500 or more. Studies through 2002 suggest that 12% to 15% of HIV-infected people remain asymptomatic with about normal T4 cell counts for at least 8 to 12 years (Conant, 1995; Levy, 1995; updated). At least two people are known to be asymptomatic now, 25 years after HIV infection! (Shernoff, 1997; updated). **The question is: How does their immune system differ from those who do not live as long?**

Some Male, Long-Term Nonprogressors

Perhaps the longest long-term nonprogressor is Robert Massie. He was infected in 1978. Ending 2003, he will have lived for 25 years with his HIV infection. Massie is the current executive director of Ceres, a coalition of environmental, investor, and advocacy groups. In 1994, he went to the Massachusetts General Hospital, urging doctors to study him. He told them that he was infected with HIV, had never been treated and that his immune system was fine. Massie first learned he was infected in 1984, when he had an HIV test as part of a research study. He was not surprised by the result, he explained, because he is hemophiliac, and, like virtually every other American with this genetic disease who was alive in the early 1980s, he was repeatedly exposed to HIV through the blood clotting factors made from pooled blood of donors (see Chapter 8). Massie kept waiting to become ill. "I would read a report saying it could be as long as five years before you come down with symptoms of AIDS and die, then it could be as long as seven years, then as long as 10 years, then 12 years. I always thought I was at the limit." When Massie's doctors looked back at his blood samples, which they had stored in hemophilia research projects, they found antibodies to HIV as early as 1979. They suspect that he was infected in November 1978 when he became gravely ill. Massie said, "One day I was sitting at my desk and I suddenly felt overwhelmingly tired, incapable of talking, I was so tired." He had a fever and symptoms that led doctors, at that time, to suggest pneumonia, tuberculosis, a cerebral hemorrhage and a seizure disorder. So, in 1994, when Massie arrived at Massachusetts General Hospital, he had been infected with HIV for 16 years. Now age 48, he has been infected for more than half his life. Since then, Massie has been meeting with Bruce Walker, an infectious disease specialist in HIV infection. The first question for Walker was what was Massie's T4 or CD4+ cell count? He found Massie had near normal levels of T4 cells. Walker said, "This was the first evidence that HIV followed the rules that other viruses follow." It meant that his body's immune system could control HIV. Massie, in fact, had the AIDS virus under such exquisite control that Walker and Eric Rosenberg, who joined him in the research, could not find HIV in his bloodstream. There were, however, antibodies to HIV in his blood. This left no doubt that he was HIV infected. For Walker and Rosenberg, Massie is a very unusual case!

The second longest documented case of a long-term nonprogressor to date is that of a gay male who in retrospect was infected 23 years ago. His T4 count remains normal.

In 1983, at age 71, a man became HIV positive. He received a contaminated blood transfusion while undergoing colon surgery. Unlike most long-term HIV survivors, he has suffered no symptoms and no loss of immune function. He celebrated his 81st birthday. He is one of five patients who came to the attention of an AIDS researcher as he was preparing a routine update on transfusion-related HIV infections. He has since died of natural causes. All five people were infected by the same donor. And 10 to 14 years later, none of the remaining four has suffered any effects.

The blood donor was a gay male who had contracted the virus during the late 1970s or early 1980s and gave blood at least 26 times before learning he was infected. After locating the donor it was found that the man was just as healthy as the people who got his blood.

A 39-year-old San Francisco artist has beaten the odds by living with the virus that causes AIDS for 18 years. He has only routine medical complaints: the stuffiness of an occasional head

BOX 7.3 *(continued)*

cold or the aches and pains of a flu. He has never taken an anti-HIV drug. His own immune system seems to have held the virus at bay.

Susan Buchbinder and colleagues (1992, 1994) reviewed 588 HIV-infected gay men. Thirty-one percent were still AIDS-free 14 years after infection. They attempted to determine why these men lived while others died of HIV/AIDS. Some long-term survivors have low T4 cell counts, some have never taken antiviral therapy, and some have high T4 cell counts. The question is, what is keeping them healthy? If it can be determined why or how their bodies have delayed the progression of HIV disease, then perhaps new approaches to treating all HIV-infected persons will follow. Understanding their defense may help in preventing HIV infection per se.

Buchbinder and colleagues have found that three aspects of the healthy survivors' immune system appear to delay HIV disease progression: Survivors have strong cytotoxic lymphocyte activity, or T8 cell activity, and have higher levels of antibodies against certain HIV proteins.

It is also possible that long-term nonprogressors carry a less pathogenic virus or that these men have not been reexposed to HIV through unprotected sexual activities. Nicholas Deacon and colleagues (1995 updated) have sequenced HIV DNA from a blood donor and a group of six recipients who have not shown HIV disease symptoms despite being infected for 14 to 18 years. Deletions were found in the *nef* gene. Because the lack of disease progression appears to depend on the virus instead of the host immune system, these results suggest a possible use of such HIV strains in live vaccines. However, in July of 1998, it was reported that the HIV donor and two of the six blood recipients experienced a drop in their T4 cell counts. Physicians who treat HIV/AIDS persons do not notice any trends that would lead one to recognize the type of patient or factors that would lead to long-term survival. It was concluded that, at the moment, there is a lack of advice for longer life for persons who have become HIV-infected. No one can tell them how to live longer. AIDS investigators at the National Institute of Allergy and Infectious Diseases are studying the immune systems of 14 people who have been HIV positive for 13 or more years.

Some Female, Long-Term Nonprogressors

For years, some 18 women have intrigued AIDS investigators because they have remained HIV-free despite having frequent, unprotected sex with an infected partner. Researchers at the University of Medicine and Dentistry of New Jersey found that in most of the women, key immune cells worked in various ways to block HIV from multiplying in their bodies. During the study, only one became infected with HIV, and that took nine years of frequent, unprotected sex. The 17 uninfected women had unprotected sex with their HIV-positive partners for periods ranging from one year to 11 years dating as far back as the mid-1980s. Tests on their blood focused on two types of immune cells, cytotoxic or CD8+ and T4 or CD4+ cells, which kill invading organisms and rev up the rest of the immune system. The CD8+ cells and the CD4+ cells separately were mixed with HIV proteins in laboratory dishes mimicking how they would interact in a person's body and researchers watched for reactions. In many samples, the CD4+ cells rapidly reproduced, as if stimulating the rest of the immune system and the CD8+ cells. Also, they produced two different substances that stopped the virus from reproducing. The research team expected to find one immune response protecting the women from HIV infection, but instead found different types of immune responses spread among the 17 women (Skurnick et al., 2002).

In the Pumwani district of Nairobi, a group of 100 women have become well known to HIV researchers around the world by offering evidence that the immune system can, in rare cases, fight off HIV. The evidence derives from a group of women sex workers (prostitutes) established in 1984 by Elizabeth Ngugi and colleagues from the University of Nairobi and the University of Manitoba for the purpose of studying sexually transmitted diseases (STDs). Despite an estimated 60 or more unprotected exposures to HIV every year, one of the highest documented exposure rates in the world, 100 of the 2000 women enrolled in the study have tested negative for HIV infection for at least three years, and for some women up to 15 years. Studies of these highly exposed persistently seronegative (HEPS), also referred to as exposed seronegative (ESN), women convinced many skeptics that immunological resistance to HIV and by extension that an HIV vaccine is possible.

Current evidence suggests that between 5% and 10% of HIV-infected people will live up to 20 or more years. It should be mentioned that if the average time from infection to AIDS is 11 years, statistically speaking, survivors at 20+

BOX 7.3 *(continued)*

years are expected to occur. Time will tell! For other accounts of long-term survivors, see the articles by Cayo (1995), Pantaleo (1995), Kirchhoff (1995), Baltimore (1995), Gegeny (2000) and Migueles (2000).

IMMUNE CELL RECEPTORS, MOLECULES THAT BIND TO THESE RECEPTORS (LIGANDS), AND T4 OR CD4+ AND CTL CELL INFLUENCE ON SURVIVAL

Chemokine Receptors: An Association of Coreceptors to Progression to AIDS As discussed in Chapter 4, the **chemokine receptors** [the four most familiar are CCKR5 (R5), CXCKR4 (X4), CCKR3 (R3), and CCKR2 (R2)] reside on immune system cell membranes. The receptors act as host sites for a variety of chemokines that need entry into such cells. But scientists recently learned that these chemokine receptors also act as **coreceptors** to the CD4 receptor, the receptor to which HIV first attaches. That is, HIV anchors to the cells CD4 receptor, but also needs to bind with a coreceptor, one of the chemokine receptors, in order to complete its entry into the cell. **Genetic mutations** that inhibit given chemokine receptor formation and/or **reduce** the numbers of such receptors on the immune cell membrane offer such cells a complete or partial resistance to HIV infection. A double or homozygous mutation at R5 makes a person completely resistant to HIV infection, but the R2 mutation only slows the progression of HIV disease to AIDS. Such mutations **contribute** to some people's long-term survival. Both CCKR5 and CCKR2 receptor mutations offer this protection (Balter, 1998; Collman, 1997; Cocchi et al., 1995; Feng et al., 1996). Exciting research published in 1998 reports that the genetic mutation that interferes with the X4 receptor actually interferes with the **production** of the **specific chemokine** that attaches to the R4 receptor. It appears that this mutation causes the **overproduction** of a chemokine called **S**tromal **D**erived **F**actor-1 (SDF-1). With an excess in the environment, SDF-1 fills available R-4 receptor sites blocking HIV attachment. So, those persons carrying an SDF-1 mutation, although HIV infected, progress through HIV disease at a much slower pace, delaying the onset

of AIDS as much as 7 to 10 years later than average (Winkler et al., 1998; Balter, 1998). Thus it appears that the progression rate to AIDS is linked to the types of coreceptors people carry on their T4 cells and macrophages. (Reynes et al., 2001).

CHILDREN

Micheline Misrashi and colleagues (1998) reported that children carrying one copy (heterozygous) of the **mutant** R5 gene demonstrate a substantial reduction in progression of HIV disease to AIDS.

T4 OR CD4+ AND CYTOTOXIC LYMPHOCYTE (CTL) CELLS

One notable immunologic problem that occurs after HIV infection is that most people show no evidence of altered T4 cell activity. But an abnormality in immune function is present, long before a significant decline in T4 cell number is seen. In order to be able to kill off HIV-infected cells, cytotoxic T lymphocytes (CTLs) require the assistance of T4 cells—the very T4 cells that HIV infects. These T4 cells must also be able to recognize HIV antigens in order to direct the cytokine signals that will activate CTLs to kill. During the initial (acute) stage of HIV infection, even before seroconversion when antibodies are generated, the T4 cell population is devastated by HIV. Without sufficient T4 cells capable of recognizing HIV, the killer CTLs cannot in turn learn to recognize HIV antigens and kill off infected cells. Recently, it has been shown that some long-term nonprogressors with low viral loads have high amounts of HIV-specific T4 cell activity, while some patients with rapidly progressive disease have no detectable HIV-specific T4 cell activity. This suggests again that T4 cell responses play an extremely important role in containing infection.

Studies in long-term nonprogressors show that they have a persistent, vigorous, virus-inhibiting CTL response, and that this response is broad and adaptable. Rapid progressors, on the other hand, appear to have a narrowly directed CTL response that is unable to adapt to changes in the virus (Hay, 1998).

of a person's age, the time of day a measurement is taken, and even whether the person smokes (Sax et al., 1995).

Performing T4 or CD4+ Cell Counts in HIV-Infected People Continues To Be Essential

A major player in the body's immune system is the T4 or CD4+ cell. By binding with CD4+ cells, HIV can kill them and stop associated production of antibodies, leaving the immune system weakened and vulnerable to opportunistic disease. Doctors gauge the health of the immune system by counting T4 or CD4+ cells. A healthy, HIV-negative adult has between 600 and 1,200 CD4+ cells per cubic millimeter of blood. If the count falls below 350, the immune system has become weakened. Further loss leads to immune suppression and the onset of opportunistic diseases.

Thus, accurate and reliable measures of T4 or CD4+ lymphocytes are essential to the assessment of the immune system of HIV-infected persons. The progression to AIDS is largely attributable to the decrease in T4 lymphocytes. Progressive depletion of T4 lymphocytes is associated with an increased likelihood of clinical complications. Consequently, the Public Health Service (PHS) has recommended that T4 lymphocyte levels be monitored every three to six months in all HIV-infected persons. The measurement of T4 cell levels has been used to establish decision points for initiating *Pneumocystis carinii* pneumonia prophylaxis and antiviral therapy and to monitor the efficacy of treatment. T4 lymphocyte levels are also used as prognostic indicators in people who have HIV disease and recently have been included as one of the criteria for initiating prophylaxis for several opportunistic infections that indicate an HIV infection. Moreover, T4 lymphocyte levels are a **criterion** for categorizing HIV-related clinical conditions by CDC's classification system for HIV infection and surveillance case definition for AIDS among adults and adolescents (*MMWR*, 1997).

Levels of HIV RNA in the Blood: VIRAL LOAD

David Baltimore (Figure 7-9) the Nobel Prize-winning retrovirologist, and coworkers have found a useful clinical predictor of HIV disease progressors, **levels of HIV RNA in the blood. More RNA means more HIV**, and that makes patients get sicker sooner. HIV RNA is a more sensitive measure than other assays and may detect the virus earlier than it would be seen otherwise.

Since the reported work of Baltimore and others on the levels of HIV RNA in the blood, Dennis Henrard and coworkers (1995) have concluded that the stability of HIV RNA levels suggests that an equilibrium between HIV replication rate and efficacy of immunologic response is established shortly after infection and persists throughout the asymptomatic period of the disease (Figure 7-4). Thus, a defect in immunologic control of HIV infection may be as important as the viral replication rate for determining AIDS-free survival. Because individual steady-state levels of HIV RNA were established soon after infection, HIV RNA levels can, as Baltimore suggests, be useful markers for predicting clinical outcome. **Viral load measurements indicate the amount of current HIV activity. T4 cell counts indicate the degree of immunologic destruction**. Thus, the best

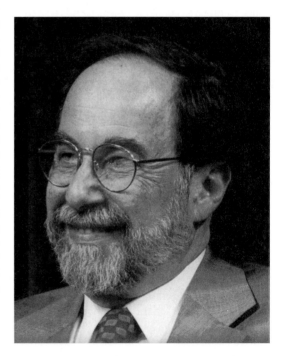

FIGURE 7-9 David Baltimore, 1975 Nobel Prize molecular biologist. President of the California Institutes of Technology. *(Photograph courtesy of AP/Wide World Photos)*

VIRAL LOAD AND T4 CELL COUNTS: THEIR USE IN CLINICAL PRACTICE

VIRAL LOAD

Viral load assays measure only viral RNA present in the plasma. They do not account for **intact virus** in the lymph system or other tissues. Individual measurements are a good surrogate (substitute) for virus replication. Although the relationships among viral replication, T4 cell count, and disease progression are not entirely clear, viral load correlates fairly well with all of them. Viral load measurements can be effectively used to monitor therapy or the effectiveness of a given drug.

HIT EARLY, HIT HARD?

The level of plasma HIV RNA at 6 months after primary infection is called the **SET POINT,** but treatment should be considered regardless of **set point** RNA values. The idea is to stop HIV replication **early rather than later.** (In February 2000 the previously NIH-recommended HIT EARLY, HIT HARD was changed to HIT HARD, HIT LATER, see referenced material and Chapter 4 for reasoning.)

T4 OR CD4+ CELL COUNTS

T4 cell counts remain helpful in determining the stage of the disease. But, T4 counts are highly variable, even from hour to hour in some HIV-infected people. They are also significantly influenced by other current viral infections. Although T4 cell counts function well as reliable markers of disease progression and antiretroviral drug efficacy in large populations, they are less reliable for prescribing therapy for the individual. Viral load determinations present a better basis on which to present therapy. Until viral load determination costs fall and until physicians become more familiar with them and insurance companies pay for them, the T4 tests will remain the more practical determinant of disease stage and when to begin therapy. (Medicaid, Medicare, and some HMOs do cover HIV RNA determinations.)

It is suggested that HIV RNA levels be used as a means to prescribe medication. RNA levels should be determined after exposure, at 6 weeks, 12 weeks, and at 6 months—the **set point.**

SUMMARY

The level of circulating RNA in plasma is a direct reflection of ongoing HIV replication in the host. The T4 lymphocyte, a **target** of HIV replication, is an **indirect** marker of antiretroviral therapy. The T4 count itself is a measurement of the relative production and destruction of the T4 cell population. For example, if there is a production problem, either due to nutritional, toxicity, or other factors, the T4 count may not rise proportionately to the **decrease** in viral load. Thus, the change in viral load is more precisely measuring the effect of antiretroviral therapy and, therefore, is the best marker of how well drugs are working.

---

monitor of disease progression is the use of both, the T4 cell count and viral load (Merigan et al., 1996; Katzenstein et al., 1996; Voelker, 1995; Goldschmidt et al., 1997).

No current viral or immunological markers adequately reflect drug toxicities caused by therapy.

HIV INFECTION OF THE CENTRAL NERVOUS SYSTEM

A wide variety of central nervous system (CNS) abnormalities occur during the course of HIV infection. They result not only from the opportunistic infections and malignancies in the immunodeficient individual, but also from direct HIV infection of the CNS. It was believed that because some brain cells contain CD4-like receptors they were receptive to HIV infection. In

---

Table 7-4 Neurological Manifestations Associated with Direct HIV Infection of the Nervous System

AIDS dementia complex
Asymptomatic infection
Acute encephalitis
Aseptic meningitis
Vacuolar myelopathy
Inflammatory demyelinating polyneuropathy
Radiculopathy
Mononeuropathies
Distal sensory neuropathy

addition, other brain cells contained a glycolipid that allowed for HIV infection (Ranki et al., 1995). However, more recent research shows that after HIV-infected monocytes migrate to the brain, become tissue macrophage, and release HIV, the virus **does not infect brain cells; rather HIV resides in brain spaces, in the cerebral spinal fluid**. HIV investigators believe that HIV may invade the brain within a few weeks to months after HIV infection. Although the precise mechanisms by which HIV produces nerve cell dysfunction are still undetermined, infection of the brain is an integral component of the biology and natural history of HIV infection; the resulting clinical manifestations are summarized in Table 7-4.

Genetic analysis and clinical studies have revealed that HIV in the cerebrospinal fluid (**CSF**) of some people with AIDS-related dementia evolves **independently** of the HIV in their blood, leading **to two genetically distinct forms of the virus**. This finding poses a new challenge for treatment of these patients, suggesting that drugs effective against HIV in their blood may not do the job in the central nervous system, and vice versa. Why HIV evolves independently in the CSF of the demented patients is not clear. It may reflect a separate viral subpopulation thriving in their central nervous system, or maybe those with dementia have progressed further in immunodeficiency that may allow HIV to become more virulent. Scientists at Gladstone Institute of Virology and Immunology also found preliminary evidence that in some AIDS dementia patients HIV in the CSF compartment is more resistant to antiretroviral drugs than as HIV in the blood. This can cause rebound of virus levels in the CSF while the viral load in the blood is suppressed. Ongoing studies of resistant mutations should clarify this pattern (Haas et al., 2000).

AIDS Dementia Complex

In addition to cancers and opportunistic diseases, a progressive dementia (mental deterioration) due to HIV infection of the central nervous system develops in 55% to 65% of AIDS patients. Pathological changes in the CNS are observed in up to 80% of those autopsied (McGuire, 1993). But the mystery remains as to why some HIV-infected people develop dementia while others do not. Some people with high viral loads were not demented, while others with low viral loads had

AIDS dementia. A study by Johnson and colleagues (1996) suggests that factors other than viral load lead to dementia. Investigators have found that this dementia is solely associated with HIV infection and progression to AIDS. HIV-caused dementia has a unique set of clinical and pathological features. Some authorities estimate that 90% of AIDS patients in the terminal stages of the disease have AIDS Dementia Complex (ADC) (Hanley et al., 1988). Information presented by the National Institute of Allergy and Infectious Diseases in June 1989 indicated that **asymptomatic HIV-infected persons do not demonstrate mental impairment** (Figure 7-10). Therefore, the onset of mental impairment must begin sometime after the HIV-infected person becomes symptomatic (1989, Updated). Initially, investigators thought that OIs caused ADC, but it was later discovered that HIV is carried into the brain by HIV-infected macrophages, the Trojan Horse.

Early Symptoms— Early symptoms of cognitive dysfunction include forgetfulness, recent memory loss, loss of concentration and slowness of thought, social withdrawal, slurring of speech, loss of balance (inability to walk a straight line), deterioration of handwriting, and impaired motor function. An early diagnosis of ADC in AIDS patients is difficult because the early signs of neurological disease are very similar to those symptoms used to identify emotional depression. However, neurological symptoms may be the first sign of illness in about 10% of adult AIDS patients.

Late Symptoms— These symptoms are characterized by loss of speech, great fatigue, muscle weakness, bladder and bowel incontinence, headache, seizures, coma, and finally death. About 95% of patients with ADC have HIV antibodies in their cerebral spinal fluid.

PEDIATRIC CLINICAL SIGNS AND SYMPTOMS

Currently over 90% of pediatric AIDS cases are newborns and infants who received HIV from mothers who were injection drug users or from the sexual partners of IDUs. For those who become HIV-infected during gestation, clinical symptoms usually develop within 6 months after birth. Few children infected as fetuses live beyond

BOX 7.4

SCIENTISTS NEED A SMALL ANIMAL MODEL IN WHICH TO STUDY HIV DISEASE—WHY ISN'T THERE ONE?

To date, scientists do not really know how HIV kills cells that carry the CD4 protein on their outer membranes—mostly those cells of the human immune system, the T lymphocytes. But, that is not all that is unknown about how this unique virus attacks, inserts itself into human DNA, replicates, and exits the cell. To learn more about the devastation HIV brings to humans after cellular infection, replication, and release into the blood stream, scientists must use chimpanzees and rhesus macaque monkeys. HIV does not cause AIDS in these animals. HIV evolved in humans and to date, only causes AIDS in humans. But, there are no other animals that are closer to the human system in which to study the infection and disease process. So scientists have routinely infected these primates with an HIV/SIV (human/simian or monkey virus/hybrid virus called SHIV). This hybrid virus will cause AIDS-like symptoms in these primates. But, these primates are scarce and expensive. Chimpanzees cost up to $50,000 each. Rhesus macaque monkeys, more abundant than chimpanzees, but still short in supply, cost up to $5,000 each. Breeding of either species takes years. Scientists in a number of laboratories have, for years, been trying to develop specific strains of mice and rats to use as animal models to study HIV. To date, all attempts to develop rodent models have failed. HIV just won't adapt to the biology of species other than humans! Intense research shows that (a) HIV will not infect cells other than human or (b) if HIV enters a cell it will not replicate or (c) if it replicates it will not have the proper proteins produced to create new HIV or (d) if the products are made they cannot be assembled into a new virus. Many steps in HIV's life cycle require the presence of human—and only human—molecules. This may explain why chimpanzees and monkeys don't die from HIV infections. After all these obstacles are overcome, there is first, the problems of mouse or rat immune responses that is still not understood—so how does one make observations about HIV in non-primate models and make critical decisions on drug use or vaccine trials in humans? Second, viruses are most often species specific. At the moment, however, there are no promising alternatives to using the scarce and expensive primates and hoping that to some degree, lady luck will appear.

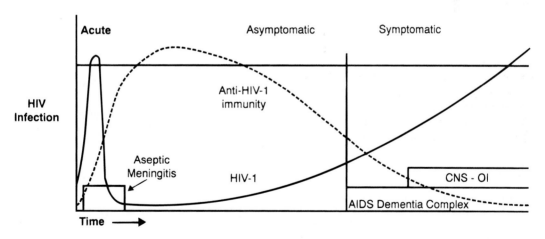

FIGURE 7-10 Central Nervous System Events After HIV Infection. Note that aseptic meningitis (an inflammation of the membrane of the brain and spinal cord in the absence of viral or bacterial infection), when it occurs, occurs early after HIV infection. Although usually apparent later, AIDS dementia complex may begin during the early-late phase. The late phase represents the period during which major AIDS-defining opportunistic infections occur. The headings acute, latent, early-late, and late refer to periods after HIV infection. It appears that OI infection of the brain occurs after the onset of ADC. *(Adapted from Price et al., 1988)*

2 years and survival past 3 years used to be rare; but with the use of anti HIV drugs and therapy for opportunistic diseases, some children born with HIV are still alive at 5, 10, and 15 years of age.

The clinical course of rapid HIV disease progression in infants diagnosed with AIDS is marked by failure to thrive, persistent lymphadenopathy, chronic or recurrent oral candidiasis, persistent diarrhea, enlarged liver and spleen (hepatosplenomegaly), and chronic pneumonia (interstitial pneumonitis). Bacterial infections are common and can be life-threatening. Bacterial infection and **septicemia (the presence of a variety of bacterial species in the bloodstream)** was the leading cause of death in one group of affected infants in Florida. An excess of gamma globulin and depressed cell-mediated immunity and T cell function are frequently encountered.

Less than 25% of AIDS children express the kinds of OIs found in adult AIDS patients. Kaposi's sarcoma occurs in about 4% of them. Young AIDS children experience delayed development and poor motor function. Older AIDS children experience speech and perception problems.

SUMMARY

The clinical signs and symptoms of HIV infection and AIDS have been addressed in the previous chapters. However, there are two major classification systems used to diagnose patients as they progress from HIV infection to AIDS. The first is the Walter Reed System. It recognizes six stages of signs and symptoms that a person passes through to AIDS. The CDC uses four groupings that identify the stage of illness from infection to AIDS. Both systems revolve around the recognition of a failing immune system, persistent swollen lymph nodes, and opportunistic infections. Mysteries still to be resolved are exactly why and how HIV attacks the body cells, and why some people stabilize after the initial symptoms of HIV infection while others move directly on to AIDS.

One disorder that was not immediately recognized in AIDS patients is AIDS dementia complex (ADC), a progressive mental deterioration due to HIV infection of the central nervous system. ADC develops in over 50% of adult AIDS patients prior to death. Research has shown that some of the symptoms of this dementia can be reversed with the use of the drug zidovudine.

REVIEW QUESTIONS

(Answers to the Review Questions are on page 489.)

1. Name the two major AIDS classification systems in use in the United States.

2. What percent of HIV-infected individuals will progress to AIDS in 5 years; in 15 years?

3. What is the neurological set of behavioral changes in AIDS patients called?

4. Name three body organs and their associated AIDS-related diseases.

5. True or False: Currently the single most important laboratory parameter that is followed to monitor the progress of HIV infection is the T4 cell count.

6. True or False: The average time from infection to seroconversion is two weeks. Explain.

7. True or False: Being infected with HIV and being diagnosed with AIDS are the same thing. Explain.

8. True or False: The average length of time from infection with HIV to an AIDS diagnosis is approximately two years.

9. Write a brief essay on: (a) In general, about how long HIV can reside in the body before one shows signs of HIV infection. (b) In general, about how long it takes the body to generate antibodies to HIV after infection.

10. The general signs and symptoms associated with HIV/AIDS include:

   A. recurrent fever

   B. weight loss for no apparent reason

   C. white spots in the mouth

   D. night sweats

   E. all of the above

Epidemiology and Transmission of the Human Immunodeficiency Virus

---

When a population becomes infected with a contagious disease, an epidemic results. **Epidemic** is derived from Greek and means "in one place among the people." To understand how an infectious disease can spread or remain established in a population, investigators must consider the relationship between an infectious disease agent and its host population. The study of diseases in populations is an area of medicine known as **epidemiology.**

We learned the danger of complacency from earlier epidemics. Complacency about HIV infection is especially dangerous because the infection can remain hidden for years. Because many infected people remain symptom-free for years, it is hard to be sure just who is infected with the virus. The more sexual partners, the greater the chances of encountering one who is infected and subsequently becoming infected.

With regard to HIV infection, it is your behavior that counts. The transmission of HIV can be prevented. HIV is relatively hard to contract and can be avoided.

The presence of HIV/AIDS is not isolated—the transmissibility of HIV between individuals

197

and across borders and populations is what drives this global pandemic and makes it imperative that nations work together to prevent the continued transmission of HIV. On an individual level, IT IS NOT IMPORTANT HOW YOU GOT HIV, WHAT IS IMPORTANT IS HOW YOU LIVE YOUR LIFE WITH THE VIRUS.

HIV AS A COMMUNICABLE DISEASE

HIV is a communicable disease in a limited sense. A communicable disease is one in which the causative agent passes from one person to another. The modes of transmission for communicable diseases include: direct contact with body fluids, contact with inanimate objects, and contact with vectors, including flies, mosquitoes, or other insects capable of spreading disease. HIV is communicable only in the first of the three modes, that is, through direct contact with certain body fluids. The ways in which HIV can be transmitted have been clearly identified. However, some information that conflicts with scientific findings had been widely dispersed. Information in this chapter should correct these misperceptions. HIV transmission requires close contact. **HIV is transmitted in human body fluids by three major routes: (1) sexual intercourse through vaginal, rectal, oral, or penile tissues; (2) direct injection with HIV-contaminated drugs, needles, syringes, blood, or blood products; and (3) from HIV-infected mother to fetus in utero, during childbirth, or during breast-feeding.** Additional body fluids that may transmit the virus health care workers may come in contact with are: cerebrospinal fluid surrounding the brain and the spinal cord, synovial fluid surrounding bone joints, and amniotic fluid surrounding a fetus.

How HIV Enters the Body

In all cases, HIV is transmitted in one of two ways. **First,** it can be transmitted as the virus itself, or **second,** as the cell associated with HIV. The virus is held within the white blood cells of the immune system and are carried Trojan horse-style within the fluid of one person into the body of another.

HIV and Sexual Transmission

Epidemiological data suggest that sexual transmission, in general, is relatively inefficient, in that exposure often does not produce infection. HIV is transmitted more efficiently intravenously than through sexual routes. However, worldwide the predominant mode of transmission of HIV is through exposure of mucosal surfaces, of the vagina, vulva, penis, rectum, or mouth, to infected sexual fluids (semen, cervical/vaginal, rectal) and during birth. Sexual transmission of HIV accounts for more than 75% of infections worldwide.

Factors Driving Sexual Transmission

There is evidence from around the world that many factors play a role in initiating a sexually transmitted HIV epidemic or driving it to higher levels. Among the **behavioral** and **social factors** are (a) little condom use, (b) large proportion of the adult population with multiple partners, (c) overlapping (as opposed to serial) sexual partnerships—individuals are highly infectious when they first acquire HIV and thus more likely to infect any concurrent partners, (d) large sexual networks (often seen in individuals who move back and forth between home and a far-off workplace), (e) age mixing, typically between older men and young women or girls, and (f) women's economic dependence on marriage or prostitution, robbing them of control over the circumstances or safety of sex.

Biological factors include (a) high rates of sexually transmitted infections, especially those causing genital ulcers, (b) low rates of male circumcision, and (c) high viral load HIV levels in the bloodstream which are typically highest when a person is first infected and again in the late stages of illness.

While all these factors help spread the virus, it is not known exactly how much each of them contributes and to what extent they need to be combined in order to spread the epidemic. The issue of male circumcision is a good example. Many countries in which all boys are circumcised before puberty have very limited epidemics, and even in some countries with wider epidemics, circumcised men have lower HIV rates than uncircumcised men.

HIV: Other Routes of Transmission?

HIV is not communicable through contact with fomites (inanimate objects) or through vectors. Thus **people do not "catch" HIV in the same way that they "catch" the cold or a flu virus.** Unlike colds and flu viruses, HIV **is not,** according to the CDC, spread by tears, sweat, coughing, or sneezing. The virus **is not** transmitted via an infected person's clothes, phone, or toilet seat. HIV **is not** passed on by eating utensils, drinking glasses, or other objects that HIV-infected people have used that are free of blood.

HIV **is not** transmitted through daily contact with infected people, whether at work, home, or school. Insects do not transmit the virus. Kissing is also considered very low risk: **There is only one documented case to prove that HIV is transmitted by kissing.** Paul Holmstrom and colleagues (1992) report that salivary HIV antibodies are detected regularly in HIV seropositive subjects. This suggests that these antibodies neutralize HIV, producing the negative results of HIV cultivation or antigen detection in the saliva. The route of HIV into saliva is not fully understood. Both salivary glands and salivary leukocytes have been shown to harbor HIV. Gingival fluid (fluid seeping out of the gums) has been regarded as the main source of salivary HIV antibodies and infectious HIV.

In its 1990 supplemental guidelines for cardiopulmonary resuscitation (CPR) training and rescue, the Emergency Cardiac Care Committee of the American Heart Association (AHA) noted that there is an extremely small theoretical risk of HIV or hepatitis B virus (HBV) transmission via cardiopulmonary resuscitation (CPR). To date **NO** known case of seroconversion for HIV or HBV has occurred in these circumstances.

LOOKING BACK 8.1

PUBLIC OPINION ON HOW THE DISEASE—AIDS—WAS TRANSMITTED JUNE 1983

A *Newsweek* poll found that nine in ten (90%) Americans over 18 had heard of AIDS, but also found that four in ten (40%) believed it was possible to contract the disease through casual contact. From 1983 to 1985, AIDS stories made regular appearances in newspapers and on television news broadcasts. Over 150 AIDS stories were broadcast by the three major TV network evening news programs in 1985—more than double the combined totals of AIDS stories broadcast in 1983 and 1984 (source: the Vanderbilt Television Archives). These initial years of AIDS press coverage were marked by stories that often focused on the dramatic aspects of the disease (for example, its progressive nature), the death toll among higher-risk groups, and its potential to spread to the public at large.

WE MUST STOP HIV TRANSMISSION NOW!

Education and advocacy for risk reduction remain important tools for preventing HIV infection, but alone they will never accomplish the objective of slowing the speed and extent of the virus's spread. This can only be achieved by combining educational and early intervention efforts with specific measures guiding those resources to the people who need them most: those who are already infected and to their sex and drug partners.

Beginning year 2003, there were about 850,000 AIDS cases in the United States. Figure 8-1 breaks this number down according to means of HIV infection—sexual behavior, drug use, medical exigencies, and undetermined causes. Figure 8-2 gives a breakdown by transmission category for 38,000 AIDS estimated cases for 2002.

EPIDEMIOLOGY OF HIV INFECTION

The first scientific evidence of human HIV infection came from the detection of HIV antibodies in preserved serum samples collected in **Central Africa in 1959.** The first AIDS cases appeared there in the 1960s. By the mid-1970s HIV was being spread throughout the rest of the world. The earliest places to experience the arrival of HIV were Central Europe and Haiti. Transmission into the United States may have been by tourists who had vacationed in the area of Port-au-Prince, Haiti (Swenson, 1988).

On entry into the United States the virus first spread among the homosexual populations of large cities such as New York and San Francisco. The first **recorded** AIDS cases in the United States occurred in 1979 in New York. The first CDC-**reported** AIDS cases were in New York, Los Angeles, and San Francisco in 1981. In all cases, the diagnosis of AIDS was based on clinical descriptions.

According to the CDC's first clinical AIDS definition, at least one case of AIDS occurred in New York City in 1952 and another in 1959. Both males demonstrated opportunistic infections and *Pneumocystis carinii* pneumonia, today a hallmark of HIV infection. This early evidence of AIDS suggests that the virus might have been in the United States, Europe, and Africa at about the same time (Katner et al., 1987). If HIV has been present for decades as

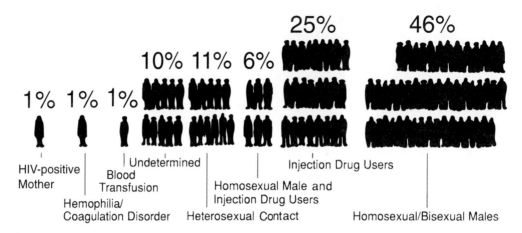

FIGURE 8-1 Cumulative AIDS Cases by Route of Transmission. Beginning year 2003, there were about 850,000 AIDS cases in the United States. This diagram gives the percentage of adults and adolescents in each group through 2002. Groupings are according to sexual preference, drug use, medical conditions, and others not associated with any of these. *(Courtesy of CDC, Atlanta—updated)*

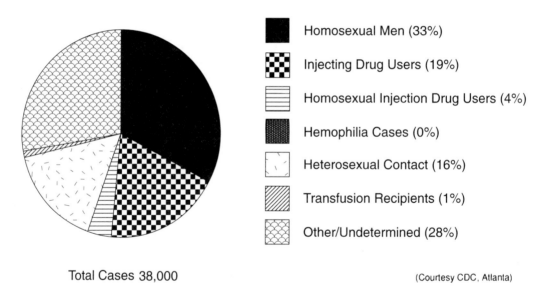

Total Cases 38,000   (Courtesy CDC, Atlanta)

FIGURE 8-2 Adult/Adolescent AIDS Cases by Transmission Category Estimated for 2002, United States.

suggested, its failure to spread may reflect a recent HIV mutation, a major change in social behaviors conducive to HIV transmission, or both. For example, the sexual revolution and the widespread use of birth control pills, which began in the 1960s, and the subsequent decrease in the use of condoms may be involved with the transmission of HIV.

TRANSMISSION OF TWO STRAINS OF HIV (HIV-1/HIV-2)

The spread of HIV-1 is global. The clinical presentation of AIDS caused by HIV-1 is similar regardless of geographical area.

HIV-2 is a genetically distinct strain. HIV-2 was first discovered in 1985 in West Africa. It is believed to have been present in West Africa as early as the 1960s. Clinical data demonstrate that HIV-2 has a reduced virulence compared to HIV-1 (Marlink et al., 1994).

What appears certain is that HIV-2, like HIV-1, will spread worldwide. HIV-2 has already spread from West Africa to other parts of Africa, Europe, and the Americas. Both HIV-1 and HIV-2 are transmitted or acquired through the same kinds of exposure.

BECAUSE OVER 99% OF GLOBAL AIDS CASES ARE CAUSED BY THE TRANSMISSION OF HIV-1, ONLY DATA THAT PERTAIN TO HIV-1 (HIV) WILL BE PRESENTED UNLESS OTHERWISE STATED.

IS HIV TRANSMITTED BY INSECTS?

In spite of convincing evidence of the ways in which HIV can be transmitted, it remains difficult for the general public to believe that a virus that appears to spread as rapidly as HIV is not either highly contagious or transmitted by an environmental agent. After all, there are many viral and bacterial diseases that are highly contagious and transmitted by insects. **The question was asked: Is this virus being transmitted by insects?**

Necessary data to resolve the question were available. Epidemiological data from Africa and the United States suggested that AIDS was not transmitted by insect bites. If it were, many more cases would be expected among school-age children and elderly people, groups that are proportionally underrepresented among AIDS patients. In one study of the household contacts of AIDS patients in Kinshasa, Zaire, where insect bites are common, not a single child over the age of 1 year had been infected with the

AIDS virus, while more than 60% of spouses had become infected.

In 1987, the Office of Technology Assessment (OTA) published a detailed paper on the question of whether blood-sucking insects such as biting flies, mosquitoes, and bedbugs transmit HIV (Miike, 1987). The conclusion was that the conditions necessary for successful transmission of HIV through insect bites and the probability of their occurring rule out the possibility of insect transmission as a significant factor in the spread of AIDS. Jerome Goddard reported (1997) that blood-sucking arthropods (for example, **mosquitoes** and **bedbugs**) for good biological reasons, **cannot** transmit HIV. Insects inject their own saliva as a lubricant to assist feeding. They do not inject their own or a previously bitten person's blood. Malaria and yellow fever are transmitted through insect saliva—HIV isn't. The virus has to overcome many obstacles. It must avoid digestion in the gut of the insect, recognize receptors on the external surface of the gut, penetrate the gut, replicate in insect tissue, recognize and penetrate the insect salivary glands, and subsequently escape into the lumen of the salivary duct. Webb and colleagues (1989) inoculated bedbugs intraabdominally (belly) and mosquitoes intrathoracically (chest) with HIV to enable the virus to bypass gut barriers. The virus failed to replicate in either.

HIV TRANSMISSION

If most HIV-exposed people can become HIV-infected, can most infected people **transmit** HIV to others? This is a difficult question to answer. Infection with HIV appears to depend on a large number of variables that involve the donor, recipient, and portal of entry. The most important variables are mode of transmission, viral load, which subtype and variant of HIV is present, and the recipient's genetic resistance.

A report in the 1998 12th International AIDS Conference stated that for the first time strains of HIV resistant to all protease inhibitors and other widely used anti-HIV drugs are being transmitted from one person to another! Prior to this announcement, scientists did not believe that such highly mutant forms of HIV could be transmitted. It is becoming increasingly clear that, although almost every country is touched by HIV, the virus spreads very differently in different parts of the world. Across the globe, depending on the developing nation, IDU may be associated with the highest incidence of HIV transmission; in other countries it may be via men having sex with men, or heterosexual sex among males and females.

HIV TRANSMISSION IN FAMILY/HOUSEHOLD SETTINGS

Several studies of the family members of AIDS patients have failed to demonstrate the spread of

HIV through household contact. The only cases in which family members have become infected involved the sexual partners of AIDS patients or children born to mothers who were already infected with the virus. Even individuals who bathed, diapered, or slept in the same bed with AIDS patients have not become infected. In one study, 7% of the family members shared toothbrushes with the infected person and no one became infected.

Perhaps the best evidence **against** casual HIV transmission comes from studies of household members living with blood-transfused AIDS

BOX 8.1

A NEIGHBOR'S STORY: PUBLIC IMAGE, PUBLIC FEAR

We have over the last 21 years witnessed educated people offer misrepresentation and fantasy about HIV infection and AIDS. We have listened to them distort the truth by presenting false perceptions rather than facts. If education is to become a major player in prevention of the spread of HIV, the mix of myth and fantasy must be replaced by reality—and this can be done by giving the proper respect to a new disease in our lifetime.

The Neighbor

A neighbor was having a garage sale. Their friend came over and asked them a question about AIDS. They mentioned that he should talk to me and he came over to the house. He said, "I'm looking for the truth about who is, and who isn't HIV infected and how I can tell people that are HIV-infected from those who are not?" I asked if he cared to share the reason for the questions and he immediately told me that he divorced three years ago and has been so frightened by the information he has seen on TV, heard on the radio, and read in the paper that he has remained celibate for three years and that it has truly affected his quality of life. He said, "I'm afraid to have sex with any woman I date because I believe almost every woman in Jacksonville and elsewhere carried HIV. It's driving me insane. My male friends are still having sex. Are they crazy or am I the fool?" I took the second question first. I assured him that his worst fears were correct. You can't tell the HIV positive from the HIV negative just by their appearance. Infected and noninfected all look alike—at least in the early and middle stages of

the disease. For the second question of who is and who is not HIV-infected, I gave him some details relating to people's behavior, the particular behavioral risk groups and I said that if he did not belong to such groups or did not have a blood transfusion before 1985–1986, and that if he had some information about his sexual partner and did not change sexual partners too frequently and always used a condom, he could feel as safe as one can. The expression on his face went from concern to relief. He shook my hand repeatedly. He thanked me profusely and he said, "I feel like the media, the government, the gays, and everyone else has cheated me out of three years of my life. I can never get that back." I said, "Yes, to some degree that is true, but here you stand after three years still HIV negative. Would you like to exchange three years of free-wheeling sexual encounters for an HIV infection?" He agreed that he would not, but we both understand his point. We all need to understand his point. Misinformation—data skewed by ignorance or lack of education causes fear. And failure to give an accurate representation of a disease, from both the medical and social vantage points, can cause a great deal of harm—in ways that most of us would not begin to contemplate. Did I give him the right advice? No, because I did not give him advice at all. I simply attempted to put things in their proper perspective. He did not leave me less afraid of dying of AIDS. He left me with the idea that he could have his sex life restored without dying from AIDS, provided he maintains his low-risk behavior.

The Author

---

patients (Peterman et al., 1988). Transfusion infection cases are unique because their dates of infection are known retrospectively. Prior to the onset of AIDS symptoms, the families were unaware that they were living with HIV-infected individuals. Family life was not altered in any way, yet family members remained uninfected. In some cases, the transfusion patients were hemophiliacs who received weekly or monthly injections of blood products and became HIV-infected. From the combined studies of these households, only the sexual partners of infected hemophiliacs became infected. In some cases, the sexual partners of hemophiliacs remained HIV free after three to five years of unprotected sexual intercourse.

Although contact with blood and other body substances can occur in households, transmission of HIV is rare in this setting. Through 2002, at least nine reports have described household transmission of HIV not associated with sexual contact, injection drug use, or breast-feeding. Of these nine reports, five were associated with documented or probable blood contact. In one report, HIV infection was diagnosed in a boy after his younger brother had died as the result of AIDS; however, a specific mechanism of transmission was not determined.

Home Nursing Exposure

Three reports involved home nursing care of terminally ill persons with AIDS in which a blood exposure might have occurred but was not documented; in these reports, skin contact with body secretions and excretions occurred.

In another reported case in the United States, a mother apparently became infected with HIV as a result of extensive, unprotected exposure to her infected child's blood, body secretions, and excretions. The child, who underwent numerous surgical procedures to correct a congenital intestinal abnormality, had become infected through multiple blood transfusions. **The mother did not wear gloves when performing procedures such as drawing blood, removing intravenous lines, emptying ostomy bags, changing diapers, and changing surgical dressings.** On numerous occasions her hands became contaminated with blood, feces, saliva, and nasal secretions. Although she reported no accidental needlesticks or open

wounds on her hands, she often failed to wash her hands immediately after such exposures.

In a similar case, a woman in England developed AIDS after caring for a man who died of AIDS. Again, the care involved frequent contact with body secretions and excretions. The woman reported that she had some small cuts and eczema on her hands during the time that she cared for the man.

NONCASUAL TRANSMISSION

The routes of HIV transmission were established **before** the virus was identified. The appearance of AIDS in the United States occurred first in specific groups of people: homosexual men and injection drug users. The transmission of the disease within the two groups appeared to be closely associated with sexual behavior and the sharing of IV needles. By 1982, hemophiliacs receiving blood products, as well as the newborns of injection drug users, began demonstrating AIDS. By 1983, heterosexual female partners of AIDS patients demonstrated AIDS. **Twenty-two years** of continued surveillance of the general population has failed to reveal other categories of people contracting HIV/AIDS (Table 8-1). It became apparent that the infectious agent was being transmitted within specific groups of people, who by their behavior were at increased risk for acquiring and transmitting it (Table 8-2). Clearly, an exchange of body fluids was involved in the transmission of the disease.

With the announcement that a new virus had been discovered, further research showed that this virus was present in most body fluids. Thus, even before there was a test to detect this virus, the public was told that it was transmitted through body fluids exchanged during intimate sexual contact, contaminated hypodermic needles, contaminated blood or blood products, and from mother to fetus. In addition it was concluded that the widespread dissemination of the virus was most likely the result of multiple or repeated viral exposure because the data from transfusion-infected individuals indicated that they did not necessarily infect their sexual partners. In other words, it was concluded early on and later confirmed that this viral infection did not occur as easily as other blood-borne viral diseases such as hepatitis B, or viral and bacterial sexually transmitted diseases.

Table 8-1 HIV Transmission and Infection

CHAIN OF HIV INFECTION

Agent causing the disease	HIV
Major reservoirs (source of HIV in the body)	Lymph nodes, blood, genitals
Replication site of HIV	Mostly inside T4+ or CD4-bearing lymphocytes
Portal of exit (how does HIV leave the body)	Mucosal openings, skin breaks, bleeding, or expulsion of body fluids
Transfer or transmission of HIV (from one human to another)	Via body fluids
Portal of entry (how does HIV enter the body)	Mucosal openings, skin breaks, areas of bleeding, injection

TRANSMISSION ROUTES

Blood Inoculation

Transfusion of HIV-infected blood and blood products
Needle sharing among injection drug users
Needlesticks, open cuts, and mucous membrane exposure in health care workers
Use of HIV-contaminated skin-piercing instruments (ears, acupuncture, tattoos)
Injection with unsterilized syringe and needle (mostly in undeveloped countries)

Sexual Contact: Exchange of semen, vaginal fluids, or blood

Homosexual, between men
Lesbian, between women
Heterosexual, from men to women and women to men
Bisexual men and women

Perinatal

Intrauterine
Peripartum (during birth)
Breast-feeding

Table 8-2 Adult/Adolescent AIDS Cases by Sex and Exposure Categories, Estimated Through 2002, United States[a]

Male Exposure Category (80%)	Total No.
1. Men who have sex with men	282,482
2. Injecting drug use	235,401
3. Men who have sex with men and inject drugs	67,256
4. Hemophilia/coagulation disorder	6,726
5. Heterosexual contact:	26,903
a. Sex with injecting drug user	9,954
b. Sex with person with hemophilia	53
c. Sex with transfusion recipient with HIV infection	215
d. Sex with HIV-infected person, risk not specified	16,545
6. Receipt of blood transfusion, blood components, or tissue	6,726
7. Other/undetermined	47,080
Total male AIDS cases	672,575

Female Exposure Category (20%)	
1. Injecting drug use	77,346
2. Hemophilia/coagulation disorder	
3. Heterosexual contact:	82,391
a. Sex with injecting drug user	33,293
b. Sex with bisexual male	4,036
c. Sex with person with hemophilia	572
d. Sex with transfusion recipient with HIV infection	807
e. Sex with HIV-infected person, risk not specified	42,036
4. Receipt of blood transfusion blood components, or tissue	5,044
5. Other/undetermined	3,363
Total female AIDS cases	168,144
Total male/female cases	840,719

[a]Pediatric cases, 9281.

Table 8-3 lists the means of HIV transmission worldwide. Table 8-4 lists the means of HIV transmission in the United States.

Mobility and the Spread of HIV/AIDS

Mobility is an important epidemiological factor in the spread of communicable diseases. This becomes particularly obvious when a new disease enters the scene. In the early stage of the HIV/AIDS epidemic, for example, the route of the virus could be associated with mobility.

The first HIV-infected people in some Latin American and European countries reported a his-

Table 8-3 How HIV Is Transmitted Worldwide, 2002

Exposure	Efficiency, %	% of Total
Blood transfusion/ blood products	>90	3
Perinatal	20–40	9
Sexual intercourse[a]	0.1–1.0	80
Injection drug use	0.5–1.0	8

[a]Heterosexual intercourse 70%

(Source: WHO/Global Programme on AIDS and UN-AIDS, 1999, Updated)

Table 8-4 An Approximation of How an Estimated 850,000 Americans Became Infected with HIV, through 2002

85	health care workers got infected from the blood or body fluids of patients;
11,475	children infected through their mothers;
18,275	people got HIV from infected blood or blood products;
59,500	people did not know how they were infected, did not report their risk, or died before anyone could find out;
55,250	people were infected who had both unprotected sex and shared needles;
212,500	people were infected who shared needles;
493,000	people were infected through unprotected sex.

(Based on data from HIV/AIDS Surv. Rpt, CDC, Year-End Edition, 2001)

tory of foreign travel. In some African countries, spread of the virus could be traced along international roads. Today, increasing numbers of HIV infection have been observed to be associated with the relaxation of travel restrictions in Central and Eastern Europe.

Few countries are **unaffected** by HIV/AIDS. This has made it clear that restrictive measures such as refusal of entry to people living with HIV/AIDS and compulsory testing of mobile populations are inappropriate and ineffective measures to stop spread of the virus. In times of increasing international interdependency, it is an illusion to think that the disease can be stopped at any border.

HIV/AIDS Immigration Laws for America

The Immigration and Naturalization Service (INS) requires HIV antibody testing as part of the medical examination required for all nonimmigrants over the age of 15 who apply for visas.

Nonimmigrants applying for permanent residence who test HIV positive are considered "excludable and deportable." Although travelers applying for a nonimmigrant visa (temporary stay) are not required to take a medical exam, HIV antibody testing may be required at the port of entry if there is reason to believe an individual is infected (for example, the presence of antiretroviral medications). Nonimmigrants infected with HIV who wish to visit the United States may apply for a 30-day waiver to see relatives, conduct business, attend conferences, or seek medical treatment. For additional information about HIV/AIDS and immigration, you may wish to contact: National Immigration Project, National Association of People With AIDS, 1413 K Street, NW 7th Floor, Washington, DC 20005-3476, (202) 898-0414.

Number of HIVs Required for Infection

Robert Coombs and colleagues (1989) calculated the dose of HIV necessary to cause an HIV infection. They reported that **"one infective dose"** of 1,000 HIV particles is necessary to establish HIV infection in human tissue culture cells. To establish HIV infection in the body, it was reasoned that it would take **10 to 15 infective doses.** Their study indicated that a pint of blood from an AIDS patient contains 1.8 million infective doses, or about 2 billion HIV particles per pint of blood, or about 4.2 million HIV particles per milliliter.

Body Fluid Transmission

High levels of HIV have been isolated from blood, semen, vaginal fluids, saliva, serum, urine, tears, and breast milk. Lower levels of HIV are found in lung fluid and cerebrospinal fluid (Friedland et al., 1987). HIV has not been found in sweat.

In cases of low levels of HIV in cell-free body fluids and within the cells of these fluids does not mean that HIV cannot be transmitted via these fluids or cells—it can, but the dose (number of viruses) is so small that the risk of infection is minimal; thus the reason for the low number of health care workers contracting HIV infection after touching, being splashed by, or needlesticking themselves with blood containing HIV.

HIV is found in greatest numbers **within T4 or CD4+ cells, macrophage, and monocytes of blood, vaginal fluids, and semen.** Laboratory findings, along with overwhelming empirical observations, support the scientific conclusion that the major route of HIV transmission is through human blood and sexual activities involving exchange of semen and vaginal fluids. Semen carries significantly larger numbers of HIV than vaginal fluid. It appears that of all body fluids, these three contain the largest number of infected lymphocytes (Figure 8-3), which provide the largest HIV concentration in a given area at a given time.

Presence of HIV-Infected Cells in Body Fluids

Blood— Recent observations indicate that both latent and HIV-producing cells are present throughout the course of infection. Considerable numbers of HIV and HIV-infected cells can be detected in the blood. Thus it is probable that HIV-infected people harbor substantial numbers of HIV-infected cells in their blood from soon after the initial infection through the terminal stage of the disease.

Semen— A single specimen of ejaculate contains between 1 million and 10 million nonspermatozoal cells, and many leukocytes including

FIGURE 8-3 Electron Micrograph of an HIV-Infected T4 Lymphocyte. The T4 or CD4+ cell has produced a large number of HIVs that are located over the entire lymphocyte. **Each HIV leaves a hole in the cell membrane.** The photograph shows part of the convoluted surface of the lymphocyte magnified 20,000 times. *(Courtesy of The National Biological Standards Board, South Mimms, U.K. and David Hockley)*

T4 cells. But the number and type of all mononuclear cells in the semen of a healthy man differs considerably from day to day (Kiessling, 1999).

Reducing the numbers of T4 cells (lymphocytes and macrophages) in semen could decrease the chances of infection. In one study on 94 semen samples from HIV-infected men, HIV DNA was found in 35% of the mononuclear cells (Bagasra, 1996). It has been suggested that **vasectomy** could reduce the infectivity of HIV-infected men because it would eliminate mononuclear cells or cell-free virus in semen originating from the testes and epididymis. The work of John Krieger and colleagues (1998) shows that sperm can exist in semen for up to three months after vasectomy (see **sperm** below) and that there was **no significant** difference in **pre-** and **post-vasectomy** in HIV RNA levels (viral load). Robert Coombs and colleagues (1998) reported that viral load in semen may not correspond to the viral load in blood. Seth Kalichman reported in 2001 that 53% of men with undetectable levels of HIV in their blood had measurable HIV in their semen. Ann Kiessling has provided evidence that HIV is compartmentalized in the body—and this makes it more difficult to treat HIV infection (Zhang et al., 1998). However, Lee Harrison and colleagues (2000) reported on 93 HIV-positive men on antiretroviral drugs. Before drug treatment 74% had detectable levels of HIV in their semen. After six months on therapy 33% had detectable HIV in their semen. Collectively, it would appear that a **vasectomy does NOT stop HIV transmission!**

With regards to the presence of HIV in semen and actual transmission, investigators at the University of North Carolina at Chapel Hill have used HIV RNA in semen samples from several hundred men to estimate the effects of semen in viral burden on heterosexual transmission. They concluded that when HIV RNA in semen was low (<5000 copies/mL) transmission was unlikely to occur, at 1 per 10,000 episodes of intercourse. Conversely, when the concentration of HIV in semen was high (e.g. 1 million copies/mL) the probability of transmission rose to 3 per 100 episodes of intercourse.

Sperm— Omar Bagasra (1996) reported that 33% of sperm samples, from 94 HIV-positive men, contained HIV RNA. Many investigators have now reported that the **mitochondria** of various tissue types are infected with HIV. The sperm midpiece contains large numbers of mitochondria.

Sperm Washing— Sperm washing is a procedure for separating sperm from seminal fluid. Sperm washing has been used for years in fertility clinics and sperm banks to increase the odds of fertilization by selecting the healthiest, most active sperm for artificial insemination. However, the use of sperm washing to reduce or eliminate transmissions like HIV to a mother or baby has only emerged over the last decade. The CDC has twice recommended against insemination with semen from HIV-infected men because there was no evidence that any procedure could reliably eliminate HIV from semen. Part of their concern was based on a 1990 Virginia sperm-washing case. The woman failed to become pregnant but was infected with HIV. The couple claimed to have used condoms consistently, suggesting that the infection was caused by the insemination attempt.

Sperm Washing Research in Europe— In contrast to the widespread institutional resistance to sperm washing for HIV positives in the United States, European fertility clinics have widely experimented with sperm washing. At Milan's Sao Paolo Hospital, Augustus Semprini has reported over 1000 insemination attempts in 350 couples using sperm washing and artificial intrauterine insemination. As of 1998, more than 250 women became pregnant and 187 gave birth. None of the women tested positive before or after delivery. While these successes are encouraging, American researchers have questioned whether Semprini's results can be duplicated among other HIV-infected donors because little information is given about the donor's disease state (viral load or CD4+ cell counts). Researchers in Spain, France, the United Kingdom, and Switzerland have also reported successes using sperm washing.

Saliva— There continues to be some concern over the presence of HIV in saliva because of the exchange of saliva during **deep kissing,** the saliva residue left on eating utensils, and saliva on instruments handled by health care workers, especially in dentistry. Results of studies on hundreds of dental workers, many of whom have cared for AIDS patients, have shown no evidence of HIV infection (Friedland et al., 1987 updated). Also, in a CDC study, none of 48 health care workers became infected after parenteral (IV) or mucous membrane exposure to the saliva of HIV-infected patients (Curran et al., 1988). Studies by Fox (1991), Archibald (1990), and Pourtois (1991) showed that human saliva contains factors that inhibit HIV infectivity. Crombie and colleagues (1998) reported that the glycoprotein **thrombospondin** is concentrated in saliva and blocked HIV infection of human cells in the **test tube!**

In 1999, Baron and colleagues at the University of Texas Medical Branch reported a provocative theory regarding a powerful protective effect from saliva. Baron's test-tube studies found that saliva, due to its **low level of salt, inactivates more than 90 percent of the HIV-infected leukocytes**

LOOKING BACK 8.2

FEDERAL STUDY COMMITTEE ADVISES THE FOOD AND DRUG ADMINISTRATION ON THE ACCEPTANCE OF BLOOD DONATIONS IN THE TIME OF AIDS, JULY 1983

The Seattle Times reported that a federal study committee faced a tough task in advising the Food and Drug Administration regarding blood donations and transfusions in relation to the mysterious disease called Acquired Immune Deficiency Syndrome, or AIDS. The committee recommended that the government not have an automatic policy of destroying a large reserve of blood just because one donor is suspected of having AIDS. We're not sure how helpful that recommendation will be to the FDA. Not having an automatic policy could mean anything from destroying 99% of suspect blood reserves to destroying none. But the committee did base its recommendation on three seemingly sound factors. **First,** although a few people have contracted AIDS after receiving blood transfusions, it is unclear what the cause-and-effect relationship is. **Second,** any contaminated blood from a potential AIDS victim would be diluted in a large pool. **Third,** widespread destruction of blood pools could put people who suffer bleeding diseases at a great risk. Two other advisory-committee recommendations to the FDA are of unquestioned validity. The committee called for a public education campaign and the screening of blood donors who are in the high-risk categories. The latter point can scarcely be overemphasized. The government should take every possible step to ensure the screening is thorough and that it is so perceived by a concerned public.

(blood cells) that may be the main transmitter of HIV on mucosal surfaces, thereby blocking HIV transmission by more than 10,000-fold. This happens, Baron says, because salt is needed to keep cells alive. If you put red blood cells (that contain salt) in a glass of water, for example, they quickly pull in the liquid, swell up, and burst. The absence of salt in saliva causes HIV-infected cells to do the same thing. That's why kissing appears so safe in many instances. Saliva, concludes Baron, "is breaking down the infected cells." When asked why saliva did not protect people during oral sex or children during breast-feeding, Baron stated that "If you add HIV infected cells in the presence of a large amount of blood, semen, or breast milk and then add saliva, those three fluids cancel out the low salt protection effect. Semen and breast milk are seven times saltier than saliva. That coincides with the epidemiological evidence that those three fluids can transmit HIV. But in the absence of those three fluids, there appears to be only rare transmission of HIV."

First Documented Kissing Transmission Case

Although over 70 million people around the world have been HIV-infected, there are remarkably few reports of its spread by kissing, dental treatment, biting, or coughing. Even among those people whose bodies are actively shedding HIV, their saliva usually contains only noninfectious components of the virus.

In July of 1997, the first documented case of HIV transmission via deep kissing was reported on by the CDC. In this **one** case, the man was HIV positive, via IDU in 1988. Both he and his female partner had serious gum (periodontal) disease. His gums routinely bled with brushing or flossing. Investigators at the CDC believe that the HIV was transmitted via blood within the man's

---

POINT OF INFORMATION 8.2

DANGER OF HIV INFECTION VIA ARTIFICIAL INSEMINATION

By early year 2003, 15 women were reported to have been HIV-infected through the use of anonymous donor sperm to initiate pregnancy; one in Germany, two in Italy, four in Australia, two in Canada, and six in the United States. Thirty recipients of semen from HIV-infected donors refused to be HIV tested. (Guinan, 1995 updated). All cases except Germany occurred **before** the availability of HIV antibody testing. About 80,000 women each year are artificially inseminated with donor sperm. But 22 years into the AIDS epidemic, the increasingly popular fertility business remains largely unregulated and unmonitored, even though it traffics in semen, long known to be one of the two main HIV transmission routes.

Only a few states (New York, California, Ohio, Illinois, and Michigan) require HIV testing of semen donors. **There are no federal regulations.**

Medical and public health experts agree that artificial insemination is an HIV risk that somehow fell through the cracks of public education and health regulations. They insist, however, that the risk is low.

In January of 1996 Washington State's top educator announced that she had AIDS. She received the virus trying to become pregnant through artificial insemination with donor sperm. This announcement once again focused national attention on the problem, the lack of federal regulations for this industry.

Omar Bagasra and colleagues (1994, 1996) state unequivocally that there is a risk of HIV transmission during artificial insemination. To quote Bagasra, "As we have shown, the sperm easily penetrates other cells—and when this occurs, the midpiece also penetrates. A single ejaculation contains [millions of] sperm. We have data to show that the mitochondria in the midpieces of HIV-infected sperm are loaded with HIV. If 1 in 1,000 of these mitochondria contains HIV, that is a significant viral load. The viral load transmitted from a man to a woman in this manner is quite likely to be high."

Lack of federal and state regulations means you must protect yourself! (1) Stay away from private physicians unless you know they are using only certified sperm banks to get their products. **(2)** Review a doctor's or clinic's testing and record-keeping procedures and demand to see donor medical records, which can be shared even if the donor's identity is protected. **(3)** Accept only frozen donor semen that has been HIV tested at least twice at 3- to 6-month intervals.

---

oral cavity due to oral lesions onto the mucus membrane of the woman (*MMWR*, 1997).

Spitzer and colleagues (1989) reported that a male became HIV-infected during unprotected fellatio with an HIV-infected prostitute. A second similar case has also been reported. The mechanism of transmission, saliva, in these cases may be suspected, but it is not conclusive!

The precise risk of oral sex is difficult to assess because most couples engage in other sexual practices.

Mother's Milk— Several studies have shown that HIV can be transmitted by breastfeeding. Van de Perre and coworkers (1993 updated) found that infection of babies via breast milk was most strongly correlated with the presence of HIV-infected cells in the milk, suggesting that infection might be cell-mediated. However, infection was also correlated with low levels of antibodies to HIV, suggesting that infection was initiated by cell-free virus.

Dentist with AIDS Infects Patient During Tooth Extraction?

In July of 1990, the CDC reported on the possible transmission of HIV from a dentist with AIDS to a female patient (*MMWR*, 1990a). This case, like no other before it, sent chills through many. But why this case? Because the vast majority of people go to dentists! They don't inject drugs and are not gay. This case, however, is difficult to resolve. For example, two years had elapsed from the time of the dental work to when the patient, Kimberly Bergalis (Figure 8-4), was diagnosed with AIDS. Both patient and dentist, David J. Acer of Stuart, Florida, were uncertain of exactly what happened.

FIGURE 8-4 Kimberly Bergalis, age 23. Bergalis is being comforted by her mother after their train trip from their home in Florida to Washington, D.C. She made the trip to testify before a congressional committee on September 26, 1991. Bergalis favored mandatory HIV testing for health care personnel. She died December 8, 1991. *(Photograph courtesy of AP/Wide World Photos)*

Some of the pertinent factors in this case are (**1**) review of dental records and radiographs suggest that the two tooth extractions were uncomplicated; (**2**) interviews with Bergalis and the dentist did not identify other risk factors for HIV infection. Bergalis, age 22, stated over national TV in 1990 that she was still a virgin. This point was disputed on June 19, 1994, during the TV program *60 Minutes* (with Mike Wallace). Yes, she did engage in sexual foreplay, but not intercourse. Yes, she was infected with the human papilloma virus, which can be sexually transmitted, but this is not at all uncommon in immune-suppressed AIDS patients with no history of sexual intercourse; (**3**) nucleotide sequence data indicated a high degree of similarity between the HIV strains infecting her and the dentist; and (**4**) the time between the dental procedure and the development of AIDS was short (24 months), and Bergalis developed oral candidiasis 17 months after infection. At this time, only 1% of infected homosexual/bisexual men and 5% of infected transfusion recipients develop AIDS within two years of infection.

David Acer, a bisexual, was diagnosed with symptomatic HIV infection in 1986 and with AIDS in 1987. He died on September 3, 1990. Since then, 1100 of his 2500 patients were contacted for HIV testing. In January of 1991, the test results of 591 of these patients revealed that five were HIV positive: a 68-year-old retired school teacher, a middle-aged father of two, a 37-year-old carnival worker, an unemployed drifter, and a 19-year-old student. As with Bergalis, infection in these patients may have come from some other source. All six patients denied having sexual contact with the dentist or with one another (*MMWR*, 1991a). **If an absolute case can be made that Acer transmitted the virus to Bergalis, this will be the *first documented case of a health care professional infecting a patient.***

Bergalis died of AIDS on December 8, 1991. She was 23 years old and weighed 48 pounds.

There is no shortage of ideas as to how Acer might have infected his patients. For example, he could have used the same dental instruments on himself or his sexual partners that he used on his patients without sterilizing them.

The actual route of HIV transmission in the Acer–Bergalis case will most likely never be known. There have been suggestions that the dentist did not wish to die alone and chose certain people to infect. It was suggested that he may have attempted to infect still others, but was unsuccessful. A friend of the dentist said that he believed that Acer intentionally infected his patients to call attention to the HIV/AIDS problem in the United States. Acer felt that mainstream America was ignoring the problem.

A CDC estimate put the theoretical risk of HIV transmission from an HIV-infected dentist to a patient during a procedure with potential blood exposure at 1 chance in 260,000 to 1 chance in 2.6 million (Friedland, 1991).

Point for Discussion: Is this last point, one of revenge against society, reasonable?

(Read: Denis Breo (1993). The dental AIDS cases—murder or an unsolved mystery? *JAMA*, 270:2732–2734.)

Conclusion— Beginning 2003, two of the six patients believed to have been infected by Acer have progressed to AIDS but are still alive: Kimberly Bergalis, Richard Driskill, John Yecs, and Barbara Webb have died. To date, the six people have received $10 million from Acer's insurance company.

Sexual Transmission

The predominant mode of HIV transmission is through sexual contact. Not all sexual practices are equally likely to result in HIV transmission. HIV usually gains access to the immune system at mucosal surfaces. Such surfaces include the oropharynx (throat area), rectum and genital mucosa. Mucosal surfaces are rich in Langerhans cells, dendritic cells that trap antigens and virus particles. In addition, lymphoid aggregates are found throughout the tissue immediately below the mucosal surface.

Sexual transmission of HIV occurs when infected blood, semen, or vaginal secretions from an infected person enter the bloodstream of a partner. This can happen during anal, vaginal, or oral penetration, in descending order of risk. Unprotected anal sex by a male or female appears to be the most dangerous, since the rectal wall is very thin. Masturbation or self sex is the safest. In general, a person's risk of acquiring HIV infection through sexual contact depends on (**1**) the number of different partners, (**2**) the likelihood (prevalence) of HIV infection in these partners, and (**3**) the probability of virus transmission during sexual contact with an infected partner. Virus transmission, in turn, may be affected by biological factors, such as concurrent sexually transmitted disease (STD) infections in either partner. If there is a genital ulcer caused by syphilis or chancroid or herpes, the risk of getting HIV increases 10- to 20-fold. If there is gonorrhea or chlamydial infection, which are more common, the risk increases probably 3- to 4-fold. Behavioral factors, such as type of sex practice and use of condoms, or varying levels of infectivity in the source partner (for example viral load) related to clinical stage of disease also increase the risk of HIV transmission/infection. Based on these factors, the risk for HIV infection is highest for an uninfected partner of an HIV-infected person practicing unsafe sex. In February 2001 researchers at the University of North Carolina, Chapel Hill reported that HIV could be transmitted via unprotected sex between 5 and 13 days after infection. Persons who have sex partners with risk factors for HIV infection or who themselves have multiple partners with high rates of injection drug and "crack" cocaine use, prostitution, and other STDs are also at increased risk.

Circumcision and HIV Transmission

The issue of circumcision as it relates to HIV transmission is hardly trivial. In 1989, Bill Cameron and colleagues published the results of a prospective study demonstrating a greater than eight-fold increased risk of HIV infection among uncircumcised men. There have also been a number of reports illustrating that the foreskin provides a vulnerable portal of entry to HIV and other pathogens. As summarized in an editorial authored by Daniel Halperin of the University of California, San Francisco, and Robert Bailey of the University of Illinois at Chicago in a recent issue of *The Lancet*, the highly vascularized prepuce contains a higher density of Langerhans cells—the primary target cells for sexual transmission of HIV—than cervical, vaginal, or rectal mucosa (Halperin, 1999). They also note research finding the foreskin is more susceptible to traumatic epithelial disruptions during intercourse, which allows additional vulnerability to ulcerative STDs and HIV.

Personal Choice–Personal Risks

Ray Bradbury wrote that "living at risk is jumping off a cliff, and building your wings on the way down." About 90% of the HIV infections that occur within the heterosexual noninjection drug use population occur through one or more sexual activities. Some 90% of the HIV infections that occur among gay males occur through anal intercourse (Kingsley et al., 1990). In any sexual activity, HIV is transmitted via a body fluid. Transmission may occur between men, from men to women, women to men, and possibly from women to women (see Chapter 11).

Heterosexual HIV Transmission

Heterosexual HIV transmission means that the virus was transmitted during heterosexual sexual activities. As such, the **proportion** of HIV infection and AIDS cases among the heterosexual population in the United States is now increasing at a greater rate than the proportion of HIV infections and AIDS cases among homosexuals or IDUs (Friedland et al., 1987). Persons at highest risk for heterosexually transmitted HIV infection include adolescents and adults with multiple sex partners, those with sexually transmitted diseases (STDs), and heterosexually active persons residing in areas with a high prevalence of HIV infection among IDUs. In 1985, fewer than 2% of AIDS cases were from the heterosexual population; by year 2002 the incidence of heterosexual AIDS cases is over 10% of the total number of reported AIDS cases in the United States. Of the number of the **heterosexual AIDS cases** reported in the United States, about two-thirds (66%) of cases occur among women and one-third among men.

Key Factors in Heterosexual HIV Transmission

The key factors involved in the transmission of HIV heterosexually are: frequent change of sexual partners, having unprotected sexual intercourse, the presence of sexually transmitted infections, the lack of male circumcision, the social vulnerability of women and young adults or adolescents, and the amount of poverty or economic instability in a given community.

Heterosexual HIV Transmission Outside the United States— Heterosexual intercourse is the most common mode of transmission of HIV in poor countries. In Africa, over 80% of infections are acquired heterosexually, while mother to child transmission (5–15%) and transfusion of contaminated blood account for the remaining infections. Homosexuality and injection drug use occurs, but at a very low incidence. Heterosexual contact and injection drug use are the main modes of HIV transmission in South and South East Asia. Studies in Haiti, and other Caribbean and Third World countries indicate that HIV transmission is most prevalent among the heterosexual population. The HIV infected male-to-female ratio in Africa is about even. In late 1991, the World Health Organization stated that 75% of worldwide HIV transmission occurred heterosexually. By the year 2004, up to 90% will occur heterosexually. The high frequency of AIDS cases in Third World countries is thought to be due to poor hygiene, lack of medicine and medical facilities, a population that demonstrates a large variety of sexually transmitted diseases and other chronic infections, unsanitary disposal of contaminated materials, lack of refrigeration, and the reuse of hypodermic syringes and needles due to supply shortages.

Vaginal and Anal Intercourse— Among routes of HIV transmission, there is overwhelming evidence that HIV can be transmitted via anal intercourse. In vaginal intercourse, male-to-female transmission is much more efficient than the reverse. This is believed to be due to (1) a consistently higher concentration of HIV in semen than in vaginal secretions, and (2) abrasions in the vaginal mucosa. Such abrasions in the tissue allow HIV to enter the vascular system in larger numbers than would occur otherwise, and perhaps at a single entry point.

The same reasoning explains why the **receptive** rather than the **insertive** homosexual partner is more likely to become HIV-infected during anal intercourse. It appears that the membranous linings of the rectum, rich in blood vessels, are more easily torn than are those of the vagina. In addition, recent studies indicate the presence of receptors for HIV in rectal mucosal tissue. A recent report by Richard Naftalin (1992) states that human semen contains at least two components, collagenase and spermine, that cause the breakdown of the membrane that supports the colonic epithelial cell layer of the rectal and colon mucosa. This leads to the loss of mucosal barrier function allowing substances to penetrate the rectal and colon mucosa.

Homosexual Anal Intercourse— Today about 60% of homosexual men in San Francisco are infected, probably the highest density of infection anywhere in the developed world. "It colors everything we do out here," said a gay activist. "The gay community, to a large extent, is about

---

BOX 8.2

HIV/AIDS ROULETTE

Case I: The Woman Executive

I am a successful executive woman. A year ago I applied for life insurance. I was required to take an HIV antibody test. It came back positive.

I am not a prostitute or promiscuous. I am not and have never been an injection drug user. I am not a member of a minority group, indigent nor homeless, and I have not slept with a bisexual male (?).

I don't fit any of the stereotypes that people have designated for those infected with HIV. I got HIV from a man I love and have been seeing for five years. He is not homosexual or bisexual. He has never used injection drugs. He had no idea he was carrying the virus. He believes he may have been infected about six years ago by a woman with whom he had a brief, meaningless relationship. For that one indiscretion we will both pay the ultimate price.

Case II: The HIV-Infected Male

In February of 1994, a 21-year-old man walked into a sexually transmitted disease clinic and told the doctor he had "the clap," or gonorrhea, but he carried HIV.

When a counselor inquired about his sex partners, he told them about several, including a 12-year-old girl. The girl had gone elsewhere to be treated for gonorrhea and tested positive for HIV.

The man admitted to sleeping with 27 women, including 13 teenagers. Ten of the partners couldn't be found. Of the 17 others, 12 tested positive for HIV.

The man has since died, and the clinic has not been able to track all of his sexual partners.

There is a message to be found in these two cases: People with HIV are much more dangerous to a community than someone with AIDS. On average, the HIV-infected are asymptomatic for 11 years. Those with AIDS and not treated, are symptomatic. They are losing weight. They are sick. They have little or no sexual appetite. Those with HIV are healthy and vigorous. That's where the sexual roulette begins.

---

addressing AIDS. It has to be, because it's literally a war: Your entire community is under siege."

In a single year, 1982, 21% of the uninfected gay male population became infected, and for some reason not yet known, many of those infected early, died early. "Soon everyone, and I mean everyone, had a friend who was dying" (Science in California, 1993). During 1995 through mid-1997, three gay men died of AIDS each day. From mid-1997 through 2002, using aggressive anti-HIV drug therapy, daily deaths from AIDS dropped to two per week! (Conant, 1995 updated).

It appears that of all sexual activities, anal intercourse is the most efficient way to transmit HIV (DeVincenzi et al., 1989). Information collected from cross-sectional and longitudinal (cohort) studies has clearly implicated receptive anal intercourse as the major mode of acquiring HIV infection. The proportion of new HIV infections among gay males attributable to this single sexual practice is about 90%.

Major risk factors identified with regard to HIV transmission among gay males include anal intercourse (both receptive and insertive), active oral-anal contact, number of partners, and length of homosexual lifestyle (Kingsley et al., 1990).

Heterosexual Anal Intercourse— A number of sexuality-oriented surveys of the heterosexual population indicate that between one in five and one in ten heterosexual couples have tried or regularly practice anal intercourse. Bolling (1989) reported that 70% to 80% of women may have tried anal intercourse and that 10% to 25% of these women enjoyed anal sex on a regular basis. He also reported that 58% of women with multiple sex partners participated in anal sex. James Segars (1989) reported that the highest rates of anal sex occur among teenagers who use drugs and older married couples who are broadening their sexual experiences.

Although it may increase the risk of HIV infection, it must be emphasized that anal intercourse is not necessary for HIV transmission among heterosexuals. In fact, most HIV-infected heterosexuals say they have never practiced anal intercourse.

Risk of HIV Infection; Number of Sexual Encounters— The risk of HIV infection to a susceptible person after one or more sexual encounters is very difficult to determine. In some cases, people claim to have become infected after a single sexual encounter.

In some reported transfusion-associated HIV infections, the female partners of infected males remained HIV-negative after 5 or more years of unprotected sexual intercourse. Television star **Paul Michael Glaser** said that he had normal sexual relations with his wife Elizabeth for 5 years prior to her being diagnosed as HIV-infected (Figure 8-5). He was not HIV-infected. She received HIV during

a blood transfusion, but was not diagnosed until after their first-born child was diagnosed with HIV. In other studies of heterosexual HIV transmission, many couples had unprotected sexual intercourse over prolonged periods of time with no more than 50% of the partners becoming HIV-infected. There are many instances of heterosexuals and homosexuals who remained HIV negative after having repeated sexual intercourse with HIV-infected partners.

The fact that not all who are repeatedly exposed become infected suggests that biological factors may play as large a role in HIV infection as behavioral factors. For biological reasons, some people may be more efficient transmitters of HIV; while others are more susceptible to HIV infection, that is, require a smaller HIV infective dose. Some people carry genes that may make them resistant to HIV infection (see "Mutant CKR-2 and CKR-5 Genes" in Chapter 5).

Number of Sexual Partners and Types of Activity— One relatively large risk factor for HIV infection in both homosexuals and heterosexuals is believed to be the number of sexual partners. The greater the number of sexual partners, the greater the probability of HIV infection.

FIGURE 8-5 Paul Michael and Elizabeth Glaser. Elizabeth died of AIDS on Dec. 4, 1994. *(Photograph courtesy of AP/Wide World Photos)*

DISTRIBUTION OF HIV-CONTAMINATED BLOOD: FRANCE, GERMANY, THE UNITED STATES, AND OTHER COUNTRIES

Near the end he could not bring himself to visit his youngest brother, to see him dying of AIDS. He too was dying of AIDS. Their deaths would close out a family of four HIV-infected hemophiliac brothers, all diagnosed with AIDS. The first died at age 24, the second committed suicide at age 33, the last two brothers died in 1993. The four brothers became HIV-infected about 1985 from using HIV-contaminated blood-clotting factor.

FRANCE

The French National Center of Blood Transfusions (CNTS) knowingly distributed HIV-contaminated blood products to hemophiliacs in 1985. The scandal, which broke in 1991, prompted the center's director to resign and an official government investigation.

In the confidential minutes of a 1985 CNTS meeting, agency officials concluded that 100% of the concentrated blood-clotting factors used to treat French hemophiliacs were contaminated with HIV. The agency, which has a monopoly on blood for transfusions, kept its secret and ignored a 1984 recommendation from the U.S. Centers for Disease Control and Prevention that blood products be heated in order to kill the deadly virus (Dorfman, 1991).

Whatever the reasons, the secrecy and delay produced catastrophic results. Nearly half of France's 3000 hemophiliacs were infected with HIV; subsequently beginning 2003, about 1000 have died. Bowing to public and media pressure, the French government will provide compensation for some 7000 French citizens who have been infected with HIV through blood products and transfusions (Aldhous, 1991, updated).

French Ministers To Face Poisoning Charges

Formal charges of "collusion in poisoning" were made in October 1994 against Laurent Fabius, the former Socialist prime minister, and four of his colleagues—Edmond Hervé, then deputy health minister, and Georgina Dufoix, then minister of social affairs, Francois Gros, scientific advisor to Fabius, and Claude Weisselberg, physician and advisor to Fabius—over their role in France's HIV-contaminated blood scandal in the mid-1980s. In 1995, Gerard Jacquin, former director of bioindustry at CNTS, was charged with poisoning and Louis Schweitzer and Patrick Baudry, advisors to Fabius and Dufoix, respectively, were charged with delaying the screening of blood products

(Reichhardt, 1995). The charge carries a maximum sentence of 30 years in prison. In addition to these three men, the charge of collusion to poison were also brought against Jean-Pierre Allain (just released from prison) and Michel Garretta (released from prison) (Butler, 1994a, 1994b, updated).

In 1999, former Prime Minister Laurent Fabius, former Health Minister Edmond Hervé, and former Social Affairs Minister Georgina Dufoix are accused of keeping a U. S. HIV test off the market while the Pasteur Institute completed its own test. They are charged with involuntary homicide related to the deaths of seven hemophiliacs infected with HIV after blood transfusions. They went to trial in February 1999. Conviction could bring each a five-year jail term and a $130,000 fine.

Conclusion to the Nine-Year-Old Blood Transfusion Case

In March 1999, Laurent Fabius and Georgina Dufoix were acquitted of all charges in the French contaminated blood scandal. Edmund Herve was found guilty but **received no penalty.** During the case, several dozen scientists, physicians, administrators, and politicians testified on behalf of the former prime minister and two former cabinet ministers.

GERMANY

The German blood scandal began with two questions. The **first** question was how to explain several unexpected cases of HIV infection. The **second** question, associated with the first, was how could 7000 units of blood have been screened for HIV using 2500 HIV blood testing kits (it takes one kit/unit of blood screened)? The search for the answers led investigators to a blood supply company called UB Plasma in the city of Koblenz. The investigators concluded that either the firm had failed to test thousands of units, or it had "pooled" units from multiple donors before conducting the test, an illegal practice that reduces the chances of detecting HIV contamination.

Investigators discovered that after UB Plasma began running into financial trouble in 1991, technicians were told to pool units to save money on the $2 test kits. After German kit manufacturers stopped deliveries (UB Plasma failed to pay its bills) technicians switched to an unauthorized and less reliable test. There was also evidence that the firm may have distributed blood that was not screened at all.

Because of the extent of blood banking violations, German authorities closed UB Plasma. They arrested the manager and three employees on charges of fraud and "negligent bodily harm." The current health minister disbanded the German Federal Health Bureau, and the Director of Pharmaceuticals was relieved of his duties relating to the control of blood and blood products. In stark contrast to the HIV blood scandals in France and the United States, German investigators attribute the distribution of HIV-contaminated blood and blood products to incompetence rather than company greed—UB Plasma did not attempt to distribute known HIV-positive blood until current stocks were used up!

In 1995 the director and the head of product testing of Haemoplas, a German blood products company, were charged with murder on the grounds that they had been motivated by greed. They are alleged to have conspired in the early 1980s to economize by not testing blood samples, and to have persisted after testing was made compulsory in 1985.

Fourteen people became infected with HIV through Haemoplas products between 1986 and 1987, and three have since died.

Both men have also been charged with 5837 counts of attempted murder—corresponding to the number of batches distributed—infringing legislation on the control of pharmaceutical products, and fraud (Abbott, 1995).

THE UNITED STATES

In late 1993, a class action suit was filed on behalf of 9000 hemophiliacs who became infected with HIV after using HIV-contaminated blood products, called Blood Factor 8, which is essential for proper blood clot formation following an injury. In the case of severe hemophilia, many persons spontaneously bleed into their joints. Blood Factor 8 is sometimes referred to as Anti-

Hemolytic Factor or AHF. Hemophiliacs are now dying of AIDS at the rate of one a day.

The suit charges that five manufacturers of AHF and the National Hemophilia Foundation continued to pursue aggressive advertising and marketing of AHF while downplaying the risk of viral infection. In 1995, the United States Supreme Court disallowed the suit.

By the mid-1970s, the dangers of viral infection from blood products was well known and methods had been provided for blood viral inactivation. Such methods were patented and available by 1977. In 1981, Donald Francis, an epidemiologist then with the CDC (Figure 9-4), and Max Essex, a retrovirologist at Harvard Cancer Biology Laboratory, were convinced that AIDS, then referred to as Gay Related Immune Deficiency or GRID, was caused by an infectious agent, most likely a virus. But others thought GRID was related to the gay male lifestyle. The disease was spreading rapidly among gay males through sexual contact. But the evidence continued to mount that the disease, or agent causing the disease, was being transmitted by blood. In that same year, the president of an AHF-producing company stated the agent was in the blood supply. He said he thought it was a 100% fatal retrovirus. At this time, a major part of blood stocks came from paid donors, mostly from poor neighborhoods. To offset taking in contaminated blood, this single company began questioning donors face-to-face: Are you homosexual? In the first two weeks of new guideline operations, 308 donors said yes and their blood was not taken. Another 500 refused to answer and left.

The American Association of Blood Banks (AABB) and the American Red Cross issued a joint statement that "Direct or indirect questions about a donor's sexual preferences are inappropriate." Clearly, they kept open the door to high behavioral risk blood donors. The FDA went along with the joint statement and against the CDC recommendations for screening blood donors.

According to Milton Musin, former medical research director of Cutter Laboratories, by the end of 1983 he knew that the hemophiliacs clotting factor could transmit AIDS. Virtually all lots of the concentrate were contaminated with the AIDS virus. "You'll never convince me that profit margins and fear of the product liability and fear of losing a very lucrative business did not drive the CEOs and leaders of these companies."

In 1985, the FDA announced a blood test. "This test adds a major dimension of protection to our present safeguards. Its use will keep our blood supply safe and indeed make them even safer."

The HIV antibody test, called the ELISA test, would help make the blood supply, in large part, safe. But it came at a cost to the blood banks. Technicians had to be hired and trained. Donors had to be checked and every new unit of blood tested and logged. **But, astonishingly, the blood banks were not required to go back to the inventories on their shelves.** In hindsight, the current head of the AABB says that was a mistake.

But perhaps the worst was yet to be learned. While the AABB was stalling testing, it convinced the FDA to reduce the number of blood bank inspections at the very time HIV was entering the blood system of the country.

It wasn't until 1988 that the blood banks began recalling HIV-positive blood. FDA reports were discovered that told of errors and accidents. Between 1985 and 1987 thousands of units of potentially contaminated blood had been released and officially recalled. But recalling blood that was released for transfusion is a bit misleading because, depending on when and how you are trying to recall it, the chances of being able to get it all back are almost zero. Once it is released, it is used. Potentially contaminated blood had been used, most of it quickly, in emergency rooms. The FDA now had no choice but to take action. In September 1988, the FDA and the Red Cross entered into what is known as a voluntary agreement to comply with all FDA regulations. From now on there would be yearly inspections! But that did not work. The Red Cross kept poor records at local blood banks and the FDA constantly had to threaten license revocations.

Finally, in 1993, FDA commissioner Dr. David Kessler went to federal court and obtained an injunction against the Red Cross for failure to fulfill its promise under the 1988 voluntary agreement.

It is now estimated that as many as 30,000 Americans were infected with AIDS through blood. It is a tragedy that has exposed critical weaknesses in the rules and practices in blood banking. It's also a story of missed opportunities, vested interests, and lax regulations stretching back more than a decade when a mysterious virus entered America's bloodstream. In November 1993, Donna Shalala, secretary of health and human services, asked for a high-level investigation of how thousands of American hemophiliacs became HIV-infected from contaminated blood products. As a result of the investigation and other political action, the Ricky Ray Hemophilia Relief

Fund of 1998 was passed by the House on May 19, 1998, the Senate on October 21, 1998, and became Public Law 105-369 when signed by President Clinton on November 12, 1998. The law authorizes payments of $100,000 to each of 7200 hemophiliacs who were infected using HIV-contaminated blood or blood extracts, to compensate them or their survivors. In October 2000, the U.S. Department of Health and Human Services began notifying such AIDS patients and their families that they will begin receiving those checks.

In April 1997—The four major producers of blood-clotting factors made a $640 million offer to hemophiliacs of the United States. In the summer of 1997 over 6000 hemophiliacs or their families received $100,000. Some refused and went to court to settle.

Class Discussion: Do you feel this saga of delayed and controlled misuse of blood in the United States is equal to or greater than the French and/or German scandals? Explain.

USE OF HIV-CONTAMINATED BLOOD OR BLOOD PRODUCTS IN OTHER COUNTRIES

Canada and Nova Scotia

The royal Canadian Mounted Police have launched a full-scale criminal investigation into Canada's tainted blood scandal in which about 2000 people became HIV infected. To date, over 800 Canadian hemophiliacs tested positive for transfusion-associated HIV infections. About 265 have died of AIDS.

A flood of lawsuits is expected to follow the decision to award more than half a million Canadian dollars to the HIV-infected wife of a man who died of AIDS after receiving a transfusion of HIV-contaminated blood. The outcome of this case was announced on the eve of a deadline set by all except one of Canada's provinces and territories for acceptance of a compensation package by more than a thousand recipients of HIV-infected blood. To obtain the money, victims had to sign waivers promising not to sue Ottawa, the provinces or territories, hospitals, the Red Cross, and pharmaceutical and insurance companies. Compensation was set at C$515,000 per case or per person plus interest and legal fees.

The Canadian compensation is less generous than the province of Nova Scotia, which, as well as making annual payments of C$30,000 to the HIV-infected, pays for expensive AIDS drugs, as well as funeral costs and post-secondary education for their children (Spurgeon, 1994, 1996).

In late 1998 the Canadian Blood Services agency started operations, replacing the Canadian Red Cross as the country's national blood service.

Switzerland

In mid-1994, Alfred Haessig, the former head of the Swiss Red Cross Central Laboratory in Bern was charged with causing "grievous bodily harm" by allowing HIV-tainted blood-clotting factors to be distributed to Swiss hemophiliacs in 1985 and 1986.

The Swiss case resembles the French scandal. In both cases, a national lab continued to distribute blood products that were known to be potentially infected with HIV. France stopped using such products in October 1985, but in Switzerland they were marketed through May 1986.

The suspect Swiss factors were made with blood collected some months before July 1985, when HIV testing became routine. The trial centered on his failure to stop production of the factors in July 1985, when the New York Blood Center identified one HIV-positive sample among 3375 units of donated Swiss blood. But the Swiss Red Cross insists that no alternative supplies were available: "If these products would not have gone out, the hemophiliacs would have bled to death." (Holden, 1994)

Results of Swiss Case: Alfred Haessig Found Guilty

In December of 1998, the former director of the Swiss central laboratory of the Red Cross, was found **guilty,** by a Geneva court, of supervising the distribution of HIV-infected blood products to hemophiliacs. The 77-year-old man was given a one-year suspended sentence. The prosecutor in the case argued that Haessig should have been aware of the risk of transmitting HIV through blood products in 1982, but that he supervised the manufacture of the blood products until November 1995 and distribution through May 1996, failing to implement safer options. Haessig, who retired in 1987, asserts that he did not use pasteurization because he thought the process was less efficient in the treatment of hemophiliacs. The case was brought following complaints by eight Swiss hemophiliacs who were infected with HIV.

Japan

In July of 1993, 92 Japanese hemophiliacs filed suit against the Japanese government and blood product manufacturers. They are seeking compensation for failure to protect them from blood products contaminated with HIV. Blood product manufacturers continued to advertise untreated blood products in Japan without warning until late 1985; Japanese hemophiliacs used them into 1986. They sought $1 million each in compensation.

During 1983–1985, Japan dramatically increased its imports of untreated U.S. blood products and, as a result, about 2000 of Japan's 5000 hemophiliacs were infected with HIV. Through 2000 over 500 have died and another 500 have AIDS. (Swinbank, 1993, 1994 updated).

In 1996, after a seven-year court battle, Japan's hemophiliacs and their families reached an out-of-court settlement. Each HIV-affected hemophiliac received about $430,000. Those with AIDS will receive an additional $1,400 a month for life (Abbott, 1996).

In September of 1996, the president and two former presidents of Green Cross Corporation (Midori Juji), Japan's leading blood product manufacturer, were arrested in connection with the infection of thousands of Japanese with HIV through the use of non-heat-treated blood products in the 1980s. They were being held on suspicion of negligence in promoting the continued sale of non-heat-treated blood coagulants in 1986, after safer heat-treated products, including those of the Midori Juji Company, were approved for sale by the government in 1985.

Update—The Japanese HIV blood scandal is over, with three drug company executives being convicted. Renzo Matsushita, former president of Green Cross Corporation, which supplied blood products, was given two years in jail for his role in a patient's death from HIV, while two other Green Cross officials were handed sentences of up to 18 months.

India

A blood bank in Bombay operated by the India Red Cross Society (IRCS) has been closed down following a government decision to conduct an inquiry into charges that the center had supplied blood infected with HIV to hospitals in the city between 1992 and 1994.

The medical officer in charge of the blood bank has already been removed from his post, and more officials are expected to lose their jobs. The affair has caused concern throughout India, as the IRCS is intended to set national standards for blood safety.

The affair came to light when the chairman of the IRCS subcommittee on blood transfusion services examined the records of the blood bank. These showed that HIV-positive blood had been supplied to at least 10 city hospitals, including one that specializes in transfusion services.

In addition, there have been suspicions that employees of the blood bank, rather than discarding infected blood, have been selling it on the black market created by an overall shortage of blood supplies (Jayaraman, 1995).

China

In October of 1996, China's Ministry of Public Health ordered thousands of state-run medical institutions to stop using a certain brand of serum albumin, a common blood product produced by a military-run factory.

Two years after Chinese journalists in Hong Kong and the United States first published reports that the blood product was contaminated with HIV, China's Foreign Ministry acknowledged that tests of some samples of the blood product indicated the presence of HIV. But, at the Department of Medicine Administration and Control, a Mr. Liu said: "No, no, it has never happened. Some people outside China and some foreign journalists just made their reports on the basis of rumors."

In October of 1998, in an effort to reduce the spread of HIV, the Chinese government created a law requiring that all blood products come from volunteers. Many countries banned the practice of payment for blood donation long ago, since there were concerns that the people who would be most likely to be strapped for money—such as drug users—would also be at high risk for blood-borne diseases. However, in China it can be hard to get donors because there is a cultural aversion to blood donation. Traditionally, the donation of blood is considered disrespectful to ancestors and parents; the culture also equates blood levels with health. Because China has a chronic blood shortage, many experts believe it will take several years for the illegal blood trade to die down. The government is trying to confront this problem by actively encouraging officials, students, and soldiers to donate blood.

Chinese health officials now believe that 20% of over 1 million HIV-positive Chinese contracted HIV through the blood trade.

The Secret of China's Henan Province, 2001

Hints of a secret AIDS epidemic in China's countryside first began to surface in 2000. The depth of the tragedy and the unusually high incidence and impact of HIV/AIDS on villages in the Henan Province are now emerging, as disparate, dying farmers have begun to tell their stories of illness and death. All their stories begin with their willingness to sell their blood, money necessary for their economy. Because of the plasma collection methods routinely used at the time throughout China, even those who donated only a few times ran a high risk of becoming ill. Blood from dozens of sellers was pooled and put into a huge centrifuge where it was spun at a speed sufficient to separate out the desired plasma. The remaining fraction, mainly red cells, was divided up and **transfused back into the sellers**, who felt the process to be healthful because it limited the blood loss. The process was highly unsanitary. The result was once one blood seller in a village was infected with HIV or hepatitis, the rest were quick to become ill because the viruses from other people's bodies rode along with the red cells back into their veins. Because the sellers did not lose enough red cells with any donation to result in anemia, using this method meant that people could sell their blood frequently—raising their chance of infection.

In the village of Donghu, population 4500, every family has one or more members who suffer from fevers, chronic diarrhea, mouth sores, unbearable headaches, weight loss, racking coughs, and boils that do not heal. Residents estimate that more than 80% of adults carry HIV and more than 60% are already suffering debilitating symptoms. That would give this village, and the others like it in the province, localized rates that are the highest in the world.

Physicians who have worked in the Henan province said more than a million people had probably contracted the virus from selling their blood. They add that while the sale of blood has stopped in the most severely affected villages, it continues elsewhere to a lesser extent, both in Henan and other provinces.

Beginning 2003, China continues to downplay the effect of returning blood cells to paid donors in the Henan province. Officials have stopped villagers from traveling outside of Henan province or from speaking to the media. The epidemic in Henan province is still shrouded in silence because local officials were often involved in the profitable blood business. So while the authorities in Beijing held a big international conference in November of 2001 and aired television dramas on the subject, repression and concealment continues into 2003.

Iran

Court proceedings began in June 1999 in Tehran to deal with the complaints lodged by 170 hemophiliac and thalassaemia patients against the former head of the Blood Transfusion Organization, Mohammad Farhadi, and other officials in a blood-processing laboratory. The patients' lawyer read the complaint in three sections, calling on the court to deal with the case. The lawyer accused Blood Transfusion Organization officials of being negligent in screening the blood, buying contaminated blood factors from Merieux company of France in 1994, and using outdated blood-testing equipment. Case is pending.

Ireland

In September 1999 an Irish Tribunal began hearings into the HIV infection of over 300 hemophiliacs of which 79 have now died of AIDS. There are some 400 hemophiliacs in Ireland. The Irish Hemophiliac Society has been battling for years to get an inquiry into how the state's Blood Transfusion Services Board failed to screen out the infected products. The inquiry is investigating the manufacture and purchase of the infected blood products.

A just monetary compensation is expected for the affected (mid-2002). The case is in the court system for final judgment.

OTHER BLOOD SCANDALS IN BRIEF

In Columbia, a drug-addicted bisexual who knew he had AIDS sold his blood 12 times to a laboratory. Twelve patients received the blood between 1989 and 1990 and went on to infect an additional 200 people through sexual contact.

In Romania during the Communist era, HIV-contaminated blood infected 2376 children.

Currently developing countries must rely on paid donors, who may include gay and bisexual men, prostitutes, and drug addicts needing money. Countries like India, Pakistan, and Russia have an open paid donor system.

Parts of Africa and Latin America use family replacement donors—a scheme that allows paid donors to pose as relatives of the patient. Paying unquestioned donors without HIV screening is an invitation for HIV transmission. But developing countries do not have the capital nor sufficient trained personnel to do anything else at the moment.

SUMMARY

The issues cited were delays in institution of donor screening, delays in screening donated blood with HIV antibody testing, and failure to withdraw contaminated factor from use and replace it with heat-treated factor for economic reasons—after it was known that these actions would protect individuals from infection.

According to the World Health Organization (WHO), the majority of nations are using **unsafe blood** with regard to HIV and hepatitis. The use of unsafe blood is most common in developing countries, home to 80% of the world's population, or some 4.8 billion people. Because of the high cost of blood testing, between $40 to $50 per unit, more than 13 million pints of blood annually are not checked for transmissible infections including HIV, malaria, and syphilis. **Globally, transfusions of contaminated blood are thought to have infected up to 10% of AIDS patients.** Moreover, unsafe transfusions and injection practices are estimated to cause up to 160,000 new HIV infections, 16 million new cases of hepatitis B, and 4.7 million new hepatitis C infections each year. In response to these findings, the WHO, in cooperation with the International Federation of Red Cross and Red Crescent Societies, launched a global campaign to promote blood safety.

For the United States, the CDC states that over the past 18 years of blood screening for HIV (1985–2003) 45 adults and two children have developed AIDS after receiving an HIV-negative blood transfusion. This blood was taken in the window period before antibodies were made against HIV (Klein, 2000 updated). The majority of over 9000 HIV-contaminated blood transfusions occurred prior to 1985, the year when HIV blood screening began. It is estimated that about 50 new HIV-contaminated blood transfusions continue to occur each year in America. For additional information on blood scandals, read *Blood Feuds: AIDS, Blood and the Politics of Medical Disaster*, edited by Eric Feldman and Ronald Bayer, Oxford University Press, 1999.

BOX 8.3

GAY MEN PUTTING THEMSELVES AT HIGH RISK FOR HIV INFECTION

Gordon Mansergh reported at the 12th International AIDS Conference (June–July 1998) that of gay men in Denver, Chicago, and San Francisco, almost two-thirds engaged in **unprotected anal sex** in the previous 18 months and that 56% of gay men **under age 25 had unprotected receptive anal sex** in the same time frame.

Experts believe one reason risky behavior continues among the young is that they have not yet seen their friends die of the disease.

Another is simply the kind of risk-taking common among the young—the same impulse that prompts teenagers to drive fast or take up smoking. Indicators of increased risky sex among gay men included: gay men having **unprotected sex** increased from 35% in 1994 to 55% in early 1999. Thirty percent of 3000 gay men surveyed in four large American cities had **unprotected sex**—7% of them were HIV positive. In three large American cities, 66% of gay men surveyed had **unprotected sex** in the last 18 months. **One in five** gay men in San Francisco and New York City said they had **unprotected sex** with an HIV-negative partner or with a partner who's HIV status was unknown. In 1998 the CDC surveyed about 22,000 gay men in San Francisco. Over 39% said they have **unprotected sex**—this is a 30% increase since 1994. Linda Valleroy and colleagues at the CDC reported at the 8th Conference on Retroviruses, February 2001, on testing and interview results of 2400 gay men ages 23 through 29. The men were from Baltimore, Dallas, New York, Los Angeles, Miami, and Seattle. Over 12% or 293 of the men were HIV positive. **Twenty-nine percent** knew they were HIV positive before testing! Forty-six percent said they had unprotected oral sex during the previous six months. These data shocked the researchers.

On January 29, 1999, the *San Francisco Chronicle* carried a story about an $8 admission for a night of communal sex—the rules: no clothes, no condoms, no discussion of HIV. The article also covers an internet link offering gay men the **extreme sex party** where becoming infected or HIV-infecting another is the erotic allure of the party. Still another twist is the **Russian Roulette Party** where three noninfected men have sex with five others, one of the five being HIV positive!

UPDATE 2002— Mitchell Katz and colleagues (2002) examined the data from interviews from

over 26,000 men having sex with men (MSM) conducted between 1995 and 1999. They found that although the use of HAART reduced the risk of HIV transmission, the success of that therapy might have caused MSM to be less cautious and more likely to engage in unsafe sex. The interviews indicated that, as a result of the availability of HAART, HIV negative men who have sex with men (MSM) are less concerned about contracting HIV; HIV positive MSM are less concerned about transmitting HIV; and both groups are more likely to engage in unsafe sex. Also because HAART decreases mortality and improves the quality of life of persons with AIDS, it has increased the number of persons living with HIV/AIDS who are engaging in sexual relations.

Circuit Parties—Circuit parties got their name from those who travel to various cities— the circuit—to attend several parties each year. The parties, which began in 1986, essentially are the gay version of raves, parties that are popular among some young people. There are two or three circuit party weekends a month. Among the cities where they are held: Montreal, San Francisco, Atlanta, Palm Springs, Miami, and Washington. The parties are not universally popular among gay men, although many say they have attended one. The parties generally attract professionals ages 21 to 35. The parties began with the intention of fund raising and community building. But somewhere along the way, the original intent of the party has become diluted. Now, circuit parties have become weekend long bashes in cities across the United States and Canada. They attract thousands of mostly young gay men who dance until dawn and whose admission fees raise millions of dollars for AIDS prevention groups and gay charities. But, according to Ronald Johnson, an official of the circuit party organization, "It (circuit parties) became a social phenomenon above and beyond what (we) intended and beyond what (we) could control." Health officials say the parties have become a reflection of the risky behavior that is contributing to rising rates of HIV infection among gay men. Drugs are so prevalent at the parties that organizers often hire medical teams to treat overdoses. Troy Masters, publisher of a gay newspaper in New York, who now opposes these parties said, "You wouldn't find the American Cancer Society throwing a smoking party." Gay Men's Health Crisis, which was founded in

BOX 8.3 *(continued)*

1981 and serves 11,000 clients annually in the New York area, stopped holding its party in 1998 after it became known for drug use and sex. Two Philadelphia couples said they attend up to eight parties a year and usually take Ecstasy pills with a liquid shot of GHB or some ketamine, which can be liquid or powder. They agreed that "if you don't do drugs, you're not going to enjoy it as much."

BAREBACKING: CHASING THE BUG—INTENTIONALLY SEEKING HIV INFECTION

It has recently been observed that a minority of both HIV positive and negative men have begun to consciously, willfully, and proudly engage in unprotected anal sex. The new phenomenon, referred to as raw, skin-to-skin, or bareback sex. Such behavior in this group leads to the intentional transmission and reception of HIV! This form of barebacking is referred to as "bug chasing" or "chasing the bug." HIV-negative gay men seek to become HIV infected. According to Yvonne Abraham of the Boston Globe Online, and DeAnn Gauthier (1999), health professionals are seeing something unexpected in the gay community: a small group of men who want to contract HIV in the belief that it offers community and kinship. Increasing numbers of chat rooms and websites approach the subject of men who want to convert from HIV negative to positive. Marshall Forstein, medical director of mental health at Fenway Community Health Center in Boston, says some of the men feel lonely or shunned and believe that HIV will bring them attention from friends and caregivers. One California activist who stopped using condoms and later contracted HIV also noted, "When I was entering the gay community at the height [of the epidemic], I felt like I'd joined the war. And that somehow transformed HIV into this rite of passage as opposed to something to be reviled and avoided." Some websites even discuss conversion parties, where uninfected men can have unprotected sex with HIV positive men to try to contract the virus. The groups refer to HIV infection as a rebirth and a way to bond with a new family. According to Gautheir, bug chasing as a form of bareback sex actually involves two categories of participants. There are the HIV-negative men who seek to become infected with the virus (bug chasers), and there are the gift givers, HIV positive men who seek to share their gift of HIV to others. Chasers typically advertise for partners with statements such as: "Will let you ____ me raw only if you promise to give me all your diseases like AIDS/herpes, etc. Let's do it." Gift givers, on the other hand, typically make comments such as: "Attention neg men! Why stay locked in a boring world of sterile sex when you can join the ranks of the AIDS Freedom Fighters? Let me give you my gift and set you free." Becoming "bug brothers" may occur one-on-one but is just as likely to result at special marathon group sex parties that are held for the purpose of seroconverting as many HIV-negative participants as possible. That individuals would knowingly participate in such events is shocking not only to some members of the gay community, but also the community at large (Gauthier, 1999).

THE HIGH RATE OF HIV INFECTION AMONG GAY MEN ON SOUTH BEACH, MIAMI, FLORIDA

Miami's South Beach—hot music, hot spots, hot sun, hot bodies. The once sagging tip of Miami Beach has been turned into the playground of the beautiful, the rich, and the chic. South Beach is also a growing mecca for young gay men. In a world where homosexuality is often confined to the closet, it is a place to be out and to be open. But behind the perfect tans, there is the dark reality! According to a new study one in every six gay men between the ages of 18 and 29 in South Beach has tested HIV positive.

William Darrow, AIDS researcher who surveyed 87 gay men ages 18 to 29 and 70 gay men age 30 and older, said, "People seem to think they're on a holiday there from everything—including AIDS." Darrow's survey showed that about 75% of gay men in both age groups had **unprotected anal sex** in 1996.

Testimonial—One gay male living at South Beach said he fell victim to **love.** "I was in a relationship, and we both got tested together and we tested negative, so we started having unprotected sex. But during the relationship, my partner was cheating on me and he was infected and in turn infected me."

A majority of young gay men have grown up thinking they won't reach middle age; for those who aren't positive, the specter of AIDS haunts them. For many of those who have grown up with the safer sex message, the words of warning

BOX 8.3 *(continued)*

are often lost. In addition, the media covering anti-AIDS drugs, protease inhibitors, are generating **hype and new hope,** but there is a downside: Young gay men may be letting their guards down because of the hype. Another contributing high-risk behavioral factor is the growing number of gay bathhouses and sex clubs cropping up across the country. People come to South Beach to have anonymous sex; they pay to use the facility and condoms are free. Safer sex posters are everywhere. But, some argue that bathhouses are centers for HIV infection; others argue that shutting down bathhouses will drive men in search of sex to public parks or other unmonitored settings.

The scale of multiple-partnering during the late 20th century is unprecedented. With over 6 billion people on Earth, an ever-increasing percentage of whom are urban residents; with air travel and mass transit available to allow people from all over the world to go to the cities of their choice; with mass youth movements advocating, among other things, sexual freedom; with a feminist spirit alive in much of the industrialized world, promoting female sexual freedom; and with **47% of the world's population made up of people between the ages of 15 and 44**—there can be no doubt that the amount of worldwide urban sexual energy is unparalleled.

The amount of protection one actually obtains from limiting one's number of partners depends mainly on who those partners are. Having one partner who is in a high-risk group may be more dangerous than having many partners who are not. An example of this is seen in prostitutes, who may be more likely to be infected by their regular injection drug-using partners than by customers who are not in a high-risk group. The risk status of a person who remains faithful to a single sexual partner depends on that partner's behavior: If the partner becomes infected, often without knowing it, the monogamous individual is likely to become infected (Cohen et al., 1989).

Sexual Activities— In addition to a high-risk partner or a number of sexual partners, the types of sexual activities that occur are also significant (Table 8-5). Any sexual activity that produces skin, anal, or vaginal membrane abrasions prior to or during intercourse increases the risk of infection. Recent studies show that men who have been circumcised are at less risk of infection. Foreskin of the penis tears as it is forced back over the glans, providing a direct route for HIV to enter the blood stream.

Orogenital Sex— Orogenital sex may be a greater risk factor for becoming HIV-infected than previously thought. The risk of transmission is related to the presence of HIV at the sexual sites (oral, vaginal, penile, and anal), the amount of HIV present, and whether there are physical openings such as tissue tears or open sores (Rothenberg et al., 1998; Kahn et al., 1998).

After reviewing over 100 research reports Sara Edwards and colleagues (1998) concluded that HIV can be transmitted through oral sex. In a very rigorous study, Beth Dillon and colleagues (2000) appear to have clearly pinpointed oral transmission in approximately 7% of primary infection cases. By mid-2000, strong evidence for at least 30 cases of oral HIV infection were reported in the United States (Dillon, 2000). In Britain, Barry Evans, director of Public Health Laboratory Service, reported that oral sex may account for up to 8% of HIV infections among gay men. He said that oral sex leads to 30 to 50 new HIV infections annually in the United Kingdom. Evans states that the risk of HIV infection via oral sex is greater than previously thought.

Susan Buchbinder and colleagues in 2001 calculated that the odds of acquiring HIV from any single act of oral sex with an infected partner are roughly 4 in 10,000 (1 in 2500) compared with odds of 4 in 1000 (1 in 250) for anal sex with a condom. Jorge del Romero and colleagues (2002) reported on 135 uninfected or HIV-negative men and women whose only risk of HIV exposure was through **unprotected** orogenital sex with their HIV-infected partners. Collectively, the 135 people had over 19,000 unprotected oral genital contacts with their HIV-infected partners. None of the 135 HIV-negative partners became infected! The authors of this study conclude that the probability of HIV transmission via oral sex is very low.

It should also be recognized that one can get other sexually transmitted diseases from oral sex, such as gonorrhea, syphilis, chlamydia, and herpes.

Prostitution (Sex Worker): United States

There is little if any evidence that prostitutes in the United States and other **developed** nations

Table 8-5 Sexual Activity According to Degree of Risk for Transmitting HIV

Lowest risk	1.	Abstinence
	2.	Masturbating alone
	3.	Hugging/massage/dry kissing
	4.	Masturbating with another person but not touching one another
	5.	Deep wet kissing
	6.	Mutual masturbation with only external touching
	7.	Mutual masturbation with internal touching using finger cots or condoms
	8.	Frottage (rubbing a person for sexual pleasure)
	9.	Intercourse between the thighs
	10.	Mutual masturbation with orgasm *on*, not *in* partner
	11.	Use of sex toys (dildos) with condoms, or that are not shared by partners and that have been properly sterilized between uses
	12.	Cunnilingus
	13.	Fellatio without a condom, but never putting the head of the penis inside mouth
	14.	Fellatio to orgasm with a condom
	15.	Fellatio without a condom, putting the head of the penis inside the mouth and withdrawing prior to ejaculation
	16.	Fellatio without a condom with ejaculation in mouth
	17.	Vaginal intercourse with a condom correctly used and spermicidal foam that kills HIV and withdrawing prior to orgasm
	18.	Anal intercourse with a condom correctly used with a lubricant that contains spermicide that kills HIV and withdrawing prior to ejaculation
	19.	Vaginal intercourse with internal ejaculation with a condom correctly used and with spermicidal foam that kills HIV
	20.	Vaginal intercourse with internal ejaculation with a condom correctly used but no spermicidal foam
	21.	Anal intercourse with internal ejaculation with a condom correctly used with spermicide that kills HIV
	22.	Brachiovaginal activities (fisting)
	23.	Brachioproctic activities (anal fisting)
	24.	Use of sex toys by more than one partner without a condom and that have not been sterilized between uses
	25.	Vaginal intercourse using spermicidal foam but without a condom and withdrawing prior to ejaculation
	26.	Vaginal intercourse without spermicidal foam and without a condom and withdrawing prior to ejaculation
	27.	Anal intercourse with a condom and withdrawing prior to ejaculation
	28.	Vaginal intercourse with internal ejaculation without a condom but with spermicidal foam
	29.	Vaginal intercourse with internal ejaculation without a condom and without any other form of barrier contraception
Highest risk	30.	Anal intercourse with internal ejaculation without a condom

(Source: Shernoff, 1988)

play a large role in heterosexual HIV transmission (Cohen et al., 1989).

A consequence of the attention prostitutes or sex workers have attracted in relation to AIDS in the United States and other developed countries, is that they tend to be seen as responsible for the spread of HIV—an attitude reflected in descriptions of prostitutes as reservoirs of infection or high-frequency transmitters. But, the sex worker is only the most visible side of a transaction that involves two people: For every sex worker who is HIV positive there is, somewhere, the partner from whom she or he contracted HIV. Given the fact that the chance of contracting HIV during a single act of unprotected sex is not high, infection in a sex worker is likely to mean that she or he has been repeatedly exposed to HIV by clients who did not or would not wear condoms. Thus the more useful way of reading the statistics of HIV infection in prostitutes or sex workers is to view them as an indication of how strong a foothold the epidemic has gotten within a community.

Prostitution—Developing Countries

In a garbage-strewn alley in the city's red-light district, a 24-year-old prostitute slumps on a string bed, weak from tuberculosis and diarrhea. She knows she has AIDS but she has never heard of the multidrug "cocktail" that curbs the progress of the disease. Even if she had, she could never afford to buy it. Nobody wants the girls once they get sick, explains a health counselor who visits the alley each week. She says prostitutes with AIDS are shunned by many hospital doctors, brothel operators, and their own families. "We feel helpless; all we can do is comfort them and find them a place where they can go to die." This true vignette is happening in small towns, the suburbs, and in every large city in every country in the developing nations. Many of the prostitutes are housewives out to make the difference between starvation and existence for her family. The prostitutes sell their bodies for money or drugs to anyone who can afford their services. In some towns in Africa, Vietnam, and India between 50% and 90% of the prostitutes are HIV positive. Prostitution in developing countries is a large contributing factor to the spread of HIV/AIDS.

In Chennai, India, Mobile brothels manned by cell-phone toting operators are proving profitable. For those in the trade, running a mobile unit makes sound business sense as it cuts down on operational costs of renting a building and paying bribes. As for the client, it promises "pick and drop" facility of sex workers at a place of his

---

BOX 8.4

SPORTS AND HIV/AIDS: EARVIN "MAGIC" JOHNSON AND OTHER ATHLETES

HIV-INFECTED ATHLETES AND COMPETITION

The question regarding whether HIV-infected athletes should be allowed to compete has two facets:

1. Should these athletes be banned from competition to avoid the risk of spreading HIV infection?
2. Does the exercise that is demanded in competition accelerate progression of HIV disease?

There is no hard, fast, scientifically supported answer to either question. However, beginning 2003, there has not been a single reported case of HIV transmission in any sporting event worldwide! (Drotman, 1996 updated).

Magic Johnson: Professional Basketball Player, Los Angeles Lakers, HIV Positive

On November 7, 1991, Magic Johnson age 32 appeared at a nationally televised press conference and said, "Because of the HIV virus I have obtained, I will have to announce my retirement from the Lakers today." He admitted having been "naive" about AIDS and added, "Here I am saying **it can happen to anybody,** even me, Magic Johnson." He also assured the world that his wife, Cookie Kelly, two months pregnant, had tested negative for the virus.

The National AIDS Hotline lit up with 40,000 phone calls on the day of Johnson's announcement, instead of the usual 3,800. At the Centers for Disease Control and Prevention in Atlanta, AIDS-related calls, which usually average 200 per hour, jumped to 10,000 in a single hour. Prior to Magic's announcement, the black community lacked a focal point for action: No leader of national stature had claimed a prominent space from which to address HIV disease. Few black politicians, entertainers, civil rights leaders, or sports figures had tackled the issue of AIDS either through public service announcements, television talk shows, radio addresses, church pulpits, theaters, or school auditoriums. Magic's announcement—at least for a time—changed that.

Some Events Since Magic's Announced Retirement

June 4, 1992—Earvin the III is born *without* antibody to HIV. As of August 14, 2002, Magic is age 44. His wife, age 44, and son, age 12, are HIV negative (Figure 8-6).

BOX 8.4 *(continued)*

FIGURE 8-6 Earvin "Magic" Johnson, wife Cookie, and son Andre arrive for a special ceremony of *Hoodlum* at a Magic Johnson-owned theater. Magic has become a spokesman for those struggling against HIV/AIDS. *(Photograph courtesy of AP/Wide World Photos/Michael Caulfied)*

Magic announced in April 1997 that his AIDS drug combination, which included a protease inhibitor, has reduced his viral load to unmeasurable blood levels!

February 16, 2000—Magic Johnson joined the AIDS Healthcare Foundation (AHF), the largest direct provider of HIV/AIDS care in the United States, in *unveiling Thrive Magazine,* a new national magazine targeting minorities living with and impacted by HIV and AIDS. *Thrive Magazine* seeks to address the severity of the impact of AIDS among people of color by providing minority communities a unique, multicultural perspective on resources and information concerning HIV education and treatment. In August of 2001, *Sports Illustrated* reported that Magic takes Combivir (AZT+3 TC) and a protease inhibitor. Magic said "I never thought I would die from AIDS." He believes he owes his good health to "keeping stress out of my life."

In July 2001, Magic played in a basketball game in a Summer Pro League in Los Angeles, nearly 10 years after he announced that he was HIV positive. His September 2002 checkup confirms he's still asymptomatic after 11 years.

OTHER SPORTS, OTHER ATHLETES

Basketball players are not the only athletes whose behavior may place them at risk for HIV infection. In 1996 there were 6114 professional athletes in the United States involved in boxing (3500), National Football League (1590), National Hockey League (676), and the National Basketball Association (348). Of these professionals, the CDC estimated 30 to be HIV positive.

John Elson (1991) wrote a revealing article for *Time* magazine just after Magic Johnson revealed his HIV status. Elson tells of groupies that follow athletes in all sports. They are usually college-age or older. Mainly they seek money, attention, and the glamour of associating with celebrated and highly visible "hard bodies." According to a 31-year old who has had affairs with athletes in two sports, "For women, many of whom don't have meaningful work, the only way to identify

BOX 8.4 *(continued)*

themselves is to say whom they have slept with. A woman who sleeps around is called a whore. But a woman who has slept with Magic Johnson is a woman who has slept with Magic Johnson. It's almost as if it gives her legitimacy."

The Girls

Baseball players call them **"Annies."** To riders on the rodeo circuit, they are **"buckle bunnies."** To most other athletes, they are **"wannabes"** or just **"the girls."** They can be found hanging out anywhere they might catch an off-duty sports hero's eye and fancy, or in the lobbies of hotels where teams on the road check in. To the athletes who care to indulge them—and many do—these readily available groupies offer pro sport's ultimate perk: free and easy recreational sex, no questions asked. Recently, an HIV-infected female stated publicly that she had had sex with at least 50 Canadian ice hockey players. She could not recall their names. **The sex may be free, but now there is a price for the lifestyle—HIV/AIDS.**

Sports/Injuries/Blood

Concerns over the transmission of HIV are shared throughout sports, particularly those sports that cause blood-letting injuries—football, hockey, and boxing. In football Jerry Smith, a former Washington Redskin, died of AIDS in 1986; no others are known at this time. In 1996, the National Football League officials estimated that there was the **possibility** of one HIV transmission from body fluid exchange in 85 million football games played. In boxing, Esteban DeJesus, WBC lightweight champion, died of AIDS in 1989. Four other boxers are known to be HIV positive.

Tommy Morrison

In February of 1996 Tommy Morrison, age 27, a heavyweight boxing title contender (Figure 8-7) said, on announcing that he was HIV positive, "I honestly believed I had a better chance of winning the lottery than contracting this disease. I've never been so wrong in my life. I'm here to tell you I thought that I was bulletproof, and I'm not." Morrison went on to describe his promiscuous sexual lifestyle and ignorance about AIDS. Former heavyweight champ Floyd Paterson, former chairman of the New York State Athletic Commission, who was asked why his organization waited until the Tommy Morrison case to institute HIV testing for boxers, said

FIGURE 8-7 Tommy Morrison. Las Vegas, June 7, 1993—Tommy Morrison raises his right hand after being declared the new WBO heavyweight champion. Morrison won the 12-round bout against former heavyweight champion George Foreman at the Thomas & Mack Center. *(Photograph courtesy of Archive Photos)*

"AIDS just came out, I go back to the '50s. I fought for 23 years. There was no AIDS. **I just heard of AIDS a few weeks ago."** Just heard of AIDS? Since Morrison's announcement, 12 states have banned HIV-positive professional boxers from the ring. In November 1996, Morrison fought in Japan. He knocked his opponent out in 1:38 (1 minute, 38 seconds). The fight would have been stopped at the first sign of Morrison's blood.

Update July 1997 POZ Magazine Interview— Tommy Morrison now believes that HIV is not a disease-causing virus! **"AIDS has been here since creation, but it doesn't do anything"** and as for AIDS, he says, **"Acquired Immune Deficiency Syndrome is something that's easily cured."** With regard to taking anti-HIV drugs, he "fired" his

BOX 8.4 *(continued)*

physician who prescribed them for him (Dr. David Ho, *Time Magazine* **Man of the Year 1996**). He points to an HIV-infected friend and says **"this kid was perfectly healthy until he started taking medication."** He says that he and his wife have **unprotected** sex because **"HIV can't hurt you. There is no way you can get HIV from sex. It's scientifically impossible."**

Morrison refers to himself as the most educated person he knows regarding HIV (he read Peter Duesberg's book, *Inventing the AIDS Virus* and Richard Wilner's *Deadly Deception*). "I don't know how I know the things I know, I just know I'm right—I have not been sick in 5 years—if it ain't broke don't fix it." Fighting weight about 240 pounds—early 1998 he weighed about 185.

By early 1998, nine states, (Oregon, Indiana, Washington, Pennsylvania, Nevada, Arizona, Maryland, New Jersey, New York) and Puerto Rico required all professional boxers to be HIV tested. There are no known cases of HIV transmission via a boxing match. In late 1998 Morrison began taking antiretroviral medications.

There is a certain irony in all of this because as part of his probationary terms of a suspended sentence for weapons violation and assault charges, he gives speeches to high school and college students on HIV/AIDS!

UPDATE 2001 According to the *Kansas City Star* newspaper, the ex-boxing champ is being incarcerated in a southwest Arkansas Correctional facility near Texarkana. Morrison is serving a 10-year sentence (eight of which have been suspended) for felonies that include possession of cocaine, firearms, and drug paraphernalia. An *Arkansas Democrat-Gazette* reporter who interviewed Morrison revealed that "Morrison is requesting clemency from Governor Mike Huckabee so he can receive treatment from his HIV specialist in Fayetteville. Or so he can go to San Diego and sit in a chamber that will flood his body with oxygen, hoping it eradicates the HIV in his system. He wants to talk about HIV and AIDS education and treatment, which he calls 'the biggest government conspiracy since who shot JFK'.

Ice Skating

In professional ice skating, the *Calgary Herald* reported that by 1992, at least 40 top U.S. and Canadian male skaters and coaches have died from AIDS (among them, Rob McCall, Brian Pockar, Dennis Coi, and Shawn McGill).

Swimming

In February 1995, Greg Louganis, the greatest diver in Olympic history, announced that he had AIDS (Figure 8-8).

FIGURE 8-8 Greg Louganis. *(Photograph courtesy of Archive Photos)*

Race Car Drivers

It was reported in 1996 that Tim Richmond, race car driver, age 34, died of AIDS. He won 13 Winston Cup races on the NASCAR racing circuit. One report states that Richmond may have infected up to 30 women (Knight-Tribune Service, March 27, 1996, A-1). His physician estimated that he was HIV positive for at least eight years. During this time, according to accounts of friends he was sexually promiscuous. (Richmond actually died in 1989 but his story was kept silent until 1996.)

Ice Hockey

Bill Goldsworthy, five-time NHL All-Star, age 51, died of AIDS. He played 14 seasons in the NHL. He was diagnosed with AIDS in 1994. Goldworthy said his health problem was caused by drinking and sexual promiscuity.

choice. More than 17 mobile units operate in the city, according to Chennai-based NGO Indian Community Welfare Organization (ICWO), which works with Commercial Sex Workers (CSWs). According to estimates, there are 6300 women sex workers operating throughout the city. Thirty percent said they couldn't use condoms with regular clients. Another 30% said, at times, they would forget to have their clients wear condoms and 10% felt that condom usage would prolong sexual activity. Another 10% said some clients would object to it. About 20% said they knew better techniques to avoid infection! As for reasons why they chose to be sex workers, 31% respon-

dents said they entered the profession due to family debts and 29% said their husbands deserted them. About 29% said their lovers had ditched them.

***Risk Estimates for HIV Infection During Sexual Intercourse in the Heterosexual Population*—** Norman Hearst and Stephen Hulley of the University of California, San Francisco calculated that the odds of heterosexual HIV transmission range from **one in 500 for a single act of sexual intercourse with an HIV-infected partner when no condom is used to one in 5 billion if a condom is used and the sexual partner is HIV negative at the time.**

Table 8-6   Risk of HIV Infection for Heterosexual Intercourse in the United States

	Estimated Risk of Infection at Random	
Risk Category of Partner	1 Sexual Encounter	500 Sexual Encounters
HIV SEROSTATUS UNKNOWN		
Not in any high-risk group		
Using condoms	1 in 50,000,000	1 in 110,000
Not using condoms	1 in 5,000,000	1 in 16,000
High-risk groups[a]		
Using condoms	1 in 100,000 to 1 in 10,000	1 in 210 to 1 in 21
Not using condoms	1 in 10,000 to 1 in 1000	1 in 32 to 1 in 3
HIV SERONEGATIVE		
No history of high-risk behavior[b]		
Using condoms	1 in 5,000,000,000	1 in 11,000,000
Not using condoms	1 in 500,000,000	1 in 1,600,000
Continuing high-risk behavior[b]		
Using condoms	1 in 500,000	1 in 1100
Not using condoms	1 in 50,000	1 in 160
HIV SEROPOSITIVE		
Using condoms	1 in 5000	1 in 11
Not using condoms	1 in 500	2 in 3

[a]High-risk groups with prevalences of HIV infection at the higher end of the range given include homosexual or bisexual men, injection drug users from major metropolitan areas, and hemophiliacs. Groups with prevalences at the lower end of the range include homosexual or bisexual men and injection drug users from other parts of the country, female prostitutes, heterosexuals from countries where heterosexual spread of HIV is common (including Haiti and central Africa), and recipients of multiple blood transfusions between 1983 and 1985 from areas with a high prevalence of HIV infection.
[b]High-risk behavior consists of sexual intercourse or needle sharing with a member of one of the high-risk groups.
(Source: Adapted from Hearst and Hulley, 1988.)

Table 8-6 presents estimates of the risk of HIV infection from a single heterosexual encounter and after five years of frequent heterosexual contact for various types of partners. Risk depends on the following: (1) the probability that the sexual partner carries the virus; (2) If one of the sexual partners is HIV positive, the height of their viral load (suppression of viral load reduces the risk of HIV transmission); (3) the probability of infection given a single sexual exposure to an infected partner; and (4) the reduction in risk by using condoms and spermicides.

The most striking feature of the table is the large variation in the risk of HIV infection under different circumstances. The most important cause of this variation is risk status of sexual partners (Figure 8-9). Choosing a partner who is not in a high-risk group provides almost 5000-fold protection compared with choosing a partner in the highest-risk category.

Condoms are estimated to provide about a 10-fold protection. A negative HIV antibody test provides about 2500-fold protection against false negatives.

The implication of this analysis is clear: **Choose sex partners carefully and use condoms.**

Other Studies on Heterosexual HIV Transmission

Nancy Padian and colleagues (1991) reported that women are 17.5 times more likely to become HIV-infected from an infected male than men are to contract the disease from an infected female.

In a follow-up study, Padian and colleagues (1997) reported that it took an average of 1000 sexual acts with an HIV-positive male for an HIV-negative female to become HIV positive, and 9000 sexual acts for an HIV-negative male to become HIV positive through sex with an HIV-positive female.

Viral Load and Heterosexual Transmission

Recent data from two separate HIV investigations shed light on the issue of gender transmission. Thomas Quinn and colleagues (2000) reported that the lower the level of HIV in the blood, the less likely HIV-infected persons will transmit the virus to their heterosexual sexual partner. This research team studied 400 heterosexual couples over 2.5 years. In each couple, only one person was HIV positive. **No one with less than 1500 copies of HIV/milliliter of**

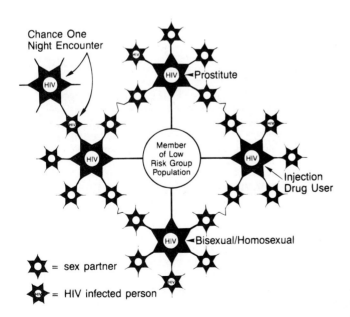

Risk Group Activities May Place You In The Middle Of HIV Being Distributed Among Sexual Partners.

Chance One Night Encounter

HIV

Prostitute

Member of Low Risk Group Population

Injection Drug User

Bisexual/Homosexual

★ = sex partner

★ = HIV infected person

FIGURE 8-9 Risk Transmission of HIV. Sexual transmission can occur among homosexuals or heterosexuals. Prostitutes can be either male or female. The diagram shows possible bridges for transmission of HIV from high-risk groups into low-risk groups. To be safe, *you* must not become part of the chain. Be sure your sexual partner is free of HIV.

blood infected his or her partner. In those cases where one partner became infected, 80% of the time the viral load of the other partner was over 10,000. Such data confirms the benefit of lowering HIV levels in the blood via antiretroviral therapy.

Injection Drug Users and HIV Transmission

HIV entered injection users during the mid-70's and spread rapidly through 1983 largely unrecognized and unidentified. HIV transmission via IDU is the second most frequent risk behavior among adults/adolescents, for becoming HIV-infected in the developed world (Table 8-7). Illicit drug injection occurs in at least 121 countries and HIV infection has been reported in IDUs in over 100 of these countries. Beginning year 2003, of 850,000 cases of AIDS reported to CDC, 306,000 (36%) were directly or indirectly associated with injecting-drug use. Injecting-drug-user-associated AIDS cases include persons who are IDUs $n=266,000$, their heterosexual sex partners $n=34,000$, and children $n=6000$ whose mothers were IDUs or sex partners of IDUs. About half the

females and about one-third of the heterosexual males who were diagnosed with AIDS had a sex partner who was an IDU *(HIV/AIDS Surveillance Report,* 1998 updated). It is estimated that half the 50,000 new HIV infections in the United States, or 68 people per day through the year 2003 will be associated with IDUs. The epidemic among injection drug users in New York City is an example of a very large, high-seroprevalence HIV epidemic. More than 100,000 injection drug users have been infected with HIV, and more than 50,000 cases of AIDS are reported among injection drug users, their sexual partners, and their children in New York City (DesJarlais et al., 2000).

UNITED STATES: HETEROSEXUAL IDU

Over ninety percent of injection drug users in the United States are heterosexuals. Thirty percent are women, of whom 90% are in their child-bearing years. From 1988 beginning year 2003, female IDUs made up about 40% of all AIDS cases in women. Of the 41% of women infected

---

Table 8-7 Population[a] Risk of HIV Transmission Based on Type of Activity[b]

Activity	Risk
Vaginal sexual intercourse	1 infection per 1,000 acts with HIV-positive partner (0.1%)
Receptive anal intercourse	5 to 10 infections per 1,000 acts with HIV-positive partner (0.5%–3%)
Intravenous drug injection with infected needle	10 to 20 infections per 1,000 needle uses (1%–2%)
Accidental stick in medical setting with infected needle	3 infections per 1,000 sticks (0.3%)
Transfusion of screened blood[c]	1 infection per 450,000 to 650,000 donations (0.0002%–0.00015%)

[a]Rough estimates of the relative risks in the United States and Western Europe of the more risky activities that can transmit HIV. **THESE CALCULATIONS CANNOT BE USED AS A GUIDE TO INDIVIDUAL BEHAVIOR.** Risk to any one person depends on many factors that cannot be reduced to a single number. Recent research, for example, suggests that the infectiousness of HIV can vary greatly over the life of an infected person; infectiousness is likely to be high both at the very outset of the infection, before symptoms have appeared, and several years later. Also, women may be several times more likely than men to be infected during vaginal intercourse, a distinction that the overall risk figure obscures. (Adapted from Bennett et al., 1996)

[b]Risks vary because of differences in genital, anal, and oral mucous membranes. Sex is risk free, with or without a condom **if the partner is known to be uninfected.** Nonpenetrative sex such as mutual masturbation is nearly risk free. Sex involving penetration with fingers is low risk. Sex involving unshared sex toys is risk free. Receiving oral sex is less risky than other penetrative behaviors. Penile-receptive sexual behavior is more risky than its penile-insertive counterpart. Anal or vaginal sex without a condom is far more risky than performing oral sex without a condom. (Source: Voelker, 1996)

[c]With the implementation of nucleic acid testing (NAT) in late 2002, the risk in transfusion of screened blood should drop to 1 in about 1 million donations.

by **heterosexual** contact 38% were infected by having sex with a male IDU! During this same period over 7,700 new cases of AIDS in children occurred—37% were from IDU mothers and 18% were from mothers whose sex partners were IDUs (*MMWR*, 1992; *HIV/AIDS Surveillance Report*, 2001, updated). Women IDUs and sexual partners of male IDUs represent the largest part (61%) of the estimated 100,000 HIV-infected women of childbearing age. Thus, there is a direct correlation between HIV perinatal transmission and pediatric AIDS cases and injection drug use.

Over 80% of reported adult **heterosexual** AIDS cases in America are associated with people who have a history of injection drug use or have sex with IDUs. Twenty-five percent of *all* AIDS cases in the United States occur in IDUs; 21% of these cases occur where IDU is the only risk factor (*HIV/AIDS Surveillance Report*, 2001 updated). In New Jersey, about 45% of IDUs are now HIV-infected. Because 70% to 80% of IDUs have sex with non-drug users, IDUs are a major source of heterosexual and perinatal HIV infection in the United States and Europe. HIV is also spreading rapidly among IDUs in developing countries such as Brazil, Argentina, and Thailand (Des Jarlais et al., 1989 updated).

Injection Drug Use and HIV Infections in Other Countries

Worldwide there may be as many as 2 to 3 million past and current injecting drug users (IDUs) living with HIV/AIDS. Accordingly, in many countries, IDUs represent a significant proportion of those individuals who are in need of antiretroviral drugs. The dual epidemic of injecting drug use and HIV particularly affect resource poor countries where there is limited access to HIV prevention measures such as needle and syringe exchange programs.

It appears that IDU is the major mode of HIV transmission in Kazakhstan, Malaysia, Vietnam, China, North America, Eastern Europe, The Newly Independent States, and the Middle East. Additionally, it is becoming more of an issue in West Africa and Latin America. The greatest problem has been seen in the Newly Independent States, in Eastern Europe, and in China.

Eastern Europe and the Former Soviet Union

The countries of Eastern Europe, countries of the former Soviet Union, and Russia are currently ex-periencing the most rapid spread of HIV anywhere in the world. Previously characterized by very low prevalence rates, the region now faces an extremely steep increase in the number of new infections, up from 420,000 ending 1999 to over 1.5 million beginning 2003. Russian health officials estimate there may be as many as 5 million people taking drugs. They say up to 60% of them are between ages 18 and 30 with precollege teenagers accounting for another 20%. Vadim Pokrovsky, head of the official AIDS prevention center, told a news conference broadcast on Internet site www.presscentr.ru. that, "We are currently going through the peak of an epidemic among drug users. Currently about 90% of HIV infections are associated with IDU. In two or three years there will be another upsurge from sexual transmission of the disease."

The hotbed of the disease had moved from the tiny Baltic enclave of Kaliningrad to Moscow and its suburbs. In some parts of Moscow, up to 5% of the young people are already HIV positive. If counted as a percentage of the population, Russia will reach U.S. levels. About 80% of the infected are aged 15 to 25. They will be lost in 10 years, just after they have finished their education. It means one gets infected at 20, graduates at 30, starts working, and dies. Murray Feshbach, a specialist in Russian demographic trends, estimates that 5 to 10 million people will die of AIDS in Russia after year 2015.

At the 2002 14th International AIDS Conference, Pokrovsky said, "The spread of HIV in Russia is the fastest in the world, there is an average 2000 to 5000 new cases each week." He also said that "his government allocated less than $5 million in 2002 to fight AIDS, when $65 million is needed immediately, plus a further sum of up to $15 million per year." In contrast, he said, "While the United States in 2002 is spending $500 million on AIDS-related research, Russia had put aside just $190,000 for that purpose."

The Ukraine's AIDS epidemic, the worst of all the former Soviet Union nations is causing alarm among Ukrainian physicians and other neighboring countries. In a nation of 50 million people, about 250,000 (5%) are HIV positive, and the level of infection continues to rise.

China

The lifting of a ban on AIDS-related reporting in 2000 in the state-run media appears to have fed a public panic through alarmist reports that China is on the verge of an epidemic. The government recently projected that the number of people infected with HIV could rise to 20 million by 2015 from an estimated 1 million now if preventive measures are not enforced. The current estimate provided by the Chinese health officials is believed, by the WHO and UNAIDS, to be several times that high. By 2001 HIV infections were found in every province with prevalence rates of 77% among injection drug users, ages 20 to 29, and 11% among prostitutes.

Caribbean HIV/AIDS: Big Problems Among Small Islands

In the Caribbean, an estimated 60,000 adults and children became infected in 2000, 2001 and again in 2002 bringing the total number of infected to over a half million. The Caribbean has the highest rate of HIV infection in the world after sub-Saharan Africa and AIDS is already the single greatest cause of death among young men and women in this region. The rate of HIV infection in the Caribbean is about four times that of North America, Latin America, and South and Southeast Asia. The rate is 35 times that found in East Asia and the Pacific and almost 10 times the rate in Western Europe (Figure 8.10). According to UNAIDS, if left unchecked HIV/AIDS will, by year 2020, cause 75% of deaths in the Caribbean. Such a scenario mimics what is happening in some parts of Africa. In some countries of Africa as much as 35% to 40% of the population is infected. Once

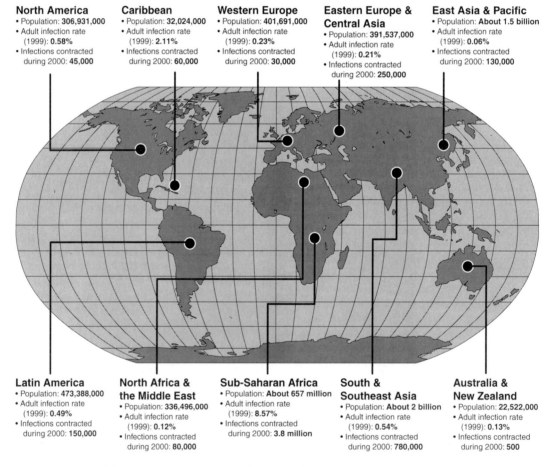

North America
- Population: **306,931,000**
- Adult infection rate (1999): **0.58%**
- Infections contracted during 2000: **45,000**

Caribbean
- Population: **32,024,000**
- Adult infection rate (1999): **2.11%**
- Infections contracted during 2000: **60,000**

Western Europe
- Population: **401,691,000**
- Adult infection rate (1999): **0.23%**
- Infections contracted during 2000: **30,000**

Eastern Europe & Central Asia
- Population: **391,537,000**
- Adult infection rate (1999): **0.21%**
- Infections contracted during 2000: **250,000**

East Asia & Pacific
- Population: **About 1.5 billion**
- Adult infection rate (1999): **0.06%**
- Infections contracted during 2000: **130,000**

Latin America
- Population: **473,388,000**
- Adult infection rate (1999): **0.49%**
- Infections contracted during 2000: **150,000**

North Africa & the Middle East
- Population: **336,496,000**
- Adult infection rate (1999): **0.12%**
- Infections contracted during 2000: **80,000**

Sub-Saharan Africa
- Population: **About 657 million**
- Adult infection rate (1999): **8.57%**
- Infections contracted during 2000: **3.8 million**

South & Southeast Asia
- Population: **About 2 billion**
- Adult infection rate (1999): **0.54%**
- Infections contracted during 2000: **780,000**

Australia & New Zealand
- Population: **22,522,000**
- Adult infection rate (1999): **0.13%**
- Infections contracted during 2000: **500**

FIGURE 8-10 Global Impact Of HIV/AIDS. About 42 million adults and children worldwide were living with HIV/AIDS by the end of 2002, according to UNAIDS estimates. *(UNAIDS; World Health Organization; U.S. Centers for Disease Control and Prevention)*

an epidemic reaches its tipping point—that threshold from which it grows exponentially—it is almost impossible to stop. For example, bodies are routinely stacked up in morgues in Nigeria, where only a few years ago those dying from the virus were largely invisible. The disease has spread over the African continent through mobility. Long-haul truck drivers having sex with prostitutes along their routes have brought it home to wives and girlfriends. Likewise, throughout the Caribbean, tourists, truck drivers, shipmates, and soldiers have been important male agents of the spread of HIV as is the use of injection drugs. In Puerto Rico, for example, over half of 30,000 AIDS cases were/are associated with IDU. Between 35% and 50% of injection drug users are HIV-infected. According to the CDC, Puerto Rico has the fourth highest HIV infection rate of American states and territories, behind Washington D.C., New York City, and the U.S. Virgin Islands. Puerto Rico plays a special role as a global border town in the transmission of AIDS because it is a central transportation and commerce hub for the Caribbean. It is a favorite location for both trafficking drugs and smuggling people, especially from the Dominican Republic.

The Sex Trade, Women and Children: Two Examples, The Caribbean and South East Asia

Overall, in the Caribbean, the majority of HIV infection is sexually transmitted (Figure 8-11). According to a 2000 UNAIDS report, the spread of HIV is partly driven by older men who have numerous sex partners, seek out young women for sex, and infect them. They in turn pass the virus on. If Caribbean women in general refuse unsafe sex and insist on the use of a condom— they often risk spousal abuse because it creates a suspicion of infidelity. Ten years ago there were seven times more infected men than women in the Caribbean. By 2003 that ratio changed to 2 to 1.

South East Asia, The Golden Triangle

There are no reliable statistics on the number of children working in the sex industry worldwide, but the lowest figure cited is 1 million. The United Nations Children's Fund estimates that one-third of sex workers in Southeast Asia are 12 to 17 years of age. The smuggling of vast quantities of heroin

FIGURE 8-11 A sex worker solicits a tourist in Boca Chica, a well-known beach for prostitution about 20 minutes from Santo Domingo. About 100,000 women in the Dominican Republic are engaged in sex work. Most sex workers will tell you they will not have sex without a condom, but sometimes clients think that insistence on using a condom is a bargaining tactic based on economics. Since its first appearance in the Caribbean, AIDS has been a mobile epidemic closely linked to the region's underground sex trade and has altered the economy in many regions of the Caribbean and Latin America. *(Photo by Hilda M. Perez/South Florida* Sun-Sentinel*)*

and amphetamines from Burma and China through Thailand has given the region its infamous tag, "The Golden Triangle," but it's the explosion in the recruitment of girls into the lucrative Thai sex industry that has put this border town on the map. Every year, hundreds of young girls from Mae Sai, town of 80,000 inhabitants on Thailand's northern most border with Burma, are spirited away to brothels in Bangkok where they feed the insatiable appetite of the $20 billion commercial sex industry. Mae Sai has two main trades, drugs and daughters. A non-governmental organization in Mae Sai that works with local girls who are at risk of being sold, estimates that of Pa Tek's 800 families, 7 in every 10 have sold at least one daughter into the trade.

When a Burmese migrant in Pa Tek sold his 13-year-old daughter into prostitution for $114, his wife had one regret—they didn't get a good price for her. She said, "I should have asked for $228. He robbed us." The mother earns about $100 a year selling bamboo bowls in the local market and lives in a thatched hut in Pa Tek village on the outskirts of Mae Sai. With prices varying from $114 to $913 per daughter, the latter figure is equal to almost six years' wages for most families. Parental bonds in impoverished households are easily broken. In fact, child prostitution is so established that many brothel agents live in the village, and are often friends or relatives of the family from whom they buy the children. The director of the Child Protection and Rights Center in Mae Sai said, "Agents will come to the village with orders to fill so people in Bangkok, Thai men, and foreigners, mostly Europeans, can order girls like they order pizza. If they want a girl with thin hips and big breasts, the agents will come here and find her. They always deliver."

The cross-border movement of women who are trafficked from country to country for prostitution is furthering the dispersion of the HIV. For instance, outbreaks in Europe of traditionally African strains of the disease have been traced to the import of sex workers from Africa. Due to the nature of the virus, there is the potential for these new geography-jumping strains to recombine with the other versions of the virus found in other parts of the world. This could create wholly new subtypes of the virus that would not only be untreatable by current successful antiviral treatment regimes, but could also be unaffected by vaccines now under development.

Additional Reasons for the Spread of HIV

Political disarray and poverty are also important factors. The poorest country in the region—Haiti—has the highest infection rate, and the country most isolated from tourism in the epidemic's early years—Cuba—has the lowest. In Haiti, the epidemic was concentrated mainly in urban areas until the early 1990s, but attacks on the urban poor by the country's military juntas drove refugees back into the countryside and the epidemic traveled with them.

Caribbean Connection to America: South Florida

Five nations in the Caribbean with the highest infection rates have HIV infections in all segments of their populations. During the last 22 years over 300,000 Haitians have died of AIDS. UNAIDS estimates that Haiti, with 12% of the urban and 5% of the rural population infected (about 350,000), has the highest rate of HIV infection in the Caribbean. Next is the Bahamas at over 4% and 3% for Barbados. Guyana and the Dominican Republic are each at 2% with about 8% of their pregnant women HIV-infected.

The Connection

The cruise ships and planes that leave and return to Fort Lauderdale and Miami weekly depend on the allure of tropical beaches, exotic ports, and lusty streets in the islands. Discount department stores depend on shirts sewn in Haitian textile plants, and increasingly, much of the low- and high-tech workforce essential to South Florida comes from Haiti, the Dominican Republic, and other Caribbean countries. In short, there is no way that South Florida can be spared the effects of the AIDS calamity in the Caribbean. The region is so tightly linked through culture, race, ethnicity, and economics that any public health crisis in the islands is felt here. In a highly mobile, global age, there are few boundaries that cannot be crossed. The disease, carried unknowingly among tourists and workers every day throughout the region, respects no borders.

Other Means of HIV Transmission

Other means of HIV infection have been documented. There has been a reported case of HIV transmission via **acupuncture**. It is believed that HIV-infected body fluids contaminated the acupuncture needles (Vittecoq et al., 1989). Also, **artificial insemination** can be a means of HIV transmission (Point of Information 8.2). Unlicensed and unregulated **tattoo** establishments may also present an unrecognized risk for HIV infection to patrons. If the operator does not use new needles or needles that have been autoclaved (steam sterilized), the possibility exists that infection with HIV or a number of other blood-borne

BOX 8.5

HIV TRANSMISSION: PREPARATION AND USE OF INJECTION DRUGS

Group use of drug paraphernalia and the type of substance used are factors in transmission of HIV from person to person.

Drugs in powdered form are usually placed in a bottle cap, or **"cooker,"** an item often found on streets or in garbage cans. Water is added and heated to dissolve the powder into a solution.

The solution is withdrawn by needle through a "cotton," or a filter through which the drug solution is drawn into the syringe. Cotton swabs, lint from clothing, cigarette filters, and a variety of other materials are used.

The needle then punctures a vein wherever there is one that can be used. Blood is drawn up into the syringe to mix with the drug solution and the blood-solution mixture is injected into the vein. If the vein is missed, the drug injected subcutaneously (under the skin) hurts and may cause an abscess. Small quantities of a drug may be injected repeatedly—each time blood is drawn up into the syringe. Then, following drug injection(s), the syringe is refilled several times with blood from the vein to wash out any heroin, cocaine, or other drug left in the syringe after the injection(s). If even a tiny, invisible amount of HIV-infected blood is left on the needle or in the syringe, the virus can be transmitted to the next user.

The **"works,"** as the syringe and needle are referred to, are shared and the amount of sharing depends on the number of users present. Everyone after the first user in the "shooting gallery" line receives potentially HIV-infected lymphocytes from all those with HIV infection who used the equipment before them.

It should be noted that in the injection drug culture, the sharing of needles is a sign of comradery, a sign of mutual trust. An unwillingness to share needles may cause others in the group to become suspicious of possible police connections.

Drug paraphernalia are commonly rented in **shooting galleries** by users who lack the equipment. A set of works is usually rented out until the needle is too dull to penetrate the skin. By then the needle has been sharpened often on whatever was available to give it a penetrating edge. Thus, not only is HIV transmitted among those in a shooting gallery but other bacteria and viruses that contaminate their surroundings are also shared.

The world of injection drug use is designed to transmit infectious agents. However, **it is not the drug that is responsible for HIV transmission, rather it is the infected blood shared by each of the users of an HIV contaminated works.** The practice of sharing works appears to be equally common among homosexual and heterosexual drug users. Thus it provides a common link between the homosexual and heterosexual population, placing both at risk for HIV infection.

Cocaine vs. Heroin—The use of injected cocaine is rising as is exposure to HIV in cocaine IDUs. One major difference between cocaine and heroin abuse is that IV cocaine abusers are binge users or repeat injectors, while the heroin abuser falls asleep after one injection. Studies in New York and San Francisco show that IV cocaine abusers are more likely to test HIV positive.

FIGURE 8-12 An Injection Drug User. Note that the arm is tied to force veins to fill with blood, making them easier to reach. A candle is used to heat the drug into a solution. This is referred to as "cooking" the drug. *(Photograph courtesy of the author)*

pathogens may take place. In addition, single-service or individual containers of dye or ink should be used for each client.

Human Bites— Brazilian investigators reported at the 2002 9th Annual Retrovirus Conference that a woman was infected with HIV when her HIV-positive son, who was suffering from an AIDS-related brain seizure, accidentally bit her on the hand. This case is one of only a relatively few worldwide to show that HIV can be transmitted through human bites. The infection from son to mother was confirmed through sophisticated DNA tests showing the virus in both patients to be virtually identical. In the United States, according to police reports, a Florida woman with a history of arrests for prostitution and who has tested HIV positive, bit a 93-year-old man on his arm, head, and leg while robbing him. The bites required stitches. The man initially tested HIV negative but a test several months later was HIV positive. A complete investigation into his personal life ruled out previous HIV infection.

The CDC also confirmed that a 91-year-old male became HIV-infected when, **being robbed**, he was bitten deeply, inflicting extensive tissue damage to the hand by a prostitute with bleeding gums. The man tested HIV negative shortly after the bite but tested positive eight weeks later. There have been eight other reports, according to police files, in which HIV appears to have been transmitted by a bite. Severe trauma with extensive tissue tearing and damage and presence of blood were reported in each of these instances. Biting is not a common way of transmitting HIV. In fact, there are numerous reports of bites that did not result in HIV infection (see Box 8.6).

Sexual Assault— **UNITED STATES** The subject of sexual assault, in all its forms, of children by adults or adult on adult is beyond the scope of this text. However, each time there is a date rape or any other type of rape there is the chance that the rapist may be HIV positive. One in five adult American women has been the victim of a completed rape at some time in her life (Koss et al., 1991). A **conservative estimate** of the **risk of transmission** of HIV **from sexual assault** (that involved anal or vaginal penetration and exposure to ejaculate from an HIV-infected assailant) is greater **than two infections per 1000 contacts,** given a variety of factors, such as clinical stage of the assailant's HIV infection, strength of the strain of HIV, and repeated exposure. The per contact risk is higher if there was violence producing trauma and blood exposure or the presence of inflammatory or ulcerative sexually transmitted diseases (Gostin, 1994; Zierler et al., 2001).

Beginning 2003, there were at least 200 reported cases of purposeful HIV infection of males by HIV-infected females or vice versa. This too should be looked on as a form of **sexual assault—** one partner is being sexually deceived by the other. In some of these cases the jury found the HIV-positive persons who kept this knowledge from their sexual partner guilty of attempted murder.

FEAR Many rape victims who know their attacker has HIV are left living in fear and are taking all necessary precautions to protect family and friends from possibly contracting the virus. In other cases the raped woman has no idea whether her assailant is HIV infected and will continue to worry even though her first or second test is negative! In some cases, people who have been raped cannot be told their attacker's HIV status because laws prevent states from releasing HIV test results; however, some states—including Arizona and Hawaii—have changed their laws in recent years to give victims access to records.

Sexual Assault— **AFRICA** In at least 10 countries in Africa, 20% to 25% of the adults/adolescents are HIV positive. These countries have been reported to have an unusually large number of rape cases. In South Africa, it is estimated that one in three women are raped during their lifetime. In Johannesburg, South Africa, about 40% of men between the ages of 20 and 29 are HIV positive. *Time Magazine,* in 1999, estimated that there are 50,000 women raped each year in South Africa. Peter Hawthorne, who wrote the *Time* article, reported that only 1 in 35 rapes is reported; suggesting that there are over 1.6 million rapes annually. Are such numbers credible? If so it will be most difficult to show the transmission of HIV in South Africa. The high rate of HIV infection in these countries means there is a significant possibility that the assailant is HIV positive. Because of culture norms, the rapes are unlikely to be reported. In addition, these women do not have access to counseling or necessary antiretroviral therapy. They suffer and die in silence from AIDS due to sexual assault.

BOX 8.6

ASSAULT WITH HIV

Reflecting a growing frustration and fear about AIDS, legislators around the country are passing an increasing number of laws intended to protect the public. This latest wave of legislation shifts the focus from earlier laws that protected the civil liberties of HIV-infected people to laws that seek to identify, notify, and in some cases punish people who intentionally place others at risk of contracting the virus. At least 38 states now make it a crime to knowingly transmit or expose others to HIV, the virus that causes AIDS, with a third of those states enacting laws within the last two years. In 1998, 16 state legislatures introduced such bills.

According to Richard Lacayo (1997), Darnell McGee, age 28, **through 1995 and 1996,** had sex with at least 61 women ranging in age from **12 to 29.** According to a Missouri public health report in February 1998, McGee had sex with at least 101 females, including four whose ages were 13 or 14. It is reported that McGee infected 18 women but Missouri officials believe he infected 30 women. Some are pregnant. At least one has given birth to an infected infant. State public health officials, who are trying to track down and notify his sex partners, expect the tally to climb as more women come forward to be tested.

McGee knew what he was doing. According to the *St. Louis Post-Dispatch,* which broke the story, state records show that he tested positive in 1992 and was told the results.

On January 15, 1997, he was shot and killed, assailant unknown!

Darnell "Bossman" McGee is just one of a number of men who recklessly and in some cases, even willfully transmitted HIV to their sex partners. Nineteen years ago it was Gatean Dugas, or patient zero, a gay male who, over three years knowingly infected an untold number (probably 50) of gays across the United States. Thirteen years ago it was Fabian Bridges, a gay prostitute in Texas who was followed from city to city in the last months of his life by cameras from PBS's Frontline, as he continued to have unsafe sex.

In January 1997 James Wallace Jones, a convicted sex offender with HIV, faced charges in Michigan for failing to notify four sex partners (including a 15-year-old girl) of his infected status. There is no evidence that he infected anyone, but he faces **nondisclosure charges.**

FIGURE 8-13 Nushawn Williams. Chautauqua County officials issued posters like this one in October 1997, for hanging on restroom walls in Jamestown, New York. The poster was to alert the public to his sexual activities throughout the county that may have exposed many to HIV infection. *(Photograph courtesy of AP/Wide World Photos/Bill Sikes)*

In April 1997, an HIV-positive African American rap artist was sentenced to 14 years in prison after having infected at least five women in Finland. And there was Nushawn Williams (Figure 8-13), age 21, who in mid-1997 admitted to having **unprotected sex** with 50 to 75 women after he was told he was HIV positive. Most of them were teenagers ages 13 and up living in New York's Chautauqua County and in New York City. To date, 13 in Chautauqua are infected, the youngest was age 13; others were ages 15, 16, 18, and 21. Ten are positive in New York City but it is not known if Williams was the

BOX 8.6 *(continued)*

source of their infection. After the newspaper and TV carried this story, 625 people showed up at the county health department for HIV testing. Williams told authorities that **he did not believe health officials** when they told him he was HIV positive in September 1996. Early in 1998, **two** of the women who had unprotected sex with Williams gave birth to HIV-positive babies. There are now 16 HIV-positive people who are linked to Williams. In April 1999, Williams was sentenced to 4 to 12 years in prison. Only two women agreed to testify against him.

In January 1998, a drifter in Michigan who just got out of prison, kept his infection secret while having sex with 10 mostly teenage women. Two of the women directly asked him about HIV and he denied his infection. The drifter received a maximum penalty of 15 to 22 years in prison for **failing to notify a sex partner he had HIV** and for having sex with a minor. To date, **none** of the women has tested HIV positive.

In the same month, a 23-year-old HIV-infected woman in Louisiana failed to disclose her infection to a man even though he asked her prior to sexual intercourse! If convicted she can receive up to 10 years in jail.

Also, in January, in Orlando, Florida, a judge ordered a man who failed to disclose his HIV infection, **a misdemeanor in Florida** that could have resulted in a four-year prison term, to have any women who he is going to have sex with to sign a form. It reads, "I____, being fully informed of the fact that Jerrime Day is positive with HIV, do consent to have sex with him." Day also had to take an AIDS awareness class. However, now his two-year probation is over he does **not** have to get written permission.

In March 1998, an HIV-positive army soldier received a dishonorable discharge, loss of pay, reduction in rank, and prison for having unsafe sex (no condom) with eight women. Four of these women became pregnant; two of them are HIV positive! Also, in **Melbourne,** Australia, in a first of a kind, a man was sentenced to a **nonparole** five-year prison term for endangering the lives of three men. He knew he was HIV positive, did **not** tell his sexual partners, and did **not** use a condom. Two of the three men are now HIV positive.

In May 1998, a 47-year-old HIV-positive male received seven years in jail because he did **not** tell a 13-year-old prostitute that he was in-fected. She tested HIV positive about three months after their sexual encounter.

In July of 1998 residents of Lewisberg, Tennessee, were shocked when a woman, age 29, told the police chief that she became angry and wanted revenge when a former boyfriend infected her with HIV. Knowing she was HIV positive, she had sex with up to 50 men she met at bars. She said she told the men she was HIV positive but they did not care. She faces two counts of criminal exposure to HIV and could face more. At the moment, if convicted it means up to 12 years in jail.

In July 1998, the Supreme Court of Arkansas sentenced Pierre Weaver to 30 years in prison for knowingly transmitting HIV to a woman through unprotected sex.

In September 1998, a Mississippi man age 45 was accused of having sex in 1993 with a man who was unaware he had tested positive for HIV in 1991. He denied having sex with the man. The Mississippi Department of Health met with him in January 1992 and told him to inform any potential sexual partners that he was HIV positive. The department later learned that he failed to inform his ex-wife of his condition. He was sentenced to five years in prison for failure to disclose and failure to use a condom with spermicide when having sex—a direct violation of a Mississippi Health Department quarantine order. Also in that month, an Ohio man, age 38, faced attempted murder for attempting to infect his sexual partner **through rape** because she was introduced him to the woman that he claims gave him the virus. The prosecutor said, "He's talking to her throughout the rape and telling her she's going to die. He's telling her he's got the AIDS virus and he's going to give it to her."

In October 1998, in Lafayette, Louisiana, a jury convicted a 52-year-old doctor of attempted second-degree murder for injecting his former 34-year-old lover with blood from an AIDS patient, infecting her with HIV. She broke off a 10-year relationship with him. He was sentenced to 50 years of hard labor. Also in October, Swedish police reported they were looking for an HIV-positive California man suspected of having unprotected sex with women he picked up in Stockholm nightspots. The man, **who is aware of his infection,** has reportedly been in Sweden since 1992. Police are currently trying to contact 190 women listed in the man's address book.

BOX 8.6 *(continued)*

In January 1999, in St. Charles, Missouri, a 32-year-old father was sentenced to **life in prison** for injecting his son with HIV because he wanted to avoid paying child support. The father was convicted of injecting AIDS-tainted blood into the boy, who was then 11 months old, during a hospital visit in 1992. The child, now 9 was diagnosed with AIDS in 1996. If the boy dies, Stewart could be tried for murder. Prosecutors said the father, who worked as a hospital technician at the time, stole the HIV-infected blood from his workplace. Also in **January 1999,** a female Army private in Maryland pleaded guilty to aggravated assault charges for having unprotected intercourse, knowing that she was infected with HIV. She was sentenced to three years in military jail and will receive a bad conduct discharge from the service. The woman had been ordered by her commanding officer to use a condom and to inform her partners that she was HIV positive; however, she disobeyed and had **unprotected** intercourse with four men and protected intercourse with five other men. None of the nine men with whom she had sex has tested positive for HIV.

In March 1999, police charged a Gainsville, Florida, male with a felony for not telling his sex partners that he was HIV positive. The man signed a statement in 1996 recognizing his legal obligation to inform potential sex partners. He admitted to having sex with 13 men without disclosing his HIV status—he said he did not tell because he was afraid that no one would have sex with him.

In May 1999, a U.S. major in the armed forces was fired from the military after receiving a six-year prison sentence for failure to obey an order by a superior officer. The major, who is HIV positive was ordered to **inform** his sexual partners of his infection and to use methods, including condoms to prevent their infection. The major was convicted in 1994 of having unprotected sex with two women, willfully disobeying the "safer-sex" order. On completion of this sentence he returned to active duty and was fired by President Clinton (the case is *Clinton vs. Goldsmith*, 98–347).

In July 2000, a man in Skagit County, Seattle, Washington received a 13-year jail sentence for infecting two women with HIV. The 27-year-old male knew he was HIV positive and did not tell.

In November 2001, an HIV-positive California man was sentenced to 17-and-a-half years in prison for planning to meet a boy for unprotected sex, marking the **first time** that a federal defendant has received this length of prison sentence for knowing he or she was HIV positive while planning to engage in unprotected sex with a minor. The man tried to arrange a sexual encounter with a person he believed was a 12-year-old boy whom he met online. In online chat rooms, he "indicated that he intended to leave his condoms at . . . home" when he flew to New York to have sex with the boy. However, the boy was a fictional creation of investigators, and he was arrested. He was sentenced on federal child sex charges and could have faced as little as five years for the indictment. But the district judge said that the man "poses a significant risk to children" because he "knew he was infected with HIV but nonetheless intended to engage in unprotected sexual acts with a minor."

In February 2002, the San Francisco Superior Court Commissioner ordered a former San Francisco health commissioner to pay his ex-lover $5 million in damages for knowingly exposing him to HIV and lying about his HIV status. This civil suit judgment is one of the largest awards to date for this kind of damage. The suit also alleged that the commissioner, who was appointed by Mayor Willie Brown to the health commission in 1997, in part to represent people with HIV, was suffering from symptoms of AIDS but told his lover that he had cancer.

In April 2002, an HIV-positive rapist in Florida received three consecutive life sentences, one for each of his victims, who so far have tested negative for HIV. Also, an HIV-positive rapist's life sentence in Louisiana will begin after he finishes a 78-year sentence for raping a teen-age girl in Tennessee.

In May 2002, a child molester with HIV in Kansas City, Missouri, was sentenced to three consecutive life terms, plus 52 years. He pleaded guilty in December to 13 counts, including statutory rape, sodomy, child molestation, and exposing others to HIV. His victims were ages 9, 11, and 14. Authorities said at the sentencing that he found out he had HIV in August 1997, but continued to attack children regardless. Also, in May 2002, an inmate was sentenced to 8 years in prison for an assault that prompted an Anne Arundel County, Maryland corrections officer to undergo treatment to prevent a possible HIV infection. The sentence is thought to be the longest ever imposed for an assault on an officer

BOX 8.6 *(continued)*

at a county jail. The inmate threw a bloody gauze pad that hit a guard in the face.

In September 2002, a 19 year old basketball player at Si Tanka-Huron University, was the first person charged under South Dakota's two-year-old law making it a felony to deliberately expose someone to HIV. The circuit judge sentenced him to five years in state prison, but suspended the sentence ordering him to spend 120 days in the regional correction center and complete 200 hours of community service, addressing high school and college students. "If you quit school, I will look hard at sending you to the penitentiary," the judge said.

Between 1987 and 2003 at least 15 HIV-infected men and three HIV-infected women were incarcerated in nine states because they **bit another person.** One of the 14 bitten people became HIV positive. The charges in these cases varied from assault with a dangerous weapon, assault with a deadly weapon, attempted murder, aggravated assault with intent to murder, felony, reckless endangerment, and assault and reckless endangerment. Prison terms varied from 18 months for reckless endangerment to 27 years for attempted murder. In eight cases within six states, one HIV-infected woman and seven HIV-infected men went to jail for periods of one to five years for **spitting on other people.** In a seventh case of spitting, in Texas, at trial, a court-recognized AIDS expert testified that HIV could be transmitted through the air! The man got a life sentence and an appeals court **upheld** the sentence. This man died in prison. None of the people that were spit upon contracted HIV.

Sex and HIV: If you have the first without disclosing the second, you can go to prison! In some states sex crimes and sex work can be elevated to attempted murder if the perpetrator (criminal) is HIV-infected. Disclosing one's HIV status to a sexual partner may exempt one from prosecution. But not telling—even if you do pro-

tect and don't infect—is still a crime in most states in America.

These cases of having unprotected sex after being told they were HIV positive and not informing their sexual partners raise several important issues.

Class Discussion: What is your response to these issues?

1. **Should the reckless or intentional transmission of HIV be a crime? If yes, how severe the penalty?**

2. **Do the cases bolster arguments for more aggressive partner notification and contact tracing? Why?**

3. **Do HIV confidentiality protections help or hinder efforts to alter the course of the epidemic? Why?**

4. **Would more ready access to condoms have helped avert these tragedies? How?**

5. **Who is responsible when an HIV-infected person knowingly continues to have unprotected sexual relations with others? Should the infected person be warned another time, assuming that the educational message was not heard? If so, how many times should warnings go forth? Are public health officials responsible for protecting susceptible spouses or long-term lovers of those who are infected and knowingly refuse to use condoms? Should the police become involved if protective advice is not followed, or should confidentially remain in effect while educational messages go out that untold persons in the community are infected and all should use condoms? Such issues are currently being debated in the United States, and likely in many nations.**

6. **Do such incidences support calls for more sex education, or less? Or perhaps different approaches to sexuality education? What approach might work? Why?**

Transplants— On any given day, about 20,000 Americans are waiting for a transplant. There is a small but present risk of receiving HIV along with the transplant tissue. A CDC report revealed that a bone transplant recipient became HIV-infected from an HIV-infected donor. HIV transmission has also occurred in the transplantation of kidneys, liver, heart, pancreas, and skin (*MMWR*, 1988a). In May of 1991, the CDC reported on 56 transplant patients who received organs

and tissues from an HIV-infected donor in 1985. A transplantation service company supplied tissues to 30 hospitals in 16 states. All tissues came from a single young male who was shot to death during a robbery. **He twice tested HIV negative before his heart, kidneys, liver, pancreas, cornea, and other tissues were removed for transplant.** By mid-1991, three recipients of these tissues had died of AIDS and six others were HIV positive. As of mid-1991, 32 other recipients had been located, 11 of whom tested HIV negative. It is unknown whether the others have ever been tested.

In May 1994, the CDC published guidelines for preventing HIV transmission through transplantation of human tissue (*MMWR*, 1994b).

Since then, at least 88 liver and kidney transplant cases have involved the use of human organs that were HIV positive. Of the 88 transplant cases, 66 of the patients were HIV negative prior to transplant and received organs that contained HIV. All became HIV positive. The average time for progression to AIDS was 32 months. The 22 people who were HIV positive prior to receiving an HIV-positive organ progressed to AIDS, on average, within 17 months (Horn, 2001).

AIDS Patients and Organ Transplants

According to published reports, Larry Kramer, age 66, who cofounded the Gay Men's Health Crisis in 1981 and the AIDS Coalition to Unleash Power (ACT UP), suffered from endstage liver disease. Kramer said his situation was similar to that of a growing number of patients who live long enough with HIV to suffer from a second infection. After being rejected by other health centers, Kramer received a new liver at the Thomas E. Starlz Transplantation Institute in Pittsburgh on December 21, 2001. The University of Pittsburgh Medical Center transplant facility has performed 10 transplants on patients with HIV/AIDS since 1997. Art Kaplan, director of the Center of Bioethics said that the medical community has yet to debate the ethics of transplanting organs into people with HIV/AIDS. This is largely because centers like

Starlz are just beginning to create possibilities. Beginning 2003, about 40 HIV-positive people have received liver transplants.

Class Discussion: Debate the ethics of giving an HIV-positive person an organ transplant in light of the fact that thousands of young and old noninfected people die each year while waiting for a transplant.

Nosocomial

Nosocomial (nos-o-ko-mi-al) refers to hospital-acquired infections. A chain of nosocomial HIV transmission has occurred in southern Russia and among children in Romanian orphanages. In Romania between 1988 and 1990, over 250 children were infected with HIV after exposure to nonsterile needles. By June 1994, 43 of these children had died of AIDS (Bobkov, 1994). Instances of nosocomial HIV transmission have also been reported from industrialized countries such as the United States, where transmission occurred from patient to patient. While nosocomial transmission accounts for a very small fraction of HIV transmission, nosocomial HIV transmission in any country at this time is unacceptable, and underscores deficiencies in present medical practices (Heymann et al., 1994).

Influence of Sexually Transmitted Diseases on HIV Transmission and Vice Versa

Sexual intercourse occurs more than 100 million times daily around the world. Results: 910,000 conceptions and over 600,000 cases of sexually transmitted disease. In the United States about 15 million new cases of sexually transmitted diseases occur each year. By age 21, about one in five people has received treatment for an STD. At current rates at least **one American in four will contract an STD at some point in his or her life.** More than 50 organisms and syndromes are transmitted or occur as a result of sexual activity (Hooker, 1996). Regardless of these facts, data from the CDC in 2001 revealed that one in four physicians do not screen their patients for STDs. In addition, a GayHealth.com online survey conducted in May 2001 found four in ten gay and lesbian patients have physicians that don't ask about their sexual practices. The survey included 184 women and 724 men. Over 40% of the men surveyed said they have not been vaccinated against either hepatitis A or B, potentially fatal viral liver infections spread through sexual activity. Men who have sex with men are at higher risk than the general population for these diseases. Annually, worldwide, there are about 180 million new cases of STDs. The majority of infections occur in those ages 20–24 followed by those ages 15–19.

Association of STDs of HIV Infection

STD researchers have long recognized that the behaviors which place individuals at risk for other STDs also increase their risk of becoming infected with HIV.

STDs are associated in several ways with HIV. Because STDs and HIV are spread by similar types of sexual activity, people who engage in behaviors that transmit HIV are also more likely to contract STDs, and vice versa. Epidemiological evidence shows that populations and geographical regions in the United States with the highest STD rates also tend to have the highest rates of HIV. According to the CDC, "The geographic distribution of heterosexual HIV transmission closely parallels that of other STDs." In the past decade, high HIV incidence rates have shifted toward women infected through heterosexual activity, young adults, African Americans, and people living in the southeastern United States, all populations with disproportionately high rates of STDs.

Infection by sexually transmitted diseases usually occurs through the **mucosal surfaces** of the male and female genital tracts and rectum. The mucosal route also accounts for a large percentage of heterosexual and homosexual transmission of HIV. It is known that STDs increase the number of T4 cells (HIV target cells) in cervical secretions, thereby increasing the chance of HIV infection in women.

Most AIDS researchers agree that treating STDs, which cures genital sores and reduces inflammation, can raise the body's barriers against HIV infection. According to a study by Grosskurth and coworkers (1995), researchers working in rural Tanzania saw the number of new HIV infections plummet by 42% after they improved STD health care.

Because HIV can be sexually transmitted, the association between HIV and other sexually transmitted diseases can be in part attributed to the shared risk of exposure and shared modes of transmission.

For the purpose of understanding which STDs best promote HIV transmission, the sexually transmitted diseases can be divided into **genital ulcer** and **genital nonulcerative diseases.**

Genital Ulcer Disease (GUD)— Signs of genital ulcer disease appear as open sores on the penis, vagina, other genital areas, and at times elsewhere on the body. The most widespread genital ulcer STDs are syphilis, genital herpes, and chancroid. About 60 million people in America over age 12, have chronic genital herpes. There are about 1 million new herpes infections and 70,000 syphilis cases annually.

In early 1997, researchers from the University of Washington showed for the first time that herpes sores contain high levels of HIV, which they believe makes the virus especially easy to spread during sexual contact. Additional research by Timothy Schacker and colleagues (1998) also showed that HIV can be consistently found in herpes genital lesions of HIV-infected people. Such data suggests that genital herpes infection likely increases the sexual transmission of HIV.

HIV Shedding

The prevalence of HIV shedding in the genital tracts of both men and women increases substantially in the presence not only of accelerating immunosuppression but also of other STDs. Furthermore, the quantification of **viral load** in genital secretions indicates that the concentration of HIV shed may increase as much as 7-fold among men who are coinfected with HIV and STDs such as gonorrhea. Most importantly, both the prevalence and the concentration of HIV shedding can

PROBABLY THE NUMBER ONE RISK COFACTOR FOR HIV IS A SEXUALLY TRANSMITTED DISEASE (STD)

TIME FOR A WAR ON STDS

According to a report, "The Hidden Epidemic," released in November 1996 by the Institute of Medicine, it is time for a national campaign against sexually transmitted diseases (STDs).

More than 12 million people in the United States, one-fourth of them teenagers, are infected with STDs such as chlamydia, genital herpes, and pelvic inflammatory disease **each year.** The situation is "a national embarrassment," said David Celentano of the Johns Hopkins University School of Hygiene and Public Health. Some of the facts:

♦ The United States has the highest rate of STDs of any developed country.

♦ Direct costs of STDs, not including AIDS, are over $10 billion annually.

♦ Women and infants bear a disproportionate burden of complications from STDs, which include infertility and various types of cancers.

♦ In 2001, it was established that over 50 million Americans, over the age of 12, have genital herpes but only about 20% (1 in 5 infected people) are aware that they are infected!

♦ Close to 22% of people over the age of 15 harbor the herpes virus.

♦ Teens are at an ever-increasing risk: By the 12th grade, 70% have had sexual intercourse—double the rate reported in the early 1970s—and close to 40% of them have had four or more partners.

Celentano said AIDS is playing a big part in bringing STDs out of the closet: **"Probably the number one risk [factor] for HIV is an STD."**

To order the $45 report, call 1-800-624-6242. (Source: *Science,* 274:1473, November 1996).

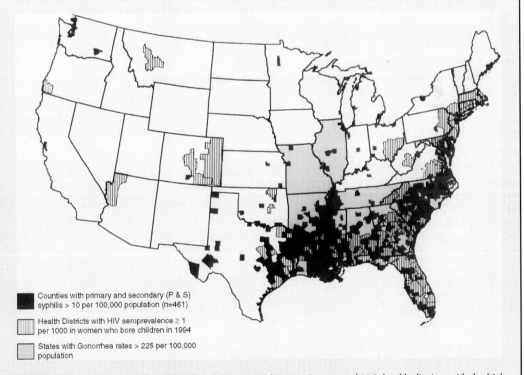

Counties with primary and secondary (P & S) syphilis > 10 per 100,000 population (n=461)

Health Districts with HIV seroprevalence ≥ 1 per 1000 in women who bore children in 1994

States with Gonorrhea rates > 225 per 100,000 population

FIGURE 8-14 HIV, Syphilis, and Gonorrhea Rates: United States. Continental U.S. health districts with the highest HIV seroprevalence among childbearing women (1994), counties reporting the highest primary and secondary syphilis rates (1993), and states reporting the highest gonorrhea rates (1993). *(Source: St. Louis et al., 1997)* be reduced rapidly to baseline levels with appropriate STD treatment. Together with observations suggesting that HIV susceptibility is increased in women by nonulcerative STDs through recruitment of endocervical CD4 lymphocytes, these data provide a biologically plausible mechanism for the markedly increased risk of HIV transmission associated with other STDs, estimated to range between 3-fold and 50-fold depending on the STD involved (St. Louis et al., 1997).

William Cameron and colleagues (1990) reported on the bidirectional biological interactions between HIV and STDs, especially the genital ulcerative STDs. Bidirectional interaction between HIV and STDs occurs with respect to both transmission and virulence. HIV transmission is a consequence of both infectivity and susceptibility, both of which can be increased by genital ulcer disease.

HIV and Virulence

Virulence, the capacity of a pathogen to produce disease, is a consequence of both pathogen and host factors. Thus, HIV infection and associated immune deficiency disease may account for the increased prevalence of genital ulcer disease; and this in turn may further amplify HIV transmission in a network of social contacts.

Worldwide the estimated number of new STD infections for 2002 includes 12 million new cases of syphilis, 62 million new cases of gonorrhea, 89 million new cases of chlamydia, and 170 million new cases of trichomoniasis. Although trichomoniasis does not increase the risk of acquiring HIV as much as does syphilis, the huge number of trichomoniasis infections makes it at least equally important in the context of HIV transmission. **All four of these STDs are curable**—and examples from high- and low-income countries show that it is feasible and affordable to achieve a significant reduction of the STD burden everywhere.

Nonulcerative Disease— The nonulcerative STDs include gonorrhea, about 650,000 new cases annually, chlamydia, about 3 million new cases annually, and trichomonal infections, about 5 million new cases annually (also called discharge diseases), and genital warts. There are over 30 million people in the United States infected with genital wart virus, with about 5 million new cases annually. In most populations, these are much more common than genital ulcer diseases. None causes the noticeable open sores that occur in the ulcer diseases but they do cause microscopic breaks in affected tissue, and are associated with HIV transmission (Laga et al., 1993). The most common symptoms are warty growths on the genitals, discharge from the penis or vagina, and painful urination.

Collectively, worldwide there are over 250 million cases a year of just seven major STDs: syphilis, herpes, and chancroid, which cause ulcers; and trichomoniasis, chlamydia, warts, and gonorrhea, which do not (Figure 8-15).

HIV infection and other sexually transmitted diseases (STDs) share the same risk factors. The major difference between HIV/AIDS and the other STDs is the degree of cell and tissue destruction and the mortality of HIV/AIDS.

HIV is transmitted most often during sexual contact with an infected partner. There is abundant evidence that if a sexual partner has an active STD, especially one that causes an ulcer, he or she is at greater risk of becoming HIV-infected (Laga, 1991).

The types of blood cells, lymphocytes, or macrophages most likely to become infected if exposed to HIV tend to collect in the genital tract of people with STDs. This makes an STD-infected person both more likely to transmit HIV and more vulnerable to it (Laga, 1991).

Pediatric Transmission

Children can acquire HIV from their mothers in several ways. A pregnant HIV-infected woman can transmit the virus to her fetus in utero (**during gestation**) as the virus crosses over from the mother into the fetal bloodstream (Jovaisas et al., 1985; St. Louis et al., 1993). At least 50% of newborn infections occur **during delivery by ingesting blood or other infected maternal fluids** (Scott et al., 1985; Boyer et al., 1994; Kuhn, et al., 1994). If breast-fed, the newborn may also become **infected from breast milk** (Zigler et al., 1985; deMartino et al., 1992; Van DePerre et al., 1993). In case reports, three women who contracted HIV by blood transfusions **immediately after birth** subsequently infected their newborns via breast-feeding (Curran et al., 1988). Other studies suggest that the risk of HIV transmission through breast-feeding is increased if the mother becomes HIV-infected during lactation (Hu et al., 1992).

The relative efficiency of these three routes of infection is unknown. However, the data on mothers' milk add to the urgency of learning more about mucosal transmission. The most like-

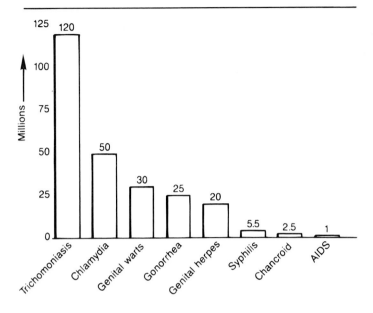

Annual Number of 8 STDs Worldwide

FIGURE 8-15 Global Incidence of Eight Sexually Transmitted Diseases. For 2002, ages 15 to 49.

ly explanation for HIV transmission through breast-feeding is that the virus penetrates the mucosal lining of the mouth or gastrointestinal tract of infants. If this occurs in newborns, then what of older children, adolescents, and adults? Does the mucosal lining change with development and become HIV-resistant?

HIV-Infected Babies— One major problem in perinatal transmission is how to determine which babies are truly HIV-infected as opposed to just carrying the mother's HIV antibodies (which would produce a false-positive test). HIV transmission can occur during pregnancy (in utero), as well as at the time of delivery (**intrapartum**) and through breast milk. HIV transmission is more likely if virus can be cultured from the mother's blood, or if she has later stage HIV disease, or if her T4 counts are low; and is more likely to occur in the firstborn than in the secondborn of twins. **A baby automatically acquires the mother's antibodies and may carry them for two or more years. Usually by 18 months of age, most of the mother's antibodies will be gone.** The babies may then begin to show signs of clinical AIDS-related illness. But, even at 18 months, a child cannot be unequivocally diagnosed. The most commonly used HIV antibody test is not sufficiently accurate until the

child is at least two years old. A new antibody test in development shows promise in recognizing newborn infection by examining the **type of HIV antibodies** the infected mother is producing.

Although the rate of perinatal and breast milk HIV transmission is unknown, evidence from 1986 into year 2003 indicates that over 90% of pediatric AIDS cases acquired the virus in utero from an HIV-infected mother after the first trimester or during the birthing process. In 1990, researchers concluded that a fetus can become infected as early as the eighth week of gestation (Lewis et al., 1990). HIV has been isolated from a 20-week-old fetus after elective abortion by an HIV-positive female and from a 28-week-old newborn delivered by Caesarean section from a female who was diagnosed with AIDS (Selwyn, 1986).

Reports on the probability of a fetus becoming HIV-infected when the untreated mother carries the virus vary widely. The most often quoted estimate in the United States is from 30% to 50%.

There is little documented information on maternal factors that influence vertical transmission. As with other congenital infections, only one of a pair of twins may be HIV-infected (Newell et al., 1990; Ometto, 1995). A mother's clinical status during pregnancy and the duration of her infection (stage of disease) may be important, but evidence remains circumstantial (see Chapter 11 for update information). Studies to determine mother-to-fetus transmission relative to stage of disease are in progress.

According to the CDC classification, children under 13 years of age are considered pediatric AIDS cases. They make up about 1.3% of all AIDS cases in the United States. Through 2001, about 5% of reported pediatric male AIDS cases occurred due to blood transfusions, 3% received HIV-contaminated blood factor VIII used in treating hemophiliacs, and in 2%, the cause was undetermined.

The largest numbers of pediatric AIDS cases through 2002 were in New York, Florida, California, and New Jersey, in that order. The highest incidence of all pediatric cases occurs in minority populations. By early 2003, there were over 9300 pediatric AIDS cases in the United States. Blacks and Hispanics make up 12% and 6% of the United States population, respectively, yet make up 55% and 20%, respectively, of all pediatric AIDS cases. Thus 75% of pediatric AIDS cases occur within two minority populations.

HIV-Infected Childbearing-Age Women

Over 100,000 women of childbearing age are estimated to be infected with HIV in the United States. The majority of these women may not know they are infected; they are identified as infected only after their children are diagnosed as having an HIV infection or AIDS. It is not uncommon for HIV-infected women to go through several pregnancies before expressing HIV disease. Also, there are women who become pregnant knowing they are HIV positive. They want to have a baby regardless (see Chapter 11).

Mother-to-fetus infection or **vertical infection** could be avoided by avoiding pregnancy, but this is possible only in cases where the female is aware of her infection and takes measures to prevent pregnancy (birth control or tubal ligation). In many cases, pregnancy occurred before the mother knew she was carrying the virus. In other cases, the mother has become infected after she has become pregnant.

Antiviral Therapy Decreases Perinatal HIV Transmission

Probably the most important step forward in the use of antiviral agents has been the discovery that antiretroviral drugs can decrease the rate of peri-natal transmission of HIV. In a landmark study by Edward Connor and colleagues (1994) and the interim results of the AIDS Clinical Trials Group (ACTG) Protocol 076 (*MMWR*, 1994d; Goldschmidt et al., 1995; *MMWR*, 1995), the intensive use of zidovudine beginning in the second trimester of pregnancy, including intravenous zidovudine during delivery, and six weeks of oral therapy in the neonate, **decreased the rate of transmission from 25% to 8%.** (See Chapter 11 for updated information.)

CAESAREAN SECTION

The time-honored surgical maxim, **"A chance to cut is a chance to cure,"** takes on new meaning in the debate now raging about **caesarean section** as a means of reducing perinatal HIV transmission. From 1998 through 2002, clinicians have shown that the use of **caesarean section** to deliver a newborn from an HIV-infected mother is a significant help in reducing HIV infection of the newborn (Riley et al., 1999; Read et al., 1999).

Possible Antiretroviral Drugs To Prevent Maternal HIV Transmission

Current concepts on the prevention of vertical transmission now focus on the appropriate antiretroviral therapy of infected pregnant women. Despite the data from ACTG 076, zidovudine monotherapy alone can no longer be considered adequate for pregnant women because some newborns are still HIV positive. Some HIV/AIDS experts recommend the use of combination therapy that includes a protease inhibitor. In March 1999, five important studies were published regarding the use of combination antiretrovirals to reduce mother-to-infant transmission. The conclusion to be drawn from the studies is that antiretroviral prophylaxis of mother and her infant is **very effective.** With many women on HAART therapy during pregnancy, there were less than 200 HIV-infected infants born in the United States in 2002. However, in developing countries, despite recent progress, there is still a great need for shorter, inexpensive, effective regimens. But the debate continues on when to begin therapy—first, second, or third trimester?

(For an excellent review of mother-to-child transmission of HIV, see the article by Peckham and College, 1995.)

WHEN THE WONDERFUL NEWS "YOU'RE PREGNANT" BECOMES A TRAGEDY

First Case: Amy Sloan

In 1982, AIDS was a homosexual disease. Amy Sloan became HIV-infected from a blood transfusion. She received the blood because of ulcerative colitis (ulcers in the colon). In 1985, three years after her transfusion, and two days *after* she learned she was pregnant, Amy was told she had AIDS. She was 24 years old.

By 1985, the general public was being educated to the devastating effects of AIDS; the virus had been named and it was known that blood transfusions were a major route of HIV transmission. Amy Sloan had become pregnant not knowing that she was carrying the AIDS virus. Amy delivered an uninfected son in 1986. She died in January 1987.

Second Case: Elizabeth and Paul Michael Glaser

On March 13, 1990, Elizabeth and Paul Michael Glaser, former star of *Starsky and Hutch,* testified before the House Budget Committee's Human Resource Task Force arguing for increased funding for pediatric AIDS research, education, and treatment.

Elizabeth Glaser was infected with HIV in 1981, after she was given a blood transfusion while giving birth to daughter Ariel. At that time, AIDS did not have a name, and the reporting of cases was just beginning. No one knew about the risk of contracting the virus through transfusions. Elizabeth breastfed Ariel, unknowingly passing the virus to her daughter. Three years later, Paul and Elizabeth had a son, Jake, who later also tested positive for HIV. Paul is the only one in the family not infected.

Elizabeth testified that she watched her daughter suffer from symptoms that did not seem to affect adults. She watched her daughter's central nervous system atrophy as she became, at age 6, unable to walk, talk, or even sit up.

Ariel Glaser died in 1988, just after her seventh birthday. Elizabeth Glaser died on December 4, 1994.

In November 1996, Jake's viral load began to increase—a sign of a failing immune system. Although the FDA had not yet approved protease inhibitors (PI) for use in children, Paul Glaser took the risk; Jake received PI. Within two weeks his viral load dropped below measurement! Jake, now age 18 (2002), is on therapy, and is asymptomatic.

HIV Infection in Older People

In 1998, of 48,159 persons aged 13 and over reported with AIDS, 6083 (11%) were aged 50 and over, this proportion has remained stable since 1991. Of those aged over 50, 48% were aged 50–54, 26% were aged 55–59, 14% were aged 60–64, and 12% were aged 65 and over. Males accounted for 84% of the cases, and blacks accounted for the highest proportion (43%) by race/ethnicity. Men who have sex with men (MSM) accounted for the highest proportion of cases by exposure category (36%). For all AIDS cases beginning 2003, 94,000 are age 50 and above, of which about 10,000 are age 65 and over.

Many seniors feel that HIV infection is just a problem for young people, homosexuals, and injection drug addicts. Now, the use of Viagra compounds the problem. With the use of Viagra, seniors are much more sexually active and few practice safe sex. The manufacturer of Viagra is trying to incorporate safe sex messages in their advertisements.

HIV Transmission in the Workplace

The idea of contracting HIV from a fellow employee generates fear in many employees regardless of their jobs. Most people in the United States have been exposed to information on the routes of HIV transmission and on how to practice safer sex, but remote possibilities remain worrisome to many in the job force. In 1999, about one in six companies offered employee HIV/AIDS education. Many people still believe that HIV can be transmitted casually via handshakes, coffee cups, and food handling.

It is the anxiety of **uncertainty** that engenders suspicion about the possibility of HIV infection in the workplace—an anxiety that HIV/AIDS scientists could be wrong about the routes of HIV transmission. As Judith Wilson Ross states, **"We have spent our lives in a culture in which infectious disease does not represent a significant threat. And thus we had consigned living in fear of life-threatening contagious diseases to the pages of history books."** But today, HIV/AIDS

IS BREAST FEEDING POLICY FOR WOMEN IN UNDEVELOPED NATIONS CHANGING?

Problem—The reality is that most of the undeveloped nations cannot afford the cost of alternative feeding. Therefore, in countries like Zimbabwe, breast-feeding will continue. In many of these countries there is no access to testing facilities and people could not afford them even if they existed; nor are drugs like zidovudine available to help reduce the incidence of maternal HIV transmission to the newborn. Also, many of these countries **do not have safe water** to use in making baby formula—even if free formula is available. As a result many of the children will die of diarrhoeal and respiratory diseases.

13th International Conference on AIDS, Durban, South Africa, July 2000

There was much debate at this conference on the pros and cons of breast feeding. The majority of controversy was sparked by the report by Anna Coutsoudis and colleagues (1999) who suggested that infants who were exclusively breast fed had similar HIV transmission rates to those infants who received only formula feeds. New data on HIV transmission rates for infants at 15 months emphasized the superiority of exclusive breast feeding over mixed (breast and formula) feeding (25% versus 36%, respectively). They concluded that there was no significant difference in HIV transmission rates between infants exclusively breast fed and infants only given formula (25% versus 20%). Coutsoudis recommended that exclusive breast feeding should be the feeding option of choice for HIV-infected women in developing and developed countries. In follow-up investigations, Contsoudis and colleagues (2001) reported that infants exclusively breast fed for three months or more had no excess risk of HIV infection over six months than those never breast fed. These findings can influence public health policies on feeding choices available to HIV-infected mothers in developing countries.

---

forces us to reexamine our faith in the certainty of science. We want to believe, we want to accept— but the fear of death prevents complete surrender to education.

PUBLIC CONFIDENCE: ACCEPTANCE OF CURRENT DOGMA ON ROUTES OF HIV TRANSMISSION

One living legacy is the distrust arising from the Tuskegee syphilis experiments. Over 30 years after the study was publicized, its impact on black Americans' view on the medical establishment remains strong, experts say. For example, a recent survey of black Americans tested for HIV in a street outreach program found that 80% reported conspiratorial believes about the virus. The Tuskegee study has never died and that distrust is continuously there and needs to be dealt with.

Since the start of the epidemic in 1981, lawmakers have championed proposals ranging from quarantines to criminal prosecution for infecting others with HIV. Beginning 2003, at least 38 states have some type of law stating that it is unlawful for anyone who knows they are infected with HIV to transmit or expose others to the virus without their knowledge and consent. Public support for such measures is high. Results of one 1997 poll show that 79% of Americans believe that an individual who knowingly infects another person with HIV should face criminal charges, and half of those surveyed said that people who knowingly transmit the virus should be charged with murder. Critics of criminal penalties say such laws will not help to control the HIV/AIDS epidemic and will likely do more harm than good.

A national telephone survey suggests that the public has **become more suspicious** of people who contract the virus, and **less knowledgeable about the disease.** Gregory Herek and John Capitano completed a survey in 1997 of 1712 people randomly picked from across America. They presented their findings at the 12th International AIDS Conference, Summer 1998. They reported that 55% of Americans believed in 1997 that they could become infected by sharing a drinking glass with an infected person, compared with 48% in 1991. Forty-one percent believed that

---
BOX 8.8

HIV AND SENIOR CITIZENS

Looking at the majority of safer sex workshops and street outreach programs, one would get the impression that only the young are at risk of contracting HIV. It's true that most people with AIDS are under 49. But, according to the CDC, now about 14% of Americans who test positive for the virus are over the age of 50. It's not just with regard to prevention that over-50s are left behind. Older people with HIV are often misdiagnosed and typically learn they have the virus only later in the disease process. Medical treatment is more difficult, both because of the later diagnosis and factors related to age. Few practitioners are expert both in HIV and the health problems associated with aging. When it comes to social support services aimed at their particular needs, older HIV-infected people are all but invisible. Attitudes about HIV/AIDS and aging reflect misconceptions about how people behave in the second half-century of their lives.

1. Old people are no longer interested in sex;
2. If they are interested, no one's interested in them;
3. If they do have sex, it's within a monogamous, heterosexual relationship;

4. They don't do drugs;
5. If they ever did, it's so long ago it doesn't matter.

It isn't hard to see how these misconceptions help erect barriers to effective HIV/AIDS prevention efforts, medical care, and social services for the late middle-aged and elderly. After all, if they're not doing anything risky, there's nothing to worry about, right? **WRONG,** older adults refuse to conform to the stereotypes.

Gender and Age

Older women are becoming HIV-infected at a higher rate than older men. No longer afraid of becoming pregnant, the postmenopausal woman who is uninformed of the danger of HIV transmission may become more sexually active, with more partners, and may give up a decades-old habit of using condoms. Even her biology increases her risk: After menopause, the vaginal walls thin and vaginal lubrication decreases. Thus, the vaginal membranes are more likely to tear during intercourse, providing easier access to HIV.

AIDS might be contracted from a public toilet, compared with 34% in 1991, and 54% believed that HIV might be transmitted through a cough or a sneeze compared to 47% in 1991. Twenty-seven percent said they would be less likely to wear a sweater that had been worn, only one time, by a person with AIDS—even if the sweater had been cleaned and sealed in a new package. Twenty-eight percent said they would be uncomfortable drinking out of a glass in a restaurant if a person with AIDS had used the same glass a few days earlier regardless that it had been washed and sterilized! Finally, compared to 1991, more respondents agreed that people who get AIDS through sex or drug use have gotten what they deserve (29%, compared to 20% in 1991). When the issues of blame and responsibility were posed in less negative terms, 55% of respondents agreed that most people with AIDS are responsible for having their illness, 51% agreed that it's their own fault if people get AIDS these days, and 26% agreed that most people with AIDS don't care if

they infect other people with HIV. (Also see Herek et al., 2002)

Public Confidence UPDATE 2000

The December 2000 issue of *Morbidity/Mortality Weekly Report* carried a public survey by Research Triangle Institute on beliefs about HIV. The survey was run using the **Internet.** The research team analyzed the responses from 5641 people. The findings:

> **18.7%** strongly agreed that "people who got AIDS through sex or drug use got what they deserve."
> **40.2%** said that HIV infection (transmission) could occur through sharing a glass.
> **41.1%** said one could get HIV by being coughed on or sneezed on by an HIV-infected person.

Compare these data with the 1997 data presented. After over 21 years into this pandemic, a significant number of people still believe one can contract HIV from casual contact!

Telephone HIV/AIDS Survey Conducted in Russia

Having reviewed what Americans feel and believe about HIV/AIDS transmission, a Russian telephone poll revealed an equal lack of effective education. Uri Amirkhanian and colleagues at the Medical College of Wisconsin presented the results of their study, which they believe to be the first population-based, random-digit telephone AIDS survey conducted in Russia. They found that significant proportions of respondents believed that HIV could be spread through mosquito bites (56%), kissing (48%), or cigarette sharing (29%).

Education Survey in The United Kingdom

Forty percent of boys in the United Kingdom have never heard of HIV or AIDS, according to the "Young People in 2000" survey conducted by the Schools Health Education Unit. The survey polled 42,000 people between the ages of 10 and 15 and found that in addition to not knowing about HIV/AIDS, more boys than girls said they would "not take care" to prevent contracting HIV. Lisa Power, head of policy for the Terrence Higgins Trust, said, "Teen-agers today were babies when the "Don't die of Ignorance" advertisements and leaflets were used in the mid-1980s, so HIV awareness among today's younger generation is low. We don't want young people to think that HIV is around every corner—but they should be aware of the genuine risks of HIV and other sexually transmitted diseases." The survey also found that 57% of older males did not know where to go to receive free condoms.

CLASS COMMENTS?

CONCLUSION Although no new routes of HIV transmission have surfaced over the last 22 years of this pandemic, **many people still do not believe that's all there is.** People still make the arguments that: (1) Scientists do not yet know enough about this disease to be certain there are no other routes of transmission; and (2) scientists know other routes exist but are either too frightened to tell the truth, or are under political pressure not to do so for fear of creating a public panic. Many thousands of people in the United States firmly believe that in a few years they will look back and say "I told you so": You can get HIV from HIV-infected people if they breathe on you or if you touch their sweat and so on.

CLASS QUESTION: How do you get everyone to believe what medical and research scientists say? Should we get everyone to believe scientific dogma?

FREQUENTLY ASKED QUESTIONS (FAQS) ABOUT HIV AND AIDS

Since the beginning of the AIDS epidemic in the United States, the CDC has taken the lead in responding to requests from the U.S. public for information. This section of the NPIN Web site provides responses from CDC to frequently asked questions (FAQs) about HIV and AIDS.

How is HIV passed from one person to another? HIV transmission can occur when blood, semen (including pre-seminal fluid, or "pre-cum"), vaginal fluid, or breast milk from an infected person enters the body of an uninfected person.

HIV can enter the body through a vein (**e.g., injection drug use**), the anus or rectum, the vagina, the penis, the mouth, other mucous membranes (e.g., eyes or inside of the nose), or cuts and sores. Intact, healthy skin is an excellent barrier against HIV and other viruses and bacteria.

These are the most common ways that HIV is transmitted from one person to another:

♦ by having sexual intercourse (**anal, vaginal, or oral sex**) with an HIV-infected person
♦ by sharing needles or injection equipment with an injection drug user who is infected with HIV
♦ from HIV-infected women to babies before or during birth, or through breastfeeding after birth

What is the probability of transmission from one HIV exposure? The risk for HIV transmission per episode of receptive penile-anal sexual exposure is estimated at 0.1%–3%; the risk per episode of receptive vaginal exposure is estimated at 0.1%–0.2%. No published estimates of the risk for transmission from receptive oral exposure exist, but instances of transmission have been reported. The risk for HIV transmission per episode of intravenous needle or syringe exposure is estimated at 0.67%.

Can HIV be transmitted from other animals to humans? No. HIV is a uniquely human disease. The chimpanzee is the only animal that has developed antibody to HIV. There are other retroviruses (HIV is but one in this family) that infect animals, such as monkeys, sheep, horses, goats, including feline leukemia virus and feline immunodeficiency virus found in cats. However, all of these animal retroviruses are specific to their hosts and have not been shown to be transmitted to humans. Similarly, HIV cannot be transmitted from a person with HIV to any of these animals.

Can I get infected with HIV from mosquitoes? No. From the onset of the HIV epidemic, there has been concern about transmission of the virus by biting and bloodsucking insects. However, studies conducted by researchers at CDC and elsewhere have shown no evidence of HIV transmission through insects—even in areas where there are many cases of AIDS and large populations of insects such as mosquitoes. Lack of such outbreaks, despite intense efforts to detect them, supports the conclusion that HIV is not transmitted by insects.

The results of experiments and observations of insect biting behavior indicate that when an insect bites a person, it does not inject its own or a previous victim's blood into the new victim. Rather, it injects saliva. Such diseases as yellow fever and malaria are transmitted through the saliva of specific species of mosquitoes. However, HIV lives for only a short time inside an insect and, unlike organisms that are transmitted via insect bites, HIV does not reproduce (and, therefore, cannot survive) in insects. Thus, even if the virus enters a mosquito or another sucking or biting insect, the insect does not become infected and cannot transmit HIV to the next human it feeds on or bites.

There is also no reason to fear that a biting or bloodsucking insect, such as a mosquito, could transmit HIV from one person to another through HIV-infected blood left on its mouth parts. Two factors combine to make infection by this route extremely unlikely—first, infected people do not have constant, high levels of HIV in their bloodstreams and, second, insect mouth parts do not retain large amounts of blood on their surfaces. Further, scientists who study insects have determined that biting insects normally do not travel from one person to the next immediately after ingesting blood.

Can HIV be transmitted by wound to wound contact? Transmission via wound-to-wound contact, although theoretically possible is highly unlikely given the improbability of such a scenario and the small concentration of virus that is likely to be present. However, persons with open wounds who are likely to have occupational contact with blood and other potentially infectious body fluids, e.g. health-care workers, are urged to comply with universal precautions for the prevention of transmission of HIV and other bloodborne pathogens.

Evidence also indicated that bloodborne and sexually transmitted pathogens such as HIV are not transmitted during the preparation or serving of food or beverages, and no instances of HIV transmission have been documented in this setting. If such transmission readily occurred, we would expect to see an increase in the proportion of AIDS cases outside of recognized high-risk groups; no evidence of this has been found for any of the U.S. AIDS cases reported to the CDC. However, the Public Health Service recommends that all food service workers take care to avoid injury to their hands when preparing food. Should such an injury occur, food contaminated with blood should be discarded.

Can I get HIV from casual contact (shaking hands, hugging, using a toilet, drinking from the same glass, or the sneezing and coughing of an infected person)? No. HIV is not transmitted by day-to-day contact in the workplace, schools, or social settings. HIV is not transmitted through shaking hands, hugging, or a casual kiss. You cannot become infected from a toilet seat, a drinking fountain, a doorknob, dishes, drinking glasses, food, or pets.

Can HIV be transmitted in swimming pool water? HIV cannot be spread by sharing washing facilities or swimming in the same pool with an HIV-infected person. The body secretions which would normally be washed off in a swimming pool (e.g., sweat or saliva) are not body fluids that transmit HIV. Blood, semen, and vaginal secretions would only enter a swimming pool under exception circumstances. Any virus that did get into a swimming pool would be greatly diluted, making it non-infectious. Most swimming pools also contain disinfective agents, such as chlorine, that inactivate HIV.

Can HIV be transmitted between women during sex? There have been several reports in the medical literature indicating possible female-to-female sexual transmission of HIV. AIDS surveillance data indicate that women with AIDS who are reported to have had sexual contact only with other women have also been reported to have injected drugs or to have received blood transfusions or blood components. Although these risk factors do not preclude the possibility that the mode of transmission of HIV for these women was female-to-female sexual contact, the absence of cases in lesbian women without other established risk factors is striking. We interpret this observation to mean that these women likely acquired their infection through injection drug use or receipt of blood transfusion or blood components.

Can I get HIV from preforming oral sex? Yes, it is possible for you to become infected with HIV through preforming oral sex. There have been a few cases of HIV transmission from performing oral sex on a person infected with HIV. While no one knows exactly what the degree of risk is, evidence suggests that the risk is less that that of unprotected anal or vaginal sex. Blood, semen, pre-seminal fluid, and vaginal fluid all may contain the virus. Cells in the mucous lining of the mouth may carry HIV into the lymph nodes or bloodstream. The risk increases:

- if you have cuts or sores around or in your mouth or throat;
- if your partner ejaculated in your mouth; or
- if your partner has another sexually transmitted disease (STD).

Can I get HIV from someone performing oral sex on me? Yes, it is possible for you to become infected with HIV through receiving oral sex. If your partner has HIV, blood from their mouth may enter the urethra (the opening at the tip of the penis), the vagina, the anus, or directly into the body through small cuts or open sores. While no one knows exactly what the degree of risk is, evidence suggests that the risk is less than that of unprotected anal or vaginal sex.

To obtain a complete listing of the Frequently Asked Questions concerning HIV & AIDS, go to: **http://www.cdcnpin.org/hiv/faq/start.htm**

NATIONAL AIDS RESOURCES

AIDS ACTION COUNCIL	1-202-547-3101
COALITION FOR LEADERSHIP ON AIDS	1-202-628-4160
GAY MEN'S HEALTH CRISIS	1-212-807-6655
MOTHERS OF AIDS PATIENTS	1-619-234-3432
NATIONAL AIDS INFORMATION CLEARINGHOUSE	1-301-762-5111
NATIONAL AIDS NETWORK	1-202-546-2424
NATIONAL ASSOCIATION OF PERSONS WITH AIDS	1-202-483-7979
PROJECT INFORM (ALTERNATIVE AIDS INFO)	1-800-822-7422
PUBLIC HEALTH SERVICE HOTLINE	1-800-342-2437
CENTERS FOR DISEASE CONTROL AND PREVENTION TECHNICAL INFORMATION	1-404-639-2070
AMERICAN RED CROSS, NATIONAL AIDS EDUCATION	1-202-639-3223
GUIDE TO SOCIAL SECURITY AND SSI DISABILITY BENEFITS FOR PEOPLE WITH HIV INFECTION	1-800-772-1213

(You can write or call for this Social Security brochure: Social Security Administration, Public Information Distribution Center, P.O. Box 17743, Baltimore, MD 21235.)

SUMMARY

The World Health Organization began keeping records of AIDS-like cases in 1980. Beginning 2003, there were an estimated 28 million AIDS cases in 194 reporting countries and territories. About 3% of these cases have occurred in the United States. Beginning 2003, of the 42 million living with HIV infection worldwide, about 2.3% or about 950,000 live in the United States. It has been reported that the first cases of AIDS entered the United States via homosexual men who had vacationed in Haiti in the late 1970s. However, there is evidence of AIDS cases in the United States as early as 1952. While testing West Africans for HIV infection, a second strain of HIV was discovered: HIV-2. Both are transmitted in the same manner and both cause AIDS. However, HIV-2 appears to be less pathogenic than HIV-1.

Nearly all Americans are aware that HIV can be transmitted through unprotected intercourse (99%), the sharing of intravenous (IV) needles (99%), and unprotected oral sex (91%). Fewer than half (42%), however, know that having another sexually transmitted disease (STD) increases a person's risk for HIV. In addition, even after years of public education, unwarranted fears of infection through casual contact persist. For example, one in five (22%) Americans incorrectly believes that sharing a drinking glass can transmit HIV, or are unsure about the risk of this activity. Sixteen percent believe that touching a toilet seat can transmit HIV or are unsure about the risk. Such views contribute to discrimination and stigma, which can interfere with public health efforts to encourage early testing and care.

There are two major variables involved in successful HIV transmission and infection. First is the individual's genetic resistance or susceptibility, and second is the route of transmission. Not all modes of HIV exposure are equally apt to cause infection, even in the most susceptible individual. There have been a number of studies and empirical observations that demonstrate that HIV **is not casually acquired**. HIV is difficult to acquire even by means of the recognized routes of transmission.

HIV is transmitted mainly via sexual activities involving the exchange of semen and vaginal fluids, through the exchange of blood and blood products, and from mother to child both prenatally and postnatally (breast milk). Besides a few cases of breast milk transmission, no other body fluids have as yet been implicated in HIV infection.

The current belief is that anal receptive homosexuals have a higher risk than heterosexuals of acquiring HIV because the membrane or mucosal lining of the rectum is more easily torn during anal intercourse. This allows a more direct route for larger numbers of HIVs to enter the vascular system.

Others at high risk for acquiring and transmitting HIV are injection drug users. They infect each other when they share drug paraphernalia. Changes in sexual and injection drug use behavior can virtually stop HIV transmission among these people.

REVIEW QUESTIONS

(Answers to the Review Questions are on page 489.)

1. True or False: Africa makes up the largest percentage of **reported** AIDS cases worldwide. Explain.

2. What evidence is there that HIV may have evolved in the United States and Africa at the same time?

3. Are HIV-1 and HIV-2 related? Explain.

4. True or False: HIV-1 and HIV-2 are transmitted differently and therefore are located in geographically distinct regions of the world. Explain.

5. True or False: HIV is **not** believed to be casually transmitted. Explain.

6. Name the routes of HIV transmission.

7. True or False: Deep kissing wherein saliva is exchanged is a direct route for **efficient** HIV transmission. Explain.

8. True or False: Insects that bite or suck have been claimed to be associated with HIV transmission. Explain.

9. True or False: Among heterosexuals, HIV transmission from male to female and from female to male are equally efficient. Explain.

10. True or False: If a person has unprotected intercourse with an HIV-infected partner he or she will become HIV-infected. Explain.

11. What is the percentage of risk that a developing fetus with an HIV-positive mother in America, will be born HIV positive, with and without zidovudine therapy? With zidovudine and "C" section?

12. Despite the warnings, groups that continue to engage in high-risk sexual activity include:
    A. high school students
    B. black women
    C. injection drug users
    D. prostitutes
    E. all of the above

13. True or False: Prior to 1985, use of blood component therapy put the hemophiliac at risk for contracting HIV.

14. True or False: Relapse to risky sexual behavior can be an important source of new HIV infection in the homosexual community.

15. True or False: The body fluids shown most likely to transmit HIV are blood, semen, vaginal secretions, and breast milk.

16. True or False: Participation in risky behaviors and not identification with particular groups puts an individual at risk of acquiring HIV infection.

17. True or False: Unprotected receptive anal intercourse is the sexual activity with the greatest risk of HIV transmission.

18. True or False: Women who are HIV-infected always transmit the virus to their fetus during pregnancy or delivery.

19. True or False: A person infected with HIV can transmit the virus from the first occurrence of antigenemia throughout the rest of his/her life.

20. True or False: Women constitute the fastest growing segment of the population with HIV infection.

21. True or False: The majority of HIV-infected women whose source of infection is known became infected through vaginal intercourse.

22. True or False: HIV infection in children is now a leading cause of death in children between the ages of 1 and 4.

23. True or False: Sexual contact is the major route of HIV transmission among black Americans.

24. True or False: Urine is one body fluid that remains an unproven route of HIV transmission.

25. Which of the following is **NOT** a recognized mode of HIV transmission?

    A. unprotected sex with an infected partner

    B. mosquito bite

    C. contact with infected blood or blood products

    D. perinatal transmission

26. HIV/AIDS word scramble

ABMETARUTS	_ _ _ _ _ _ _ _ _
ACIPMDEN	_ _ _ _ _ _ _
AERIBRR	_ _ _ _ _ _
AGSEASM	_ _ _ _ _ _
ANLA	_ _ _ _
ATOUNITM	_ _ _ _ _ _ _
BENSTCENIA	_ _ _ _ _ _ _ _ _
BLAUEXSI	_ _ _ _ _ _ _
BLMSKRITAE	_ _ _ _ _ _ _ _ _
BYUDILSFOD	_ _ _ _ _ _ _ _ _
CDRLSAIIMEP	_ _ _ _ _ _ _ _ _ _
DBOOL	_ _ _ _ _

DEIPCIME	_ _ _ _ _ _ _
EGEIVTAN	_ _ _ _ _ _ _
FOCTNEINI	_ _ _ _ _ _ _ _
HEHALIIMPO	_ _ _ _ _ _ _ _ _
HREUSALXEOET	_ _ _ _ _ _ _ _ _ _ _
IAVLNAG	_ _ _ _ _ _
IDSA	_ _ _ _
IVH	_ _ _
LSNCMIAOOO	_ _ _ _ _ _ _ _ _
MEENS	_ _ _ _ _
MNTSNAOISISR	_ _ _ _ _ _ _ _ _ _ _
MREPS	_ _ _ _ _
NCEIALBCUMMO	_ _ _ _ _ _ _ _ _ _ _
NITSARS	_ _ _ _ _ _ _
NOEUTESRIRC	_ _ _ _ _ _ _ _ _ _
OEULXMASOH	_ _ _ _ _ _ _ _ _
OMODNC	_ _ _ _ _ _
PESREH	_ _ _ _ _ _
PRLIATANE	_ _ _ _ _ _ _ _
RSNIAUVONET	_ _ _ _ _ _ _ _ _ _ _
SAXELU	_ _ _ _ _ _
SDT	_ _ _
SILAAV	_ _ _ _ _ _
SIPEN	_ _ _ _ _
SNRISEGY	_ _ _ _ _ _ _
TFYELSEIL	_ _ _ _ _ _ _
TLACER	_ _ _ _ _
UNOASNISFTR	_ _ _ _ _ _ _ _ _ _ _
VPIETISO	_ _ _ _ _ _ _ _
VSURI	_ _ _ _ _

Preventing the Transmission of HIV

The best time to plant a tree is 20 years ago. The second best time is now.

African Proverb

PREVENTION, NOT TREATMENT, IS THE LEAST EXPENSIVE AND MOST EFFECTIVE WAY TO STOP THE SPREAD OF AIDS

GLOBAL PREVENTION

Because we live in a global village, the public health of Africa, Asia, and elsewhere affects the public health of the United States. As there is one global economy, there is one global public health. **Prevention of infectious diseases in any country is prevention for all.** In each of the years from 1998 through 2002 an estimated 2.5 million to 3 million people died from AIDS. Worldwide ending year 2003, over 26 million people will have died of AIDS.

Over 80% of these deaths will be in Africa where AIDS is now causing one in five deaths. While waiting for an effective vaccine, how can the out of control spread of HIV be slowed? How can people everywhere be saved from HIV infection? In a word, **PREVENTION** is the only hope short of a vaccine.

Stop, listen and learn all you can about HIV/AIDS. Prevention and life—it's your choice!

Types of HIV/AIDS Prevention

Worldwide prevention efforts focus on **two** types of prevention: **primary** prevention—preventing HIV exposure among **uninfected** individuals, and **secondary** prevention—preventing HIV transmission by those who are **infected**.

255

After 22 years and many billions of dollars of prevention allocations, there remains an imbalance of primary and secondary prevention efforts. Yet, it was the public health strategy of secondary prevention that freed the world from smallpox and greatly reduced the incidence of syphilis and a number of other diseases worldwide.

Invest in Prevention

Spending money on prevention is a smart investment. For example, in America, adding $500 million to HIV prevention targeted to high-risk behavorial groups would yield total medical care savings of $1.25 billion. The potential for HIV prevention interventions to save lives and dollars emphasizes the need to spend money now rather that later, and to maintain consistent, if not increasing, funding for those at high-risk. At the 2002 14th International AIDS Conference, Michael Saag reported that in the United States, health care for each patient in the advanced stages of AIDS costs an average of $34,000 a year. Antiretroviral medicines make up the largest part of the cost. The cost of treating a well patient with HIV averages $14,000. Overall, medication costs were about $11,000–$24,000. Hospital costs were second, ranging from an average of $1,700 for early stage patients to $7,800 for those with advanced AIDS. Taking the average between $14,000 and $34,000 or $24,000 times 950,000 people living with HIV/AIDS in America comes to $22,800,000,000! Estimates are that about 400,000 people in 2002 are receiving some measure of care for their HIV infection. At 400,000 receiving HIV/AIDS health care, the cost would be estimated to be $9,600,000,000 a year which is in line with the federal dollars allocated for HIV/AIDS health care for 2002 or $10.3 billion (see Figure 13-6 for year 2002 federal dollars allocated to HIV/AIDS). America's prevention budget for 2002 was $1 billion. By preventing 3995 HIV infections, one theoretically saves the budget. In reality, the savings would be used to prevent others from being infected. The bottom line is prevention, regardless of the means of assessment.

Globally, it is estimated that $5 billion is required annually for HIV prevention efforts—less than 1% of the world's yearly military spending. To date however, the money for effective prevention programs globally is just not available.

What is an Effective HIV Prevention Program?

An HIV prevention program is one that is comprehensive and that addresses a community's prevention, care and treatment needs. Essential components of a comprehensive program include HIV testing and voluntary counseling, prevention of mother to child transmission, clinical care and antiretroviral treatment. Testing combined with voluntary counseling is an effective, pivotal strategy in HIV prevention and care for people with the virus, providing many benefits for people who test positive as well as for those who remain HIV negative. For example, a recently randomized controlled trial in Kenya, Tanzania and Trinidad showed that voluntary counseling and testing significantly reduced high-risk sexual behavior among individuals and couples.

The Challenge

Prevention is a hard sell. It is easier to get thousands of dollars to rescue a baby down a well than it is to get a few hundred dollars to cover old wells.

The fact that there is no cure for AIDS, and that the drugs are costly and cause severe side effects, makes it crucial to prevent people from contracting the virus. CDC researchers reviewed 83 studies from 1978 through 1998. They found that as soon as prevention education began in the early 1980s, the rate of new HIV infections plummeted and that it has remained relatively stable, at about 40,000 new infections a year (see Figure 10-7).

The means of preventing HIV infection exists. They must be used effectively to make an impact on this escalating pandemic. **HIV prevention does not have to be perfect to be effective!** The existing methods of HIV prevention are presented in this chapter.

UPDATE 2002 Robert Smith of HIV Edmonton, Canada, and Michael Yoder, chairman of the Canadian AIDS society reported at the 14th International AIDS Conference that North American prevention programs are failing. They believe it's back to the drawing board for the AIDS community that has discovered, to its horror, that no one seems to care about safer sex anymore. "None of the youth are listening. None of the youth are getting tested. It's a marketing nightmare. Canada spends $42 million a year on HIV/AIDS awareness and prevention programs. The United States spends about 25 times that. After 22 years of being bombarded with safer sex messages, you'd think everyone in North America would know how to protect themselves from HIV and other sexually transmitted diseases (STDs). As health professionals are becoming increasingly aware, getting the facts out is one thing—doing it in a way that changes people's behavior is another."

Among the depressing reports out of the 2002 International AIDS Conference in Spain is a study showing that most of the young, gay, HIV-positive men in major U.S. cities are unaware that they're infected. More than half the HIV-positive men who didn't know they had the virus considered themselves at low risk of HIV infection and nearly half of them reported they didn't use condoms.

They concluded that in North America, young people seem to be fed up with hearing about AIDS.

PREVENTION OF INFECTIOUS DISEASES: HIV/AIDS

While the hope of eradicating HIV is universal, the universe of AIDS comprises many worlds, and the goal can only be achieved if methods of prevention are designed and implemented in the context of each of these worlds. Infectious agents have persisted over the centuries through transmission from one infected person to another. To combat these infections, **prevention programs have attempted to interrupt the chain of transmission.** While some methods focus on stopping transmission from person-to-person contact by using vaccines or prophylactic (preventative) therapy, other methods focus on stopping the transmission that occurs through environmental contamination by sanitary improvements.

With regard to HIV infection, there is no available vaccine against the virus, but there is a **virtual vaccine** (meaning a **procedure** as effective as a preventative vaccine): **education.** Thus, the leading primary preventative is education: teaching people how to adjust their behavior to reduce or eliminate HIV exposure. Because the vast majority of HIV infections are transmitted through consensual acts between adolescents and adults, the individual has a choice as to whether to risk infection or not.

Despite widely supported educational efforts at both institutional and street levels, a large number of gay males, drug abusers, and heterosexuals continue to participate in *unsafe sexual* practices. Un-

safe sex is defined as having sex without using a condom. This allows the exchange of potentially infectious body fluids such as blood, semen, and vaginal secretions. Unsafe sex most often occurs with injection drug users, bartering sex for drugs, and

FIGURE 9-1 Photograph of Joseph O'Neill. In July 2002, President Bush appointed Joseph O'Neill, M.D., M.S., M.P.H., to serve as the Director of the White House office of National AIDS Policy. O'Neill, who is also a member of the White House Domestic Policy Council, leads an expanded AIDS office that is responsible for both domestic and international HIV/AIDS issues. The Office of National AIDS Policy also serves as the Executive Secretariat for the President's Cabinet Task Force on HIV/AIDS, which is co-chaired by Secretary of State Colin Powell and Secretary of Health and Human Services Tommy Thompson. Prior to his appointment, Dr. O'Neill served as Acting Director of the Office of HIV/AIDS Policy in the Department of Health and Human Services (HHS). In this role, he was responsible for coordination of policy and management of the entire HHS HIV/AIDS portfolio. O'Neill, who replaces Scott Evertz, holds a faculty appointment at the Johns Hopkins University School of Medicine and maintains a clinical practice in the Johns Hopkins Hospital HIV/AIDS program. *(Courtesy of the White House Office of National AIDS Policy, Washington D.C.)*

having sex with multiple partners. The sharp increase in the use of crack cocaine and its connection to trading sex for drugs has led to a dramatic rise in almost all sexually transmitted diseases. **The idea of *safer* sexual practices began in the early 1980s and now refers almost exclusively to the use of a latex or plastic condom with or without a spermicide.**

Among the severely drug addicted, concerns about personal safety and survival are secondary to drug procurement and use. Thus, their range of unsafe behaviors leads to random sex and sex without condoms. These behaviors are in part responsible for the increased incidence of HIV and other sexually transmitted diseases (Weinstein et al., 1990).

Comparing HIV/AIDS Prevention to Cancer

AIDS prevention is, in a sense, more essential than, say, cancer prevention. Preventing one HIV infection now will not simply prevent one death from AIDS, as preventing one incurable cancer would prevent one cancer death. Preventing an HIV infection now will help break the chain of transmission, averting the risk that the infected person will knowingly or unknowingly pass the virus on to others who in turn might infect a still wider circle of people.

PREVENTING THE TRANSMISSION OF HIV

HIV/AIDS: The News Is Mostly Bad

We are now into the twenty-second year of an epidemic that has touched—directly or indirectly— virtually every person on the planet. We know so much about the virus, yet despite our knowledge, our only option is to **prevent** the initial infection. Prevention is foremost because there is **no vaccine, no cure,** and, even using the best AIDS drug cocktails available, long-term survival remains questionable, even for those who can afford the drugs. **MOST HIV-INFECTED PEOPLE WORLDWIDE CANNOT AFFORD THESE DRUGS!** As we face this realization, alarming statistics continue to emerge about the spread of HIV infection.

In San Francisco, estimates suggest that at least 50% of homosexual African-American men are infected with HIV. Unsafe sexual practices that could lead to HIV transmission are common among adolescents and young adults, as evidenced by the epidemic of other sexually transmitted diseases in this population. Tens of millions of persons in developing countries will become HIV-infected and most likely die. Entire generations are threatened with extinction in these countries.

The Hard Questions

How can reputable HIV/AIDS scientists, anywhere, explain to the public that the world is being consumed by a disease that is preventable and have it make sense?

The political, social, cultural, economic, and biological factors that have led to the HIV pandemic seem overwhelming. How can a drug user be convinced to use clean needles to prevent an infection that may kill him in 10 years, when he faces an immediate struggle in a violent environment every day? How can condom use be promoted in countries with inadequate supplies of condoms or resources to provide even basic immunizations? Why should young women on the streets of New York, San Francisco, New Delhi, or Bangkok who depend on the sex industry for daily survival care about safer sex when it might lead to rejection by their customers and an end to their livelihood?

Class Discussion: Your answers to the hard questions are?

Gender Power

In many societies, there is a large power differential between men and women. Socially and culturally determined gender roles bestow control and authority on males. The subordinate status of women is reinforced by the fact that men are the main or only wage earners in the majority of families. This is compounded further by age differences: In most heterosexual relationships, the man is the older partner.

Wives in many cultures are expected to tolerate infidelity by their husbands, while remaining totally faithful themselves. **But AIDS has raised the price of such tolerance, as it puts women at great risk of infection by their husbands.** Many women feel powerless to ask their husbands to use condoms at home. Even when they can do this, their need to protect themselves may conflict with a social or personal imperative to have children.

BOX 9.1

HIV/STD PREVENTION EDUCATION—UNITED STATES

Eliminating all unsafe sex is not a reasonable goal. Preventing all future HIV and STD infections is impossible, but striving for anything less is unacceptable.

Since 1988, CDC has provided fiscal and technical assistance to state and local education agencies and national health and education organizations to assist schools in implementing effective HIV and STD prevention education for youth. These agencies and organizations develop, implement, and evaluate HIV/STD prevention policies and programs and train teachers to initiate effective prevention efforts and implement curricula in classrooms. As a result of these and other efforts, school-based HIV/STD education is widely implemented in the United States. From 1987 through 2002, the number of states requiring HIV/STD prevention education in schools increased from 13 states to 36 states plus the District of Columbia. This high level of policy support is consistent with public support; 95% of U.S. residents in a 1996 survey reported that information about AIDS and STDs should be provided in school.

The findings in this survey indicate that, despite wide implementation of HIV/STD prevention education in U.S. schools, improvements in HIV/STD prevention programs are still needed. In particular, efforts are needed to increase the percentage of teachers who teach HIV/STD prevention in a health education setting and who receive inservice training on HIV/STD prevention. A national health objective for the year 2000 was to increase to at least 95% the proportion of schools that provide age-appropriate HIV/STD curricula for students in fourth through twelfth grades, preferably as part of comprehensive school health education, based on scientific information that includes the way HIV and other STDs are prevented and transmitted. Based on the findings, an 11% increase is needed in the percentage of middle/ junior and senior high schools that implement HIV and STD prevention education programs.

AIDS REPORT CARD DELIVERS "F" FOR PREVENTION

In January of 2002 AIDS ACTION, or AIDS advocacy organization with 3200 national AIDS service groups presented the Bush administration their fourth annual report card (1998 through 2001) on the federal government response to the AIDS pandemic. The grades over the four years have *not changed*. Grades were given in four areas: Research, A–; care and treatment, B; global initiative, C; and F for HIV prevention. The failure in prevention is based primarily on the lack of effective education of young people who from 1999 through 2002 accounted for half of all new HIV infections, about 22,000 each year.

UPDATE 2001

In 1999 the Kaiser Family Foundation asked secondary school principals across America about their sex education programs and found 35% had abstinence-only. While 95% of public school principals reported that AIDS and other sexually transmitted diseases were discussed in sex education classes, less than 50% provided information on where to get birth control or how to use condoms. What kids learn—or don't learn— about sex seems to depend on where they live. More than half of Southern school districts use abstinence-only sex education programs compared with less than 20% in the Northeast.

UPDATE 2002

A 26-member Presidential Advisory Council on HIV and AIDS (PACHA) was formed in 1995 to advise the sitting president and federal agencies about the prevention, treatment and cure for AIDS. In March 2002, PACHA met for the first time since George W. Bush became president with members promising to go beyond politics and fight harder to prevent, treat and cure the HIV pandemic. President Bush appointed Louis Sullivan, former U.S. Secretary of Health and Human Services and Tom Coburn, former Oklahoma congressman as co-chairman for PACHA. Panel members agree that "either this pandemic gets us or we get it." To date there is a division among members of this committee over the use of condoms for the prevention of HIV transmission. Some of the panelists are pushing strongly for abstinence-only education, while others are strongly opposed to this position. The Bush administration announced its priority support for abstinence and education! Colin Powell, Secretary of State rebukes President Bush's Abstinence-Only Education Policy. In remarks aired in February 2002 on MTV rebroadcast around the globe, Secretary of State Colin Powell

BOX 9.1 *(continued)*

strongly advocated condom use to prevent the spread of AIDS, setting himself apart from President Bush's views on sex education and angering some of the president's closest supporters on the political right. Powell said, "It is important that the whole international community come together, speak candidly about it, forget about taboos, forget about conservative ideas with respect to what you should tell young people about. It's the lives of young people that are put at risk by unsafe sex. And, therefore, protect yourself." During the broadcast, Powell took questions from young people in a Washington studio and in six other satellite-linked studios around the world. Nineteen-year-old Daniela Satori in Milan asked,

through an interpreter, "As a young Catholic woman, I would like to know from the secretary of state what he thinks of the Catholic position on condoms, which are prohibited, and therefore this condemns anyone who might be exposed to the virus." "I certainly respect the view of the Holy Father and the Catholic Church. In my own judgment, condoms are a way to prevent infection. Therefore, I not only support their use, I encourage their use among people who are sexually active and need to protect themselves."

CLASS QUESTION: What is right and who is wrong? Your position on abstinence-only education is? Support your position with factual information—not just opinion.

Is There Hope?

Hopelessness threatens reason, but there is reason to believe that education may reduce the number of new HIV infections. In San Francisco, gay men organized grassroots efforts to educate themselves about HIV transmission, and the results are impressive: Less than 1% of the gay male population was infected with HIV after 1985, compared to 10% to 20% in the preceding years. People can change their behavior when educated about the risks of transmission (Clement, 1993).

Educators Given the Job of Prevention

HIV has just as much potential to kill someone infected in 2003 as it did in 1983, but are today's sixth graders and higher hearing about HIV/AIDS half as much as did students from the late 1980s through the late 1990s? The great irony is that our fear of HIV now stands in inverse proportion to the damage it does. AIDS is killing millions of people a year—"but those people are in Africa and Asia, so they don't count." To dismiss AIDS as someone else's or some other countries' problem is to deny the fundamental reality: sex is one of the few things that can link you to anyone else on this planet. Remember the 1990s bromide, *If you have sex with someone, you're having sex with everyone they ever had sex with?* It's still true.

Misinformation and Prevention

Millions of people globally have been exposed to a lot of HIV/AIDS misinformation. Because just

about everybody thinks they know how HIV/AIDS is spread, they may think they are not at risk because they are not in some specific category, or they may be denying their risk. For example, some may think, "Yes, I sleep with men, which is risky behavior, but I only sleep with men who are married, and they are clean." There is a whole category of people who don't think they are at risk for one reason or another. It is not understood why! Misinformation, denial and carelessness seriously hamper prevention efforts.

The importance of prevention is especially clear as one comes to understand the limitations in HIV/AIDS therapy. Regardless of what can be medically done for patients with HIV disease, there is no cure. Thus officials from the Centers for Disease Control and Prevention (**CDC**), the World Health Organization (**WHO**), the United Nations Joint HIV/AIDS Program (**UNAIDS**), and the American Health Organization (**AHO**) have placed the responsibility of prevention in the hands of the educators, which include health care professionals, parents, and teachers.

Current Success of Education Prevention Programs

A growing number of countries have documented the success of their prevention efforts through careful program evaluations and well-designed surveys. There should be no doubt in anyone's mind that prevention programs can reverse a major epidemic, as has been seen in Uganda and Zambia; can contain an emerging epidemic as has occurred in Thailand and Brazil; and can avoid an epidemic all together, as has been well documented in Senegal.

Complacency: The Success of Highly Active Antiretroviral Therapy—HAART

The success of HAART is good news for the people living longer, better lives because of it, but the availability of treatment may lull people into believing that preventing HIV infection is no longer important. This complacency about the need for prevention adds a new dimension of complexity for both program planners and individuals at risk. **First,** while the number of AIDS cases is declining, the number of people living with HIV infection is growing. This increased prevalence of HIV in the population means that even more prevention efforts are needed, not fewer. For individuals at risk, increased prevalence means that each risk behavior carries an increased risk for infection. This makes the danger of relaxing preventive behaviors greater than ever. **Second,** past prevention efforts have resulted in behavior change for many individuals and have helped slow the epidemic overall. However, many studies find that high-risk behaviors, especially unprotected sex, are continuing at far too high a rate. This is true even for some people who have been counseled and tested for HIV, including those found to be infected. **Third,** the long term effectiveness of HAART is unknown. HIV develops resistance to these drugs. If the development of drug resistance is coupled with a relaxation in preventive behaviors, resistant strains can and are being transmitted to others and spread widely. **Fourth,** despite medical advances, HIV remains a serious and usually fatal disease that requires complex, costly, and difficult treatment regimens. These treatments don't work for everyone. Sometimes when they do work, they have unpleasant or intolerable side effects. Some people can't take them because the interaction with their other drugs causes serious problems. Still others find it extremely difficult to maintain the drug treatment schedules. As we continue working to develop better treatment options, we must not lose sight of the fact that preventing HIV infection in the first place precludes the need for people to follow these difficult regimens.

Prevention Works—Pay Attention!

Sustained, comprehensive prevention efforts begun in the 1980s have had a substantial impact on slowing the HIV/AIDS epidemic in developed countries. While it is difficult to measure prevention— or how many thousands of infections did not occur as a result of efforts to date—in the United States the epidemic was growing at a rate of over 80% each year in the mid-1980s and has now stabilized. While the occurrence of approximately 40,000 to 50,000 new infections annually is deeply troubling, tremendous progress has been made. Also, there is now scientific evidence on which prevention programs are most effective. There is no question that prevention works and remains the best and most cost-effective approach for bringing the HIV/AIDS pandemic under control and saving lives.

Grim Reality

Steven Findlay (1991) wrote that burying those who have died from AIDS has become almost routine. With a 21-year death toll estimated at 480,000 beginning the year 2003, most Americans are indeed becoming accustomed to HIV/AIDS-related deaths. But how many will have died, say, ending the year 2010 or 2020 in America or world wide? Will a cure or preventive and therapeutic vaccines be produced? Will our health care system become swamped and ineffective? The best guess by scientists is that neither an effective vaccine nor cure will be found in the near future. Through the year 2003 it is projected that worldwide about 26 million people will have died of AIDS, about a half million of them in the United States. San Francisco may lose 4% of its population; New York 3%; Central Africa 15% to 20%. To avoid the realization of these projections, people of the world must work on HIV/AIDS **PREVENTION.**

What We Know

Based on over 20 years of intensive epidemiological surveys, scientific research, and empirical observations, it is reasonable to conclude that **HIV is not a highly contagious disease.** HIV transmission occurs mainly through an exchange of body fluids via various sexual activities, HIV-contaminated blood or blood products, prenatal events, and in some cases postnatally through breast milk. **Since 1981, no new route of HIV transmission has been discovered.**

THE "MAGIC" EVENT: A FORCE FOR PREVENTION, NOVEMBER 1991

While scientists, the public and vocal AIDS groups argued that more needed to be done to encourage people to protect themselves from HIV infection, it was not simply a matter of the media providing more information—something had to happen to capture the public's attention. That event occurred in 1991 when Earvin "Magic" Johnson made the stunning announcement that he was HIV positive and was immediately retiring from the National Basketball Association. It resulted in an unprecedented volume of AIDS coverage by the media—259 stories focused on AIDS, that week, compared with less than 100 within any other week analyzed.

Johnson's decision to become a spokesperson to promote AIDS awareness and safe sex provided a means to directly link background stories on prevention with the week's major news story. The 1995 Kaiser Family Foundation/Princeton Survey Research Associates survey identified Johnson and Elizabeth Taylor as the two individuals most recognized by the public as national leaders in this area (5% each); and among black Americans, Johnson is particularly likely to be cited as a leader (14%). After this major news event, AIDS coverage was never the same. Celebrity activities, including fundraisers, became an integral part of the AIDS story. AIDS became an issue for reporters on the sports beat as well as those in national affairs or health and science.

HIV Is a Fragile Virus: Life Span of HIV in Different Environments

The virus is fragile and, with time, self-destructs outside the human body.

The most recent data show that HIV remains active for up to five days in dried blood, although the number of virus particles (titer) drops dramatically. But it is dangerous to assume that there are no infectious viruses remaining in the dried blood or stored body fluids from an HIV/AIDS patient. In cell-free tissue culture medium, the virus retains activity for up to 14 days at room temperature (Sattar et al., 1991). According to a recent study, HIV was found to survive between two and four days in glutaraldehyde, a lubricant used to clean surgical instruments. This finding has serious implications for instruments too delicate to be autoclaved: (high-pressure steam sterilization), such as endoscopes. (Lewis, 1995).

Joseph Burnett (1995) reported that HIV can survive 7 days storage at room temperature, 11 days at 37° C in tissue culture extracellular fluid, and can still be infectious in refrigerated postmortem cadaver tissue for 6 to 14 days. Nadia Abdala and colleagues (1999 updated) reported that HIV recovered in the blood from used syringes can remain active up to at least six weeks. The bottom line is HIV is more resistant to the environment than originally believed. Chemical agents such as household bleach can be used to destroy or inactivate the virus.

BEHAVIORAL CHANGE

Perhaps the most difficult area of HIV/AIDS prevention lies in the area of behavior change. Behavior change is certainly difficult to inspire and extremely hard to measure. Furthermore, the theoretical basis for behavior change has been difficult to characterize.

It appears that HIV transmission can be prevented by individual action but it will require change in social behaviors. The best way to protect against all sexually transmitted diseases is *sexual abstinence.* The next best way is a mutually monogamous sexual relationship. Following these two options is the use of a barrier method during sexual activities—male and female condoms or rubber dental dams.

Over 90% of **new** HIV infections now occur in the developing world. For the foreseeable future, prevention through behavioral change is the only way to slow this epidemic. In fact, **history shows that prophylaxis and immunization for most infectious diseases are only partially effective in the absence of behavioral change.**

Sexual transmission accounts for the majority of HIV infection in the developing world, but this is the most difficult type of transmission to prevent. The use of condoms, reducing numbers of partners and abstinence remain the mainstays of preventing sexual transmission of HIV, but they will not be enthusiastically adopted just because health authorities tell people to do so.

Behavior has changed in many populations: among gay men in San Francisco, among injecting drug users in Amsterdam and New Haven, Connecticut, and among sex workers and their clients in Nairobi, to name a few. In none of these examples is it clear how the behavioral change took place. Even so, success stories in HIV/AIDS prevention seem to have some elements in common, including consistent and persistent intervention measures over a period of time, a clear understanding of the realities of the target population, and involvement of members of that population in prevention efforts. Successful interventions do far more than provide information: They teach communication and behavioral skills, change perceptions of what is **preventive behavior,** and ensure that the means of prevention, such as condoms or clean needles, are readily available (Hearst et al., 1995).

Table 9-1 provides a number of recommendations for preventing the spread of HIV. These recommendations place the responsibility for avoiding HIV infection on both adults and adolescents. **Lifestyles must be reviewed, choices made, and risky behavior stopped.** The public health service and the CDC have established guidelines that, if followed, will prevent HIV transmission while still allowing individuals to be somewhat flexible in their personal behaviors (*MMWR*, 1989).

UPDATE 2002 In June 2002 the results of the Global HIV Prevention Working Group were released. The group of 40 of the world's leading HIV prevention experts were sponsored by the Bill and Melinda Gates Foundation and the Henry J. Kaiser Foundation to review scientific evidence on HIV prevention and assess the status of global prevention efforts.

The report, Global Mobilization for HIV Prevention: A Blueprint for Action, was released in conjunction with a new study in The Lancet (Stover et al., 2002), which projects that there will be 45 million new HIV infections by 2010 without an expanded prevention effort. The study states, however, that 29 million of these infections could be prevented with the aggressive scaling up of existing prevention strategies. The study was conducted by UNAIDS, WHO, The Futures Group International, the U.S. Census Bureau and the Imperial College, London. The working group's blueprint strongly affirms the importance of a comprehensive approach to fighting the epidemic—one that combines both prevention and treatment. The study in Lancet by researchers examined 126 countries. It divided them into two groups: those where transmission of

HIV was mainly through heterosexual contact and spread through the general population (41 countries); and those where it was transmitted mainly in concentrated groups such as gay men, drug users and prostitutes (85 countries). The researchers then looked at 12 widely used interventions, studied 86 scientific studies on the success of the interventions and ran three computer models to come up with their projections. The interventions included mass media campaigns, voluntary counseling and testing, peer counseling, school-based programs, workplace programs, condom marketing, treatment for sexually transmitted diseases and efforts to prevent mother-to-child transmission of the virus. A separate study, also released in June 2002, gave a blueprint for boosting current prevention programs and starting new ones, estimating that such an effort would cost $4.8 billion annually by 2005. Up to 2010, an additional $27 billion would be needed to adequately pay for the initiative.

Quarantine

With few exceptions, proposals to quarantine all individuals with HIV infection have virtually no public support in the United States. Given the civil liberties implications of quarantine, its potential cost, and the realization that alternative, less repressive strategies can be effective in limiting the spread of HIV infection, quarantine proposals in most countries have been dismissed. Despite claims that HIV/AIDS is similar to other diseases for which quarantine has been used, public health officials have insisted on distinguishing between behaviorally transmitted infections and those that are airborne. HIV/AIDS is not airborne.

Through early year 2003, HIV prevention methods in the United States and other developed nations are education, counseling, voluntary testing and partner notification, drug abuse treatment, and syringe exchange programs. To date, the power to quarantine, for any disease, has rarely been used in the United States. In fact, only one country, Cuba, officially used the power of quarantine in 1986 to stem the spread of HIV. Data to date indicate that the use of quarantine of HIV-infected and AIDS persons in Cuba had been very effective. Cuba had 14 sanatoriums holding some 900 persons of which about 200 have AIDS. Cuba stopped the quarantine of HIV-infected persons in mid-1993. Controversial as

Table 9-1 Guidelines for Prevention of HIV Infection

I. For the General Public:

1. Sexual abstinence

2. Have a mutual monogamous relationship with an HIV-negative partner (the greater the number of sexual partners, the greater the risk of meeting someone who is HIV-infected).

3. If the sex partner is other than a monogamous partner, use a condom.

4. Do not frequent prostitutes—too many have been found to be HIV-infected and are still 'working' the streets.

5. Do not have sex with people who you know are HIV-infected or are from a high-risk group. If you do, prevent contact with their body fluids. (Use a condom and a spermicide from start to finish.)

6. Avoid sexual practices that may result in the tearing of body tissues (for example, penile–anal intercourse).

7. Avoid oral–penile sex unless a condom[a] is used to cover the penis.

8. If you use injection drugs, use sterile or bleach-cleaned needles and syringes and *never* share them.

9. Exercise caution regarding procedures such as acupuncture, tattooing, ear piercing, and so on in which needles or other unsterile instruments may be used repeatedly to pierce the skin and/or mucous membranes. Such procedures are safe if proper sterilization methods are employed or disposable needles are used. Ask what precautions are being taken before undergoing such procedures.

10. If you are planning to undergo artificial insemination, insist on frozen sperm obtained from a laboratory that tests all donors for infection with the AIDS virus. Donors should be tested twice before the sperm is used— once at the time of donation and again six months later.

11. If you know you will be having surgery in the near future and you are able to do so, consider donating blood for your own use. This will eliminate the small but real risk of HIV infection through a blood transfusion. It will also eliminate the more substantial risk of contracting other transfusion blood-borne diseases, such as hepatitis B.

12. Don't share toothbrushes, razors, or other implements that could become contaminated with blood with anyone who is HIV-infected, demonstrates HIV disease, or has AIDS.

II. For Health Care Workers:

1. *All* sharp instruments should be considered as potentially infective and be handled with extraordinary care to prevent accidental injuries.

2. Sharp items should be placed into puncture-resistant containers located as close as practical to the area in which they are used. To prevent needlestick injuries, needles should not be recapped, purposefully bent, broken, removed from disposable syringes, or otherwise manipulated.

3. Gloves, gowns, masks, and eye coverings should be worn when performing procedures involving extensive contact with blood or potentially infective body fluids. Hands should be washed thoroughly and immediately if they accidentally become contaminated with blood. When a patient requires a vaginal or rectal examination, gloves must always be worn. If a specimen is obtained during an examination, the nurse or individual who assists and processes the specimen must always wear gloves. Blood should be drawn from all patients—regardless of HIV status—only while wearing gloves.

4. To minimize the need for emergency mouth-to-mouth resuscitation, mouthpieces, resuscitation bags, or other ventilation devices should be strategically located and available for use where the need for resuscitation is predictable.

III. People at Risk of HIV Infection:

1. See recommendations for general public.

2. Consider taking the HIV antibody screening test.

3. Protect your partner from body fluids during sexual intercourse.

4. Do not donate any body tissues.

5. If female, have an HIV test before becoming pregnant.

6. If you are an injection drug user, seek professional help in terminating the drug habit.

7. If you cannot get off drugs, do not share drug equipment.

IV. People Who Are HIV Positive:

The prevention of transmission of HIV by an HIV-infected person is probably lifelong, and patients must avoid infecting others. HIV seropositive persons must understand that the virus can be transmitted by intimate sexual contact, transfusion of infected blood, and sharing needles among injection drug users. They should refrain from donating blood, plasma, sperm, body organs, or other tissues. HIV-infected people should:

Table 9-1 *(continued)*

1. Seek continued counseling and medical examinations.
2. Do not exchange body fluids with your sex partner.
3. Notify your former and current sex partners, and encourage them to be tested.
4. If an injection drug user, do not share drug equipment and enroll in a drug treatment program.
5. Do not share razors, toothbrushes, and other items that may contain traces of blood.
6. Do not donate any body tissues.
7. Clean any body fluids spilled with undiluted household bleach.
8. If female, avoid pregnancy.
9. Inform health care workers on a need-to-know basis.

V. Practice of Safer Sex:

Safer sex is body massage, hugging, mutual masturbation, and closed mouth kissing. HIV seropositive patients must protect their sexual partners from coming into contact with infected blood or bodily secretions. Although consistent use of latex condoms with a spermicide can decrease the chance of HIV transmission, condoms do break. If engaging in sexual intercourse with an HIV-positive person use two condoms. Even this is no guarantee. (Also see 1 through 6 under "For the General Public" in this table.)

[a]Tests show that HIV can sometimes pass through a latex condom. Experts believe that natural-skin condoms are more porous than latex and therefore offer less effective protection. Never use oil-based products such as Vaseline, Crisco, or baby oil with a latex condom because they make the latex porous, causing latex deterioration and breakage, thus nullifying the protection the condom provides against the virus. The use of condoms containing a spermicide is recommended.

the sanatoriums were, involving serious violations of civil liberties, the measures worked. Cuba has screened all blood donors for HIV since 1986, well ahead of other Caribbean countries. In 1987, it began screening all pregnant women, people diagnosed with sexually transmitted diseases and just about anyone else who showed up at a government health center. Jorge Perez, who diagnosed the country's first AIDS patients and helped shape the policies of the Santiago sanatorium as its director for 11 years said, "The Cuban point of view is that you have the right to be sick, but not to transmit it to anyone else." Currently, Cuba has the distinction of having one of the smallest HIV infection rates in the world in a region with one of highest. It also is the most populous country in the region and according to surveys, has some of the most liberal attitudes toward sex. Beginning 2003 there were about 1300 AIDS cases of which 950 have died.

NEW RULES TO AN OLD GAME: PROMOTING SAFER SEX

The use of barrier methods is one of the few behavioral strategies that individuals can adopt to protect themselves against sexually transmitted diseases. Male, and in some countries female, condoms are currently the only barrier methods widely available. However, there are many cultural, gender, economic and service-delivery barriers that impede the wide scale and consistent use of barrier methods for preventing STDs.

Barriers to HIV Infection

The two most effective barriers to HIV infection and other sexually transmitted diseases are **(1) abstinence,** which can be achieved by saying *NO* emphatically and consistently; and (2) **forming a no-cheating relationship with one individual, preferably for life.** These solutions to the danger of HIV infection may not be "cool," but they do work. These two apparently safe approaches are endorsed by the Surgeon General as the preferred methods. For those who do not practice abstinence, barrier methods are necessary to prevent HIV infection/transmission.

The barrier methods used to prevent HIV infection are the same methods used to prevent other sexually transmitted diseases (STDs) and often pregnancy. They include latex condoms, plastic condoms (new in 1995), and latex dental

SAN FRANCISCO PREVENTION PROGRAM FAILING

Despite $20 million spent each year on prevention in San Francisco, many in the AIDS community say HIV prevention strategies are not working, and the growing number of infections seems to support their claim that more men are having unsafe sex. The latest figures from the Department of Public Health show that estimated rates of new HIV infections in the city's gay community doubled in 2001 to 800 from the reported 400 per year in the late 1990s. A recent Centers for Disease Control and Prevention study found that 14% of gay men intentionally engaged in sex without a condom in the past two years. The CDC reports have put AIDS prevention workers in a quandary. While they struggle to find a solution, the majority of prevention workers agree that the current policy is a failure. In the early days of the epidemic, many in the gay community were confronted daily with the prospect of death. Now, with the aid of medications, many HIV-positive people are living relatively healthy lives, but there is a downside. Marcus Conant, head of the Conant Foundation, and one of the first doctors to work with AIDS patients said, "The messages didn't make it work, only fear made HIV prevention work in the first place." Michael Siever, director of the Stonewall project and advisor to the Castroguys prevention program said, "AIDS prevention has gotten so professional, so slick, and there are so many posters and ads that people don't listen to them. The disease isn't in your face anymore, so people aren't as careful. They are tired of getting tested and they're tired of hearing the same old campaigns to scare them about having sex." AIDS prevention specialists say the urgency to stop infections was removed after 1996 when HIV drugs began to combat the disease. But

that's not the only shift. Steven Gibson, Stop AIDS Project spokesman, said beyond the evaporation of urgency is the plain fact that sex without a condom feels better. Tom Coates, director for the Center of AIDS Prevention Studies at the University of California at San Francisco said, "We have all these programs and HIV prevention people are scratching their heads saying, 'How can we help people with HIV?' When all is said and done it's up to the community to say we just don't want HIV to spread." At its peak in the Castro district a decade ago, over 1800 people with AIDS died annually. In 2001, that figure was 218. The sharp decline is a profound relief, but San Francisco is still far from winning its long battle with the disease. In fact, some of the troubles the city thought were over are returning. Cases of syphilis, a disease that significantly increases the risk of being infected with HIV, have quadrupled in the past three years. Cases of HIV infection have doubled in the past five years. The same trends are apparent in other cities with large numbers of gay men. In 2001, a federal study concluded that young, gay men across the country were contracting HIV at a rate not seen in more than a decade. In May 2002, the CDC recommended that all gay and bisexual men be tested for HIV exposure at least once a year. Previously, the CDC had recommended screening only for patients with risky lifestyles. In 2002, gay men in the Castro district were saying, "It is easier than it has been in decades to hide a sexually transmitted disease. Or to forget to ask sexual partners whether they have any illnesses. Or to stop wearing condoms. Everybody around here looks so good now that nobody thinks they're going to catch anything bad."

dams and diaphragms used in conjunction with a spermicide. Barrier dams or dental dams are thin sheets of latex or similar material placed over the vagina, clitoris, and anus during oral sex. (Ask your dentist to show you a dental dam.) **Spermicides are chemicals that kill sperm.** These same chemicals have also been shown to kill some bacteria and inactivate certain viruses that cause STDs. Spermicides are commercially available in foams, creams, jellies, suppositories, and sponges. **Use of these products may provide protection**

against the transmission of STDs, but the only recommended barrier protection against HIV infection is a condom with a spermicide. National Condom Week is February 14–21. National Condom Day is always on Valentine's Day.

Condom—A Medical Device?

Condoms are classified as medical devices. Every condom made in the United States is tested for defects and must meet quality control guidelines

BOX 9.2

HIV/AIDS PREVENTION WORKS?

Prevention works was the most frequently used phrase at the 13th International AIDS Conference. But are the prevention interventions widely referred to as successful really understood? Twenty-two years into the pandemic, do we actually know what works and what doesn't in controlling the spread of HIV? **If HIV prevention is working, why are infection rates still rising around the world?** Although prevention strategies have been known for over two decades, very few countries or their international partners have taken sufficient action to slow the spread of HIV. **Prevention methods work, yet prevention isn't working.** This pandemic is washing the globe in human suffering and death! Experience in a number of countries has taught that HIV infection can be prevented through investing in information and life skills development for young people. Promoting abstinence, the use of condoms, and ensuring early treatment of sexually transmitted diseases are some of the steps needed. Also needed is an expanded political response and the individual and global acceptance that HIV does cause AIDS.

Undifferentiated Prevention Strategies

All HIV prevention guidelines function as if the same **"safer sex"** mantra applied to every individual in all populations. The basic message being—protect yourself, use a condom every time. But this has not worked for many reasons including economics, religion, education, poverty, denial, and legal and political will among the global population. In virtually every country people are afraid to take an HIV test or reveal their HIV status because they fear stigma, ostracism, and violent retribution.

In the 1960s there was the peace symbol; it promoted love and loosened sexual attitudes in America. In the 1990s and 2000s, the symbol is a square or round foil-wrapped condom. AIDS revived and catalyzed the use of condoms in developed countries. The dilemma, however, is that the longer the sexual relationship between couples, the less likely they will continue to use the condom—they assume they know each other. But no one knows where their sexual partner is 24 hours a day. In many underdeveloped countries, condoms are either not available, not affordable, or simply shunned by cultural standards. Another problem is that in many poor countries that allow the use of condoms, their pool of many millions of donated condoms is dropping due to donor fatigue. Some governments are asking, where is the honor in continuously supplying multimillions of condoms when they do not appear to be working?

Rate of Condom Usage

Prevention, despite numerous programs around the world, is in its infancy stages. The use of condoms, the cheapest and most effective form of protection against AIDS during sexual contact, is rare in most regions in the developing world. In nearly all African countries condom use rate is less than 5%. Entering 2003, in sub-Saharan Africa, the estimated total condom supply was sufficient to supply three condoms per man, per year! These data include the purchase of 300 million condoms in Kenya in year 2002 at a cost of $7.5 million. In Russia, from the results of a telephone survey in 2001, 8 out of 10 respondents said they rarely or never used a condom. Only 6% reported regular condom use. One in three believed that condoms provided protection against HIV transmission. In Vietnam in 2002, condom sales of 40 million amounted to a third of their estimated needs. In countries like Iran, Iraq and other countries in the Middle East, their religious teachings do not allow the use of condoms. Only four countries in Asia and four in Latin America and the Caribbean have condom use rates of 10% or more. The highest rate of condom use is in Japan with 46%, and Singapore 24%. In Europe, Denmark, Finland, Sweden, Spain, and Slovakia all show a rate over 20%. The U.S. condom usage rate is 13% and Britain in 18%.

Currently, the United States and other developed countries, the World Bank, and other global organizations have committed billions of dollars to distribute antiretroviral drugs in underdeveloped nations. But this does not, in itself, promote prevention. Short of an effective vaccine, billions of dollars more will have to be committed to prevention methods if this pandemic is to be brought under control.

PREVENTION IN THE UNITED STATES

Over the last 14 years the number of new HIV infections has remained stable at about 40,000 to 50,000 a year. For the last five years the number of AIDS-associated deaths has stabilized at about

BOX 9.2 *(continued)*

16,000–18,000 a year. In February 2001, the CDC, recognizing that such levels of new HIV infections and AIDS deaths are unacceptable, announced a new program to **half** the number of new HIV infections by year 2005. The CDC's primary strategy has now shifted to identifying people already infected and encouraging them not to spread HIV. The CDC's **Serostatus Approach to Fighting the HIV Epidemic,** or **SAFE** program, is based on the assumption that "Most HIV infections are spread by outwardly healthy people who do not realize they have HIV." The CDC, which already spends over $700 million a year on AIDS prevention, estimated that it will need to

increase its budget to $900 million a year to cover the campaign. Within the SAFE program, the CDC also wants to increase the proportion of persons who know they are HIV-infected from the currently estimated 70% up to 95% and to increase the proportion of HIV-infected people who are linked to appropriate treatment services from 50% up to 80% by 2005. Currently about 320,000 Americans are infected but do not know it. For years 2001 and 2002, about 85,000 HIV infections were discovered in the United States. This number comes from the 50,000 new infections annually and 35,000 of previously infected but newly discovered infections.

---

enforced by the federal Food and Drug Administration (FDA).

Condoms are intended to provide a physical barrier that prevents contact between vaginal, anal, penile, and oral lesions, secretions and ejaculate.

At least 50 brands of condoms are manufactured in the United States. They are produced to fit every fancy. There are colored condoms—pink, yellow, and gold; flavored condoms; and condoms that are perfumed, ribbed, stippled, and phosphorescent (glow in the dark). This assortment of condoms exposes the user and his partner not only to rubber but also to a variety of different chemicals—some that can cause allergic skin reactions **(contact dermatitis).** One to two percent of people are sensitive to latex rubber and demonstrate contact dermatitis.

Condoms are also called rubbers, prophylactics, bags, skins, raincoats, sheaths, and French letters. They can be lubricated or not, have reservoir tips or not, and can contain spermicide.

Condoms: Barriers to Bad News

Over the years people have been told to use condoms to prevent STDs and pregnancy. Today people are told that an additional use of the condom is to save lives.

History of Condoms

It has been reported that early Egyptian men used animal membranes as a sheath to cover their penises (Barber, 1990). Animal intestines were flushed clean with water, sewn shut at one end and cut to the length of the erect penis. In 1504,

Gabriel Fallopius designed a medicated linen sheath that was pulled on over the penis. A Japanese novel written in the 10th century refers to the uncomfortable use of a tortoise shell or horn to cover the penis.

It is interesting to note that condoms were used far more often throughout history as protection against STDs than as contraceptives. For example, an 18th-century writer recommended that men protect themselves against disease by placing a linen sheath over the penis during intercourse.

The term condom came into common usage in the 1700s. According to accounts in the early 1700s, condoms were sold and even exported from a London shop whose proprietress laundered and recycled them in a back room (Barber, 1990). Condoms became more widely available after 1854 when the method for making rubber was invented by Charles Goodyear (as in Goodyear tires). The latex condom was first manufactured in the 1930s.

Condoms have been available in the United States for over 130 years, but have never been as openly accepted as they are now. Their sale for contraceptive use was outlawed by many state legislatures beginning in 1868 and by Congress in 1873. Although most of these laws were eventually repealed, condom packages and dispensers until only a few years ago continued to bear the label **"Sold only for the prevention of disease,"** even though they were being used mainly for the prevention of pregnancy.

After the advent of nonbarrier methods of contraception during the 1960s (mainly the use of the birth control pill) there was an ensuing epi-

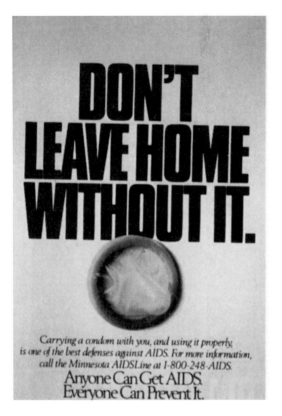

Carrying a condom with you, and using it properly, is one of the best defenses against AIDS. For more information, call the Minnesota AIDSLine at 1-800-248-AIDS.

Anyone Can Get AIDS. Everyone Can Prevent It.

FIGURE 9-2 Advertisement for Condoms. A common theme centered around the use of a condom to protect against sexually transmitted diseases. *(Photograph courtesy of the Minnesota AIDS Project, Minneapolis)*

demic increase in most sexually transmitted infections. Condoms once again are being marketed for the prevention of disease (Judson, 1989) (Figure 9-2).

Safer Sex, the Choice of Condom

Although a variety of preventative behaviors have been recommended (Table 9-1), the responsibility of **safer sex,** with a condom, is a personal choice. If one decides to use a condom, then the choice is what kind, and whether or not to use a spermicide.

The Male Condom— The American-made condom most often sold is made of latex, is about 8 inches long, and in general, one size fits all. About 500 million condoms are sold annually in the United States. Seven to ten billion are sold annually worldwide (Grimes, 1992 updated).

Intact latex condoms provide a continuous mechanical barrier to HIV, herpes virus (HSV), hepatitis B virus (HBV), *Chlamydia trachomatis*, and *Neisseria gonorrhoeae.* A recent laboratory study indicated that latex and the **new polyurethane condoms** are the most effective mechanical barrier to fluid containing HIV-sized particles (0.1 μm in diameter) available.

Three prospective studies in developed countries indicated that condoms are unlikely to break or slip during proper use. Reported breakage rates in the studies with latex condoms were 2% or less for vaginal or anal intercourse (*MMWR*, 1993a; Spruyt et al., 1998).

Choice— The best choice for preventing STDs and pregnancy is condoms that are made of **latex** or **polyurethane (plastic)** and contain a **spermicide.** The spermicide is added protection in case the condom ruptures or spills as it is taken off. Although some laboratory evidence shows that some spermicides can inactivate HIV, researches have found that these products cannot prevent a person from becoming HIV-infected.

During the 13th International AIDS Conference held in Durban, South Africa, July 9–14, 2000, researchers from the Joint United Nations Program on AIDS (UNAIDS) presented the results of a study of a product, Col-1492, which contains nonoxynol-9 (N-9). The study examined the use of candidate microbicide, or topical compound to prevent the transmission of human immunodeficiency virus (HIV) and sexually transmitted diseases (STDs). The study found that N-9 did not protect against HIV infection and may have increased the risk of transmission. Women using N-9 gel became infected with HIV about 50% more often than women who used the placebo gel.

CDC has released a "Dear Colleague" letter that summarizes the findings and implications of the UNAIDS study. The letter is available on the Web, http://www.cdc.gov/hiv; a hard copy is available from the National Prevention Information Network, telephone (800) 458-5231. Future consultations will be held to reevaluate guidelines for HIV, STDs, and pregnancy prevention in populations at high risk for HIV infection.

Condom Advertising on American Television— On January 4, 1994, condoms danced into America's living rooms as part of the most explicit HIV prevention campaign the nation has ever seen. Previously, condoms were rarely seen or even mentioned on American television. But the Centers for Disease Control and Prevention (CDC) launched a series of radio and television public service announcements targeting sexually active young adults, a group at high risk for HIV infection.

One of the television ads, entitled *Automatic,* features a condom making its way from the top drawer of a dresser across the room and into bed with a couple about to make love. The voice-over says, "It would be nice if latex condoms were automatic. But since they're not, using them should be. Simply because a latex condom, used consistently and correctly, will prevent the spread of HIV." Another, entitled *Turned Down,* features a man and woman kissing, when the woman asks the man, **"Did you bring it?"** When he says he **forgot it,** she replies, "Then **forget it,**" and turns on the light. There is also a pair of abstinence ads, in which condom use is not mentioned. The ads feature a man and woman talking. She says, "There is a time for us to be lovers. We will wait until that time comes."

Language that was once forbidden on TV has now become routine. Will it prevent HIV infection? Will it save lives?

Beginning 1996, the CDC began another series of radio and TV public service condom announcements.

The spots reel along like MTV videos, interspersing personal advice from young people with scenes from dance clubs, Greenwich Village, and a drugstore. They are punctuated by headlines that scream, "Put It On," "Talk About It," and "It's O.K. to Wait to Have Sex."

The bottom line to the new announcements is: **"Respect Yourself, Protect Yourself."**

The advertising campaigns are hailed as a milestone, marking a high point of visibility for the condom on network television and introducing a new level of explicitness to the Centers for Disease Control and Prevention's public pronouncements about AIDS prevention.

Class Discussion: What is your opinion on condom advertising? When? Where? Why?

Buying Condoms— Women are taking a more active role in buying condoms. In 1985, women bought about 10% of the condoms sold. Now they purchase 40% to 50% of condoms sold. According to surveys, most women buying condoms are single, and their concern is about HIV infection rather than pregnancy. **The fact that more women are willing to buy condoms is evidence that HIV education is working to some degree.**

Many condoms are purchased from vending machines. The FDA recommends the following guidelines when purchasing condoms from a vending machine:

1. Is the condom made of latex or polyurethane?
2. Is the condom labeled for disease prevention?
3. Is the spermicide (if any) outdated?

EDUCATION VERSUS RISK: IT'S NOT WHAT YOU KNOW, IT'S WHAT YOU DO

Sixty-five percent of all AIDS cases in the United States have been attributed to sexual contact. HIV is transmitted from infected semen, pre-ejaculate, vaginal secretions, or blood that comes into contact with the penis, vagina, anus, or rectum of an uninfected sexual partner. Additionally, contact of the mouth with semen or pre-ejaculate has transmitted infection, but at a very low rate compared with other penetrative sexual acts (refers to penile insertion and penile receptive anal and vaginal sex, and to oral contact with a partner's vulva or penis). The likelihood that sexually active people will become infected with HIV is determined by the probability of their having sex with an HIV-infected partner, the route of exposure and viral load in body fluids during sex, and one's genetic resistance. Any sexual act with an uninfected partner is HIV-safe (but not necessarily safe from other sexually transmissible diseases). Sex with an infected partner while correctly using a condom substantially reduces the likelihood of HIV infection. It is easy to forget, however, that unsafe sex is simply ordinary human sex.

SEXUAL RISKS

The degree to which patients may be willing to consider changing or modifying risk behaviors depends on how risky they perceive their behavior. Although HIV transmission occurs through specific behaviors, emotional and psychological factors determine whether or not these behaviors occur. The importance that sexually active people place on sexual behavior has an influence on their willingness to take HIV risks, regardless of their current HIV status. People continue to be confused and concerned about their level of sexual risk. Reports from the 7th Conference on Retrovirus and Opportunistic Infections shows that the confusion about risk is becoming even more clouded in the era of antiretroviral therapy. Interviews of 1976 HIV-negative or untested at-risk persons revealed that 48% were less careful about sex and drug use because of better therapy. Sixty-five percent of gay males interviewed said they were having unprotected receptive anal intercourse. In short, the availability of antiretroviral drugs is creating false sense of security among people in the high-risk groups. They are failing to practice safer sex. To that end one might instill caution by saying, **use a little bag to prevent the use of a body bag!**

---

4. Is the machine exposed to extreme temperatures or direct sunlight?

In mid-1992, the first drive-up "Condom Hut" opened in Cranston, Rhode Island. With each purchase the customer receives a brochure on safer sex.

It is generally recommended that condoms be stored below 25° C (77° Fahrenheit; room temperature is 72° Fahrenheit or 22° Centigrade). The packaging should be impermeable to both sunlight and gas. If air, which includes ozone, enters the package, it will affect the condom very quickly—ozone is like rust to a condom. Latex is a natural product—it will go bad if you don't treat or store it properly.

Condoms in Public Schools?

Condoms are now being dispensed without charge in most college and university and public health clinics, and in at least 400 high school health offices in the United States. Some cities in Canada have been providing access to free condoms in high schools since 1984.

In December of 1999, the American Medical Association (AMA) adopted a policy that advocates handing out condoms in schools and minimizes the value of abstinence-only sex education. While some doctors and groups have called the policy medically irresponsible, it is supported by the U.S. Surgeon General. The policy, based on studies, concluded that safer sex programs are effective in delaying sex in teenagers, and that abstinence-only programs have limited value.

Are Policies or Studies Reality?

Regardless of educational programs on safer sex and condom usage, recent studies indicate that teenagers still refuse to use condoms. **What they**

CLARIFYING THE ISSUES OVER CONDOM USE

Two major issues surface in the debate over advocating condom use in the prevention of HIV infection: One concerns the concept of efficacy, the condom's ability to stop the virus from passing through, and the other, the fear that making condoms available will encourage early sexual activity among adolescents and extramarital sex among adults.

EFFICACY (DO THEY WORK?)

All condoms are not 100% impermeable; they are not all of the same quality. Investigators using different testing methods have reported that latex condoms are effective physical barriers to high concentrations of *Chlamydia trachomatis, Neisseria gonorrhoeae,* the herpes and hepatitis viruses, cytomegalovirus, and HIV (Judson, 1989). But for maximum effectiveness condoms must be properly and consistently used from start to finish (Table 9-2).

To be effective, a condom must be worn on the penis during the entire time that the sex organ is in contact with the partner's genital area, anus, or mouth. Care must be taken that the condom is on before vaginal, anal, or oral penetration, and that it does not slip off. If properly used, the condom provides protection against most of the STDs that occur within the vagina, on the glans penis, within the urethra, or along the penile shaft.

Because the condom covers only the head and shaft of the penis, it does not provide protection for the pubic or thigh areas, which may come in contact with body secretions during sexual activity.

Margret Fischel reported in 1987 that 17% of women whose husbands were HIV positive became HIV-infected while using condoms properly and consistently.

Susan Weller (1993) reported on the use of condoms as a barrier to HIV transmission. She analyzed the data from 11 studies involving 593 partners of HIV-infected people. The resulting data showed that condoms are only 69% effective in preventing HIV transmission in heterosexual couples. These data surprise people because earlier contraceptive research indicated that condoms were about 90% effective in preventing pregnancy. Thus many people assume condoms prevent HIV transmission with the same degree of effectiveness. However, transmission studies by Weller do not show that to be true. Weller states

Table 9-2 Proper Placement of a Condom[a] on the Penis

1. Open the packaged condom with care; avoid making small fingernail tears or breaks in the condom.
2. Place a drop of a water-based lubricant inside the condom tip before placing it on the head of the penis. Be sure none of the lubricant rolls down the penis shaft as it may cause the condom to slide off during intercourse.
3. Hold about half an inch of the condom tip between your thumb and finger—this is to allow space for semen after ejaculation. Then place the condom against the glans penis (if uncircumcised, pull the foreskin back).
4. Unroll the condom down the penis shaft to the base of the penis. Squeeze out any air as you roll the condom toward the base.
5. After ejaculation, hold the condom at the base and withdraw the penis while it is still firm.
6. Carefully take the condom off by gently rolling and pulling so as not to leak semen.
7. Discard the condom into the trash.
8. Wash your hands after the procedure.
9. Never use the same condom twice.
10. Condoms should not be stored in extremely hot or cold environments.

[a]Males should practice putting on and removing a condom prior to engaging in sexual intercourse.

that condom effectiveness in blocking HIV transmission may be as low as 46% or as high as 82%!

Isabelle de Vincenzi (1994) reported on HIV transmission among heterosexual sexual couples in which one partner was known to be HIV positive. Study participants were advised to use condoms during intercourse, and among the 124 (or 48% of) couples who followed that advice consistently, no seronegative partner became HIV-infected during 24 months of followup. However, despite knowledge about HIV transmission, more than 50% of the couples failed to use condoms consistently. Twelve of the seronegative individuals in that group became HIV positive during the study.

The importance of compliance is illuminated by an analogy with pregnancy prevention programs. Although typical pregnancy rates for couples who use condoms are as high as 10% to 15%, rates are estimated to be as low as 2% for couples who use condoms correctly and consistently.

In July 2001, a National Institute of Health panel of 28 experts released a review of CDC studies that evaluated the effectiveness of condoms in protecting people against diseases transmitted during heterosexual sex. The panel concluded that condoms significantly reduce the risk of HIV transmission and gonorrhea infection in men. Also, it was established that a quality, male latex condom was impermeable to the smallest viruses contained in genital secretions. The report also states that about one in four Americans have an STD. This includes almost a million people who are living with an HIV infection. The report also stated that data on the prevention of other sexually transmitted diseases neither support nor refute condom effectiveness. The bottom line to all of this is that condoms reduce some of the risks in preventing the transmission of HIV and other STDs, thus condoms are used for **safer sex** but they cannot guarantee **safe sex.**

DO CONDOMS ENCOURAGE SEXUAL ACTIVITY?

Many persons assert that those who promote condom use to prevent HIV infection appear to be condoning sexual intercourse outside of marriage among adolescents as well as among adults. Recent data from Switzerland suggest that a public education campaign promoting condom use can be effective without increasing the proportion of adolescents who are sexually active. A 3-year, 10-month study showed condom use among persons aged 17 to 30 years increased from 8% to 52%. By contrast the proportion of adolescents (aged 16 to 19 years) who had sexual intercourse did not increase over that same period. A report from Deborah Sellers and colleagues (1994) and Sally Guttmacher et al. (1997) also concluded that the promotion and distribution of condoms did not increase sexual activity among adolescents. The study involved 586 adolescents who were 14 to 20 years of age. Douglas Kirby and colleagues (1998) studied 10 Seattle high schools that made condoms available to students through vending machines and school clinics. The study measured the number of condoms students took and the subsequent changes in sexual behavior. The investigators concluded that making condoms available in Seattle schools enabled students to obtain relatively large numbers of condoms but did not lead to increases in either sexual activity or condom use.

The AIDS epidemic has brought new dimensions of complexity and urgency to the debate over adolescent sexual activity. Some have urged abstinence as the only solution while others champion condom use as the most practical public health approach. Thus a clear message about condoms may have been obscured by controversy over providing condoms for adolescents in schools while at the same time trying to discourage these same young people from initiating sexual activity.

There must be a common ground: People should be able to agree that premature initiation of sexual activity carries health risks. Therefore, young people must be encouraged to postpone sexual activity. Parents, clergy, and educators must strive for a climate supportive of young people who are not having sex. Let them know it is a very positive and intelligent decision, and so help to create a new health-oriented social norm for adolescents and teenagers about sexuality.

The message that those who initiate or continue sexual activity must reduce their risk through correct and consistent condom use needs to be delivered as strongly and persuasively as the message **"Don't do it."** Protection of the individual and the public health will depend on our ability to combine these messages effectively (Roper et al., 1993).

ANECDOTE

Presenting facts without understanding won't work! Here is a simple story to emphasize the point: A minister following his custom, paid a monthly call on two spinster sisters. While he was standing in their parlor, holding his cup of tea, engaged in their usual chit chat, he was startled by something that caught his eye. There on the piano was a condom! 'Ladies, in all the years we've known each other I have never intruded into your private lives, and never felt the need to. But now I am forced to ask what is that thing doing there?' One of the ladies replied, 'Oh, that's a wonderful thing, pastor, and they really work!' The minister was agitated: 'I'm not talking about their value or effectiveness. I just want to know what that thing is doing on your piano.'

'Well, my sister and I were watching television. We heard this lovely man, the surgeon general of the whole United States. He said that if you put one of those on your organ, you'll never get sick. Well, as you know we don't have an organ, but we bought one and put it on the piano, and we haven't had a day's sickness since!'

know is not equal to what they do! Based on their findings, the researchers said information-oriented school- and community-based AIDS prevention programs will not succeed in getting adolescents to use condoms because there is no association between knowledge and preventive behavior.

Equally discouraging are studies from the United States and several countries that show a return to high-risk practices in populations, particularly men who have sex with men, in which risk reduction had been previously observed. Surveys conducted in London gay bars, gyms and health clinics showed that at least one in five gay or bisexual men was practicing unprotected anal intercourse, and many of these men knew that they were HIV infected. In France, unprotected anal intercourse among gay men increased from 17% in 1997 to 23% in 2000. In the Netherlands, between 1996 and 2000, rates of unprotected anal intercourse with casual partners increased from 25% to 34%, with parallel increases in sexually transmitted infections. In Cape Town, South Africa, one-third of gay men surveyed had recently had unprotected intercourse with partners of unknown HIV status. In Vancouver, a study of gay men found increases in risk behaviors and HIV infection rates. In Australia, rates of unprotected anal intercourse are steadily increasing. Together, these studies also illustrate that levels of risk are ever changing within the populations in which HIV prevention efforts have been most concentrated. (Kalichman et al., 2001) Perhaps the following quote will help explain the current rise in HIV infections. "It's not just the fact that young people don't know any older people with HIV. The image of HIV itself isn't bad anymore. We don't walk through the streets like we used to and see people so sick they can hardly walk. Today, people with HIV are buffed, they have boyfriends and they are doing things. It's just not such a terrible thing anymore."

Condom Availability in Developing Nations

Access to condoms in developing nations, although crucial, is poor even though over **1 billion** condoms are distributed in developing nations each year. The World Health Organization spends some $70 million a year for male condoms distributed in 14 countries. But, it would cost $460 million to provide just Africa with an adequate condom program. In 1992, the United Kingdom purchased 66 million condoms for Zimbabwe but the country needs at least 120 million condoms per year.

In May 1999, researchers on sexually transmitted diseases started to close the gap between the number of condoms now produced and the numbers needed. It will take an additional 24 billion condoms a year to slow the transmission of STDs including HIV.

Religion Prohibits Use of Condoms. It is a teaching of the Catholic church that the conjugal act must always leave open the possibility of conception. It is the purpose of devices such as condoms to rule out impregnation. Consequently, the church holds that the use of contraceptives in order to prevent the origination of new life is immoral. Peter Piot, executive director of UNAIDS said, "Catholicism has had a major role in virtually all aspects of the global response to AIDS since the disease was identified. With its hospices and hospitals, orphanages and parish outreach, the Catholic church provides more direct care for people with AIDS and their families and communities, particularly in Africa and Latin America, than any other institution. Yet, while the UN, most governments and governmental agencies, and almost all of the international organizations working in AIDS agree that condoms are the most effective means of slowing the spread of HIV, the Vatican has remained steadfast in its opposition to their use." In December 1999 and again in November 2000, the Vatican reiterated the Catholic Church's **opposition** to condom use as a way to prevent the spread of HIV. The church promotes a moral education to protect its members. Given that 1 billion, 30 million people worldwide are Catholics and that not all are low-risk individuals, the sanction against condom use presents a difficult problem in slowing the transmission of HIV.

In July 2001, The Southern African Catholic Bishops Conference after a seven-day meeting denounced the use of condoms, which they said destroy moral fiber and encourage casual sex. The bishops regard the widespread and indiscriminate promotion of condoms as an immoral and misguided weapon in our battle against HIV-AIDS. The bishops' stance was shared by Doctors for Life, a group of some 700 doctors in South Africa. Albu van Eeden, a member of Doctors for Life said "There has to be a change in lifestyle behavior. Just distributing condoms has no effect . . . society as a whole has to change its value systems."

First Global Campaign to End Catholic Bishops' Ban on Condoms Launched on Internet, Billboards in Subway and Newspapers

The first global campaign to end the Catholic bishops' ban on condoms was being launched by Catholics for a Free Choice (CFFC) on the eve of World AIDS Day 2001. Billboards and ads in subways and newspapers carrying the message "Banning Condoms Kills" began appearing around the world on November 30. This unprecedented worldwide public education effort is aimed at Catholics and non-Catholics alike to raise public awareness of the devastating effect of the bishops' ban on condoms. It invites the public to join a global campaign to end the ban—Condoms4life at www.condoms4life.org. People who join the campaign are being asked to contact local policy makers and express their support for the availability of condoms and their concern that the bishops should not undermine responsible public health policy on HIV/AIDS. Advertising in the United States and in countries with a significant Catholic population or AIDS crisis, such as Mexico, the Philippines, Kenya, South Africa, Chile and Zimbabwe, is the first phase of a sustained mobilizing effort to change the Vatican's policy and its aggressive lobbying against availability and access to condoms, especially in areas of the world where HIV transmission and AIDS deaths are rising dramatically.

Condom Quality

Some have touted condoms as a bulletproof vest for preventing HIV infection. This is simplistic and inaccurate because condoms may break or be used improperly. Condoms have been shown to **reduce** significantly but **not eliminate** the transmission of HIV. **Condom use is a form of safer sex, but not absolutely safe sex.** The March 1989 issue of *Consumer Reports* did a rather extensive study on the quality of different brands of condoms. The reader survey revealed that one in eight people who used condoms had two condoms break in one year of sexual activity; one in four said one condom had broken. Calculated from its data, about one in 140 condoms broke, with condom breakage occurring more often during some sexual activities than others. For example, the breakage rate during anal sex was calculated at one in 105 compared to one in 165 for vaginal sex. One

in 10 heterosexual men admitted to engaging in anal sex using condoms (*Consumer Reports*, 1989).

In a separate U.S. Public Health Service study (1994), if a couple used male condoms consistently and correctly, there was a 3% chance of unintentional pregnancy. Other studies have found that condoms reduce the risk of gonorrhea by as much as 66% in men, but by no more than 34% in women. It doesn't appear as though they prevent papilloma virus infection—which causes genital warts—in either sex (Stratton et al., 1993).

In 1987, FDA inspectors began making spot checks for condom quality. They fill the condom with 10 ounces (about 300 mL) of water to check for leaks. If leaks are found in more than four per 1,000 condoms, that entire batch is destroyed. Over the first 15 months of spot inspections, one lot in 10 was rejected. Import condoms failed twice as often—one lot in five.

The New Polyurethane (Plastic) Condoms— For the 1% of the general population that is sensitive to latex and for those who have a variety of other reasons not to use a latex condom, there is now a clear, thin, FDA-approved polyurethane (plastic) condom for sale in the United States. The condoms are colorless, odorless, and **can** be used with **any** lubricant. The current cost is about $1.80 each. Manufacturers of at least five other plastic condoms are waiting FDA approval. A report by Ron Frezieres and colleagues (1999) reported that although polyurethane and latex condoms provide equivalent levels of contraceptive protection, the polyurethane condom's higher frequency of breakage and slippage suggests that this condom may confer less protection from sexually transmitted infections than do the latex condoms.

A Polymer Gel Condom?— In November 1997 Michael Bergeron of the Laval Infectious Disease Research Center in Canada created a liquid condom that is nontoxic, tasteless, and transparent. The condom, made out of a polymer gel, is spread over the vagina or anus using an applicator. It gelifies in response to body heat and surrounds the penis. According to the inventor: "It's a physical barrier, but it moves—that's the advantage." The polymer gel can be flushed out with water. Bergeron developed the gel due to patient complaints about tight condoms. A major benefit is that the gel condom is somewhat **invisible**—

either sexual partner can use it as a protective measure. Trials to determine the contraceptive's efficacy in preventing HIV, herpes, and pregnancy have begun.

Why Some Men Don't Use Condoms: Male Attitudes About Condoms and Other Contraceptives— This is the name of a study published by the Henry J. Kaiser Family Foundation (1997). The study shows that men, especially teenage males, don't use condoms mostly because of **embarrassment:** buying the condom, talking about the condom with their sexual partner, putting the condom on in front of their sexual partner, offending or scaring their sexual partner, losing an erection while putting the condom on, and the **reduction of sexual pleasure.** (This free report can be obtained at 1-800-656-4533 monograph #1319.)

UPDATE 2000–2003 Reports reveal that HIV-infected people who have successfully suppressed HIV replication, their viral load is low or unmeasurable, may be less likely to practice safer sex. People on antiretroviral therapy who answered a survey said they used condoms less than half the time while having sex.

The Female Condom (Vaginal Pouch)— The female condom was FDA approved in May of 1993, and has become available to the general public. Before giving the Reality condom final approval, the FDA asked that two caveats be put into the labeling. **First,** the agency required a statement on the package label that male condoms are still the best protection against disease, and **second,** that the label compare the effectiveness of female condoms with that of other barrier methods of birth control. According to the FDA, in a study of 150 women who used the female condom for six months, 26% became pregnant. The manufacturer contends that the pregnancy rate was 21%—and only because many women did not use the condom every time they had sex. With "**perfect use,**" company officials say, the rate is 5%, in contrast to 2% for male condoms. Both conditions were met to the FDA's satisfaction. Gaston Farr and coworkers (1994) concluded that the female condom provided contraceptive efficacy in the same range as other barrier methods, particularly when used consistently and correctly, and has the added advantage of helping protect against sexually transmitted diseases.

Design of the Female Condom

The female condom is now called the **vaginal pouch.** It is 17 cm (about 6 3/4 inches)long and it consists of a 15-cm polyurethane sheath with rings at each end (Figure 9-3). The closed end fits into the vagina like a diaphragm. The outer portion is designed to cover the base of the penis and a large portion of the female perineum (the area of tissue between the anus and the beginning of the vaginal opening) to provide a greater surface barrier against microorganisms. Studies of acceptability, contraceptive effectiveness, and STD prevention are currently underway. Potential advantages of this product are: (**1**) it provides women with the opportunity to protect themselves from pregnancy and STDs; (**2**) it provides a broader coverage of the labia and base of the penis than a male condom; (**3**) its polyurethane membrane is 40% stronger than latex; and (**4**) is more convenient; it can be inserted hours before sexual intercourse. Disadvantages are (1) not aesthetically pleasing and (2) can be difficult to insert and remove.

Because of the polyurethane used to make it, the female condom is both strong and durable. No special storage arrangements have to be made because polyurethane is not affected by changes in temperature and dampness. The expiration date on the female condom is 60 months (five years) from the date of manufacture.

Global Use of the Vaginal Pouch (Female Condom)— Female Health Company (FHC) of Chicago is the sole manufacturer of the female pouch. Under agreement between UNAIDS and FHC the female pouch is sold for between 50 and 90 cents (US) in the developing world to encourage its use and provide greater access to women. It is also marketed in the Americas and Europe for about $2.50 (US). In March of 2002, France unveiled its first female pouch (condom) machines, blue for men and pink for women. Over 4 million were sold in 1997 and 14 million in 1998 within developing nations. Beginning year 2003, over 25 million female condoms were distributed in 84 countries in Africa, Asia, and Latin America. They cost Third World governments 12 cents each. Male condoms cost 3 cents each! UNAIDS hopes to get the pouch into all developing nations by year-end 2001.

Who Uses the Female Condom? Users of the female condom are generally in their mid- to late

1

Outer ring – add extra lubricant if wanted.

Inner Ring at the Bottom

Tip of pouch – add extra lubricant if wanted.

2

INDEX FINGER

INNER RING

OPEN END

Use three fingers to steady REALITY™ for inserting.

3

The inner ring helps insert REALITY™. It also helps to hold it in place during sex.

4

It is important for the inner ring to be up by the bone. If it is not in place, you or your partner could feel it during sex.

5

6

Outside Ring Correctly Covering Lip Area for Sex

If wanted, add extra lubricant to both sides of REALITY™ for more comfort.

B

FIGURE 9-3 **A.** The Vaginal Pouch. **B.** The 7-inch female condom or vaginal pouch is made of light-weight, lubricated polyurethane and has two flexible rings **(1),** one at either end. It is twice the thickness of the male latex condom. The inner ring **(2)** is used to help insert the device and fits behind the pubic bone. The outer ring remains outside the body. Unlike the diaphragm, the vaginal condom protects against the transmission of HIV, which can penetrate the vaginal tissues. The pouch can be inserted any-time from several hours to minutes prior to intercourse. The vaginal pouch is inserted like a diaphragm and removed after sex. FDA approved in May 1993. *(Courtesy of Female Health Co., Chicago)*

QUESTIONS AND ANSWERS ABOUT THE FEMALE CONDOM

1. **Does one have to be fitted for use of a female condom?** The female condom is offered in one size and is available without prescription. Unlike using a diaphragm, the female condom covers not only the cervix but also the vagina, thereby containing the man's ejaculate.

2. **Should a lubricant be used with the female condom?** A lubricant is recommended for use with the female condom to increase comfort and ease the entry and withdrawal of the penis. The female condom is prelubricated on the inside with a silicone-based, nonspermicidal lubricant. Additional water-based lubrication is included. The lubricant can be placed either inside the female condom or on the penis.

3. **Can oil-based lubricants be used with the female condom?** The female condom is made of polyurethane, which is not reported to be damaged by oil-based lubricants.

4. **Can a spermicide be used with the female condom?** Use of a spermicide has not been reported to damage the female condom.

5. **How far in advance of sexual intercourse can the female condom be inserted?** The female condom may be inserted up to 8 hours before sexual intercourse. Most women insert it 2 to 20 minutes before engaging in vaginal intercourse.

6. **Can the female condom be reused?** No. A new female condom must be used for each act of vaginal intercourse. After intercourse, the condom must be removed before the woman stands, to ensure that semen remains inside the pouch.

7. **Should a female condom and a male condom be used at the same time?** The female condom and male condom can be used at the same time but it is not recommended because the condoms may not stay in place due to friction between the latex in the male condom and the polyurethane in the female condom.

8. **Does Medicaid cover the female condom?** Currently Medicaid covers this device in 40 states, as it does the male condom, spermicide, and other barriers. (*Information provided by the New York State Department of Health AIDS Institute Division of HIV Prevention*, Info Bulletin, *Jan. 1994, Number Five Updated*)

---

twenties, and compared to male condom users and non-users of either method, have higher levels of education and access to household resources. Among women, more users of the female condom are unmarried and are primary breadwinners in their households compared to male condom users and non-users. A higher percentage of men who have used the female condom are married compared to male users of the male condom. The vast majority of men and women used the male condom at least once prior to trying the female condom.

Redressing the Balance of Power

The symbolic importance of the female condom should not be understated: **It is the first woman-controlled barrier method officially recognized as a means for the prevention of sexually transmitted disease.** The female condom allows women to be able to deal with the twin anxieties—AIDS and unwanted pregnancy—with a method that is under their own control.

Many women become HIV-infected due not to their own behavior, but to their partner's behavior. Because of the nature of gender relations, women may have little influence over their partner's sexual behavior.

Commentary: Positive messages for women have been spread worldwide on the advantages of using the female condom. But convincing women, in large numbers, to use this relatively new device may not be so easily accomplished. For example, it took 17 years before women in developed countries accepted and began to routinely use the tampon.

Condom Lubricants

It has been demonstrated that petroleum or vegetable oil-based lubricants should not be used with latex condoms. Nick White and colleagues (1988) have reported that these lubricants weaken latex condoms. Latex condoms exposed to mineral oil for 60 seconds demonstrated a 90% decrease in strength (Anderson, 1993). There are a number of water-based lubricants that do not adversely af-

Table 9-3 Water-Based[a] and Oil-Based[b]
Lubricants Often Used with Latex Condoms

Lubricants Recommended	Lubricants Not Recommended
Aqualube	Petroleum jellies
Astroglide	Mineral oils
Cornhuskers Lotion	Vegetable oils
Forplay	Baby oil
H-R Jelly	Massage oil
K-Y Brand Jelly	Lard
RePair	Cold creams
Probe	Hair oils
Today Personal Lube	Hand lotions containing vegetable oils
	Shaft
	Elbow Grease
	Natural Lube

[a]Water-based lubricants can be used with latex condoms.
[b]Oil-based lubricants will chemically weaken latex, causing it to break.
The above lists are not exhaustive of all available lubricants used by consumers.
(Source: The STD Education Unit of the San Francisco Department of Public Health)

fect latex condoms; these should be the lubricants of choice (Table 9-3).

CLASS QUESTION: Reaching this point in the text and having just read the section on male and female condoms, do you think the danger for life, with respect to HIV and other life-threatening STDs, is high enough that condoms should be as familiar to everyone as are toothpaste and toilet paper and also as available? Yes or No—defend your view with credible information.

An Alternative to Condoms: Vaginal Microbicides

While condoms, when used consistently and correctly, are effective in preventing the sexual spread of HIV, there is an urgent need for chemical barrier methods that women can use for HIV prophylaxis, such as vaginal microbicides. Vaginal microbicides are products for vaginal administration that can be used to prevent HIV infection and/or other sexually transmitted diseases. An ideal vaginal microbicide would be safe and effective, and also tasteless, colorless, odorless, nontoxic, stable in most climates, and affordable. It must be pointed out that like condoms, microbicides will not protect injection drug users.

What are Microbicides?

Microbicides are chemical substances that, when applied in the vagina or the rectum, would substantially reduce transmission of STDs. They could be produced in many forms, including gels, creams, suppositories, films, or as a sponge or vaginal ring.

In developing a vaginal microbicide, **scientists must be sure that the substance is safe, does not kill microbes naturally present in the vagina that benefit female hygiene, and does not impair a woman's ability to conceive.** Any microbicide will have to be tested to determine whether it damages spermatozoa, which could result in birth defects.

Application

A woman can apply a microbicide vaginally or rectally to protect herself and her partner. Current techniques to prevent HIV exposure—condom use, monogamy, reducing the number of partners, and treatment of other sexually transmitted diseases—often are not feasible or available for women. Many women face cultural barriers that prevent them from requiring their partners to use condoms, as well as cultural and economic barriers to securing other types of protection and treatment. Meanwhile, nearly 6 of every 10 new HIV infections occur in women worldwide. It is estimated that in the United States, about 22 million women would use an effective microbicide. Recognizing that 90% of all new HIV infections worldwide occur through sexual contact, the Rockefeller Foundation stated at the National Press Club in 2002, that a first-generation microbicide could save 2.5 million lives over three years in developing countries.

Vaginal Microbicide Research

The identification of novel microbicidal compounds is a rapidly expanding area of HIV prevention research. The United Kingdom is sponsoring a five-year, $22 million program, working with agencies in five African countries (South Africa, Tanzania, Uganda, Cameroon and Zambia) to find an effective gel to protect women against HIV infection. In America, a total of 56 products are currently in the pipeline: 34 are in pre-clinical stages; 15 are in Phase I safety trials, four are in Phase II expanded safety and preliminary effectiveness trials (Savvy cream, Emmelle gel, Lactobacillus crispatus suppository), and three entered

Phase III trials (Carraguard get, BufferGel and Pro-2000 gel), in 2002. The candidates fall into four categories or combination of categories:

1. Products that kill or inactivate the infectious pathogens—these include detergents (like nonoxynol-9, Savvy), peroxides, lipids, plant extracts (Praneem, gossypol), antimicrobial peptides, monoclonal antibodies and acidic buffers.
2. Products that block fusion, i.e. prevent attachment to the mucosal surface of target cells—these include those that specifically target HIV surface proteins or HIV receptors and non-specific blockers that are active against multiple organisms (Carraguard, Emmelle, Pro-2000 and Usercell).
3. Products that inhibit post-fusion activity by interrupting HIV life cycle after the virus has infected the cell—these included nucleoside/nucleotide RT inhibitors; non-nucleoside/nucleotide RT inhibitors; protease inhibitors; and post-binding fusion inhibitors.
4. Products that enhance naturally occurring vaginal defense mechanisms. The natural vaginal flora of healthy women is dominated by lactobacilli, which produce a number of compounds that inhibit pathogenic microorganisms. These compounds also maintain a low, acidic pH in the vagina. Other important defenses are naturally occurring antimicrobial peptides and antibodies in the vagina. A few newly developed microbicides aim to enhance these natural defenses. They may be of particular relevance to those countries in sub-Saharan Africa where almost half the women of childbearing age have bacterial vaginosis, characterized by a lack of vagina lactobacilli. (Products include Lactobacillus crispatus suppository, BufferGel, Acidform gel, Protegrins, Plantibodies [monoclonal antibodies]). Depending on trial outcomes and adequate funding, it is likely that one or more of these products could come to market by 2007. About 35 of the products currently in research are contraceptives as well as microbicidal.

MALE TOLERANCE TO MICROBICIDES

If men are to be exposed to unknown products used to prevent HIV infection, the product should not cause open genital lesions or major discomfort. To this end, studies on the products mentioned above are in progress. The results to date are that those products, at most, cause minor itching, small lesions or minor pain upon urination. Studies continue.

INJECTION DRUG USE AND HIV TRANSMISSION: THE TWIN EPIDEMICS

About 36%, over 300,000 of the 850,000 (beginning year 2003) U. S. AIDS cases recorded since 1981 were transmitted through injection drug use. Now about half of all new HIV infections occur from IDU. About 75% of all people with IDU-related AIDS are either black (50%) or Latino (24%).

Syringes and needles used to inject drugs or steroids, or to tattoo the body, or to pierce the ears, should **never be shared.** If an individual is going to assume the risk of HIV transmission through needle sharing, the risk can be reduced by sterilizing the needle, and the syringe, if one is used, in undiluted chlorine bleach. The needle and syringe should be flushed through twice with bleach and rinsed thoroughly with water. (**NOTE: FROM THIS POINT FORWARD, NEP STANDS FOR NEEDLE EXCHANGE PROGRAMS AND INVOLVES A NEEDLE AND A SYRINGE.**)

Both injection drug use (IDU) and HIV infection are on the increase. They are twin epidemics in the United States and Europe because the virus is readily transmitted by injection drug users and then from infected drug users to their noninfected sexual partners. Stopping injection drug-associated HIV transmission in theory is easy—just avoid injection drug use. But, that is a difficult proposition for most of the estimated 6.5 million IDUs worldwide (2.5 million in the United States). The number of countries **reporting** IDU in 1989 was 80, in 2001, 135. IDUs will remain a major HIV connection to the homosexual, heterosexual, and pediatric populations (Anderson et al., 1998 updated).

HIV PREVENTION FOR INJECTION DRUG USERS

What can be done and what is being done to prevent HIV transmission by this population? Available drug rehabilitation programs are far too few. It is estimated that only 15% of injection drug users in the United States are receiving treatment at any given time. Many addicts want to quit their habit but may become discouraged because of having to wait long periods of time before getting treatment because of lack of money. Even if there were a sufficient number of treatment centers, there will always be the hard-core IDUs who will not enter a program.

A massive education program on how to clean drug equipment and not sharing such equipment has for the most part failed. IDUs have an economic motive to share equipment (Mandell et al., 1994). In addition, it takes time and effort to clean the syringe and it takes time to find and purchase cleansing chemicals (detergents or bleach). Beginning year 2002, studies continue to show that over 50% of IDUs share drug injection equipment. Also, **less than half clean their injection drug equipment!** Perhaps the most important drawback may be that IDUs have little interest in health care or changing their behaviors. In addition, there is always the problem of legality. **IDU is illegal throughout the United States** (see Box 9.2).

IDUs know this and fear incarceration without the possibility of a "fix." A "Catch-22" situation also exists for those who want to help make injection drug use safer: **Many governmental agencies and law enforcement officers interpret the intention of making drug use safer as advocating drug use.** As a result, many proponents of safer drug use have avoided becoming involved in the issue. The 2000 Kaiser Family Foundation National Survey of Americans showed that 58% of those polled were in favor of syringe exchange programs. Beginning year 2003, federal money could still **not** be used to fund **NEPs.**

Peter Lurie and colleagues (1998) state that each year, about one billion syringes would be required for IDUs to have a sterile syringe for each injection.

UPDATE 2002 After reviewing the many studies that support NEPs worldwide, the report by Steffanie Strathdee of the Bloomberg School of Public Health, Johns Hopkins University comes as a surprise. The results of a 10-year study, 1988 through 1998, revealed that the biggest predictor of HIV infection for both male and female injection drug users (IDUs) is sexual behavior, not sharing needles used to inject drugs. High risk homosexual activity was the most important factor in HIV transmission for men; high risk heterosexual activity was the most significant for women. Risky drug use behaviors also were strong predictors of HIV transmission for men but were less significant for women. Roland Foster, aid for the U.S. Congress subcommittee on Criminal Justice, Drug Policy and Human Resources said, "While needle exchange advocates have been arguing that needle distribution was the answer to ending HIV infection among drug users, it turns out their assumptions were wrong: sexual behaviors rather than needle sharing are the most significant HIV risk behaviors for drug abusers."

The Needle Exchange Program Strategy (NEPs)

The idea of syringe-needle exchange program (NEP) is based on the established public health policy of eliminating from any system potentially infectious agents or, where possible, carriers of infectious agents. The rationale of NEPs is similar, wherein active injection drug users exchange used, potentially contaminated syringes for new, sterile syringes (Figure 9-4). In general, these exchanges are done on a one used needle and syringe for one new needle and syringe basis, though some programs will add an additional number of needle and syringes on top of those already exchanged. NEPs also provide other paraphernalia and supplies including cotton, cookers, water, and sterile alcohol prep pads. In addition, NEPs offer a variety of other services to IDUs including education, HIV testing and counseling, referrals to primary medical care, substance abuse treatment, and case management.

THE WORLD'S FIRST NEP on record began in 1984 in Amsterdam, The Netherlands. It was started by an IDU advocacy group called the **Junkie Union.**

Free Needle Exchange Programs in the United States

Jon Parker is believed to be the first person in the United States to distribute free drug injection equipment publicly in North Haven, Connecticut and in Boston in November 1986.

Evaluation of Needle/Syringe Exchange Programs

Entering year 2003, NEPs operating in American cities were exchanging about 25 million syringes annually. An IDU makes about 1000 drug injections each year (*MMWR*, 1997). The San Francisco

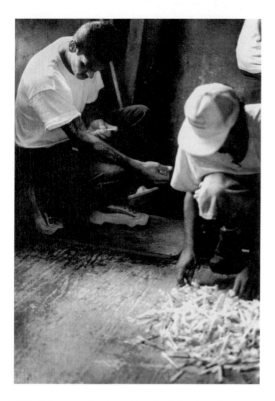

FIGURE 9-4 Getting a Fix. An injection drug user shoots up in a shooting gallery in the La Perla neighborhood of Old San Juan, Puerto Rico. Another man sorts used syringes to be exchanged for new. *(Photo by Enrique Valentin/South Florida Sun-Sentinel)*

AIDS Foundation operates the largest NEP in the United States. There are too many NEPs to list, just a few are presented.

Tacoma, Washington— Their **NEP** began in August 1988. It began as a one-man program by Dave Purchase, a 20-year drug counselor.

The NEP in Tacoma held the HIV infection rate to under 5% over a 5-year study period (1988–1992). During that same 5-year study period, the prevalence of HIV infection among IDUs in New York City, with few syringe exchange programs, increased from 10% to 50%!

New York City— In November 1988, after many delays, New York City began its NEP. The program was canceled in early 1990—the reason: because over 50% of NYC's 240,000 IDUs were HIV-infected, the program offered too little too late to have an impact. IDUs make up about 38% to 40% of NYC AIDS cases. The NEP was resumed in 1992. Beginning 1998 there were at least five NEPs operating in New York City. In May of 2000, New York State passed a law making it legal to buy needles without a prescription; the 43rd state to do so.

New Jersey— As of mid-2002, New Jersey is the only state in the northeast without NEPs. Yet, IDU is the leading cause of HIV transmission in this state. Of over 44,000 AIDS cases in New Jersey, over half are IDU associated. The belief of the objectors to NEPs is that NEP has not stemmed the spread of HIV in other states. The state governor has agreed to a pilot NEP.

New Haven, Connecticut— Their twelve-year-old program has demonstrated that NEPs dramatically slow the rate of infection without encouraging new injection drug use. Some indicators even suggest that the program has been responsible for a decrease in both crime and the amount of drugs used illegally. These results have enabled policymakers elsewhere to call for NEPs. Edward Kaplan (1993) of Yale University reported at the 8th International AIDS Conference that the New Haven syringe program cut the rate of new HIV infections by 33% to 50%. His data came from comparing the number of HIV-contaminated syringes found on the streets versus those turned in at syringe exchange points. (There is some controversy over this data.)

After passing a 1992 law permitting pharmacies to sell syringes without a prescription, syringe sharing has dropped 40% in the state of Connecticut. Seventy-five percent of AIDS cases in Connecticut occur among IDUs, their sex partners, and their children. Going into year 2003, Connecticut, North Dakota, Alaska, Iowa, and South Carolina allow nonprescription sales of syringes and have no drug paraphernalia law against their possession. Six states and the District of Columbia require prescriptions both to buy syringes and to possess them. Four of the six states (New Jersey, Illinois, Pennsylvania, and Massachusetts) have the largest numbers of IDUs and the highest incidence of AIDS among them.

California— Each year about 8000 Californians are infected with HIV and injection drug use is the second leading cause of those infections.

In October 1999 a law was passed that would allow cities and counties to establish NEPs. By early 2000 at least six cities and counties had funded NEPs! No new NEPs have opened as of late-2002.

Hawaii— In 1990, Hawaii became the first state to legalize a statewide NEP. The state legislature felt it was necessary to stem the rate of HIV infection in women and newborns.

Needle Exchange Programs (NEPs) in Other Countries

There are an estimated 7 million IDUs worldwide. Many countries are now involved in **NEPs** to lower the spread of HIV.

Needle exchange program results from England, Austria, the Netherlands, Sweden, and Scotland, presented at the 4th International AIDS Conference (1988) suggest that the European programs attracted IDUs who had no previous contact with drug treatment programs; and that IDUs were drawn from NEPs into treatment programs, thus the decrease in drug use. There was no indication in these studies of an increase in injection drug use in cities with exchange programs. Where HIV testing had been done, the rate of HIV infection showed a marked decline after the introduction of NEPs (Raymond, 1988; Hagen, 1991).

Some of the countries with active NEPs are:

Canada— In 1989, Montreal, Toronto, and Vancouver began NEPs. Beginning 1998, Vancouver has the highest rate of HIV infections among IDUs in the world with 40% of IDUs infected. Vancouver also has the largest NEP in the North America and one of the largest in the world. Over the last 10 years, their NEP distributed over one million needles annually. In Ottawa, 19% of IDUs are HIV-infected. Experts believe a shift to injecting **crack cocaine** is responsible for the rising infection rates among IDUs. While heroin users routinely use a **few** needles a day, injection cocaine users may use 30 to 40 needles a day!

England— Over 2 million syringes and needles are exchanged in 120 NEPs each year. Needles and syringes can be legally purchased throughout England. Free distribution and exchange remains a relatively nonpolitical and noncontroversial issue (Stimson et al., 1989). One problem found in England, the United States, and elsewhere is that NEPs attract IDUs who are at **lower risk** for HIV infection while **high-risk** IDUs are less likely to participate.

France— An experimental Marseille, France, program utilizing vending machines to accept contaminated needles and dispense sterile syringes has successfully attracted younger injection drug users who typically avoid NEPs and pharmacies. A survey distributed at 32 pharmacies, four needle exchange sites, and three syringe vending machines in Marseille found that 222 out of 343 respondents have used the machines citing free access and 24-hour availability as the main incentives. Primary users of the machine were more likely to be under age 30, to have no history of drug maintenance treatment, and to avoid needle sharing and other high-risk injection behaviors.

Dublin, Ireland— The Merchant's Quay needle exchange project has released a new set of recommendations. The report, titled **Making Contact: An Evaluation of a Needle Exchange,** calls for syringe vending machines, pharmacy involvement in the distribution of needles, and mobile needle exchanges. According to the study, which was based on 1300 participants in the needle exchange, one-third reported borrowing and lending syringe equipment. Also, women were more likely than men to share needles and take part in risky sex. During the 18-month study there was a 71% reduction among participants in borrowing drug injecting equipment.

Netherlands— NEPs are available in 40 municipalities. Data from these programs suggest that the staff operating the syringe exchange centers are multilingual and the centers should be operational 24 hours a day.

Australia— Australia has 10% of the population of the United States but has 2000 NEPs in five states and one territory. The remaining state and one jurisdiction may have since joined the program (Wodak, 1990 updated).

The Queensland health department says that the NEPs cost A$500,000/year but potentially saves A$279 million/year when all diseases that can be transmitted by IDU are considered.

BOX 9.3

THE CONTROVERSY: PROVIDING STERILE SYRINGES AND NEEDLES
TO INJECTION DRUG USERS (IDUS)

As the HIV pandemic enters the new century in the United States, the profile of those affected is beginning to change. HIV is slowly changing from a disease of men who have sex with men to a disease of injection drug users, their sexual partners, and children. From 1997 through 2002, 50% of all new HIV infections were associated with IDUs. **THE SYRINGE IS A TYPHOID MARY!** Accordingly, should IDUs be provided at public expense, with free syringe and needles to help stop the spread of HIV?

There has been no other HIV prevention activity, with the possible exception of condom distribution in public schools, that has generated as much controversy as needle exchange programs **(NEPs.) Pro forces** believe that it is impossible to eliminate injection drug use. Providing IDUs with free sterile equipment is an attempt at slowing the spread of HIV among drug users and their sexual partners, subsequently reducing the number of people in the general population that will become infected. In support of the Pro forces, the CDC and the National Institutes of Health reviewed many of the NEPs operating in the United States (Beginning year 2003 there were about 600 sites in 82 cities in 34 states) and others in Canada and Europe. **The most important conclusion is that NEPs are preventing HIV infections in drug users, their sex partners, and their children.** That finding was based, in part, on evidence collected in Tacoma and Seattle, Washington, and in New Haven, Connecticut, where there was a 33% reduction in the rate of new infections among NEP clients. **In another key finding, they found no evidence that distributing syringes leads to an increase in drug use.**

Gibson and colleagues (2001) analyzed 42 publications published between 1989 and 1999 that evaluated the efficacy of syringe exchange programs. They found significant evidence for the conclusion that syringe exchange is effective in preventing both risky behavior and HIV seroconversion. Twenty-eight studies reported positive effects regarding the use of needle or syringe exchange, two found negative associations, and 14 found either no association or a combination of positive and negative effects.

Besides saving lives, these NEPs deliver a huge financial payoff. Consider the case of an HIV-positive addict who infects eight others in a 1-year period (a reasonable estimate). If each turns to Medicaid to pay his or her lifetime medical costs (at an average $119,000 plus), that's about a $1 million burden for taxpayers—money that could have been saved if the one addict had been in a NEP. In addition, arguing for the availability of NEPs is *not* an argument against using police and criminal justice mechanisms to deal with drug use-related robbery, assault, or other crimes.

Con forces argue that any move to make injecting-drug use safe is a move to make it attractive or socially acceptable and thus represents a step backward in the long-declared war on drugs. Those opposing the needle exchange programs say that to provide NEPs is to condone drug addiction and perhaps promote injection drug use among those who would not otherwise participate. Some feel that free syringe programs are just a Band-Aid that attempts to prevent HIV infection but does nothing to cope with the underlying drug addiction problem. **(These people may feel it's too little, too late.)**

A side issue of course is the fact that it is **illegal to sell** needles and syringes over the counter in 4 of the 50 states and the District of Columbia through 2002. Statutes in 45 states and the District of Columbia place criminal penalties on the possession and distribution of syringes (drug paraphernalia laws) (*MMWR*, 1993b; 1997). Laws restricting these sales were intended to discourage drug use, (Fisher, 1990; Gostin et al., 1997). Law enforcement and community leaders (police, churches, businesses, parents, teachers, and residents) are concerned that allowing access to needles and syringes sends the wrong message, encourages initiation into drug use, and accelerates the disintegration of families. Residents and business owners fear increased street crime, lower property values, and health risks from discarded needles and syringes.

Middle Ground

There is a **third force** of people who take the middle ground. They advocate providing free bleach to IDUs to clean their drug equipment. People from many AIDS-action groups in metropolitan areas are involved in the free bleach dispensing program. With each bottle of bleach is a set of directions. But since many IDUs cannot

BOX 9.3 *(continued)*

read, they are given verbal instructions, though some are too "spaced out" to listen or too uncomfortable to care. Third force people have to understand that NEPs and distribution of bleach kits have to be accessible privately, off the street and out of sight, as well as publicly. Use of a public, streetcorner NEP is a statement to the entire community that the person exchanging a syringe is an IDU. This has potentially very different consequences for women than for men. Women who have children have good reason to try to conceal their addiction as they risk losing custody or contact with their children if the state finds out they are actively using drugs—and if they are using a public NEP the child welfare bureaucracy is more likely to find out than if they are not getting needles and syringes in public. Perhaps NEPs should provide some type of informal child care so that a mother doesn't have to literally exchange needle and syringes in front of her children. Addiction among women is often taken as a statement of sexual availability.

Legalize Drugs

A **fourth force** suggests that drugs be legalized so that they can be used openly, thereby reducing the threat of HIV transmission through illegal "shooting galleries." Discussion of the fourth force's position is beyond the scope of this text. However, a quasi-fourth force situation did exist in Zurich, Switzerland, until 1992.

Zurich gained notoriety for its vast amounts of gold but in 1987 it gained a new image—that of an open Needle Park. The city of 250,000 people experimented in setting aside Platz Pitz park where cocaine and heroin addicts could openly buy, sell, and use injection drugs. The park attracted up to 4000 drug users/day. In early 1992, the park was closed because the park became a magnet for professional dealers, especially Lebanese, Yugoslav, and Turkish gangs that overran small dealers in a violent price war. Some of the park's inhabitants clustered around the central train station, others headed off in search of methadone. Others went back to the alleys and shelters from which they came. With sales suddenly back underground, addicts complained that the price of heroin had doubled overnight to $214 a gram (454 grams/pound=$97,156). Health workers said efforts to prevent the spread of HIV/AIDS will now be much more difficult.

UPDATE Switzerland is currently experimenting with providing IDUs with **heroin** three times a day in 18 treatment centers across the country. So far Swiss health authorities say the program has reduced criminal activity among the participants about 60%. The program also reduced their homelessness from 12% to zero and death rate by 50%. Germany recently began the Swiss experiment.

CLASS QUESTION: The United States has a zero tolerance for such activities and will not become involved in what the Swiss term, "an innovative program." Do you think the United States should, based on the Swiss data, offer heroin to the addicted in a controlled environment similar to the Swiss? Present a credible reasons/data to support your stand.

LIFTING THE BAN ON THE USE OF FEDERAL FUNDING TO SUPPORT NEEDLE EXCHANGE PROGRAMS

Since 1990, seven national reports have reviewed the scientific evidence and recommended that the federal ban for NEP funding be lifted. Needle exchange programs are supported by the President's Advisory Council on HIV/AIDS, the American Medical Association, the National Academy of Sciences, the Centers for Disease Control and Prevention, and the American Public Health Association, as well as other prestigious medical and public health organizations. In addition, the American Bar Association and the U.S. Conference of Mayors have urged the federal government to allow states and localities to use Federal HIV-prevention funds to implement NEPs. Polls have shown that the American public supports lifting the ban on federal funding of NEPs. A recent Harris poll found that 71% of Americans believe that cities and states—and **not** the federal government—should decide whether federal HIV-prevention funds can be spent on NEPs.

On April 20, 1998, Health and Human Services Secretary Donna Shalala informed President Clinton that the scientific research has proven that NEPs effectively prevent the transmission of HIV and hepatitis, and do not lead to increased drug use. Her long-awaited action cleared the way for the president to lift the 10-year ban on federal funding for NEPs. Clinton accepted the findings, but stated that in spite of them he would continue to block the use of federal funds for NEPs. Clinton endorsed lifting the ban in his 1992 presidential campaign. HIV

BOX 9.3 *(continued)*

prevention advocates charge that the president's decision is politically motivated and will cause thousands of new and preventable HIV infections. Beginning 2003, the ban remains in effect.

Class Discussion: Do you agree with current federal policy on money for NEPs? List any scientific facts or studies that could be used to support the president's action. List any scientific facts or studies that disagree with his decision.

COMMENTARY

It is hard to avoid the suspicion that the concerns about free syringe programs have less to do with science or public health than with politics: specifically, a reluctance to **detract** or **distract** from the **"JUST SAY NO"** message. But there is another message that both sides would agree on—that no one should die needlessly! A leading University of California researcher estimates that nearly 10,000 lives could have been saved over the past few years by an aggressive expansion of syringe exchange programs. **Isn't the war on drugs supposed to be about saving lives? Isn't a part of government about saving lives? Your response is?**

In 1998 Ansett, Australia, became the world's first airline to install needle/syringe disposable bins. Ansett said the disposable bins in its 69 aircraft were installed primarily as a safety measure to avoid needle-stick injuries to staff but is intended for the use of legitimate syringe users, such as diabetics, as well as addicts.

New Zealand— A nationwide NEP began in 1988. The overall rate of HIV-infected IDUs remains low. In 1995, less than 1% of IDU men and no women tested at the syringe exchange centers were HIV positive. There have been about four to six new cases each year since 1987.

Italy— Only a few limited NEPs have been reported. However, between 1983 and 1988, the sale of syringes and needles, which is legal, increased by 50%.

Summary

Through 2002, 84% of IDUs in Glasgow, 82% in Lund, 84% in Sydney, 73% in Tacoma, and 87% in Toronto reported they had changed their behavior in order to avoid HIV/AIDS. The most commonly mentioned specific behavior change: reduced sharing of injection equipment.

PREVENTION OF BLOOD AND BLOOD PRODUCT HIV TRANSMISSION

A combined fear of disease and lawsuits have led most wealthy-developed nations to adopt a zero tolerance policy regarding HIV contamination of the blood supply. However, 10% of all new HIV infections in developing countries are now due to transfusions of tainted blood. In the early 1980s, one of every 50 bags of blood collected in San Francisco contained HIV. The chance of acquiring either HIV or hepatitis C from a blood transfusion now is about one in one million.

Blood Donors

In the United States, there are at least 52 medically related restrictions for donating your blood. Thirteen of these reasons place a person on permanent restriction from donating blood—for example, being HIV positive, having multiple sclerosis, being a hemophiliac, men having sex with other men since 1977 (even once), having used injection drugs (even once), or having had a stroke.

There should be **no risk** in the United States or in other **developed nations** of contracting HIV **by donating blood** if blood centers use a new, sterile needle for **each** donation. Yet a 1998 survey revealed that 25% of those polled believed that they could become HIV-infected by donating blood.

Over 8 million people are donating some 18 million units of blood that are transfused into about 5 million people annually in the United States. Blood can carry HIV in a cell-free state or HIV may be carried within cells of the blood. **A large dose of HIV received via blood transfusion almost universally results in HIV infection. A small dose of HIV-contaminated blood, such as the blood received by a needle stick seldom results in infection** (Francis et al., 1987). The mean volume of blood injected by a needle stick has been calculated to be 1.4 µL (1.4 millionths of a liter). It is difficult to determine exactly how large a viral dose is necessary to cause infection. However, it is known that infection is more likely to occur if blood is donated close to the time the HIV-infected donor becomes symptomatic. Entering year 2003, 6% of HIV-infected adults and 10% of HIV-infected children in the United States are believed to have become infected via blood transfusions or by the use of contaminated blood products. The majority of HIV infections occurred prior to the initiation of the blood screening program in 1985. To date **only** whole blood, blood cellular components, plasma, and blood clotting factors have been involved in transmitting HIV.

Blood Collection and Blood Screening for HIV

Testing blood for infectious diseases began with syphilis screening in the 1940s. Hepatitis-B antibody screening was added in the 1970s, HIV antibody screening in 1985, for biomedical evidence of hepatitis in 1986, the hepatitis B-core antigen in 1986, HTL V-1 and II-antibodies in 1988, and hepatitis C antibodies in 1990. Inclusion of the HIV antigen (p24) test in 1996 provided detection of HIV infection sooner than antibody testing. At least **eight tests** for infectious diseases are now routinely performed on each unit of blood collected.

No Blood Purchases for Transfusion— All blood transfused in the United States comes from volunteer donors. Blood from paid donors is used for pharmaceuticals such as Rh Ig, albumin, and intravenous immunoglobulins. Under the current standards for blood banks and transfusion services of the American Association of Blood Banks, all units must be clearly labeled **volunteer, paid,** or **autologous** (donated for self use).

Blood Screening for HIV— **If the test indicates that the blood carries antibodies to HIV, it is treated to destroy the HIV and then discarded.** In March of 1983, the major United States blood banking organizations instituted procedures to reduce the likelihood of HIV transmission through blood transfusions. People with signs or symptoms suggestive of HIV disease /AIDS, sexually active homosexual and bisexual men with multiple partners, recent Haitian immigrants to the United States, past or present IDUs, men and women who have engaged in prostitution since 1977 or have patronized a prostitute within the past six months, and sexual partners of individuals at increased risk of HIV infection **are asked to refrain from donating blood.**

United States FDA Approves Blood Screening Test for HIV— Blood screening for HIV and HIV-testing procedures are presented in Chapter 12. The risk of becoming HIV-infected from a blood transfusion has dropped by more than 99% from 1983 to 2003. Regardless, a male living in Durango, Texas, received HIV contaminated blood during heart bypass surgery in August 2000. In March 2002, he filed a $100 million lawsuit against those thought to be responsible for his HIV infection. This is reported to be the first case of an HIV positive blood transfusion since restrictive blood screening tests for HIV were put in place in April 1999. In 2002, two people became HIV infected from blood transfusions in Florida's Tampa Bay area. Tracing the infectious blood back to its donor source revealed that, in both incidents, the donors were in the window period; they were infected but the blood test failed to detect the virus.

Blood Transfusions Worldwide— Fifteen years after the industrialized world began to screen all blood used in transfusions for HIV, about one in ten people in developing countries are still being infected through this route.

A combination of the lack of screening with high levels of infected donors turns transfusion into a form of roulette. Beginning year 2003, blood transfusions accounted for 5% to 10% of HIV infections worldwide.

Blood Safety— From 1985 into 2003, about 450 million units of blood or plasma have been screened for HIV antibody in the United States. By excluding those who test HIV positive and by asking people from high-risk behavior groups not to donate blood, the incidence of HIV transmission from the current blood supply is relatively low. With faster and more accurate testing procedures now in use, the risk is becoming even lower. **However, the probability or risk of receiving HIV-contaminated blood will never be zero.** The reason a small risk still exists is because some people infected with HIV may donate blood during what is known as the **"window period." During that period, a person may be infected with the HIV, but the test cannot yet detect the infection. And, the test is not 100% accurate.**

Eve Lackritz and colleagues (1995) reported that of 4.1 million blood donations from 19 regions served by the American Red Cross, one donation in every 360,000 was made during **the window period.** They further estimated that one in 2,600,000 donations contained HIV but was not identified (**false negative**) because of laboratory error. Their report states that collectively, of 42 Red Cross regions collecting 9 million units of blood, **the risk of HIV transmission was one transmission for every 450,000 to 660,000 available units of screened blood.** Based on their data they conclude that there are about 18 to 27 infectious units of blood available for transfusion each year. This is about half the previous estimates. (The American Red Cross collects about half the donated blood in the United States annually.) With the widespread use of the recently FDA approved Nucleic Acid Test (2002) the numbers of infectious units of blood should be cut in half.

Autologous Transfusions— These are transfusions using **"self" (your own) blood.** It has been suggested that the two groups that benefit most from autologous blood storage are: expectant mothers facing Caesarean section and certain elective surgical candidates where substantial loss of blood is anticipated. A person's blood is drawn and refrigerated for transfusion back into his or her own body when needed. (**Stored whole blood remains usable for a maximum of 42 days.**) This is the safest blood available.

INFECTION CONTROL PROCEDURES

With no cure or vaccine for HIV/AIDS, prevention of infection is of paramount importance. With the advent of the HIV/AIDS epidemic, health care workers and others who are occupationally exposed to body fluids, especially blood, are understandably concerned about the risk of becoming HIV-infected. However, when precautions are observed, the risk is very small, even for those treating HIV/AIDS patients.

Two sets of infection control procedures are in use in hospitals, medical centers, physicians' offices, and units that deal with people in medical emergencies. One is called **universal precautions,** the other is **blood and body substance isolation.**

Universal Precautions

Universal precautions (Table 9-4) are standard practices that workers observe on the job to protect themselves from infections and injuries. These precautions or safety practices are called **universal** because they are used in all situations even if there seems to be no risk. Universal precautions had their beginnings in 1976 when barrier techniques were first recommended for the prevention of hepatitis B infection. Precautions required the use of protective eyewear, gloves, and

---

BOX 9.4

AMERICANS SUPPORT SEX EDUCATION AND CONDOMS IN SCHOOLS AND IN TV ADS, AND NEEDLE EXCHANGE PROGRAMS

In 1966, the Kaiser Foundation reported the following facts after reviewing the results of its **"Survey of Americans and HIV/AIDS":** Virtually all Americans (95%) think AIDS information should be provided in the schools, including 69% who think children should start receiving AIDS education **at the latest** by age 12; seven out of ten Americans think the major television networks should accept condom advertisements; two-thirds favor providing clean needles to IV drug users; and 63% say there should be more references to condom use in movies and

television. However, when asked whether they thought high schools should provide condoms or information about AIDS to teens, Americans were almost evenly divided: 49% say just AIDS/HIV information and 46% say making condoms available should be the priority. Support for AIDS prevention measures persists across demographic groups.

Eight out of ten parents with children under 21 years of age say they are concerned about their child getting AIDS, including 53% who say they are **very** concerned. When asked

BOX 9.4 *(continued)*

about the information they want most about AIDS, five out of ten parents say they need more information about "what to discuss with children about prevention." Getting information about where to go for help if exposed to HIV was the number two information needed, picked by 12% of parents.

Americans Concerned About AIDS Both Personally, for the Nation, and Worldwide

The year 2000 Kaiser Family Foundation Survey reveals how Americans feel about HIV/AIDS on a personal, national, and global level.

Personal

Twenty-two percent (over one in five) Americans say they are more concerned about becoming infected with HIV today than a few years ago. Blacks and Latinos are more likely than whites to be more concerned today (35%, 43%, and 18%, respectively). Nearly 25% of Americans say the problem of AIDS is a more urgent problem for their local community today than it was a few years ago, with 30% saying it has stayed about the same. Overall, the proportion of Americans saying that AIDS is a more urgent problem for their local community today than it was a few years ago has remained relatively stable since 1997, except for Latinos where there has been a significant decline.

National

Twenty years into the epidemic, the American public continues to view HIV/AIDS as one of the most urgent health problems facing the nation, second only to cancer. In the past five years, however, the proportion who view AIDS as the number one health problem facing the nation has declined. Nearly half (49%) of all Americans believe HIV/AIDS is a more urgent problem today than it was a few years ago, an amount roughly equal to the proportion who said that was the case in 1997 (48%).

Global

Americans rank AIDS as the number one health problem facing the world today (37%), followed by cancer (35%), heart disease (12%), the cost of health care (7%), and hunger/malnutrition (6%). Almost half (49%) of African Americans and 41% of Latinos rank AIDS as the number one health problem facing the world, compared to 35% of whites. Three-quarters (76%) of Americans say that AIDS is a more urgent problem for the world today than a few years ago.

Americans Generally Informed About HIV/AIDS, Although Some Gaps in Knowledge Persist

Minorities and those with low incomes and less education are most likely to be personally concerned about AIDS. More than a third (35%) of people with annual incomes under $10,000 say they are "very concerned" as compared with only 14% of those with incomes over $50,000 per year. Similarly, while 34% of those without a high school degree say they are "very concerned" about getting AIDS, only 14% of college graduate's say they are.

Most people (54%), however, think 100,000 or fewer Americans have died from AIDS, when in fact it's five times that number. While underestimating the number of lives lost to AIDS, many Americans (51%) overstate the impact here relative to the rest of the world, believing that half or more of all AIDS cases occur in America. In reality it's less that 2%. Half of the population (51%) incorrectly thinks a person can get AIDS while "giving or donating blood for use by others." (There are no known cases of HIV transmission as a result of **donating** blood. Some of the confusion may be related to perceived risk of **receiving** blood transfusions.

Significant Percentages of Americans Distrustful of Information About HIV/AIDS

Although most Americans believe they are receiving accurate information about the AIDS epidemic, significant percentages doubt what the government and media are telling:

♦ 34% do not believe the government is telling the whole truth about AIDS; and

♦ 25% do not believe the media is telling the whole truth about AIDS.

In addition, fewer, but still some Americans question the origins of the epidemic:

♦ 18% believe there is some truth to report that the AIDS virus was produced in a germ-warfare laboratory; and

♦ 12% believe that AIDS came from God to punish homosexual behavior.

gowns, and careful handling of needles and other sharp instruments. In 1977, hepatitis B immunoglobulin was recommended for those exposed to hepatitis B through needle sticks. In 1982, hepatitis B vaccine became commercially available and recommended for all health care workers exposed to human blood.

In 1987, the CDC published "Recommendations for Prevention of HIV Transmission in Health-Care Settings." Blood and body fluid precautions should be consistently followed for all patients regardless of their blood-borne infection status. This extension of blood and body fluid precautions to all patients is referred to as **Universal Precautions (UP).**

Under universal precautions, the blood and certain body fluids of all patients are considered potentially infectious for HIV, hepatitis B virus (HBV), and other blood-borne pathogens.

Universal precautions are intended to prevent parenteral (introduction of a substance into the body by injection), mucous membrane, and broken skin exposure of health care workers (HCWs), teachers, or any other person who may become exposed to blood-borne pathogens. **In 1987, the CDC also published a report that got the immediate attention of most, if not all, informed health care workers.** The report stated that three health care workers who were exposed to the blood of AIDS patients tested positive for HIV. What was so startling was that until that time, needle punctures and cuts were thought to be the only dangers in a clinical setting. These three cases appeared to involve only skin exposure to HIV-contaminated blood. **One** of the three cases involved a nurse whose chapped and ungloved hands were exposed to an AIDS patient's blood.

The **second** case involved a nurse who broke a vacuum tube during a routine phlebotomy on an outpatient. The blood splashed on her face and into her mouth. A blood splash was also involved in the **third** case. The worker's ungloved hands and forearms were exposed to HIV-contaminated blood (Ezzell, 1987).

The importance of these three cases of HIV infection is that they informed health care workers in the most dramatic way that they were all **vulnerable.** Perhaps these three cases produced a fear among health care workers out of proportion to the actual risk of their becoming infected. However, the fear of an individual and the actual reason he or she has for it are very difficult to

judge. **Although calculations show that the risk of HIV infection after exposure to blood from an HIV/AIDS patient is about one in 200, if you are that one, probability is meaningless.**

The universal precautions as published by the CDC currently apply to some 5.3 million health care workers at 620,000 work sites across the United States and another 700,000 Americans who routinely come in contact with blood as part of their job, for example, people in law enforcement, education, fire fighting and rescue, corrections, laboratory research, and the funeral industry.

In July of 1991, the CDC published an additional set of recommendations. These recommendations are also for preventing the transmission

Table 9-4   Universal Precautions

DEFINITION

Universal precautions (UP) are a set of infection control practices developed by the Centers for Disease Control and Prevention (CDC), in which health care workers (HCWs) appropriately utilize barrier protection (gloves, gowns, masks, eyewear, etc.) for anticipated contact with blood and certain body fluids of *all* patients.

1. The hands and skin must be carefully washed when contaminated with blood or certain body fluids.
2. Particular care is taken to prevent injuries caused by sharp instruments.
3. Resuscitation devices should be available where the need is predictable.
4. HCWs with exudative lesions or weeping dermatitis should refrain from patient care until the condition resolves.

BLOOD AND BODY FLUIDS TO WHICH UP APPLY

Blood is the single most important risk source of HIV, HBV, and other blood-borne pathogens in the occupational setting. Prevention of transmission must focus on reducing the risk of exposure to blood and other body fluids or potentially infectious materials containing visible blood.

1. UP should be used when exposure to the following body fluids may be anticipated:
   a. Blood
   b. Serum plasma
   c. Semen
   d. Vaginal secretions
   e. Amniotic fluid
   f. Cerebrospinal fluid (CSF)
   g. Synovial fluid
   h. Pleural fluid
   i. Vitheous fluid
   j. Peritoneal fluid
   k. Pericardial fluid
   l. Wound exudates
   m. Any other body fluid containing visible blood (but not feces, urine, saliva, sputum, tears, nasal secretions, or sweat, unless they contain visible blood).
2. Note: Blood, semen, and vaginal secretions have been shown to transmit HIV. The others, with the exception of fluids containing visible blood, remain a theoretical risk.

RATIONALE

1. UP reduce the risk of parenteral, mucous membrane, and skin exposure to blood-borne pathogens such as, but not limited to, HIV and HBV.
2. For several reasons, focusing precautions only on diagnosed cases misses the vast majority of persons who are infected (many of whom are asymptomatic or subclinical) and who may be as infectious as the diagnosed cases. Persons who have seen a physician and have been diagnosed with acute or active disease represent only a small proportion of all persons with infection. Infectivity always precedes the diagnosis, which often is made once symptoms develop.

(Adapted from Mountain-Plains Regional AIDS Education Training Center. *HIV/AIDS Curiculum,* Nov. 1994.)

of HIV and hepatitis B virus to patients during exposure-prone procedures.

In summary, the concept of universal precautions assumes that all blood is infectious, no matter from whom and no matter whether a test is negative, positive, or not done at all. Rigorous adherence to universal precautions is the surest way of preventing accidental transmission of HIV and other blood-borne pathogens.

Blood and Body Substance Isolation (BBSI)

An alternative, and some believe superior, approach to the CDC's universal precautions in areas of high HIV prevalence is the system referred to as **body substance precautions or Blood Body Substance Isolation (BBSI)** (Gerberding, 1991).

In practice, these precautions are similar to universal precautions, in that prevention of needle stick injury and use of barrier methods of infection control are emphasized. Philosophically, however, the two are quite different. Whereas universal precautions place a clear emphasis on avoidance of blood-borne infection, body substance precautions take a more global view. **Body substance isolation (BSI) requires barrier precautions for all body substances (including feces, respiratory secretions, urine, vomit, etc.) and moist body surfaces (including mucous membranes and open wounds).** BSI is designed as a system to reduce the risk of transmission of all **nosocomial** (hospital-associated) pathogens, not just blood-borne pathogens. Gloves are worn for any anticipated or known contact with mucous membranes, or nonintact skin and moist body substances of all patients.

PARTNER NOTIFICATION

One of the most controversial issues in HIV prevention is **contact tracing** or **partner notification** of sexual contacts mostly because HIV/AIDS is considered as an incurable disease with a great deal of stigma attached to the infected. Partner notification is the practice of **identifying** and **treating** people exposed to certain communicable diseases. The term *partner notification* is used by the CDC and some health care providers because it more comprehensively describes the process by which the physician, other health care workers such as Disease Intervention Specialists (DIS, someone who is specially trained in STD work), and the infected person may provide information to at risk partners, sometimes to family, friends or care provider.

There are two very different approaches to informing unsuspecting third parties about their potential exposure to medical risk.

Each approach has its own history, including a unique set of practical problems in its implementation, and provokes its own ethical dilemmas. The **first approach,** involving the moral **duty to warn,** arose out of the clinical setting in which the physician knew the identity of the person deemed to be at risk. This approach provided a warrant for disclosure to endangered persons without the consent of the patient and could involve revealing the identity of the patient. The **second approach**—that of contact tracing—emerged from sexually transmitted disease control programs in which the clinician typically did not know the identity of those who might have been exposed. This approach was founded on the voluntary cooperation of the patient in providing the names of contacts. It never involved the disclosure of the identity of the patient. The entire process of notification was kept confidential (Bayer, 1992).

History of Partner Notification

The concept of partner notification was proposed in 1937 by Surgeon General Thomas Parran for the control of syphilis (Parran, 1937). By tracing and treating all known contacts of a syphilitic patient, the chain of transmission could be interrupted. According to George Rutherford (1988), contact tracing has been successfully used in a number of STDs beginning in the 1950s. It is still used in cases of syphilis, endemic gonorrhea, chlamydia, hepatitis B, STD enteric infections, and particularly in cases of antibiotic-resistant gonorrhea.

In 1985, when the HIV antibody was first used in screening the blood supply, notification of blood donors and other HIV-infected individuals and their contacts became possible. **The strategy in HIV partner notification is the same as that used for the other STDs: to identify HIV-infected individuals, counsel them, and offer whatever treatment is available.** In asymptomatic HIV-infected people only counseling is given. But, symptomatic HIV-infected patients receive counseling and treatment, if available, for their signs and symptoms. Partner notification depends on HIV-positive people to give the names of their partners; but, they may be reluctant to do so fearing that their identification may result in physical abuse and loss of their jobs and housing. For a review of partner notification read the article by Kevin Fenton, et al., 1997. Those who oppose the use of partner notification call the investigators "sex police."

The Use of Partner Notification: Examples

In April 1993 an incarcerated male asked for an HIV test. The diagnosis was HIV positive. Contact tracing turned up a network of 124 persons; all were linked by syringe sharing and syringe sharing with sex. One hundred and twenty-one were contacted and offered an HIV test; 118 accepted the test; 44 were HIV positive. One hundred and thirteen of the 124 lived in the same county. The estimated cost for partner notification in this network was $13,969. (*MMWR*, 1995).

During a five-month period (February through June 1999) seven young people were diagnosed with HIV in a small rural town in Mississippi. The CDC, working with the Mississippi Health Department through partner contact investigation, defined a social network of 122 people. Persons in the network had a median age of 21 (range: 13 to 45 years). Of the 78 people tested for HIV infection, five women (median age, 16 years) and two men (median age, 25 years) were infected, all through heterosexual sex. Results of the interviews of the infected and noninfected people indicated a serious lack of HIV/AIDS prevention knowledge (*MMWR*, 2000).

Opposition to Partner Notification for HIV Disease

Currently opposition to partner notification continues on the grounds that: (**1**) it is not cost effective; (**2**) there is little evidence that those who are informed of their infection will do anything about changing the high-risk behaviors that got them infected in the first place; (**3**) the threat of social discrimination undermines the intent of contact tracing; (**4**) the unintended consequences of partner notification may include violence and even death from an abusive partner (Rothenberg, 1995); and (**5**) in 24 states homosexuality is a crime, and HIV-infected homosexuals fear prosecution if they acknowledge same-sex contacts because their sexual partner(s) may be prosecuted.

In Support of Partner Notification

The following discussion is from Stephen J. Josephs' article, "The Once and Future AIDS Epidemic," *Medical Doctor*, 37:92–104. Mr. Joseph is the past Commissioner of Health of New York City, 1986–1990.

The New York City medical examiner looked at a large sample of dead persons who were tested postmortem and found to be HIV positive, but who had no notification in their medical records of having been diagnosed as infected. Over 35% of those persons had a readily identifiable spouse or steady sexual partner. Josephs asks,

> How can one justify, on clinical, public health or humanitarian grounds, *not* notifying that surviving partner, who might be the source of the infection in the deceased, or the recipient of infection? Arguments against this procedure border on the absurd; one has to start with the premise that increased medical knowledge is more dangerous than helpful to the individual, and that the rights of the uninfected count for nothing against the rights of the infected.

POINT AND QUESTION With current life-sustaining antiretroviral treatments available, is there an overwhelming excuse not to use partner notification—especially when so many HIV/AIDS experts promote the "hit early—hit hard" approach to therapy?

What is your response to the reasons for partner notification and to the opposition's point of view?

Legality of Partner Notification

Legal Obligations To Warn Third Parties at Risk— Many state laws permit, but do not require, disclosure by physicians to third parties known to be at significant future risk of HIV transmission from patients known to be infected. Thus, if a physician reasonably believes that a patient will share drug injection equipment or have unprotected sex without informing a partner of the risk, the physician has discretion to inform the partner. Under some disclosure laws, the physician is required to first counsel the patient to refrain from the risk behavior, and, in providing the third party warning, the physician is prohibited from disclosing the patient's identity. In the absence of state laws permitting such disclosure, physicians may be held liable for breach of confidentiality for disclosing patient information to sex partners.

The **"duty to warn"** may extend to nonpatient third parties in other contexts, based on the provider's primary duty to the patient. Thus, health care professionals have a duty to inform patients that they have been transfused with HIV-contaminated blood and this duty may extend to third parties. A physician in one case failed to inform a teenager or her parents that she had been transfused with HIV-contaminated blood. When the young woman's sexual partner tested positive for HIV, the court upheld his claim against the physician based on the physician's failure to inform the patient. Similarly, courts have upheld that a health care professional's duty to inform the patient of his or her HIV infection may extend to those the patient foreseeably puts at risk, such as a spouse or family member caregiver. On the other hand, courts have ruled that disclosure is wrongful in cases in which the third party, such as a family member, is not at actual risk of infection, or the physician has no knowledge that the patient has failed to disclose to the partner (Gostin, et al., 1998).

Beginning year 2003, 39 states in America have enacted partner notification laws that provide for penalties that range from a **misdemeanor** (a crime less serious than a felony, which is a serious crime) to **attempted murder** for anyone who does not reveal to a sexual partner that he or she is HIV-positive (see Box 8.6). At least 44 states passed laws requiring or permitting workers (mostly health care workers or public safety employees) to be notified of potential exposure of HIV. In some cases, the laws allow testing of the source patient. To date, Arkansas and Missouri are the only states that require patients to notify health care providers of their HIV status before receiving care. All 50 states are now somewhere in the process of establishing the capacity for contact tracing at the request of a patient.

Class Discussion: If a law was passed that made persons who practiced high-risk behaviors and who contracted HIV/AIDS pay for their care and treatment or forego medical help—do you think these people would continue to engage in high-risk behaviors? Would this law be an effective means of HIV transmission prevention? Present examples to support your position. (Can you relate this scenario to those who smoke and develop cancer?)

For a detailed report on partner notification published by the WHO and UNAIDS see: http://www.who.int/asd/knowledge/rptngdiscl.html.

VACCINE DEVELOPMENT

Historically, vaccines have provided safe, cost-effective, and efficient means of preventing illness, disability, and death from infectious diseases through the use of vaccinations.

It is now abundantly clear that no pharmacologic agent, no educational efforts directed to safer sex (regardless of how vigorously implemented), no nutritional modification will stop this epidemic. Halting the spread of HIV requires an effective vaccine. Entering 2003, an estimated 70 million people are either living with HIV or have died from it.

A BRIEF VACCINE PRIMER

The goal of any vaccine is to teach the immune system new and, hopefully better, ways to win the battle against the intruder. There are different types of immune responses, those we were born with (innate immunity) and those the immune system learns (acquired immunity). HIV vaccines are being created to exploit the side of the immune system that is learned (acquired) by providing information to cells in new ways in hopes of enhancing their learning and making them more effective against the virus.

A Little Background

The first line of defense against nearly every new disease is our innate immune responses. It includes cells called dendritic cells (DCs) and natural killer cells (NK cells). These cells are out surveying the body, looking for things that don't belong and trying to get rid of them. They're a bit like a neighborhood watch, looking for suspicious activity but not a specific perpetrator. Our learned or acquired immune system is slower to respond at first, but it is highly specific in its activity and can respond quickly once it has learned a task. It includes specialized T4 or CD4+ T cells, T8 or CD8+ T cells and B cells. Unlike the innate immune response, these specialized cells produced against HIV will move right past other intruders or antigens (i.e. other viruses and bacteria) so if they're HIV-specific cells, they will seek out and destroy HIV-infected cells or if they are HIV-specific antibodies, they will seek out and neutralize HIV floating in the blood. Some HIV-specific cells like the T8 or cytotoxic cells chemically sense the presence of HIV and destroy the human cells that carry HIV. Other immune cells, antigen-presenting cells (APC), show T4 or CD4+ cells bits and pieces of HIV that they have found while surveying the body. Once these APC cells find a CD4+ cell that can learn about HIV (a naïve cell), the CD4+ cell communicates with other cells and provides instructions on how they should respond. Depending on how HIV is shown or presented to the CD4+ cell, the cell will send out different chemical messages to activate a response. One type of response is antibody (also called humoral) responses, which are generated by B cells. Generally these battle viruses and bacteria are free floating in the blood (outside of cells). Another type of response is cellular, which is largely carried out by CD8+ cells. These destroy HIV-infected cells (eliminate virus that is inside the cells). Both humoral and cellular responses are believed to be important in controlling HIV replication, though some scientific debate remains about which, if either, is more important.

What Vaccines Do

The process of recognizing a new intruder or antigen like HIV or other agent and responding takes at least two weeks. If the way the particle of HIV was presented to the CD4+ cell wasn't done right, the entire process of antigen presentation, recognition and response could be crippled or ineffectual. But once an effective response has been learned, the immune system specifically contains and hopefully controls or eliminates it entirely. Vaccines are used to teach these responses to the immune system so that if your immune system ever encounters the same antigen used to create the vaccine—your immune system, taught by the vaccine (memory cells) can act more quickly (in days rather than in weeks). This type of vaccine is called a preventive vaccine because it does not allow the intruder to become established in your body. A therapeutic vaccine is one in which a person is already infected and the disease (signs and symptoms) is in progress. In this case the vaccine lessens the severity of the illness, somewhat like the effect of a drug therapy.

Progress to Date on an HIV Vaccine at Press Time for this Textbook:

A. There are no proven effective therapeutic or preventive HIV vaccines.

B. We don't yet know if the ability of a vaccine to induce HIV-specific immune responses tells us, in and of itself, if the vaccine (or the immune responses) is useful in treating or preventing HIV.

C. HIV vaccines researched to date have had minimal side effects, primarily pain, redness and swelling at the injection site and sometimes transient fever, fatigue and joint stiffness.

D. New vaccines, including the Merck DNA vaccine, have garnered much interest among activists, researchers and people living with HIV. Only results of human study will tell us if this enthusiasm is warranted. Initial studies are underway.

E. Therapeutic HIV vaccine research is still in its infancy.

F. In previous studies, therapeutic vaccines were delivered monthly, by injection.

G. In the short term, it's likely anti-HIV therapy (drugs) will be required in therapeutic HIV vaccine studies.

What Is a Vaccine?

A vaccine is a suspension of whole microorganisms, or viruses, or a suspension of some structural component or product of them that will elicit an immune response after entering a host. In brief, vaccines mimic the organisms or virus that cause disease, alerting the immune system to be aware of certain viruses or bacteria. Because of this advance warning system, when the real organism or virus invades the body, the immune system marshals a response before the disease has time to develop.

Ideally, the body will make neutralizing **antibodies** that bind to and disable the foreign invader (**humoral immunity**) and trigger white blood cells called T cells to organize **attack cells** in the body to destroy those cells that have been infected by viruses (**cellular immunity**). Once the immune system's T cells and B cells, which make antibodies, are activated, some of them turn into **memory cells**. The more memory cells the body forms, the faster its response to a future infection.

Vaccines can trigger these responses in three ways. **Some vaccines, such as those against smallpox, polio (Sabins), measles, mumps, and tuberculosis, contain genetically altered or weakened organisms or viruses that are reproduced in the body after being administered but do not generally produce disease. Yet since the virus or bacterium is still alive, there is a small risk of developing the disease.**

Whooping cough, cholera, and influenza vaccines are made of inactivated whole organisms and virus or pieces of them. Because killed organisms and inactivated virus do not replicate inside the recipient, the vaccines confer only humoral immunity (the production of antibody), which may be short-lived.

Finally, vaccines can be made against toxic products produced by microorganisms. In diseases like tetanus, it is not the bacteria that kill, but the toxins they release into the bloodstream (Christensen, 1994a).

What Is an Effective Vaccine?

An effective viral vaccine usually blocks viral entry into a cell, **but vaccines are generally not 100% effective.** For example, measles vaccine is 95% effective, tetanus 90%, and hepatitis B 85%. Vaccine researchers attending the 7th Conference on Retroviruses and Opportunistic Infections in February 2000 said that they may have to **lower** their sights regarding an AIDS vaccine and settle for one that **does not** completely prevent HIV infection. Based on recent calculations, it has been estimated that a vaccine that is 30% effective against HIV can begin to eradicate the virus if it is widely admistered and accompanied by prevention education. That's why the FDA has indicated that it will approve an HIV/AIDS vaccine at this level of efficacy. David Satcher, former U.S. surgeon general, said on the twentieth anniversary of AIDS that without an effective HIV vaccine by year 2020, AIDS will kill 6.5 million Africans annually!

Because HIV, once inside the cell, is capable of integrating itself into the genetic material of infected cells, a vaccine would have to produce a constant state of immune protection, which not only would have to block viral entry to most cells, but also would continue to block newly produced viruses over the lifetime of the infected person. Such complete and constant protection has never before been accomplished in humans, but it has been accomplished to some degree in cats that are vaccinated against the feline leukemia virus, also a retrovirus (Voelker, 1995). Perhaps more pertinent explanations for why there is still no HIV vaccine nor is one likely to be available soon are the facts that scientists lack sufficient understanding of HIV infection and the biology of HIV disease/AIDS is very complex.

Scientists know that the body defends itself against HIV in the early years of infection. But the great mystery has always been why it cannot neutralize HIV completely. One possibility is that the body has trouble seeing all the variant viruses. Like a Stealth fighter plane, some HIV may have hidden parts that do not show up on the immune system scanner. As a result, the immune system may not produce the right kind of antibody to neutralize all the variant HIVs.

Requirements for an HIV Specific Vaccine

Scientists agree that blocking an infection requires the production of neutralizing antibodies. This is how standard vaccines work: they show the immune system a protein that is unique to the germ. If the germ ever gets into the body, the defenses will quickly make antibodies that latch onto that protein, blocking the germ and destroying it. HIV, however, presents a changing target. It mutates so fast that it constantly changes the proteins on its surface. So a vaccine that triggers an attack against one strain of HIV may be powerless against another. Furthermore, the virus covers its surface with sugar, which hides its proteins from antibodies.

Requirements

The requirements for a preventive HIV vaccine are to generate both humoral and cellular immunity against HIV in the host before exposure to the virus. Following initial exposure to HIV, the generation of cellular immune responses against HIV may take a while to develop, and therefore, neutralizing antibodies against free virus are important to dampen initial viral spread. Subsequently, generation of HIV specific T4 or CD4+ and cytologic T lymphocyte (CTL) cells responses become important in removing HIV-infected cells from the host and in controlling further activation and spread of the virus once established in the host. Thus, both arms of the immune system are important in the immunologic control of HIV infection. However, the amount of neutralizing antibodies and CTLs made after HIV infection are insufficient to rid the body of the virus. In short, the development of an effective vaccine may be the only way to stop the spread of HIV. However, big challenges in developing this vaccine exist: HIV has a high mutation and recombination rate,

and there is no clearly defined natural immunity to HIV. Also, HIV infects cells pivotal to the immune system, and HIV is transmitted as free virus and within infected cells.

Is There Reason for Hope?

There are scientific reasons why there is hope that an HIV vaccine will ultimately be developed. **First**, studies of non-human primates that were given candidate vaccines based on HIV or SIV (simian immunodeficiency virus) have shown either complete or partial protection against infection with the wild type virus. **Second**, successful vaccines have been developed against the Feline Immunodeficiency Virus (FIV), a retrovirus. **Third**, almost all humans develop some form of immune responses that are protective or that are able to control the viral infection over a long time period. Some people have remained free of disease for up to 25 years, often with undetectable viral loads. A group of sex workers from Nairobi and South Africa have remained HIV negative despite continuing high risk exposure; resistance to HIV infection in these people is thought to be due to their ability to mount protective immune responses to HIV. This group and long-term survivors in America have provided insights into strategies for developing a vaccine.

Vaccine Expectations

Vaccines rarely prevent infection; rather they prevent or modify disease. Most vaccines currently in use—for example those for polio, tetanus, diphtheria, measles, hepatitis B, and influenza—**prevent disease without actually preventing infection.** They reduce the number of invading microorganisms, increase the rate of clearance of the infection, prevent the secondary consequences of infection, and prevent transmission. Similarly, few of the candidate HIV vaccines appear promising for preventing infection, and current expectations that HIV vaccines will prevent infection has yielded in the scientific community to the **hope** that they can produce a vaccine that can prevent disease.

Types of HIV Vaccines

Scientists are attempting to design three types of HIV vaccines: **(1)** a **preventive** or **prophylactic**

vaccine to protect people from becoming HIV-infected (chance of success—doubtful); **(2)** a **therapeutic vaccine** (this is not a true vaccination, but a postinfection therapy to stimulate the immune system; the term vaccination is reserved for preventive strategies) for those who are already infected with HIV to prevent them from progressing to AIDS (chance of success—good); and **(3)** a **perinatal vaccine** for administration to pregnant HIV-infected women to prevent transmission of the virus to the fetus (chance of success—good). Stephen Straus and coworkers (1994) reported that researchers have developed a therapeutic vaccine for the herpes virus. The therapeutic vaccine reduces the frequency with which genital sores appear in patients infected with the herpes virus. While it fails to outperform the existing antiherpes drug, acyclovir, it sets the stage for a more effective treatment in the future.

The ability to influence the frequency of genital herpes outbreaks with this vaccine inspires optimism that similar successes may be possible with other chronic viral diseases such as AIDS.

VACCINE PRODUCTION

To make vaccines, scientists use either **dead microorganisms** and **inactivated viruses** or **attenuated viruses** and **microorganisms.** Attenuated means that viruses and other microorganisms are modified; they are capable of reproducing and invoking the immune response but lack the ability to cause a disease.

Use of Attenuated HIV Vaccine— In 1997 data from several labs revealed that a vaccine made from weakened or attenuated SIV-HIV's simian analog can cause AIDS-like symptoms in adult monkeys. These findings that an attenuated vaccine caused AIDS-like disease in monkeys have worried some investigators about attempting to use an attenuated HIV vaccine in humans. Robert Gallo, director of The Institute for Human Virology, believes that a live HIV vaccine is too dangerous. He said that "live, low-replicating retroviruses almost always cause disease; that's been our experience in all animal systems. If those vaccinated do not get disease in three years, it will not tell you what will happen in 10 years or 30 years."

Use of Inactivated Viruses

To inactivate viruses for use in vaccines, the viruses are treated with formalin or another chemical. There is a danger in using inactivated viruses— **they may not all be inactivated.** Inactivated virus vaccines have been made against hepatitis B, rabies, influenza, and polio (Salk vaccine). Salk's first vaccine killed a number of recipients in the late 1950s because not all the polio viruses were destroyed, that is, some could still replicate.

Subunit Vaccines

Subunit vaccines are made from antigenic fragments of an organism or virus most suitable for evoking a strong immune response. Specific subunits can be mass produced and used in pure form to make a specific vaccine. Vaccine against hepatitis B is made from a subunit of the hepatitis B virus and produced in quantity in yeast.

In the United States, researchers are currently basing their vaccine strategies on the use of subunit proteins found in the envelope of HIV.

POINT OF INFORMATION 9.4

HIV VACCINE: PREVENTION AND THERAPY

A LOOK BACK AT THE FIRST VACCINE

The year 1996 marked the 200th anniversary of the first vaccine, which was developed against smallpox. As vaccine researchers launch a new century of challenging disease, they might find inspiration in the early beginnings of immunology, Edward Jenner's discovery.

According to lore, Jenner was a country doctor who heard a rumor that the cowpox virus could provide immunity to smallpox. Investigating the theory, Jenner endured the ridicule of his colleagues before proving his point.

In a now-famous 1796 experiment, Jenner extracted fluid from milkmaid Sarah Nelmes's hand and used it to inoculate the arm of 8-year-old James Phipps, infecting the boy with cowpox pus. Two months later, he again inoculated James but this time he added some smallpox residue. The rest, as they say, is history: James remained healthy! A smallpox vaccine—and the field of vaccinology—was launched.

No viral epidemic has ever been conquered by drug therapy—prevention is the key, and primary prevention via vaccine inoculation is the cornerstone. But, there are enormous problems inherent in constructing an HIV vaccine. **First,** the virus has extraordinary diversity, leaving little chance that just a few subtypes could induce broadly protective immunity. **Second,** the attenuated (weakened) virus strategy that has been so successful for many infections, including smallpox, polio, and measles, will be very difficult if not impossible to implement for HIV. **Third,** HIV attacks the very immune cells that are essential in an immunization procedure, and the immune cell activation that accompanies any immunization will activate HIV replication.

With that said, immunologists are still driven to achieve a most difficult task, the production of an effective HIV-preventive vaccine. Since the first injections of an experimental HIV vaccine were given in the United States in 1987, over 8000 uninfected adults have received about 45 experimental vaccines; 18 people have become HIV-infected from the vaccines. (Bolognesi et al., 1998 updated). Only a handful of HIV vaccines have made it to the second of the three stages of the trials that are needed before any vaccine can be marketed. Beginning year 2002 only one vaccine, AIDSVAX, has reached the third stage, full-scale testing. Worldwide, beginning 2003, there are some 76 experimental vaccines in basic research or animal testing. About 35 of them have been tested in humans. To date most HIV vaccines being developed target surface proteins of HIV. The reason for this approach is that the immune system **first sees** the outside boundaries of HIV—the surface proteins. There is a problem, however: Different clades or strains of HIV carry surface proteins that differ from each other because their genes have changed to make the different strains.

Thus a vaccine made against one strain's surface proteins, say type B (United States), may not work against type C (Africa or India).

VACCINE THERAPY: AN OXYMORON

The term therapeutic vaccine has become the popular terminology when it should be called therapeutic immunization because the administration of the vaccine occurs **after** infection has occurred. Thus, it is a post-infection treatment. A vaccine, by definition, means to prevent infection.

Currently, the main growth area is in therapeutic vaccine research. Rather than using vaccines in an attempt to prevent initial infection, the idea is to vaccinate HIV-positive people being treated with HAART, then halt the drug therapy. Hopefully, the vaccine will stimulate their immune systems sufficiently to bring the infection under long-term control.

One benefit from all of the HIV-vaccine research to date is that scientists found out that they know far less than they thought they knew about producing specific prevention vaccines. For example, scientists believed that vaccines work simply by producing antibodies, right? Well, probably not. This misconception coupled with basic ignorance of how they do work is stalling the urgent quest for an HIV/AIDS vaccine. No one yet has bothered to find out how highly successful vaccines like polio, measles, and hepatitis B actually protect people from disease. Phillippe Kourilsky, director of the Pasteur Institute, said, "We've had many successful vaccines over the past decades but we've missed a chance to see how these vaccines work. Each time a vaccine works the scientific community wanders off and leaves it to the public health workers to use it—and fails to invest in the research. If we had done that we would have been in a much better position to tackle the AIDS vaccine problem." Scientists are, for the first time, learning about the mechanisms of viral-host pathologies necessary to produce preventive vaccines.

The bottom line is, without access to antiretroviral drugs and therapeutic immunization, the 44 million people living with HIV infection ending 2003 will die from AIDS.

DNA VACCINE

What Is a DNA Vaccine?

To make a DNA vaccine, a gene (or length of DNA) that is responsible for making a protein in the infectious virus or organism is inserted into a bacterial plasmid (a circular length of DNA that can replicate by itself inside a bacterial cell). Plasmids carrying the gene of choice are replicated in trillions of bacteria, the bacteria are then broken open and the trillions of plasmids, each carrying a copy of the gene, are purified. The collected plasmids are then given to a patient. **Cells of the person take up the DNA and begin to make the exact protein the gene made while it was in the virus or microorganism from which it was taken.** Such a protein is considered an antigen by the body and the immune system mounts a defense against it.

Advantages of a DNA Vaccine

DNA vaccines have several potential advantages over the traditional methods. It is inexpensive and there's no risk of infection, as there is for inactivated or attenuated vaccines. DNA vaccines are also superior to protein based vaccines because proteins, while being isolated to use an antigen in a vaccine, are easily destroyed. DNA vaccine produces the protein right in the host cell! Also, DNA is a very stable, cheap chemical, even at temperatures close to boiling, a decided advantage in developing countries where refrigeration is scarce.

In March of 1996, the FDA approved the **first** human testing of a vaccine made with pure DNA. Apollon Inc. and the National Institutes of Health tested the experimental AIDS vaccine on 15 (13 men, 2 women) healthy people at the NIH hospital in Bethesda, Maryland in mid-1996. However, these DNA vaccine experiments were not successful! New DNA vaccines are now in study (Calarota et al., 1998).

Potential AIDS vaccines have been given to healthy people before, but this marked the first time a healthy person has received the pure genetic material of any disease-causing agent as a vaccine.

Although scientists are mixing the old traditional ideas of vaccine production with the new, in general there remains the fear that the production of an effective HIV-preventive vaccine may not be possible. But, if it is, it won't be available before the year 2007 and even then it may only be 30% effective in preventing HIV infection! A successful AIDS vaccine will need to induce the formation of broad, cross-reactive neutralizing antibodies against an array of HIV antigens that encompass the majority of HIV strains active in the region of interest and at the same time confer some mucosal immunity. It should be mentioned that to date, there is only one vaccine commercially available against a sexually transmitted disease (hepatitis B vaccine) and it does not stimulate mucosal immunity.

What the World Needs NOW Is a Vaccine for HIV Disease—Why Isn't There One?

On April 24, 1984, Margaret M. Heckler, who was then secretary of the Department of Health and Human Services, announced the discovery of the AIDS virus. **She predicted an AIDS vaccine within two years.** Even though the prediction proved wrong, very wrong, research was guided by the idea that finding the virus was the hard part, and vaccines could be made by simply injecting people with crucial viral proteins. Her optimism was most likely based on the success of the polio, measles, and flu vaccines. **The approach to combating these diseases was: Isolate the virus, develop a vaccine, and prevent the disease!** Since then, in the rush to develop new vaccines, scientists have only belatedly understood that their technical ability to mass produce vaccines has failed to match their knowledge about the cellular and molecular processes used by the body to protect itself from invading pathogens.

Vaccines are designed to provoke the immune system into making antibodies against a disease-causing agent. Most are made of inactivated or attenuated (genetically weakened) viruses and, in the case of some newer vaccines, extracts of viral coat proteins. In some cases, vaccination may result in worsening the disease. The distinction between protective, useless, and dangerous responses is essential for vaccine design.

Vaccines that work well are the most cost effective medical invention known to prevent disease.

PROBLEMS IN THE SEARCH FOR HIV VACCINE

In retrospect, in the movie *Rocky*, Rocky Balboa had it easy. Downing raw eggs at 5 a.m., sprinting through the streets of Philadelphia, pummeling sides of raw beef and pumping out one-armed push-ups prepared him to go the distance against world heavyweight champion Apollo Creed. Brute force was what it took. He won! With regard to developing an HIV/AIDS vaccine, brute force is just one of the ingredients essential to winning.

HIV poses some unique problems for making a human vaccine. **First,** scientists have not established what immune responses are crucial for protecting the body against HIV infection. Studies over the last couple of years have shown that the cell-mediated arm of the immune system may be more important than the HIV antibody response. If this turns out to be true, investigators will have to regroup with respect to producing an HIV vaccine—most vaccines in field trials are geared toward producing sustained HIV antibody responses. Without this information, they cannot tailor the vaccine to produce the most essential immune response.

Second, it is too risky to use the entire weakened or inactive HIV.

Third, HIV undergoes a high rate of mutation as it replicates, and strains from different parts of the world vary by as much as 35% in terms of the proteins that comprise the outer coat of the virus. Even within an infected individual, over a period of years, the virus may change its proteins by as much as 10%. This degree of antigenic drift or variation means that a vaccine made from one strain of HIV may not protect against a different strain. To prove effectiveness, vaccines may have to be tested in geographic areas where the prevalent strains are the same as the strain used in the vaccine.

Fourth, the immune response raised by the vaccine may be protective for only a short period of time. In such cases, booster vaccinations would be required too frequently to be practical.

Fifth, it is possible that the vaccine may make people more susceptible to HIV infection, a vaccine-induced enhancement of infection. That is, vaccine producers are concerned that if they are unable to make a completely HIV-neutralizing vaccine, the vaccine when taken might make the disease worse by **boosting the number of antibodies that might enhance entry of HIV into cells.** For example, enhancing antibodies are thought to be important in a few unusual viral infections such as dengue fever, Rift Valley fever, and yellow fever, in which the antibody binds to the virus and carries it into cells. **Thus, the more**

of a certain kind of antibody you have, the worse the infection can become (Homsy et al., 1989; Levy, 1989).

Sixth, entering year 2003, no vaccine trial to date has been able to stimulate the cellular side of the immune system in the manner necessary to destroy HIV. For example, vaccines involved in current studies do not generate significant numbers of **cytotoxic lymphocytes** nor do they produce significant numbers of **memory T cells** that are necessary to recall the initial response against HIV.

Seventh, Jon Cohen, writing for the journal *Science* (1994a) reported on a *Science survey* of an international sample of over 100 of the field's leading researchers, public health officials, and manufacturers. All told, 67 people from 18 countries on six continents responded. When it came to describing the obstacles that hinder vaccine development, the respondents—be they from Russia, Indonesia, Egypt, Europe, India, or Brazil—had remarkably similar views. **The scientific unknowns are the highest hurdles,** they said, but they also stressed that the field lacks the strong leadership and funding to speed progress.

Predictably, money—or rather, lack of it—was one of the most frequently mentioned obstacles. Even though vaccines are among the most cost-effective medical interventions ever devised, they are not big money-makers. **Drug companies are traditionally reluctant to invest in any form of vaccine development that carries high costs, low profits, and big risks of costly legal suits should accidents occur.** Their current analysis of the state of HIV/AIDS vaccine research is particularly bleak. Of the estimated **$30 billion to $40 billion spent globally each year** on AIDS research, care, and prevention, less than **$500 million** goes into vaccine research. In early 2001, the Bill and Melinda Gates Foundation pledged $100 million for vaccine research.

Eighth, economics clearly isn't the only factor that is discouraging companies from entering the search for an AIDS vaccine. Another is the fact that the science is very tough. Animal models used to test AIDS vaccines have severe limitations; the genetic diversity of HIV may require an effective vaccine to be based on many viral strains; and no researcher has successfully demonstrated which immune responses correlate with protection from HIV (Cohen, 1994b.)

In March 2002, Anthony Fauci told the Presidential Advisory Council on HIV and AIDS that a "broadly effective AIDS vaccine could be a decade or more away."

UPDATE 2002 Bruce Walker of Harvard Medical School presented, at the 2002 14th International AIDS Conference, perhaps the most threatening information yet on why a vaccine may not be possible reasonably soon, if ever! One of Walkers HIV/AIDS patient's, codename ACO6, immune system was holding HIV in check without antiretroviral therapy. But then the man had unprotected sex and became superinfected—he got infected with a second strain of HIV. Even though his immune system was controlling the original HIV strain, it was unable to control the second strain, which ran rampant in his body. Many HIV/AIDS researchers fear that what happened to ACO6 could happen to someone who gets **vaccinated against one strain of HIV but gets exposed to another strain.** HIV is one of the most mutable viruses known to humanity, far more variable than the influenza virus, so the chance of encountering a strain different from the strain found in a vaccine is very high. Ronald Desrosiers, a well-known and respected veteran HIV vaccine researcher who is also from Harvard, described Walker's research as a "huge blow to vaccine development." (For those wanting additional information on HIV superinfection, see Ramos et al. 2002).

Testing HIV Vaccines

Whether a vaccine will stimulate antibody production and is **safe** can be easily determined. It will not require a long time nor will it require many volunteers. To gauge a vaccine's **efficacy** (effectiveness) will require a large number of volunteers who are free of HIV but in danger of becoming infected with it (members of behavioral high-risk groups). To determine a vaccine's efficacy, two large groups of subjects are selected, one that receives the vaccine and one that receives a placebo, to see whether the vaccinated group has a lower rate of HIV infection. In carrying out efficacy trials, the number of participants, the length of the follow-up period, the rate of HIV infection, and the presumed efficacy of the vaccine are related to each other. Because the rate of HIV infection is low, even in high-risk populations, researchers estimate they will need to study several thousand participants to determine whether an HIV vaccine is effective. The original polio vaccine trial

was completed in a year but required nearly half a million children.

An important variable in determining the parameters of the trial is whether the vaccine is prophylactic (preventative) or therapeutic. If the vaccine actually prevents infection, the trial will measure the rate at which participants develop HIV antibodies. If, however, the vaccine allows infection but prevents or greatly retards disease progression, the trial will measure the rate at which disease develops and will therefore require many more years of follow-up.

Morality of Testing HIV Vaccines

Designers of the vaccine trials are confronted with a paradox unique to HIV/AIDS. **If safer-sex and safe-needle practices are not taught,** volunteers who believe they are protected by the unproven vaccine (which may actually be a placebo) could take more risks and increase their chances of becoming infected. **If such practices are taught,** and by ethical standards, they must be, volunteers could cut their risk so effectively that they are never exposed to HIV, leaving the vaccine with nothing to fight. **In a way, the trial depends on the failure of education.** To get around this potential conflict of interest, phase III trials of an AIDS vaccine will have to rely on populations in which the number of infections remains high regardless of education, like young high-risk gay men and injection drug users. **There is also the additional problem of creating vaccine for HIV-positive persons who cannot be distinguished from those who are HIV-infected.** They, too, will be subjected to adverse social, employment, and other discrimination following a positive antibody test.

HIV Vaccine Costs

Perhaps the most difficult moral question is the cost of the vaccine. A successful vaccine that sells for a high price will be of little use to poor and uninsured Americans and most people of developing nations, who have no more than a few dollars a year to spend on health care. Fourteen years have passed since the discovery of a vaccine for hepatitis B, a viral disease that is also spread by sexual contact and the sharing of hypodermic needles. But the product has yet to reach many poor people in the United States and Third World countries largely because it costs about $120 for a series of three injections.

The United States government has spent hundreds of millions of dollars supporting vaccine research. In 2002, the government spent $357 million in vaccine research. Estimate of funds spent in 2003 will top $400 million. Funds from private foundations will add an additional $250 million.

HUMAN HIV VACCINE TRIALS

The goal in producing HIV vaccines is to destroy HIV or keep it in check so that it causes no further damage. **The ideal vaccine will stop progressive immunodefeciency and restore the immune system.** In order to determine if an HIV vaccine will meet these criteria it must ultimately be tested in human vaccine field trials.

The basic principle behind human vaccine trials has changed little since the 19th century. To test for an HIV/AIDS vaccine, several thousand people at high risk for the disease will be inoculated with the experimental agent, most likely an altered version of HIV or some portion of it. The vaccine should not be dangerous enough to cause the disease, but enough like HIV to confer immunity by triggering the production of antibodies and other virus-fighting components of the immune system. The subjects in the trial will be carefully monitored to see if they have a better rate of avoiding infection than others who were not vaccinated.

Beginning in 2003, some 40 trials using at least 39 different HIV vaccines are ongoing worldwide, **and no vaccine has completed Phase III trials anywhere!**

In February 1996 the National Institutes of AIDS and Infectious Diseases announced a joint Phase II vaccine with Pasteur-Meriuex of France and Biocine Inc. of California. Early in 1997, Pasteur Merieux tested one version of the vaccine in about 100 patients. It uses the canary-pox virus to carry HIV genes into the body, where the genes produce proteins that can trigger an immune system alarm. The vaccine and a follow-up booster shot generated antibodies in all 100, a sign the immune system kicked into gear. **It also triggered the mobilization of killer T cells,** the immune system's attack force, in 40% of the people. The canary-pox vaccine is the second AIDS vaccine to make Phase II Testing in the United States. Phase III Trials began in 2002.

In the early 1990s, the BioTechnology Company, Genentech, proceeded with a large study of its therapeutic HIV vaccine, rgp160. Results suggested that the vaccine made no impact on HIV disease progression and there was some indication that people who received the vaccine did slightly worse than those on the placebo. Genentech stopped the study and abandoned efforts in this arena. (Note: This vaccine was later sold to VaxGen, who modified it and is researching it as a preventive vaccine called AIDSVAX).

On June 3, 1998, the FDA gave **VaxGen** permission to begin phase III clinical trials using their antiHIV—**AIDSVAX**—vaccine. Donald Francis, president of VaxGen (Figure 9-5) said "Our primary goal at VaxGen is to develop a vaccine that

FIGURE 9-5 Donald Francis, Virologist and President of VaxGen, Inc. With the CDC in the early 1980s, Francis was one of the **first** people to sound the alarm about the AIDS epidemic and its possible spread through the United States' blood supply. He was instrumental in developing the **AIDSVAX** HIV Vaccine. *(Photograph courtesy of VaxGen Inc., San Francisco)*

can be used around the world and help put an end to an epidemic that already has caused untold suffering and taken more than 12 million lives." AIDSVAX is a preparation of recombinant gp120 (rgp120), the glycoprotein from HIV's envelope that binds to the surface of T4 cells. Injecting rgp120 into the body stimulates production of antibodies that, in any future exposure to HIV, would hopefully **prevent infection**. The Phase III trials in progress involve 60 sites and 5000 volunteers (high-risk women and gay men) in North America. The formulation of AIDSVAX to be used at these sites is designed to protect individuals from strains of HIV found in the Americas, Western Europe, and Australia. The Phase III clinical trials of AIDSVAX in Thailand are regulated by the Thai Health Ministry and involve approximately 2500 volunteers at 17 sites. The formulation of AIDSVAX tested in Thailand is designed to protect against strains of HIV found in Thailand, Korea, Japan, Taiwan, and Indonesia. A growing number of leading vaccine researchers believe that AIDSVAX will fail because the vaccine does not induce HIV-neutralizing antibody and does not induce the production of protective cytotoxic T lymphocytes.

Regardless, VaxGen is satisfied with its data from the first Phase III study and has slated a second Phase III study that began in Thailand in late 2002. This trial is testing whether a prime boost strategy combining two vaccines—the first containing HIV genes in a canarypox virus vector (Aventis Pasteur vCP1521 construct), followed by VaxGen's envelope (gp120) protein sub-unit—can protect against heterosexual HIV transmission. If it proceeds as planned, the trial will be the only third vaccine efficacy study worldwide, and the first to test a prime-boost strategy and to use a community-based population (rather than selected high-risk groups.) A prime boost means that the two vaccines together stimulate a better immune response then either vaccine alone. Other prime boost vaccine studies in humans are now in progress—one in the United Kingdom involving a combination of a DNA vaccine with a modified vaccina vaccine. There is also a prime boost approach now in progress at Sydney's University of New South Wales under the direction of David Cooper. This vaccine contains a DNA vaccine with a bacterial protein known to enhance immune responses

and a foulpox vector used to make several poultry vaccines.

UPDATE 2001/2002 VACCINOLOGY BREAKTHROUGH

Researchers at Harvard Medical School, Emory University, The National Institute of Allergy and Infectious Diseases, Johns Hopkins School of Medicine at Glaxo SmithKline vaccine research laboratories, at Merck research laboratories, and at Oxford University are excited about the newest round of vaccine experiments. A new vaccine, according to Harriet Robinson (Cohen, 2001), showed long-lasting immunity in monkeys. The vaccine, made from pieces of DNA, triggers a powerful antiviral response in monkeys—so strong that none of the vaccinated animals became sick after 40 weeks of the study, despite subsequent exposure to a very virulent type of the monkey form of the AIDS virus. In contrast, most of the control groups of unvaccinated monkeys exposed to the virus have fallen ill, and many have died. The difference between the current monkey vaccines and previous vaccine attempts is that the former vaccines attempted to stimulate antibodies to HIV. The new optimism comes from the fact that scientists are now focusing, with success, on the other arm of the immune system, the white blood cells called **killer T** cells or cytotoxic T8 cells (CTL) which instead of attacking HIV directly, target and destroy HIV-infected cells! **This approach has never been successfully used to create an antiviral vaccine but it does look promising against HIV.** The vaccine, basically a packet of DNA, contains three key segments: gag genes for the core proteins of HIV, genes that code for a segment of SIV (the monkey form of the virus), and genes for human immune system-activating protein called IL-2, or interleukin-2. Although the vaccine-elicited immune responses **did not prevent infection**, they did effectively control virus replication and prevent immunodeficiency, clinical disease progression, and death (Shen et al., 2000; Barouch et al., 2000).

UPDATE 2002   Seven of the vaccinated monkeys in the joint Harvard/Merck vaccine research program to date have been protected by a challenge infection. The eighth monkey died. The eighth vaccinated monkey, known as No. 798, responded differently. Six months into the trial, molecular studies showed the virus in No. 798 mutated its gag gene. Within eight months, the mutated virus levels soared within No. 798. The mutated virus rapidly replaced the original virus. Levels of killer T cell levels plummeted. No. 798 died of AIDS related complications one year after vaccination. Federal scientists who reviewed both the Harvard and Merck studies said that the SHIV strain used in the trials is very aggressive and hard to control. Therefore, the data from these studies may not reflect how vaccines will perform in humans, where HIV infection promotes a more gradual destruction of the immune system. One advantage of the Merck vaccine over others is that the gag gene is common to all strains of HIV. Hence this vaccine, if proven effective, could be used all over the world. Other vaccines, such as AIDSVAX, use gp120, a protein on the surface of HIV that mutates and varies from strain to strain. Therefore, a vaccine effective in Africa many not

work in the United States or other areas of the world.

Problems with Monkey Vaccine Research

There are two unsettling issues of science that critics point to in the recent Harvard/Merck monkey/vaccine efforts. The first is that each potential vaccine was tested in monkeys using an artificial monkey AIDS virus. The second is that none of the products to date actually prevents monkeys from getting the virus or sparks the production of antibodies to fight the virus. They do, however, seem to decrease the likelihood that the virus will progress to AIDS and death by boosting some non-antibody elements of the immune system. But even the non-antibody boosting effect may be an artifact of the way the vaccines were tested. The question of whether this monkey vaccine research will apply to humans begins with the use of the artificial AIDS virus, designated SHIV89.6p. The hybrid SHIV is so different from the natural monkey virus (known as SIV) that it produces a different disease, a different immune response, and therefore, critics charge, protection against a totally artificial phenomenon. SHIV is made from the outer envelope of HIV, the human virus, along with the genes or inner workings of a strain of SIV. This SHIV was a fairly mundane AIDS virus until it was used in monkeys and mutated. It is now so powerful that it kills rhesus macaques in weeks. David Watkins, of the University of Wisconsin in Madison said, "This SHIV became terribly pathogenic. It can obliterate vital immune system cells, called CD4s, and in two weeks (there were) no CD4 cells. That's it. That doesn't occur with HIV in people." Unlike AIDS, SHIV produces a rapidly lethal immune disintegration rather than slow immune system deterioration.

A Word of Caution

As promising as the new monkey research is, its application to humans may prove a regulatory nightmare. That's because the vaccine is made of DNA. The possibility of integration of DNA into human genome will be of regulatory concern. Nobody knows whether such DNA vaccine material would find its way inside normal human genes, and, if it does, whether this could lead to mutations or disruption of human genetics. Until researchers can prove that such potentially dire events will not occur, the Food and Drug Administration is unlikely to approve licensing of DNA vaccines.

Vaccine Testing Confidentiality

Confidentiality must be maintained for the duration of the vaccine trials because people immunized with candidate AIDS vaccines who mount effective immune responses will appear positive for HIV antibody. They may be subject to the social stigma and discrimination associated with being truly HIV positive.

Vaccine-induced seroconversion may lead to difficulties in donating blood, obtaining insurance, traveling internationally, or entering the military. Vaccine-induced antibodies may be long-lived, thus volunteers in AIDS vaccine trials must be given some form of documentation that certifies that their antibody status is due to vaccination and not HIV infection. The National Institute of Allergy and Infectious Disease has (1993) provided a tamper-proof identification card to help uninfected participants in vaccine trials. The seroconversion issue may play a major role in recruitment efforts and in the future welfare of vaccine trial participants (Koff, 1988).

So the question for anyone is: Should I enter an HIV vaccine trial when I know safeguards are limited? I know why I ought to do it . . . but! (Class Discussion)

The Future Preventative Vaccine

Although future preventative vaccine is our best long-term hope to control the pandemic, it will not be a magic bullet replacing other preventive interventions. A future HIV vaccine would have to be used in combination with other preventive interventions to ensure that they contribute efficiently to our overall HIV/AIDS prevention and control effort. In February 2002, AIDS researchers Robert Gallo and Luc Montagnier, who fought a long and bitter battle over credit for the discovery of HIV and the resultant blood test, announced plans to collaborate on developing AIDS vaccines for Africa and other impoverished regions. The goal is to run clinical trials on at least five potential vaccines to pre-

vent the spread of the disease and treat those who already suffer from AIDS. The new partnership, the Gallo/Montagnier Program for International Viral Collaboration will first work to raise $4 million to start the organization and organize the research. They will work with the United Nations to develop research programs in areas with high populations of AIDS patients. The targeted areas include Baltimore, Rome, Montreal, Nigeria, Cameroon, the Ivory Coast, Central America and Asia.

For those wanting additional information about the search for an HIV/AIDS vaccine, the following literature is recommended.

AIDS Vaccine Research
Flossie Wong-Staal and Robert C. Gallo, Eds.
Marcel Dekker, 2002

Shots in the Dark: The Wayward Search for an AIDS Vaccine
by Jon Cohen
W.W. Norton, 2001

HIV and Molecular Immunity: Prospects for the AIDS Vaccine
by Omar Bagasra
Eaton Publishing, 1999

The Search for an AIDS Vaccine: Ethical Issues in the Development and Testing of a Preventive HIV Vaccine (Medical Ethics Series)
by Christine Grady
Indiana University Press, 1995

AIDS Vaccine Resources on the Internet

www.avac.org
www.niaid.nih.gov/daids/vaccine/default.htm
www.fhi.org/en/aids/hivnet/hivnet.html
www.vaccinealliance.org
www.vaccineadvocates.org/avacsite/inde.htm

These addresses will list most of the important vaccine Internet addresses and serve as linkage to others.

An excellent reading on the problems of creating an HIV vaccine and the race to accomplish this miracle is in the book "Shots in the Dark: The Wayward Search for an AIDS Vaccine" by John Cohen, WW Norton Company, ISBN 0393050270.

SUMMARY

The key to stopping HIV transmission lies with the behavior of the individual. That behavior, if the experience of the past 22 years can be used as an indicator, has proven to be very difficult to change.

Changing sexual behavior and using a condom is referred to as **safer sex**. The latex condom is the only condom believed to stop the passage of HIV, and a spermicide should be used with the condom. Oil-based lubricants must not be used because they weaken the condom, allowing it to leak or break under stress. Water-based lubricants are available and should be used. There is at least one female condom, called a vaginal pouch, approved by the FDA and sold worldwide. It is inserted like a diaphragm. It offers protection to both sexual partners.

Over 8000 cases of HIV infection have come from contaminated blood transfusions. A test developed in 1985 to screen all donated blood in the United States has reduced the risk of HIV transfusion infection. But blood bank screening has reduced the size of the blood donor pool. Many hospitals are encouraging people who know they might need an operation to donate their own blood for later use—autologous transfusion.

Ending 2002 there was only one FDA-approved vaccine in Phase III trials, AIDSVAX: many top HIV/AIDS scientists have ruled out the use of an attenuated HIV vaccine before the year 2003. Inactivated whole virus vaccines are also being held back because there is no 100% guarantee that all HIV used in the vaccine will be inactivated.

Even if a vaccine does well in Phase III trials, will it be effective against all of the HIV mutants in the HIV gene pool? Can the threat of vaccine-induced enhancement of HIV infection be overcome? How are vaccine testing agencies going to handle the ethical question of vaccine seroconverting normal subjects to positive antibody status? The social repercussions may be devastating for those who, when tested, test HIV positive even though they are HIV-free.

There are some 5.3 million health care workers in the United States. It is crucial that they adhere to the Universal Protection Guidelines set down by the CDC, as a significant number of them are exposed to the AIDS virus annually. The risk of HIV infection after **exposure** to HIV-contaminated blood is about 1 in 200.

A few states have implemented HIV partner notification; many other states are beginning to experiment with HIV partner notification or contact tracing programs. It is too early to tell just how successful locating and testing high behavioral risk partners will be, or the cost-to-benefit ratio. One thing is certain: If these programs are to be successful, they will have to ensure confidentiality to those who are traced. Partner notification or contact tracing continues to work well for other sexually transmitted diseases.

REVIEW QUESTIONS

(Answers to the Review Questions are on page 489.)

1. Which is the better condom for protection from STDs, one made from lamb intestine or one made from latex rubber? Explain.

2. Which lubricant is best suited for condom use? Explain.

3. Briefly explain safer sex.

4. True or False: If a person has unprotected intercourse with an HIV-infected partner, he or she will become HIV-infected. Explain.

5. Yes or No: If injection drug users (IDUs) were given free equipment—no questions asked—would that stop the transmission of HIV among them? Explain.

6. What is the current risk of being transfused with HIV-contaminated blood in the United States?

7. What do you think should happen in cases where a person who knows he or she is HIV positive, lies at a donor interview, and donates blood?

8. Why do most scientists wish to avoid using an attenuated HIV vaccine or an inactivated HIV vaccine?

9. What is the advantage of using recombinant HIV subunits in making a vaccine?

10. Explain vaccine-induced enhancement. How does it occur?

11. Why is it necessary to practice strict confidentiality with respect to volunteers for AIDS vaccine tests?

12. What are universal precautions? Who formulated them?

13. True or False: Research continues to show that AIDS prevention messages are effective in causing teens to change their sexual behaviors.

14. True or False: Latex condoms eliminate the risk of HIV transmission.

15. True or False: Partner notification is usually performed by the infected individual or a trained and authorized health department official.

16. True or False: The Centers for Disease Control and Prevention estimates that as many as 1 in 100,000 units of blood in the blood supply may be contaminated with HIV.

17. True or False: The three types of vaccines that scientists are interested in developing are preventive, therapeutic, and perinatal vaccines.

18. True or False: Used disposable needles should be recapped by hand before disposal.

19. True or False: Prompt washing of a needle stick injury with soap and water is sufficient to prevent HIV infection.

20. True or False: The FDA approved the **first** vaccine for broad-scale testing in the United States in 1997.

21. HIV/AIDS is not curable, but it is **preventable**. Write a short essay on the best methods of prevention.

22. HIV/AIDS Search-a-Word (below).

HIV/AIDS SEARCH-A-WORD

H	L	C	V	V	A	L	Y	L	L	L	E	C	T
H	C	A	E	L	B	D	O	K	R	S	A	R	A
R	T	N	G	R	O	S	N	S	D	I	A	Y	C
I	N	C	U	B	A	T	I	O	N	N	I	D	Q
N	E	G	I	T	N	A	O	M	S	N	M	D	U
R	D	T	S	M	F	C	I	M	Y	Y	M	U	I
O	N	E	M	I	X	A	I	R	N	X	U	V	R
A	E	P	O	C	E	S	S	N	D	O	N	U	E
W	X	P	D	T	S	U	D	B	R	A	E	N	D
P	P	S	N	I	E	A	N	P	O	A	S	R	C
N	O	H	O	N	F	L	T	H	M	T	Y	D	C
M	S	N	C	F	A	C	M	C	E	O	S	I	D
A	U	M	I	E	S	O	O	D	O	M	T	R	C
T	R	R	M	C	N	N	H	I	V	S	E	T	R
R	E	N	M	T	M	T	I	T	I	O	M	R	D
O	M	E	U	I	N	A	C	N	H	N	H	N	T
D	H	G	N	O	M	C	U	O	C	S	I	M	I
A	G	O	O	N	A	T	A	A	D	E	N	I	I
H	M	H	S	C	R	D	V	T	R	R	H	S	T
E	O	T	U	O	N	I	C	O	M	O	O	I	R
M	C	A	P	A	D	T	S	A	A	P	C	D	I
O	M	P	P	N	I	H	I	K	A	O	I	M	I
P	O	G	R	A	D	M	N	K	H	S	I	T	A
H	R	H	E	S	N	T	O	M	E	I	C	I	V
I	R	C	S	U	O	R	I	A	I	T	I	D	A
L	G	I	S	R	T	C	S	I	C	I	R	T	R
I	L	O	E	I	D	E	N	R	D	V	O	V	O
A	T	G	D	V	A	C	C	I	N	E	X	D	R

ACQUIRED
AIDS
ANTIBODY
ANTIGEN
BLEACH
CASUAL CONTACT
CDC
CONDOMS
DISEASE
EXPOSURE
HEMOPHILIA
HIV
IMMUNE SYSTEM
INCUBATION
IMMUNOSUPPRESSED
INFECTION
IV
KAPOSI
OPPORTUNISTIC
PATHOGEN
PWA
RISK
SAFE SEX
SEROPOSITIVE
STD
SYNDROME
T-CELL
TRANSMISSION
VACCINE
VIRUS

Prevalence of HIV Infections, AIDS Cases, and Deaths Among Select Groups in the United States and AIDS in Other Countries

10

CHAPTER CONCEPTS

- ◆ AIDS is a new plague.
- ◆ Worldwide, 50 percent of new HIV infections are in people under age 25.
- ◆ Worldwide, about 16,000 new HIV infections occur daily.
- ◆ Worldwide, women represent 41% of all HIV-infected adults.
- ◆ AIDS is now the world's leading cause of death by an infectious disease.
- ◆ AIDS is now ranked fourth in causes of death worldwide.
- ◆ In the United States, men make up 80% of all AIDS cases; 20% are women.
- ◆ The majority of people with AIDS can be associated with certain **lifestyle risks.**
- ◆ AIDS can be associated with single or multiple exposure risks.
- ◆ AIDS cases can be separated by sex, age group, race, ethnicity, and sexual preference.
- ◆ Risk is strongly tied to social behavior.
- ◆ At-risk groups include homosexual and bisexual men, injection drug users (IDUs), hemophiliacs, transfusion patients, and the sex partners of these people.
- ◆ HIV infection is strongly associated with injection drug use.
- ◆ All military personnel are tested for HIV.
- ◆ Two per 1000 college students are HIV-infected.
- ◆ Thirty-nine states report HIV-infected by name.
- ◆ High rates of HIV infection have been found among prisoners.
- ◆ The greatest HIV threat to health care workers is needle stick (syringe) injuries.
- ◆ All 50 states and U.S. territories must report all AIDS cases.
- ◆ January 2003: **reported** AIDS cases in the United States reaches 850,000.
- ◆ A case can be made for national HIV reporting.
- ◆ People do not always tell the truth when completing questionnaires, especially with regard to sexual behavior.
- ◆ Ending year 2003, an estimated 70 million people worldwide will have been HIV-infected.

The World Trade Center and the Pentagon were attacked on September 11, 2001. No one expected to see commercial airliners hijacked and flown into crowded skyscrapers and government buildings. Likewise, in the early 1980s, no one expected the sudden appearance of a deadly new disease spreading across the cities and of America. It was only a few years earlier that some prominent scientists declared that the fight against infectious disease was over. The horrible damage caused by fuel-laden airliners crashing into buildings and exploding into a fiery inferno was all but beyond our imagination. Equally beyond our imagination was this new disease that appeared 22 years ago. It was a disease that appeared without warning and seemed to lead to a painful, agonizing death in just a few weeks for some, a few months for others. The depth and scope of human destruction was so unprecedented that only a few people were quick to recognize the horror that was to come. On September 11, while the image of the jetliners with their passengers exploding into the World Trade Center was still painfully fresh, we were further stunned to see these seemingly invincible structures collapse in upon themselves, crushing almost three thousand men, women and children in a vast cloud of toxic dust, rubble and fire. A week earlier, no one would have believed that such pillars of concrete and steel could possibly collapse, let alone from the top down. In the tragedy that began to unfold in the beginning of the 1980s, scientists were puzzled and bewildered as they watched a disease that led to the collapse of the human immune system. Working from the inside out, here was a diabolically clever virus that destroyed the very system that was otherwise designed to defeat it. Truly, the beginning of AIDS in America in 1981 was the greatest plague in history to cross the globe, and the 2001 attack on the WTC and the Pentagon, the largest attack on the United States, caused the greatest loss of life since the Japanese attack on Pearl Harbor. The two have much in common. Both tragedies have appeared over and again on television. Both require the best in people to set them right—to save lives. The United States and the world must not let terrorists or HIV determine our way of life. Both require acts of heroism and research. Both require sacrifice, resolve and the determination to overcome. Both have placed America and the world in a race against time.

The News Media on AIDS, Terrorism and the Economy from September 11, 2001 through September 11, 2002

AIDS has now been with us for about 22 years. The terrorist attack on America on September 11, 2001, was new; for those watching television it happened in front of their eyes in about an hour. The largest collapse of a financial empire, ENRON, followed, beginning in December 2001, and also occurring relatively quickly. Both terrorism and Enron became instant hits on the nightly news along with a large variety of daylong network coverage. Although there were other events occurring worldwide, terrorism and Enron overshadowed everything. As Danny Schechter wrote, front-page stories were stuck on stories beginning with A: Arms, Al-Qaeda, Ashcroft, Annan, Arafat,

Arthur Anderson, Anthrax and Afghanistan. But one A is, for the most part, missing: AIDS. That omission says a lot about the state of the world and the world of news.

The Result of Omission

When AIDS isn't visible in the media, it doesn't exist for many communities that rely on media to tell them what matters most. This is true not only in the West, but in Africa and in other developing nations, where stigma and discrimination against AIDS sufferers is deeply entrenched, and where silence and denial still drive many governments to cover up their frightening levels of HIV infection. Often the young people who most need to know how to protect themselves have few programs directed their way. At the same time, there are many stirring and effective responses led by unsung young heroes whose stories could inspire a greater mobilization. But who is going to tell these stories if the media doesn't? AIDS will surpass the Bubonic plague or the Black Death of Asia and Europe in the 14th century unless a vaccine is found. That plague killed about 40 million people. Ending 2003, about 26 million will have died from AIDS. The 40 million mark will be reached about 2008.

A WORD ABOUT DATA

All HIV/AIDS data, including data from the Centers for Disease Control and Prevention (CDC), Joint United Nations Program on HIV/AIDS (UNAIDS), World Health Organization (WHO), and other organizations should be treated as broadly indicative of trends rather than accurate measures of HIV/AIDS prevalence. A large number of HIV/AIDS cases in developing countries, in particular, are underreported due to a lack of adequate medical and administrative personnel, the stigma associated with the disease, or the reluctance of countries to incur the loss of trade, tourism, and other losses that such revelations might produce.

Because morbidity and mortality of HIV/AIDS cases are multicausal, diagnosis and reporting can vary significantly, thereby distorting comparisons. The WHO and other international entities are dependent on such data despite its weaknesses and are often forced to extrapolate or build models based on relatively small samples, as in the case of

HIV/AIDS. Changes in methodologies, moreover, can produce differing results; for example, the ranking of AIDS mortality ahead of TB mortality. This is partly due to the fact that HIV-positive individuals dying of TB were included in the AIDS mortality category in the most recent WHO survey. Another example is the global data on those living with HIV/AIDS. The UNAIDS global data says there are 40 million such people ending 2001 but this estimate results from a low estimate of 30 million and a high estimate of 50 million—recognizably a large margin for error. Such data comes from using a relatively simple equation that calculated low- and high-risk populations with the crude adult death rate and the HIV-infected survival rate, along with variables including the start date of HIV for that country and the demand for risky sex. The bottom line is that estimates are just that—estimates. However, estimates prove to be very useful in predicting what is occurring now and in what lies ahead. Caution must be exercised, however, because the definition of AIDS differs between countries. The criteria used to diagnose a person with AIDS varies significantly from developed nations, where an HIV test is administered, to underdeveloped nations like Africa where HIV tests are generally not available and the diagnosis is based on certain signs and symptoms.

BOX 10.1

REFLECTIONS FROM THE XIV INTERNATIONAL AIDS CONFERENCE— BARCELONA, SPAIN, JULY 7–12, 2002

In July 2001, during the 13th International AIDS Conference in Durban, South Africa, the meetings were abuzz with the sense that the worst was apparently over for Africa as far as the AIDS pandemic was concerned. Models of how many patients the virus could infect—as high as 35% of adults in the nation of Botswana—indicated the peak had been reached, and although the situation in the sub-Saharan area was grave, recovery was on the horizon. In 2002, at the 14th International AIDS Conference in Barcelona, Spain, researchers said they now realize the epidemic has, in fact, worsened in Africa. New studies foreshadow the expanding epidemic spreading into Eastern Europe, the Caribbean and the massive populations of India and China—where in numbers alone, the epidemic could double in size in just a few years.

About 16,000 physicians, scientists, patients, politicians and charity workers attended the six-day AIDS Conference in Barcelona. An American delegation led by Health and Human Services Tommy Thompson attended. He is the first cabinet-level official to attend an International AIDS Conference. At the top of the agenda was the UNAIDS report suggesting that the epidemic is still in its early stages and is spreading fast. Peter Piot, Executive Director of UNAIDS said, "We did not come to Barcelona to renegotiate promises. We are here to ignite leadership, to keep the promise. It is clear that we are only at the beginning of the pandemic, the largest pandemic in human history, and the worst is yet to come. The AIDS pandemic is expected to peak in 2060! In addition, the HIV/AIDS pandemic is worsening an impending famine in southern Africa that endangers the lives of some 12 million people. Many of those infected are agricultural workers, of which 7 million have already died from AIDS in severely infected African countries and 16 million more will die over the next 20 years." Piot continued with, "Overall, the figures speak horrors: during the six days of this conference about 48,000 people died from AIDS and some 84,000 become HIV infected. Between 2000 and 2020, 68 million people will have died of AIDS in the 45 most-affected countries—five times the number of deaths in the previous two decades. In 2001, an estimated 3 million people died of AIDS. Collectively, we have grossly, grossly underestimated how bad this was going to be." Clearly such data has catapulted AIDS into a very serious high priority global issue. About $3 billion was spent on AIDS prevention and drugs therapy in 2001 and 2002, but at least $10 billion a year is required if lives are to continue and for countries to remain solvent with their gross national product and national security intact.

During an interview, Piot said, "If Durban 2000 AIDS Conference was a wake up call, Barcelona 2002 is likely to be the 'yes, but . . .' conference, with the biggest cautionary being accountability. Will promises be kept?"

It took 21 years from the first recognition of HIV in America to a global political commitment— 180 countries signing the United Nations

BOX 10.1 *(continued)*

General Assembly Special Session (UNGASS) declaration on HIV/AIDS in 2001. How long will it take for accountability to kick in? Slowly the world is becoming aware that this disease is a global political issue and accountability is shifting to those who lead world governments! It is only since the 13th International AIDS Conference in Durban, South Africa, in 2000 that the world has awakened to the unrelenting catalogue of horrors, 14 million AIDS-associated orphans, the prediction of 68 million additional deaths worldwide, 55 million of them in Africa by the year 2020; the destruction of the economies of 45 nations; the finding that the pandemic has not yet begun to level off in Africa, even in the highest prevalence countries; that without major intervention in India more than 13 million people could be infected with HIV by 2010, and that the pandemic is now, conclusively and irreversibly, a ferocious assault on women of all ages. According to the July 2002 UNAIDS report, of the 29 million infected adults in sub-Saharan Africa, women now constitute 17 million, or 58%. Linking this data to the data from the June 2002 UNICEF report reveals a nightmare scenario for women. At the beginning of that document, there is a breakdown of the numbers of young people (defined as 15 to 24) living with AIDS in various regions of the world. For sub-Saharan Africa, the total is 8.8 million, two-thirds, or 67% of whom are young women. The ratio of young women to young men, is two to one. Put in the context that more than half the new infections now occur among young people, about 7000 a day, one recognizes what may happen in Africa. With the current infection rate of 58%, and the future rate of 67%, the unthinkable may happen . . . a cataclysm of HIV/AIDS for the women of Africa. People attending this conference as with the 13th Conference held in Durban, South Africa, were embarrassed and angered by the continued disregard by the South African government for accepted antiretroviral therapy, especially for their position against the use of drugs to prevent mother to child HIV transmission, regardless of the fact that South Africa's High Court ruled in June 2002 that the government is required to permit use of such drugs. Just one week later, at the XIV International AIDS Conference, Health Minister Manto Tshabalala-Msimang told of her unhappiness with the ruling, and her characterization of the drug nevirapine (used to prevent mother to child transmission) as "poison." She said with anger, "We will implement because we are forced to implement. The High Court has decided the Constitution says I must give my people a drug. That I must poison my people."

Barcelona HIV/AIDS Protesters

Thousands of AIDS activists took to the streets in Barcelona at the Conference's "March for Life" demanding "AIDS treatment now" for the world's HIV infected, 98% of whom do not receive life-saving treatment. One of the chants during the march was "Stop the Dying, Stop the Crying." Inside the meetings protesters began blowing whistles and shouting "Shame! Shame!" and "No More Lies!" as the U.S. Secretary of Health and Human Services, Tommy Thompson, came to the podium. They continued until he finished his address. There was no violence or attempt to stop the demonstration, and there were no arrests. Thompson declared that "no administration in any nation has ever made fighting HIV/AIDS as high a priority," but virtually no one in the huge room could hear him as a group of chanting protesters crowded onstage with him. This was a replay of a scene at the AIDS conference in San Francisco in 1990, when Louis Sullivan, health and human services secretary under President Bush's father, was drowned out by protesters using megaphones and whistles. Ironically, Sullivan was sitting in the audience in Barcelona witnessing this protest.

In other protests, Coca-Cola, the largest employer in Africa, endured AIDS activists' protests because Coca-Cola did not provide heath care coverage to all its employees. But, Coca-Cola is providing antiretroviral drugs to those workers who require them. Marchers also circled the exhibition booths of Roche and Gilead Pharmaceutical exhibitions shouting "access for all", blowing whistles, and virtually destroyed the booths with spray paints, etc. because their antiretrovirals costs too much. Protesters also stopped at the UNAIDS booth where various speakers from the region denounced the lack of commitment on the part of national governments in the region as well as the International Agencies, including UNAIDS and PAHO, whose role is to facilitate expanded access to care and treatment by dialoguing with and supporting National AIDS programs.

BOX 10.1 *(continued)*

A Summary to the 2002 XIV International AIDS Conference in Barcelona

After a week of rowdy protests, bold proclamations, serious scientific exchange and intense hand-wringing, the 14th International AIDS Conference finished on a weary note. Twenty-one years into the epidemic, AIDS has become a banker's tale: Developing nations need $10 billion a year from the rich to stop this pandemic. At best, they may get $3 billion a year. The numbers, whether billions of unavailable dollars or millions of projected deaths, are simply mind-numbing, and the lofty calls for action, repeated at these gatherings every two years, are growing shopworn. In 2004, at the 15th International AIDS Conference in Bangkok, it will be abundantly clear whether there is real progress to report, or whether the eloquence at Durban in 2000 and the Barcelona in 2002 were useless. By the time the conference closed, 10 former and current prime ministers and presidents presented their views on the global HIV/AIDS pandemic. The power politicians included former U.S. President Bill Clinton, former South African President Nelson Mandela, Rwandan President Paul Kagame and Mozambican President Pascoal Mocumbi. Barcelona ended up being largely a political meeting, filled with calls/demands for the developed nations to monetarily solve the problems of the underdeveloped nations.

THE MILLENNIUM: YEAR 2003

As we begin this third year of the new millennium and enter into the early years of the **third decade of AIDS,** it is evident that the small epidemic recognized among a handful of homosexual men in 1981 is quite different from the global pandemic of today. For developed countries, current antiretroviral regimens are allowing HIV-infected individuals to live longer, healthier lives. However, the use of these regimens may be associated with complacency and a relapse to unsafe sexual practices resulting in sustaining the HIV epidemic, as will be discussed. For developing countries the problem is far more complex. The infrastructure to support the use of antiretroviral drugs is not in place, the cost of the drugs is too high, and the vast majority of HIV-infected people do not even know they are infected. Education and condom distribution campaigns have had limited success, but they remain the primary avenues of prevention.

Developed Countries: The AIDS Crisis is Over?

In the developed nations, too many people think the AIDS crisis is over. **Think again.** UNAIDS reported that in 2000 and 2001, each year 3 million people died of AIDS and over 5 million a year became HIV infected. Beginning year 2003, the AIDS pandemic has killed about 26 million people! UNAIDS estimates that ending year 2003, 70 million people have been HIV-infected, about 44 million of them are alive. Ninety-five percent of infections are in developing nations that hold 10% of the world's wealth. There is still neither a cure nor an effective vaccine.

Entering the year 2003 there does not appear to be an immediate end to either the spread of HIV infection or the devastation caused by AIDS. Looking back over the 1980s and the 1990s, it is clear that scientists and the public have consistently **underestimated** the magnitude and the potential of the HIV/ AIDS pandemic. Who would have imagined in the mid-1980s that HIV would eventually spread to every country of the world, infecting 70 million people and resulting in about 26 million deaths ending year 2003. The numbers become so large that the individuals suffering and the personal, societal, and economic losses become impossible to measure or to even attempt to estimate. While there have been successes in slowing the epidemic in some communities and dramatic advances in survival in developed countries due to combination anti-retroviral therapy, it is very important that people do not become complacent and focus on false beliefs that the pandemic is declining, that individuals are becoming less infectious, or that HIV control will be much better in the 21st century. If anything, the limited successes in prevention should encourage a continued effort to work harder at educating more people about how best to prevent further transmission through safer sex practices, antiretroviral therapy during pregnancy, treatment of STDs, provision of condoms, screening of the blood supply, the use of sterile needles, or many of the other avenues that can help to slow the pandemic until a vaccine can be developed.

Currently, UNAIDS reports that each day about 14,000 people become newly infected with HIV, or 10 men, women, and children per minute. Eleven percent of the newly infected people are under age 15. Over 50% of new infections are now occurring in people between ages 15 and 24, primarily due to sexual transmission. Worldwide women now represent 47% of all people over age 15 living with HIV infection. Ending 1998, UNAIDS reported that AIDS had become the **world's most deadly infectious disease.** It reached this level of human devastation in just 18 years. Of all causes of death worldwide, AIDS has moved up to **fourth place.** AIDS was associated with at least 2.5 million deaths each year for the last five years. All of these data are a bit ironic because as Peter Piot, executive director of UNAIDS said, "The pandemic is out of control at the very time when we know what to do to prevent its spread."

HIV Infections: Overwhelming Numbers in the United States

It is easy to be overwhelmed by statistics in reporting on HIV infections and AIDS cases and to lose track of the human faces of the epidemic. But certain numbers, like the **first half-million documented AIDS cases reported in October 1995** and about 480,000 dead beginning year 2003, take on a compelling quality of their own. Therefore, within this chapter there are many statistics presented on all facets of the HIV/AIDS pandemic. **After reading this chapter one will have gained a deeper insight into the spread of HIV and those who are affected by HIV: those who have it, and those who don't—those who will suffer and those who won't. In reality we are all impacted by this disease in one way or another!**

Prevalence/Incidence: How Many People Are HIV Positive?

The **prevalence** of a disease refers to the percentage of a population that is affected by it at a given time. **Prevalence = total number of AIDS cases** at a given time divided by total population at the same time. The **incidence** means the number of times an event occurs in a given time frame, for example, the number of new AIDS cases each month or new HIV infections each week (events that occur within a specified period of time). The two terms are similar. Much has been learned about the prevalence of HIV infection, HIV disease, and its terminal stage called AIDS since the 1981 CDC report that awakened the world to this new pandemic.

Although cases of AIDS appear retrospectively to have occurred in the United States as early as 1952, the **AIDS pandemic** in the United States is considered to have begun with the initial report in **June 1981.** Since then, the HIV/AIDS pandemic has become the most serious pandemic to occur worldwide since the **Spanish flu** of 1918, which killed between 20 million and 50 million people but lasted less than a year!

FORMULA FOR ESTIMATING HIV INFECTIONS

A newer formula proposed by the CDC for use in determining the number of HIV-infected persons is as follows:

National Number of Persons Living With AIDS (1997)		Number of PLWA in Your City (1997)

$$\frac{258,000}{900,000} \times \frac{\text{(e.g.,) } 1,000}{x} = 258,000$$

(Estimated national number of HIV-infected persons)

$$x = 900,000,000$$

$$x = \frac{900,000,000}{258,000}$$

$$= 3,488$$

(About 3,488 persons in this sample city are HIV-infected.)

Single or Multiple Exposure Categories

In Table 10-1, the number of AIDS cases estimated through 2002 are presented with respect to adult/adolescent, **single** or **multiple** exposure categories. For example, under *Single Mode of*

Table 10-1 Total Adult/Adolescent AIDS Cases by Single and Multiple Exposure Categories, Estimated Beginning 2003, United States

| | AIDS Cases | |
Exposure Category	No.	(%)
Single Mode of Exposure		
1. Men who have sex with men	370,040	(44)
2. Injection (IJ) drug use	168,200	(20)
3. Hemophilia/coagulation disorder	8410	(1)
4. Heterosexual contact	92,510	(11)
5. Receipt of blood transfusion	8410	(1)
6. Receipt of transplant of tissues/organs	17	(0)
7. Other/undetermined	155	(0)
Single Mode of Exposure Subtotal	647,570	(77)
Multiple Modes of Exposure		
1. Men who have sex with men; IJ drug use	42,050	(5)
2. Men who have sex with men; hemophilia	170	(0)
3. Men who have sex with men; heterosexual contact	16,820	(2)
4. Men who have sex with men; receipt of transfusion/transplant	3690	(0)
5. IJ drug use; hemophilia	196	(0)
6. IJ drug use; heterosexual contact	42,050	(5)
7. IJ drug use; receipt of transfusion	1655	(0)
8. Hemophilia; heterosexual contact	106	(0)
9. Hemophilia; receipt of transfusion/transplant	812	(0)
10. Heterosexual contact; receipt of transfusion/transplant	1655	(0)
11. Men who have sex with men; IJ drug use; hemophilia	52	(0)
12. Men who have sex with men; IJ drug use; heterosexual contact	8410	(1)
13. Men who have sex with men; IJ drug use; receipt of transfusion/transplant	612	(0)
14. Men who have sex with men; hemophilia; heterosexual contact	23	(0)
15. Men who have sex with men; hemophilia; receipt of transfusion/transplant	40	(0)
16. Men who have sex with men; heterosexual contact; receipt of transfusion/transplant	272	(0)
17. IJ drug use; hemophilia; heterosexual contact	83	(0)
18. IJ drug use; hemophilia; receipt of transfusion/transplant	40	(0)
19. IJ drug use; heterosexual contact; receipt of transfusion/transplant	1112	(0)
20. Hemophilia; heterosexual contact; receipt of transfusion/transplant	38	(0)
21. Men who have sex with men; IJ drug use; hemophilia; heterosexual contact	14	(0)
22. Men who have sex with men; IJ drug use; hemophilia; receipt of transfusion/transplant	15	(0)
23. Men who have sex with men; IJ drug use; heterosexual contact; receipt of transfusion/transplant	175	(0)
24. Men who have sex with men; hemophilia; heterosexual contact; receipt of transfusion/transplant	6	(0)
25. IJ drug use; hemophilia; heterosexual contact; receipt of transfusion/transplant	24	(0)
26. Men who have sex with men; IJ drug use; hemophilia; heterosexual contact; receipt of transfusion/transplant	8	(0)
Multiple Modes of Exposure Subtotal	117,740	(14)
Risk Not Reported or Identified	75,690	(9)
Total AIDS Cases	841,000	(100)

(Source: For exposure categories. CDC HIV/AIDS Surveillance Report, through 2002, 11:1–45, updated)
Pediatric AIDS cases = 9281 (Total AIDS cases about 850,000)

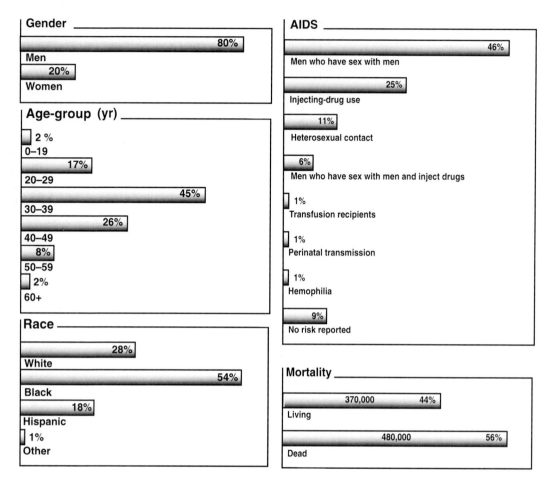

FIGURE 10-1 A Profile of 850,000 AIDS Cases: June 1981 through Beginning, 2003—United States. Four hundred and eighty thousand people died of AIDS to this point in time. Data may not add to 100% due to rounding off. *(Source: MMWR, 1995b, updated)*

Exposure, heterosexual contact accounts for 10% of all AIDS cases. Under *Multiple Modes of Exposure,* 5% of AIDS cases occurred among injection drug users who also had heterosexual contact. In other words, Table 10-1 lists the numbers and percentages of all reported AIDS cases broken down into seven categories of people who contracted HIV/AIDS from a **single risk mode of exposure** and 26 categories of people who contracted HIV/AIDS from **multiple risk modes of exposure.** Note that of the total number of adult/adolescent AIDS cases, 77% occurred from **single risk** modes of exposure. Of this 77%, 44% occurred among men who had sex with men and about 20% among injection drug users.

A composite representation of all AIDS cases by exposure category estimated beginning 2003 is shown in Chapter 8, Figure 8-1.

BEHAVIORAL RISK GROUPS AND STATISTICAL EVALUATION

Behavioral Risk Groups and AIDS Cases

As the pool of AIDS patients grew in number during 1981–1983, individual case histories were separated into **behavioral risk groups.** The early case histories of AIDS patients clearly separated people according to their social behavior and medical needs. AIDS patients were placed into the following six risk behavior categories: (1) homosexual and bisexual men; (2) injection drug users; (3) hemophiliacs; (4) blood transfusion recipients; (5) heterosexuals; and (6) children whose parents are at risk. Each of these groups is considered to be at risk of HIV infection based on some common behavioral denominator. That is, those within these groups represented a higher rate of AIDS cases than people whose needs or behaviors excluded them from these groups. However, because there is some mixing between individuals in behavioral risk groups, HIV infection has gradually spread to lower-risk behavioral groups. Over time the behavioral risk groups have been aligned and defined according to age, exposure category, and sex (see Table 10-1).

A review of AIDS cases by sex/age at diagnosis, and race/ethnicity reported through December 2001 in the United States, shows that **white, black, and Hispanic males between the ages of 20 and 44 make up 79% of all male AIDS cases. Between ages 20 and 59, they make up 97% of all male AIDS cases.** People between the ages of 25 and 44 make up over half the nation's 138 million workers! In 1998 in the United States, one in six worksites with over 50 employees and one in 16 small businesses have/had an employee with HIV/AIDS. Of the total number of male AIDS cases, 43% are white, 38% are black, and 18% are Hispanic.

Statistical Evaluation of Selected Risk Behavioral Group AIDS Cases

Adult/Adolescent AIDS Cases— On October 31, 1995, the United States reached **a half-million** (501,310) reported AIDS cases (*MMWR*, 1995a). Beginning year 2003, 850,000 AIDS cases and about 480,000 AIDS-related deaths were reported to the CDC (Figure 10-1 on the facing page). Sixty-six percent of all AIDS cases reported occurred between 1993 through 1999. Cumulative through 2002, 11% of AIDS cases have occurred among the heterosexual population, 25% occurred among injection drug users, and 52% occurred in the male homosexual/bisexual IDU population. For 1996, the first time since the United States AIDS pandemic began, more blacks were diagnosed with AIDS (41%) than whites (38%). Table 10-2 presents the total estimated number of AIDS cases for 2002 and their distribution based on race, sex, and exposure group.

BOX 10.2

THE HIV/AIDS SCENARIO

HIV/AIDS is unstoppable in the short term. Because it takes an HIV infection so long to develop into AIDS, virtually all the AIDS cases that occur during the next 5 to 20 years will be the result of existing infections. Therefore, the epidemic **cannot** be materially reduced in this time frame by any reduction in **new** HIV cases. Worldwide, millions of HIV infections will progress into AIDS into the next decade. Will some of your friends and associates *still* regard HIV/AIDS as someone else's problem? HIV/AIDS had invaded *all* segments of society worldwide! It is EVERYONE'S problem!

Table 10-2 Adult/Adolescent Behavioral Risk Groups, Race and Sex: Percent of Total AIDS Cases—United States, 2002

HIV/AIDS	No. of Cases[a]	% of Cases
Exposure Group		
Men who have sex with men	18,768	46
Injection drug user (IDU)	10,200	25
Homosexual/IDU	2448	5
Hemophiliac	82	0.2
Heterosexual contact	4488	11
Transfusion related	164	0.4
None of the above	4488	11
Total		100
Race/Ethnicity (all cases)		
White (non-Hispanic)	13,056	32
Black (non-Hispanic)	19,176	47
Hispanic	7752	19
Other	816	2
Sex (adults only)		
Male	31,416	77
Female	9384	23
Age Group (yrs)		
13–19	204	0.5
20–24	1469	3.6
25–29	5794	14.2
30–39	18,686	45.8
40–49	10,608	26
50–59	2978	7.3
60 and above	1061	2.6

[a]Cumulative estimated total = 40,800 adult/adolescent plus 190 pediatric = 41,000 = 100% of cases for 2002.

(Adapted from AIDS Surveillance Report, December 2000, updated)

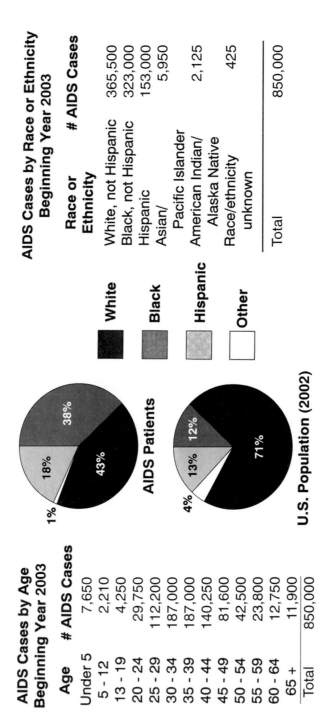

AIDS Cases by Age
Beginning Year 2003

Age	# AIDS Cases
Under 5	7,650
5 - 12	2,210
13 - 19	4,250
20 - 24	29,750
25 - 29	112,200
30 - 34	187,000
35 - 39	187,000
40 - 44	140,250
45 - 49	81,600
50 - 54	42,500
55 - 59	23,800
60 - 64	12,750
65 +	11,900
Total	850,000

AIDS Cases by Race or Ethnicity
Beginning Year 2003

Race or Ethnicity	# AIDS Cases
White, not Hispanic	365,500
Black, not Hispanic	323,000
Hispanic	153,000
Asian/ Pacific Islander	5,950
American Indian/ Alaska Native	2,125
Race/ethnicity unknown	425
Total	850,000

White

Black

Hispanic

Other

AIDS Patients

43% · 38% · 18% · 1%

U.S. Population (2002)

71% · 12% · 13% · 4%

FIGURE 10-2 AIDS Cases by Age and Racial and Ethnic Classification. Adult AIDS cases show a disproportionate percentage among blacks and Hispanics. Fifty seven percent of reported AIDS cases occur among racial and ethnic minorities. The figures reflect higher rates of AIDS in blacks and Hispanic injection drug users and their sex partners. Percentages of the population are based on the numbers of AIDS cases in the United States estimated beginning year 2003. U.S. population data about 282 million.

Figure 10-2 shows that the percentage of AIDS cases for ethnic-related adult/adolescent groups are in striking contrast to the population percentages of each group. Through year 2002 whites made up 71% of the population and represented 43% of adult/adolescent AIDS cases. Blacks made up 12% of the population but represented 38% of the adult/adolescent AIDS cases. Hispanics made up about 13% of the population but represented 18% of the adult/adolescent AIDS cases.

The CDC reported that in 2001, after seven straight years of declining AIDS cases, new AIDS cases increased nationally by about 5%. With a lapse in the practice of prevention, new AIDS cases are expected to increase through 2003.

According to 1993 data analyzed by Philip Rosenberg (1995 updated) of the National Cancer Institute, 1 in every 92 American men between **ages 27 and 39 may be HIV-infected.** The findings were especially dismal for black-American men, with 1 in 50 estimated to be HIV-infected versus 1 in 150 white men. The estimate was 1 in 60 for Hispanic men. The statistics were equally high for women of color. One in 160 black-American women and 1 in 222 Hispanic women are estimated to be infected with HIV. By comparison, the

number of white women infected with HIV was 1 in 3000. If the trends continue, Rosenberg noted, HIV/AIDS in young people and minorities must be considered "endemic in the United States."

According to the CDC, ending 2002, black Americans made up about 47% of all new AIDS cases. Latinos made up about 20% of new AIDS cases. Together blacks and Latinos represent about 67% of all new AIDS cases but they are only a quarter of the population. The two populations also represent 85% of all pediatric AIDS cases. In 2002, black women made up 65% of new AIDS cases reported among females. White women made up 18% and Latino women 17% of new AIDS cases. There are myriad factors contributing to the spread of HIV among blacks. Information about the threat of AIDS has not been disseminated widely or effectively enough, particularly among those under 21 who feel they are invulnerable. An official with the New York AIDS Coalition tells a story about a 15-year-old girl who said: "Don't tell me nothin' about no AIDS because that won't impact me. And if I was to get it, all I'd have to do is take a pill in the morning and I'll be O.K."

Figure 10-3 is a U.S. map of estimated AIDS cases through the year 2002. Note that the highest

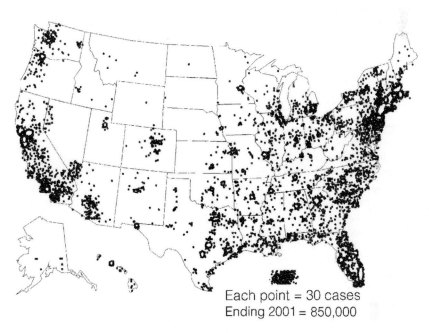

Each point = 30 cases
Ending 2001 = 850,000

FIGURE 10-3   United States: Cumulative AIDS Cases and Approximate Location. Ending 2002. *(CDC, Atlanta Surveillance Branch)*

incidence of AIDS cases occurs along the coastal regions.

Behavioral Risk Groups and Percentages of HIV-Infected People

Beginning 2003, investigators at the CDC found that HIV infection still remains largely confined to the populations at recognized behavioral risks: homosexual men, injection drug users, heterosexual partners of injection drug users, hemophiliacs, and children of HIV-infected mothers. In the general population, rates for HIV infection include 0.04% for first-time blood donors, 0.14% for military applicants, 0.33% for Job Corps entrants, 0.19% to 0.87% for child-bearing women, and 0.30% for hospital patients. Data reported by the CDC in the 1990s indicated that while the number of new AIDS cases increased by 5% in cities, it had increased by 37% in rural areas. This trend continues.

Comments on a Variety of Individual Behavioral Risk Groups

It must be kept in mind that because a group of people is at risk for HIV does not mean that these people are predestined to become infected. People are placed within these groups because of their social behavior, a behavior that has been associated with a high, medium, or low risk of becoming HIV-infected. Essentially, there is no zero-risk group because a scenario can always be formulated to show that under certain circumstances one or more members of that group could become HIV-infected.

The point of placing people in behavioral risk groups is not to offend them but to provide a warning that certain behavior might make them more vulnerable to HIV infection. It is not race or ethnic group that places people at high or low risk for infection, it is their behavior.

The fact that AIDS was first identified in 1981 in seemingly well-defined behavioral groups (homosexual men, injection drug users, hemophiliacs, Haitian immigrants) probably contributed to a false sense of security among people who did not belong to any of these groups. However, as information about HIV and AIDS accumulated, it became clear that HIV was transmitted in body fluids. This had grave implications for all social groups. On reflection, the people in the original high-risk groups simply had the bad luck of being in the way of a newly emerging infectious agent as it first began to spread. It is highly probable that in the different behavioral risk groups there are lifestyle or medical history factors that increase the efficiency with which the virus is transmitted.

Men Who Have Sex With Men (MSM)— In 1981, 100% of all AIDS cases reported to the CDC occurred in homosexual males. In the 1980s, the infection rate among gay men in San Francisco was over 60%. For 1993, 46% of the 106,618 new AIDS cases occurred in gay males. It dropped to 35% in 1997 and remained at 35% annually through 1998 (*MMWR*, 1995a; HIV/AIDS surveillance report, 1997, 1998). In the 1990s, the number of gay male AIDS cases, as a percentage of all AIDS cases, increased to over 40% per year. These findings underscore the need for community planning groups to consider culturally appropriate prevention services when addressing the HIV-prevention needs of racial/ethnic minorities. Also, there are indicators of a second wave in the HIV/AIDS epidemic among gay males.

Studies show that a significant percentage of gay men who had originally adopted safer sex behaviors are **relapsing** to unsafe sex (Stall et al., 1990; Lemp et al., 1994).

Most people who have attempted to change behavior know it is difficult to maintain new behavior patterns over a long period of time. Increasing attention and concern has been focused on the issue of relapse. High seroprevalence levels among homosexual men (estimated to be 50% in high incidence cities such as San Francisco) make relapse to risky behaviors a significant source of new infections and justify continued interventions to reinforce behavior change.

SIZE OF THE HOMOSEXUAL COMMUNITY Estimating the size of the homosexual population continues to be a problem for the CDC. Because of the lack of available information on sexual practices, the CDC has relied on the 1948 Kinsey report, *Sexual Behavior in the Human Male*, for its estimate that 2.5 million (10%) American males are exclusively homosexual, while another 2.5 to 7.5 million have **occasional** homosexual contacts. These numbers are refuted by some recent surveys like the 1992 National Opinion Research Center that reports that among males, 2.8% are exclusively gay, and among women, 2.5% are exclusively lesbian. Judith Reisman argues in her 1990

ON THE DOWN LOW

On the down low refers to men who have sex with men but do not identify themselves as gay or bisexual. They often live secretive double lives, outwardly heterosexual, sometimes even married with children, but also having sexual relations with men. The phenomenon is more common among black men than whites. In 2000, in a study of 8780 HIV-positive men who said they were infected by having sex with a man, the CDC found that one-fourth of African-American respondents identified themselves as heterosexual, compared to only 6% of white men. As an example, at the National Conference of African-Americans and AIDS in February 2000, a Columbus, Ohio, publishing executive told several hundred health care professionals, "I sleep with men, but I am not bisexual, and I am not certainly gay. I assure you that none of the brothers **ON THE DOWN LOW** like me are paying the least bit of attention to anything you have to say."

AIDS experts are worried that regardless of race, men who call themselves heterosexual but are involved in secret sexual relations with men are fueling the rising incidence of HIV infection among women. A study published in the *Journal of the American Medical Association* called young bisexual men a bridge for HIV transmission to women. In that study, one in six men who had sex with men recently had sex with women. Nearly 25% of those men had recently had unprotected sex with both men and women.

Approximately 6% of all IDU-associated AIDS cases occur in the homosexual/bisexual male population. These cases may reflect HIV transmission either by contaminated syringes or sexual activity.

Demographic Changes of HIV-Infected Men in the Gay Community

New data compiled by the CDC and reported in June 2001 reveals a striking change in the disease's demographics in America (HIV/AIDS Surveillance Report, June 2001). Year-end 2001 data shows that 74% of AIDS cases in white Americans, 37% in black Americans, and 42% in Latino Americans resulted from homosexual contacts. Beginning 2003, of the 370,000 people living with AIDS in America, 38% were white, 40% were black and 20% were Hispanic. Beginning year 2003, AIDS killed more black Americans under age 55 than heart disease, cancer, or homicide!

A 2001 report on 2000 gay men ages 23 to 29 in six major cities stated that among gay black men 30% were HIV positive, as were 15% of Hispanic gay men and 7% of white gay men. San Francisco, with the largest gay population in the United States had a rate of 1.3% in 1996. The new rate of HIV infections in San Francisco is now at 3.7%. The national level among gay men is 1%. About a third of the gay men surveyed knew they were HIV-infected (*MMWR*, 2001; Valleroy et al., 2001; Ostrow, 2001). Beginning year 2003, gay males accounted for 56% of 841,000 adult/adolescent AIDS cases in America. Ending 2002, an estimated 450,000 gay men are living with HIV infection (Wolitski et al., 2001; Catania et al., 2001 updated).

Injection Drug Users— According to the CDC, as many as 33% of the nation's 1.2 million injection drug users may be HIV-infected. This behavioral risk group contains the nation's **second largest group** of HIV-infected and AIDS patients. An association between injection drug use and AIDS was recognized in 1981, about two years before the virus was identified. **AIDS in IDUs and hemophiliacs offered the first evidence that whatever caused AIDS was being carried in and transmitted by human blood.** From the first reported IDU AIDS cases in 1981 through 2002, 31% of all adult/adolescent AIDS cases were associated with IDUs. Of IDUs, 74% listed IDU as their **only** risk factor for HIV infection; 26% were also homosexual/bisexual. The CDC estimates that

book, *Kinsey, Sex and Fraud,* that male homosexuals make up about 1% of the population. The group, Coloradans for Family Values and the Washington-based Family Research Institute believe about 3% of the male population is exclusively gay.

Using data collected from HIV testing conducted in 1986 and 1987, the CDC estimates that 20% of exclusively homosexual men are HIV-infected. This means (depending on whose numbers are used) that about 950,000 gay males in the United States have been HIV-infected. For bisexuals and men with infrequent homosexual encounters, the CDC tabulates a prevalence rate of 5%, meaning that about 90,000 of this population have been HIV-infected (Booth, 1988 updated).

through 2002 40% of infected women and 22% of infected men became HIV-infected through IDUs.

IDUs have been reported in all 50 states and the District of Columbia. Fifty-two percent of the accumulated 190,000 IDU-only AIDS cases occurred in New York and New Jersey. Among the adult/adolescent heterosexual AIDS cases over half had sexual partners who are/were IDUs.

Rates for IDU-associated AIDS varied widely by area: rates in Puerto Rico, New Jersey, New York, and the District of Columbia were greater than 10 per 100,000; in 22 states, rates were lower than 1 per 100,000 population.

About 55% of all IDU-associated cases were reported in the Northeast, which represents about 20% of the population of the United States and its territories. The South reported 20% of IDU-associated AIDS cases, 5% from the Midwest, and the West reported the remaining 20%.

The rate of IDU-associated AIDS continues to be **higher** for blacks and Hispanics than for whites. Except for the West, where rates for whites and Hispanics were similar, this difference by race/ethnicity was observed in all regions of the country and was greatest in the Northeast. Beginning 2003, overall IDU-associated **male** AIDS cases represented 9% of all AIDS cases in whites, 33% in blacks, 35% in Hispanics, 5% in Asians/Pacific Islanders, and 16% in American Indians/Alaskan Natives. For **women** it was: white, 42%; black, 40%; Hispanic, 39%; Asian/Pacific Islanders, 15%; and American Indian/Alaskan Natives, 45%.

Heterosexuals— The spread of HIV in the general population is relatively slow, yet potentially it is the source of the greatest numbers of HIV/AIDS cases. The CDC estimates there are 147 million Americans **without** an identified at-risk behavior, the general population.

Data from the CDC beginning year 2003 indicated that 11% of all the AIDS cases in the United States occurred through heterosexual contact. But this must be placed in perspective. Although 11% of anything may be a significant number, beginning year 2003 it stood for about 94,000 adult/adolescent/pediatric AIDS cases out of the total 850,000. Most of the heterosexual AIDS cases occurred in persons or the sexual partners of individuals with an identified behavioral risk. Relative to the general adult population, the number of heterosexual AIDS cases is only a fraction of 1%. Of the 50,000 plus new HIV infections occurring each year beginning 1999 through the year 2002, about 10% each year have occurred in the heterosexual population.

Global HIV/AIDS Cases and Heterosexuality

Worldwide ending year 2003, there will be an estimated 10 million people living with AIDS and about 26 million will have died of AIDS. According to a June 1999 Worldwatch Institute report, South Africa's HIV pandemic is perhaps the worst on the globe. It has engulfed the country, and "barring a medical miracle, one of every five adults will die of AIDS over the next 10 years." This unprecedented social tragedy is also translating into an economic disaster. The working-age population is being lost to AIDS. In Zimbabwe, state morgues are extending their hours to cope with the soaring death rate, mostly as a result of AIDS. An estimated 3000 people now die every week in the southern African country, nearly 70% of them from AIDS-related illnesses. The main hospital in Harare has opened its morgue around the clock and other hospital and mortuary facilities have extended closing time by four hours. At the University of Durban-Westville in Kwazulu-Natal, 255 of the students recently tested HIV positive. In 1997, 14% of the population was HIV positive—in 2001 it was about 40%.

Worldwide, ending year 2003, **heterosexuals** will make up about 75% of the estimated 44 million **living** HIV-infected people. About 70% of the 44 million infected people live in Sub-Saharan Africa (about 31 million). North America (1.7 million), Latin America (3.2 million), South and Southeast Asia (10 million), and Africa account for 97% of global HIV infections (Figure 10-4).

Of the 44 million living HIV-infected people worldwide, over 90% live in nonindustrial nations. It is estimated that through year 2003, a total of 36 million people will have/had AIDS worldwide, 77% of those cases occurred in Africa, 13% in Asia, 2.6% in North America, and 2% in Europe (UNAIDS, 1998 updated Table 10-3).

UNAIDS estimated that almost 6 million new HIV infections occurred annually from 1997 through 2003. The AIDS death toll for these seven years is estimated at 18 million of which 7.5 million were women and 3.5 million were under age 15. The United States will have about 900,000 AIDS cases by the end of 2003—worldwide

THE LATINO COMMUNITY

"In 1983, my brother died of AIDS. It infected his wife, and a year later she died. And now we had the first set of orphans in our family. Despite everything, I saw the love and unity of my family—how we pulled together and took care of my brother and loved him. My sister left another set of orphans. My uncle, who is my godfather, lost children to HIV. His son died in a prison hospital of AIDS. His daughter died at the age of 33 and left another orphan child. My uncle wasn't around to see his daughter die because he died of suffering from watching. Last year we found out my 70-year-old uncle is infected with HIV. And that's just my family. I watch the news. I watch people talk about wars in other countries and I identify with the feelings of those people. I know they have bombs thrown at them. I know they have weapons pointed at them. But we have a weapon that is killing my community. We have to silence this weapon of AIDS, which is killing us."

This was the testimony given by Marina Alvarez to 60 Latino community leaders from across the United States and Puerto Rico who had convened at Harvard University in the spring of 1998. The rate of infection among Latinos in the United States reflects an increasingly dire situation. Currently, 19% of all AIDS cases in the United States occur among Latinos, even though Latinos represent about 13 percent of the total population. For each of the years 1998 through 2002, Latinos represented 20% of new AIDS cases in America. About 65,000 Latinos are currently living with AIDS and between 130,000 to 180,000 are HIV-infected. The rate of HIV infection among Latino men is three times greater than the infection rate found among white, non-Hispanic men. Similarly, women and children in the Latino community have rates of infection that are seven times greater than the rates found among white women and children. If these trends continue, the Harvard AIDS Institute projects that by the year 2003 the percentage of total annual AIDS attributable to the Latino population will eclipse the percentage of such cases attributable to the white, non-Hispanic population.

AIDS is the fourth leading cause of death for Latinos ages 25 to 34. There are about 37 million Latino/Hispanic people in America. Ending 2003, there were about 162,000 Latino AIDS cases. The rate of new AIDS cases among Latinos is about four times the rate among white Americans but about three times lower than the rate for black Americans.

Snapshot—New York Latino Population. New York has 9% of America's Latino population but 30% (48,000) of all Latino AIDS cases. Over 55% of HIV infection occurred through IDU. Forty percent of Latino women have become infected through sex with a male IDU. Latinos make up 33% of New York's inmate population and 50% of prison AIDS cases.

The Future Threat for Latinos. The AIDS epidemic threatens not only the present generation of Latinos but also future generations. Ending the year 2000, over one-third of the members of the Latino community were under the age of 18. With rising rates of HIV infection among all youth, the implications for the Latino community are ominous. Rafael Campo, a physician at Beth Deaconess Medical Center said, "As overwhelming as this epidemic might seem to us right now, even greater devastation faces our next generation of irreplaceable young people whose future should be to lead this country into the next millennium; to take our places in medicine, business, in government; and to share with the world the tremendous brilliance and creativity of our culture" (Kao, 1999).

there will be have been 40 times that number (Figure 10-5).

Worldwide, it is estimated that one in every 100 sexually active people aged 15 to 49 is HIV-infected! In sub-Saharan Africa 7 in every 100 age 15 to 49 are HIV-infected. Overall, ending year 2003, AIDS will have orphaned about 14 million children.

The World Health Organization (WHO) projected that beginning 2002, over 90% of all new HIV infections globally will be transmitted heterosexually. In 1996, the WHO estimated that there are about a half-**billion** heterosexuals who are at moderate to high risk of exposure to HIV because of multiple sexual partners. In addition, there are about 10 million homosexuals and 5 million drug users who are also at moderate to high risk because of multiple sex partners or regular sharing of injection equipment. Most HIV infections in North America have been transmitted

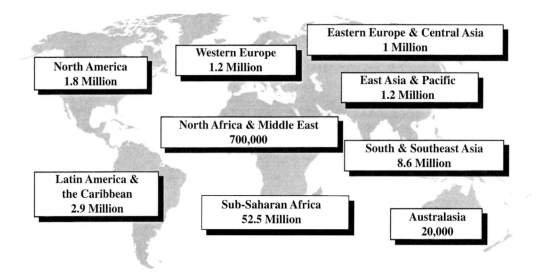

Estimated HIV Infections–Global Total: 70 Million Ending 2003

FIGURE 10-4 Estimated Number of Global HIV Infections Projected by United Nations AIDS Program and World Health Organization ending year 2003. Of the estimated 70 million HIV-infected persons, about 44 million **are living** in some state of HIV/AIDS illness. Over 5 million of these are children. Of 209 countries reporting to the WHO and UNAIDS, 194 have reported AIDS cases. World population reached 6 billion in October 1999. *(Source: Pan American Health Organization Quarterly Report, September 1996 updated; UNAIDS Report on the Global HIV/AIDS Epidemic, December 1999 updated)*

Table 10-3 Leading Cause of Death Worldwide from 1998 through 2003

Infectious Diseases	All Diseases
1. **HIV/AIDS**	1. Heart diseases
2. Diarrheal disease	2. Cerebrovascular diseases
3. Childhood diseases	3. Lower respiratory diseases
4. Tuberculosis	4. **HIV/AIDS**
5. Malaria	5. Obstructive pulmonary diseases
6. STDs excluding HIV/AIDS	6. Diarrheal diseases
7. Meningitis	7. Perinatal conditions
8. Tropical diseases	8. Tuberculosis

Data Courtesy of the World Health Organization, 1998 updated.

homosexually to men who have practiced receptive anal intercourse, whereas most of those occurring in Africa and parts of the Caribbean have been transmitted heterosexually to both women and men during vaginal intercourse. Heterosexual transmission accounts for a growing proportion of HIV/ AIDS cases in Europe and Latin America, and is proliferating at explosive rates in parts of China and India.

Hemophiliacs— There are about 16,000 to 20,000 hemophiliacs in the United States. At least

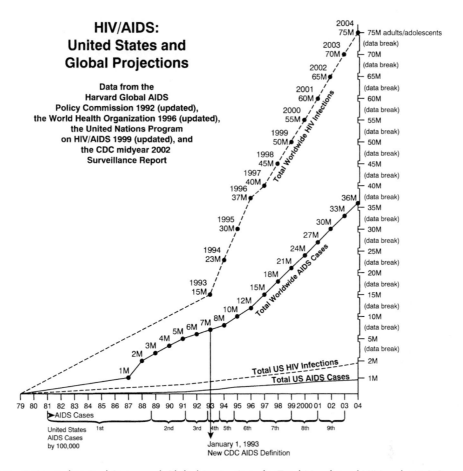

FIGURE 10-5 Estimated United States and Global Projections for Total Number of HIV and AIDS Cases. Beginning year 2003, about 850,000 U.S. AIDS cases were reported to the CDC. Most of these cases were diagnosed according to the 1987 CDC AIDS definition guidelines. On January 1, 1993, the CDC changed the definition of AIDS to include all persons with a T4 or CD4+ cell count of **less than 200.** The new definition raised the number of AIDS cases in the United States from 1992 to 1993 by about 111%. The expected number of adults/adolescent cases for 1993, 49,100, became 106,618. The new definition has raised the number of persons *living* with diagnosed and reported AIDS in the United States through 2003 to about 350,000. Worldwide, the total number of AIDS cases is expected to reach about 36 million ending 2004. Through the year 2003, about 1.4% of all HIV infections and 2.2% of total AIDS cases will have occurred in the United States. William Hazeltine, AIDS researcher formerly at the Dana Farber Institute, and now with Human Genome Sciences, Inc., said that if prevention does not work or a cure is not found, some **1 billion** people could be HIV positive by the year 2025. Global population through 2003 is projected to be about 6.5 billion people. *(Source: Harvard Global AIDS Policy Commission 1992 and World Health Organization 1993, 1994, National Census Bureau 1998, and projected data)*

half are HIV positive and through 2002, about 3000 of them have died. Of those infected, over 98% received HIV in blood products that were essential to their survival. By mid-1985, an HIV blood screening test was put into effect nationally. From that point, the risk of HIV infection from the blood supply has been significantly lowered but a small

risk still exists. **Scandals** in knowingly selling HIV-positive blood for transfusions and in production of the blood factor essential for hemophiliacs, surfaced in France, Germany, the United States, Canada, and Japan in the 1990s. (For discussion, see Chapter 8.)

From 1982 through 2002, 4,896 adult/adolescent hemophiliacs, 410 sexual partners of hemophiliacs, and 255 hemophilic pediatric AIDS cases have been reported. Almost all of these cases are the result of HIV infections that occurred prior to 1985.

American Military— The incidence of HIV infection can be measured best in groups that undergo routine serial testing. Because active duty military personnel and civilian applicants for the service are routinely tested for HIV antibody, there is a unique opportunity to measure the incidence of HIV infection in a large, demographically varied subset of the general population.

Since October 1985, all military personnel on active duty, as well as all civilian applicants for military service, have undergone mandatory testing for HIV antibody. Over the past two years, the armed forces screened over four million people for exposure to HIV. Of those tested, 0.15% were HIV positive. This total included active duty personnel, members of the National Guard, members of reserve units, and would-be recruits. The recruits who tested positive have been barred from entering the service. Those carrying HIV who are already in uniform are allowed to stay in the service as long as they remain asymptomatic. They are, however, ineligible for overseas duty and must undergo close health monitoring.

Beginning 2003, there were an estimated 1050 HIV-positive persons in the military who became HIV-positive **while serving in the military.** The Navy had the highest incidence of HIV, with 2.5 per 1000 people. The rate in the Army was 1.4 per 1000; in the Marines, 1 per 1000; and in the Air Force, 0.99 per 1000. The higher rate in the Navy may reflect that Navy personnel are based primarily on the East and West Coasts, which have the highest number of AIDS cases.

College Students— Between April 1988 and February 1989, the blood of 16,863 students enrolled at 16 large universities and three private colleges was tested for HIV antibodies. Thirty students, 28 males and 2 females, tested HIV positive for an overall rate of 2 per 1000 or 0.2%. With 12.5 million students enrolled in American colleges and universities, the rate of 2 in 1000 means there are about 25,000 HIV-infected college students.

The study was conducted by the CDC with The American College Health Association (Gayle et al., 1988). Because the samples were not identified, students who tested positive could not be informed. All blood samples from 10 of the 19 campuses were HIV negative. At five campuses the rate of HIV-positive blood ranged from four to nine samples per 1,000. In contrast, the rate of HIV in the general heterosexual population is about 0.02% and the rate for military personnel in about the same age group tested over a similar time period was 0.14%.

The question is why college students have a rate of HIV infection 10 times higher than the general heterosexual population. Are college students less well informed than the general heterosexual population?

Surveys indicate that college students are well educated about HIV/AIDS. Why, then, the higher rate of infection? Perhaps it's the age-old dilemma of information versus behavior. **They know what to do but they don't do it.** There is a difference between knowledge and action based on that knowledge. College students have always had information on drug use, alcoholism, pregnancies out of wedlock, and sexually transmitted diseases; but this knowledge has not appreciably reduced at-risk behaviors. STDs are at an all-time high in teenage and college students.

Marla Eisenberg (2001) reported that less than half of U.S. college students always use condoms during sex, and almost one-fourth never use condoms. She surveyed 8500 undergraduate students about their sexual health behavior as part of a College Alcohol Study. Although 71% of students surveyed identified themselves as sexually experienced, only 43% said they always used condoms during sex and 24% said they never used condoms. Students who lived off-campus and those more than 23 years old were least likely to use condoms. Men with higher numbers of partners also reported less frequent condom use. The survey—which for the first time asked students if they had had a sexual experience with a member of the same sex, opposite sex or both, instead of asking them to identify themselves as gay, heterosexual or bisexual—found that men who only had sex with other men were less likely to use condoms than their heterosexual peers.

Prisoners— Beginning year 2003, the nation's prison population was at an all-time high, over 2 million adults contained in 1300 state and 71 federal prisons. Ninety percent are men.

According to the U.S. Bureau of Justice Statistics, 2.1% of these people or 42,000 are HIV positive and of these, 17% have AIDS (Rubel et al., 1997 updated). The total number of **prisoners, parolees,** and **probationers** in 2002 was about 6.5 million with an HIV-positive rate of 2.1% or about 136,000 being HIV positive (DeGroot et al., 1996 updated). Beginning year 2003, about 6000 adult inmates in U.S. state and federal prisons and jails had died of AIDS. About 6000 people with AIDS were still in prisons and jails (*MMWR*, 1996c). In 2002, **four states**—New York, Florida, Texas, and California— had **more than half** the known cases of HIV in prison. Only two states and five prison systems in the United States distribute or sell condoms to male inmates: Mississippi, and Vermont, New York City, Philadelphia, San Francisco, Los Angeles, and the District of Columbia (Hooker, 1996 updated) and only two of the six distribute dental dams and condoms to female inmates. **No U.S. correctional facility distributes bleach or syringes to inmates** (Mahon, 1996, updated).

Blood testing of inmates at 10 selected prisons indicated that 1 in every 24 prisoners is infected with HIV. This study also found that incarcerated women under age 25 had a higher HIV seroprevalence (5.2%) than incarcerated young men (2.3%). The rate was comparable among older women (5.3%) and older men (5.6%). Nonwhites were almost twice as likely to be infected as whites. Rates varied widely among the 10 institutions from 2.1% to 7.6% for men, and 2.7% to 14.7% for women (Vlahov et al., 1991). Beginning 1999, 17 states tested **all** new inmates for HIV infection. Most (about 75%) prison systems will provide an HIV test on request. The House of Representatives passed legislation requiring all federal inmates serving at least six months to be HIV-tested within four months of entering the prison system.

In general, prisoners diagnosed with AIDS were infected prior to their incarceration—most are IDUs (Francis, 1987). Infected inmates most often transmit the virus to others through homosexual and drug-related activities. For that reason 21 states segregated HIV-infected and AIDS patient prisoners from the other prisoners. In September of 1989, a court order in the state of Connecticut ended their prison segregation policy. Similar antisegregation lawsuits have been filed in Alabama and Oregon. Through 1998, four states had laws that allow for isolation or segregation of HIV-infected inmates: South Carolina, Alabama, Georgia, and Mississippi.

A number of state prisons have instituted either mass screening programs or large-scale blind serological surveys for HIV infection. The Federal Bureau of Prisons tests a 10% sample of federal prisoners. Other jurisdictions conduct screening or testing programs for selected groups of prisoners, such as known injection drug users and homosexuals.

AIDS is the leading cause of death in the New York and Florida prison systems. According to the *People with AIDS Coalition Newsline*, 66% of inmate deaths in New York and New Jersey resulted from AIDS. In Florida in 2000, 24% of all deaths in the state prisons were related to AIDS. Of these, 42% were due to tuberculosis or *Pneumocystis* pneumonia (24%). Both are successfully treated complications of HIV infection if diagnosed early enough. The state of Florida spent about $19 million on HIV/AIDS inmate treatment in 1999. For years 2000 through 2002 it cost about $22 million annually.

TURNOVER IN PRISON POPULATIONS CREATES AN HIV TRANSMISSION PROBLEM FOR THE GENERAL POPULATION Large numbers of at-risk individuals cycle through prisons and jails every year. The turnover rate for some prisons is as high as 50% per year. Because the prevalence of HIV is so high among the prison population, on release from prison, they can spread HIV to others. For example, the *AIDS Quarterly Report* in May 1990 stated that in one year, 15,000 HIV-infected prisoners left the New York prison system to join the general population, and because of confidentiality laws, no one will know who they are. At Riker's Island facility in New York, of 21,000-plus prisoners, one in four are reported to be HIV-infected (National Press Release, 1989). A blinded serosurvey performed by the New York City Department of Health in 1991 determined that 26% of women and 16% of men in New York City prisons were HIV-seropositive (De Groot et al., 1996). In Florida, 3.4% of its prison population of 65,000 is HIV positive.

In April 2002, in order to stop the virus' spread to the inmates' partners outside prison, Florida passed legislation that makes HIV testing mandatory for inmates leaving Florida prisons. The purpose of the bill is to educate the inmates about the virus and their health status and to protect the public at large. Florida released about 26,000 inmates in September 2002. Now they will know which of the inmates are HIV positive and guide them into outside care facilities. The rate of AIDS in Florida's prison is 12 times higher than in the general population. Among female inmates, the rate is 60 times higher than for women of the general public.

The Elderly— The face of AIDS has changed dramatically from the 1980s into the 1990s. AIDS cases among men, in particular gay men, and IDUs predominated the 1980s. But in the 1990s the numbers of AIDS cases among women, their children, and people of color increased significantly. What did not appear to claim public or scientific notice is the ever-increasing number of **AIDS cases among the elderly.** Thus, **the face of AIDS is aging** and **wrinkling** as improved therapy keeps the HIV-infected alive longer. The numbers of elderly people with AIDS will continue to grow. The male-female ratio in the age 50 and over is about 9:1 (Ship et al., 1991). **The senior citizens of today did not grow up in the age of AIDS—they did not have sex and HIV in the same thought. They have to learn a lot of unfamiliar and scary information in a hurry.**

AIDS cases among people between the ages 50 and 90 are increasing. Nationally about **13% of the total AIDS cases occur in people over age 50.** Beginning year 2003, this represented about 110,000 people. Three percent of AIDS occurs in people over age 60 and 0.7% occurs in people over 70. One AIDS patient was 90 years old when diagnosed. He became HIV-infected from a blood transfusion during surgery at age 85. He became symptomatic after four years and died one year later of *Pneumocystis carinii* pneumonia. At least 20% or one in five people living with HIV disease are older than age 50.

In **Florida,** a state with a large retired population, the number of recorded AIDS cases among those over age 50 has risen from 6 in 1984 to 1341 in 1993 to about 10,000 beginning year 2003, or about 12% of the state's cases. In Dade County, Florida, a popular destination among retirees, almost 20% of people with AIDS are seniors—one of the highest rates in the county for the 50-plus group. Forty-four percent of senior women in Florida with AIDS, and 18% of Florida men over 50 with AIDS are known to have become infected through heterosexual sex. These numbers are predicted to grow as the more sexually liberal baby boom generation ages. Nationwide, seniors make up less that 5% of those tested for HIV at government-funded sites, according to the CDC. Seniors are much more likely than younger people to have AIDS by the time they discover they are infected with HIV. Early diagnosis is a key goal because older people tend to become sicker faster than younger people.

Age—An At-Risk Factor?

In general, Americans over 50 are potentially at risk, sometimes without realizing it, when they begin dating following a divorce or the death of a spouse. Others are at risk because they are IDUs or continue to have multiple sex partners or have a sex partner who practices unsafe sex. Individuals who acquire HIV infection at older ages progress to AIDS more rapidly, on average, than individuals infected at younger ages (excluding pediatric cases).

The majority of AIDS cases in the elderly once occurred due to HIV-contaminated blood transfusions; now the new elderly cases of AIDS most often include IDU or sexual activities (El Sadr et al., 1995; Gordon et al., 1995).

Health Care Workers— Health care workers are defined by the CDC as people, including students and trainees, whose activities involve contact with patients or with blood or other body fluids from patients in a health care setting. They represent 7.7% of the U.S. labor force.

The risk of HIV transmission from health care worker to patient during an exposure-prone invasive procedure is remote. There is a greater and well-documented risk of transmission from an infected patient to a health care worker.

As the pandemic of HIV infections continues to increase, workers in every health care field will be involved in the detection, counseling, therapy, maintenance, quantity, and quality of life for the symptomatic HIV-infected and for those expressing AIDS. Although the largest number of HIV-infected people are asymptomatic, each day many of them begin to experience signs and symptoms of HIV disease; and each day new cases of AIDS are diagnosed. As the number of patients increases, additional health care workers are required to meet their needs. As this workforce enlarges to meet the demands of the estimated numbers of AIDS cases in the coming years, precautions must be practiced to prevent health care workers, themselves, from becoming HIV-infected.

Ruthanne Marcus and colleagues (1988) reported that, across the board, health care workers exposed to HIV-contaminated blood have about a 1 in 300 chance of becoming infected. Other more recent reports place the risk of HIV infection at 1 in 250.

Health Care Workers with HIV/AIDS

A European Commission reported that worldwide, beginning year 2002, 112 health care workers (HCW) were confirmed to have acquired HIV infection on the job (**60 cases were in America**) and an additional 220 **HCWs (146 were in America)** may have become infected on the job. In the United States, nurses account for the largest number of cases.

Twenty-six of the 60 cases have developed AIDS and nine have died. These are small numbers when compared to some 7000 hepatitis B transmissions to health care workers every year in the United States (Osborne, 1993; Aiken et al., 1997 updated).

Of the 146 possible occupationally acquired HIV-infected workers, 62 have developed AIDS

(*MMWR*, 1992b; Bell, 1996 updated). The number of persons with occupationally acquired HIV infection is probably greater than the totals presented here because not all health care workers are evaluated for HIV infection following exposures and not all persons with occupationally acquired infection are reported.

Of the estimated 850,000-plus American adult/adolescent AIDS cases entering year 2003, (3.5%) are health care workers, including an estimated 119 (0.4%) physicians, 226 (0.76%) nurses, and about 164 (0.55%) dentists (Toufexis, 1991 updated). Overall, beginning year 2003, 75% of the health care workers with AIDS have died.

Like other adult AIDS patients, health care workers have a median age of 35 years. Males account for 91.6% of cases and 62% are white.

Ninety-five percent of the health care workers with AIDS were classified into known transmission categories. Health care workers with AIDS

POINT OF INFORMATION 10.1

WHERE OLDER PATIENTS WITH HIV DISEASE CAN GET HELP

ON THE SUBJECT OF SENIORS AND SEX A 12-YEAR OLD SAID, "I NEVER KNEW ANYONE OVER 50 HAD SEX."

In Orlando, Florida, a 66-year-old woman says that she gets the following reaction when she reveals she is HIV positive.

How can that be—you have four grown children and grandchildren—how could this have happened to you? "FROM SEX, IDIOT, I GOT IT FROM SEX WITH MY BOYFRIEND!"

The problem of AIDS in persons 50 and older has received little recognition. But a few organizations now provide literature or services aimed specifically at older patients and their physicians:

American Association of Retired Persons
601 E St. NW
Washington, D.C. 20049
(202) 434-2277
http://www.aarp.org

Publishes free fact sheet, "AIDS: A Multigenerational Crisis" (Stock No. D14942), that includes listings of referral services.

Senior Action in a Gay Environment (SAGE)
208 W. 13th St.
New York, NY 10011
(212) 741-2247

Provides a variety of services to gays in their 50s or older. Also offers training, education, counseling, and therapy and is a source of information for physicians and hospitals. Operates chiefly in the area surrounding New York City (NY, NJ, CT).

National Institute on Aging
Public Information Office
Federal Bldg. 31 (Room 5C27)
Bethesda, MD 20892
(301) 496-1752

Publishes fact sheet, "Age Page: AIDS and Older Adults," available as a fax transmission by calling (800) 222-2225.

Internet Addresses:
AIDS and the Elderly:
www.caps.ucsf.edu/capsweb/elderlybib.html

HIV/AIDS Treatment Information Service (ATIS): (800) 448-0440; http://www.hivatis.org

National Association of HIV over 50:
www.uic.edu/depts/matec/nahof.html

National Institute on Aging: (800) 222-2225

---

were significantly **less likely** to be injection drug users and **more likely** to be homosexual or bisexual men (*MMWR*, 1996b).

Needle stick Injuries— Health care workers are in a quandary about the possibility of becoming HIV-infected via needle sticks. Articles such as "Needlestick Risks Higher Than Reports Indicate" or "The Risk of HIV Transmission via Needlesticks Is Low" convey conflicting impressions.

The kinds of needle sticks most likely to occur in hospital or health care settings come from disposable syringes, IV line/needle assemblies, prefilled cartridge injection syringes, winged steel needle IV sets, vacuum tube phlebotomy assemblies, and IV catheters, in that order. Needle sticks and penetration of sharp objects account for about 80% of all health care workers' exposures to blood and blood products. There are about 800,000 needle stick injuries from contaminated devices in health settings each year. Of these, 16,000 devices are contaminated with HIV (Miller et al., 1997).

ESTIMATES OF HIV INFECTION AND FUTURE AIDS CASES

In 1987, Otis Bowen, then secretary of health and human services, said **"AIDS would make black death pale by comparison."**

As long as the number of newly infectious people each year exceeds the number who die, the pandemic will continue to build.

Who Reports AIDS Cases and to Whom? United States

AIDS cases are reported to the CDC through the SOUNDEX system, which involves translating names into specific sets of numbers and letters. While the resulting codes are not unique, when they are combined with other information, such as birthdates, individual cases can be followed without revealing the names. Although SOUNDEX is used at the national level, at state and local levels the names of AIDS patients are reported in all states. In states that report HIV-infected individuals by name, reporting methods parallel those used for AIDS (Colfax, et al., 1998).

The CDC considers a case of AIDS reportable when: (1) an otherwise healthy person is HIV positive and has an unusual opportunistic infection

(protozoal, fungal, bacterial, or viral) or a rare malignancy; or (2) an individual with a positive HIV antibody test has a T4 or CD4+ cell count of less than 200 per cubic millimeter of blood, which is about one-fifth the normal level; or (3) an individual with a positive HIV antibody test has been diagnosed with pulmonary tuberculosis, invasive cervical cancer, or recurrent pneumonia.

AIDS Reporting Systems

Reporting AIDS cases reveals past infections. AIDS became reportable in all 50 states, the District of Columbia, and U.S. territories to the CDC in Atlanta in 1986. AIDS surveillance has been crucial in identifying people at risk for the disease and the modes of transmission. AIDS surveillance data together with HIV surveys are important components of public health programs directed toward controlling HIV infection, and assist in providing the most accurate picture of the HIV epidemic in the United States.

By the end of 1993, all 50 states, the District of Columbia, and four territories (Guam, Pacific Islands, Puerto Rico, and the Virgin Islands) reported adult/adolescent cases. The CDC also reported the numbers of adult/adolescent/pediatric AIDS cases per 100,000 population by state. For the 10 leading metropolitan areas of at least 500,000 population for AIDS beginning year 2003, see Table 10-4. Beginning year 2003, the **10 states** and **territories** reporting the highest incidence of AIDS cases for adult/adolescents can be seen in Table 10-5.

The eight U.S. cities with the highest incidence of new AIDS cases for year 2002 were, highest to lowest: New York, Ft. Lauderdale, San Francisco, West Palm Beach, Jersey City, Newark, New Jersey, and Columbia, South Carolina.

With the widespread use of antiretroviral drugs beginning in 1996 there was a decline in AIDS cases but not in new HIV infections! Thus, it became clear that the total numbers of AIDS cases no longer accurately represent the pandemic. To track this pandemic now, it will be essential to have some form of reporting new HIV infections.

Reporting HIV-Positive Cases

Reporting HIV cases reveals current infections. Many now advocate name reporting for HIV infection from a surveillance perspective, in part because life-extending therapy is available and in

BOX 10.3

HIV/AIDS DATA COLLECTION AND DEFICIENCIES

The HIV/AIDS pandemic in the United States is monitored by state and local health departments in collaboration with the Division of HIV/AIDS Prevention Surveillance and Epidemiology of the Centers for Disease Control and Prevention. HIV/AIDS surveillance methods include unlinked anonymous HIV infection prevalence surveys, results of serologic tests from mass HIV screening programs, reporting of diagnosed HIV and AIDS cases, and reporting of deaths among persons with HIV and AIDS. Together, data from these surveillance systems provide estimates of the incidence and prevalence of infection, morbidity, and mortality from HIV/AIDS in the U.S. population.

Deficiencies

Neither the United States nor any other country has **an accurate count** of the number of people infected by HIV. Much of the testing to date comprises small samples of high-risk groups, such as prostitutes and drug addicts, and is therefore unrepresentative of entire populations. Within countries, infection rates vary widely from region to region, further complicating the problem of generalizing from a small sample. Counting the number of AIDS cases and AIDS-related deaths is also difficult, particularly since health care systems in many countries lack the required diagnostic ability. Some developing countries have AIDS rates 100 times higher than reported. Moreover, some governments suppress what information they have. **Further improvements in data collection may reveal a crisis of even greater magnitude than is portrayed in this text.**

test sites in Colorado, for instance, 11% of test seekers reported providing **false names.** While people with AIDS could similarly provide false identities, this would require considerably more effort, given their more frequent contact with medical professionals, and could also have negative consequences for them, since social services requires positive identification (Colfax, et al., 1998). Beginning 2003, only two states, Maryland and Washington, required that HIV infection reports carry only the name of persons who are **symptomatic.** Thirty-eight states and the Virgin

Table 10-4 Ten Metropolitan Areas Reporting Highest Number of AIDS Cases Beginning Year 2003

Metropolitan Area	Number of AIDS Cases
New York City	131,760
Los Angeles	47,580
San Francisco	36,600
Miami	25,620
Washington, D.C.	24,522
Chicago	23,058
Houston	21,045
Philadelphia	20,496
Newark, NJ	19,032
Atlanta	17,568
	366,000 or 43% of all AIDS cases in America.

Table 10-5 Ten States/Territories Reporting Highest Number of AIDS Cases Beginning Year 2003

State/Territory	Number of AIDS Cases
New York	155,448
California	134,640
Florida	86,904
Texas	58,752
New Jersey	47,124
Puerto Rico	28,764
Illinois	26,316
Pennsylvania	26,194
Georgia	24,480
Maryland	22,950
	612,000 or 72% of all AIDS cases in America.

part because of the success with U.S. AIDS surveillance programs. Theoretically, name reporting for HIV infection could provide more current surveillance information, since HIV infection predates AIDS. However, people with AIDS are usually reported for having a spectrum of symptoms and are often ill, or are reported from death certificate summaries, thereby ensuring high reporting rates. In contrast, those with HIV infection are reported for having a positive test result, and are more likely to find ways to remain anonymous, therefore avoiding the consequences of being reported as HIV positive. At confidential

Islands have implemented HIV case surveillance reporting HIV-infected adult/adolescents **by name** (Table 10-6). Collectively, these 38 states account for over half the nation's AIDS population. All states require some form of HIV reporting.

States that have used codes, or unique identifiers, to track HIV cases have found that such a system is flawed. Shortfalls include incomplete data, duplicate reports and difficulties ensuring access to proper care and partner notification services. States with faulty HIV reporting systems will soon be financially penalized as federal HIV/AIDS prevention care grants begin to be allocated on the basis of HIV and AIDS cases. Currently only AIDS cases are required for federal funding purposes.

NEWLY INFECTED

For the 50,000 new HIV infections occurring in 1999 through 2002 annually, 2000 and the CDC estimated that 70% of the infected were men. Of these men, 42% were infected via homosexual sex, 25% through IDU and 33% through heterosexual sex. Of these men, 54% are black, 26% are white, and 20% are Hispanics. Black American men make up 75% of new HIV infections among heterosexual cases. A small percentage are members of other racial/ethnic groups. Of the 12,000 new infections among women in the United States for 2001 and in 2002, the CDC estimated that approximately 75% of women are infected through heterosexual sex and

---

Table 10-6 Status of HIV Infection Reporting—United States, 2002

Confidential HIV Reporting Required		
Name[a] (Adults/Adolescents)		Coded/Anonymous[b]
Alabama	New Jersey	California
Alaska	New York	Connecticut
Arizona	New Mexico	District of Columbia
Arkansas	North Carolina	Georgia
Colorado	North Dakota	Hawaii
Delaware	Ohio	Illinois
Florida	Oklahoma	Kansas
Guam	Oregon	Kentucky
Idaho	Pennsylvania	Maine
Indiana	South Carolina	Montana
Iowa	South Dakota	New Hampshire
Louisiana	Tennessee[d]	Puerto Rico
Maryland[c]	Texas	Rhode Island
Massachusetts	Utah	Vermont
Michigan[d]	Virgin Islands	
Minnesota	Virginia	
Mississippi	Washington[c]	
Missouri	West Virginia	
Nebraska	Wisconsin	
Nevada	Wyoming	

All states and territories require reporting of AIDS cases by name at the local/state level to the Centers for Disease Control and Prevention.

[a]Names of HIV-infected people are provided to local or state health departments.

[b]Individual reports of people with HIV infection are provided to local or state health departments. Reports may contain demographic and transmission category information but do not record identifiers.

[c]Requires HIV reports with names for **symptomatic** HIV-infected persons **only**.

[d]Names are reported to the local health department only.

(Source: HIV/AIDS Surveillance Report, Year-end 2001, 13:1–41 updated)

25% through injection drug use. Of newly infected women, approximately 64% are black, 18% are white, 18% are Hispanics, and a small percentage are members of other racial/ethnic groups. The CDC estimates that over the next four years, over 100,000 people under the age of 25 will become HIV-infected if current trends continue. The current increases in HIV infections is a reversal of prevention program successes. **There is now a rekindling HIV epidemic in America and it is occurring mostly in the gay and black communities. The prevention messages of the past are losing their power—the safe sex ethic is losing favor. The overtly sick, the emaciated and those with visible Kaposi's sarcoma are rarely seen on the streets; antiretroviral drugs have the dying going back to work. The fear of infection and death has subsided!** According to the CDC, new AIDS cases have increased by 5% nationwide in 2001 and 2002.

Future HIV Reporting/Surveillance

In coming months, the CDC will release **HIV reporting** recommendations to states, and ultimately could tie compliance to coveted federal funding. In addition, bills are pending in Congress to make **HIV surveillance mandatory.** The California Medical Association has drafted a state HIV reporting law, and New York, Illinois, Pennsylvania, Georgia, and Massachusetts—all heavily affected states—have legislation pending or are in the process of implementation. Major advocacy organizations have come to a remarkable consensus with public health officials that AIDS-only **surveillance** puts states at risk of losing track of the changing epidemic. AIDS Project Los Angeles, the San Francisco AIDS Foundation and the Gay Men's Health Crisis have endorsed **HIV surveillance** on the condition it is done through a **"unique identifier" system** that would identify and track patients by codes. The AIDS groups and the American Civil Liberties Union are on record opposing name-based reporting. These organizations argue that HIV is different from other diseases. It still has no cure. It still is associated with stigmatized groups—gay men, drug users, prostitutes, and now ethnic minorities. Its victims, once identified, still suffer evictions, firings, hate crimes, and hostility. Regardless, whether one favors name-based reporting or unique code identifiers, **all agree** that AIDS reported data is no longer sufficient to track the spread or provide other essentials for the pandemic.

How Many People in the United States Are HIV-Infected?

How many people in the United States are HIV-infected? And just how many cases of AIDS are

---

POINT OF VIEW 10.1

JUSTIFICATION FOR HIV CASE REPORTING IN THE UNITED STATES

Reporting requirements involved an enduring conflict of values between individual rights to privacy and the collective good of society. The initial resistance to HIV case reporting may have been warranted by the sensitivity to a new and frightening disease that placed a disproportionate burden on disfavored (marginal) populations. Baffling science for years, the disease left people who had HIV infection and their partners without the benefit of effective treatment. Given the need for privacy and the near absence of effective treatments, individual rights were thought to outweigh the benefits of HIV surveillance.

1997: CDC Recommended that ALL States Implement an HIV Reporting System. With advances in **science, medicine, epidemiology,** and **law,** we are now at a very different point in the history of the epidemic. **Collective justifications for a mandatory national system of HIV case reporting are compelling.** HIV reporting would **(1)** improve our understanding of the epidemiology of the epidemic, **(2)** prevent infections by targeting scarce resources for testing, counseling, education, and partner notification, **(3)** benefit persons with HIV or AIDS and their partners by providing a link to medical treatment and other human services, and **(4)** promote more equitable allocation of government funding (Gostin et al., 1997).

Class Discussion: There is a national standard for confidential AIDS reporting, but not for reporting HIV infection. Should there be a national standard for confidential HIV reporting? Why? Why not?

expected to occur and when? Although projections have been made, the numbers are in question. **Why? They come from surveys and incidence data that lack rigorous scientific documentation.** For example, publications give information such as "researchers believe that the current number of HIV-infected people in the United States ranges from 1% to as high as 10%" (Slack, 1991). But even if this range is to be believed, the difference between 1 in every 100 versus 10 in every 100 is very significant. This range implies that the data are questionable, and that is what raises the spectrum of concern. How many people in the United States and worldwide have HIV disease and how many have AIDS? **How large a problem is the HIV/AIDS pandemic?** The answers to such questions are crucial to the allocation of funds for research and medical programs and for medical preparedness of institutions that will be hit hard as the number of cases increases.

All health care institutions and personnel will be affected by the increase in AIDS cases as will allied health service and support occupations, insurance companies, the funeral industry, and the workforce in general.

U.S. ESTIMATES LEAD TO CONFUSION. WHOSE FIGURES ARE CORRECT?: ISSUES OF CREDIBILITY

In 1992, a Harvard research group of 40 HIV/ AIDS experts estimated that by the year 2000 there would be between 38 and 110 million HIV-infected adult/adolescents and 10 million children worldwide. There would be 24 million adult and several million pediatric AIDS cases. The estimates of HIV infections by the Harvard group is over twice that of the World Health Organization. **In retrospect they were correct.** It is clear that the HIV/AIDS pandemic of the 1990s, in terms of new AIDS cases, was worse than for the 1980s.

John Karon and colleagues (1996), **based on data from three different sources and methods of calculation, estimated there are between 650,000 and 900,000 (0.3% of the population) HIV-infected people in the United States.**

According to the CDC projections in Figure 10-6, and adding in the 15% to 20% underreported AIDS cases, the estimates of the CDC fit relatively well. For 1993, before the implementation of the new AIDS definition, 65,211 cases were projected. Due to the 1993 change in the definition of AIDS, a total of 106,618 adult/adolescent cases were reported, a 37% increase over the expected and a 111% increase over the number of cases reported in 1992. The number of AIDS cases projected for 1994, 1995, and 1996 occurred. After the backlog of AIDS cases based on the new definition were reported, new AIDS cases per year as expected decreased.

Rise in HIV/AIDS Cases Among Heterosexuals

In 1989, while the number of new AIDS cases rose by 11% among gay males, it increased by 36% or more among heterosexuals and newborns. In 1993, due to the new AIDS definition, **heterosexual contact** AIDS cases increased 130% over 1992, from 4045 to 9288.

The groups most affected by the expanded 1993 definition were women, blacks, heterosexual injection drug users, and hemophiliacs. The increase was greater among women (151%) than among men (105%), and greater among blacks and Hispanic than whites. Young adults ages 13 to 29 accounted for 27% of the heterosexual contact cases. On average, women accounted for about 35% of the heterosexual contact cases from 1993 through 1997.

Will There Be a Heterosexual AIDS Epidemic in the United States?

A heterosexual epidemic on a scale similar to any developing nation is very unlikely now or in the future. Heterosexual AIDS epidemics in the developing nations result largely from conditions that do not exist in America or in other industrialized countries. These include large-scale population shifts, little information about AIDS prevention, many migrant workers, widespread prostitution, deep reluctance to use condoms, and frequent, untreated sexually transmitted diseases. Still, according to the CDC, heterosexual transmission will slowly increase in the United States largely due to low-income black and Hispanic women. Among the things that put them at increased risk: exchanging sex for crack cocaine and having sex with injection drug users and bisexual men. Also, HIV infection is a sexually transmitted disease and most people in America and other nations are heterosexual.

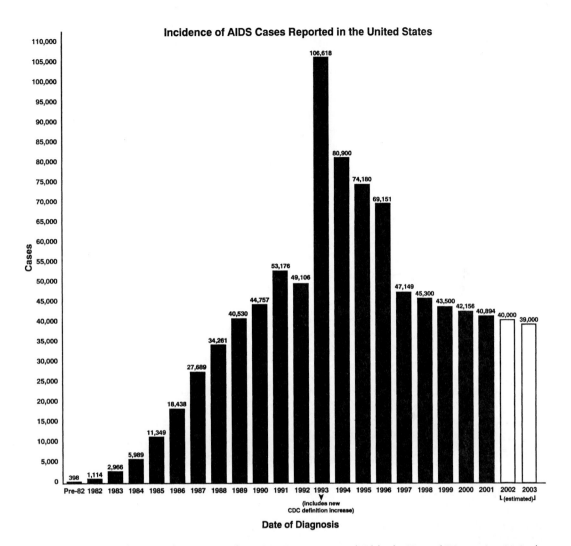

FIGURE 10-6   Incidence and Estimates of AIDS in Persons 13 and Older by Year of Diagnosis—United States, pre-1982 through 2001. The total for 1995 reflects a 9% reduction in AIDS cases from 1994 due to a drop in the backlog of persons to be identified as AIDS cases according to the 1993 definition of AIDS. Data for years 2002 and 2003 reflect expected decreases in AIDS cases resulting from better access to therapy. Throughout the American pandemic, about 85% of persons with AIDS were aged 20–49.

SHAPE OF THE HIV PANDEMIC: UNITED STATES

There is a common misconception that the AIDS epidemic is under control in the developed world. While mortality rate associated with HIV has been sharply reduced, thanks to behavioral changes and antiretroviral drugs, they are imperfect solutions.

Drug therapies are expensive, often toxic, and not a cure. AIDS education programs have impeded but have not stopped the epidemic. The United States has the highest rate of HIV infection among the world's most highly industrialized countries, in spite of the fact that it serves as a leader in AIDS **education** and **prevention.** About 1 in 300 people in the United States is HIV infected. The ratio in some sub-Saharan countries is 1 in 5 and in some African villages the ratio is 1 in 2 women of child-bearing age.

Reviewing Figure 10-7 one can extrapolate backward and see that there were about 19,000 people HIV-infected in 1977; ending 1978, 40,000; ending 1979, 60,000; 1980, 90,000. These people were all infected and relatively few had died—32 prior to 1981.

Based on the HIV presentation of HIV infections in Figure 10-7 during the years 1981 through 1983, HIV infections reached their peak and then rapidly declined. No one can say exactly which factors have been responsible for bringing the annual new HIV infection rate down from some 190,000 people in 1982 to 40,000 a year each year from 1988 to 1998. From 1999 through 2002 there were 50,000 new infection per year. For a breakdown of new HIV infections, see Figure 10-8. These figures are an estimate because new cases of HIV infection are not reportable by federal law and there is no blood-testing program that measures infection rates nationally.

The populations that are encompassed in the numbers of new infections are different from the past: HIV is now reaching younger people, it's reaching more women, it's reaching more communities of color. Forty-two percent of new infections are occurring in gay men, 33% in heterosexuals in-fected during sex, and 25% in injecting drug users. Infections in heterosexual women are increasing more rapidly than in any other group. Unless a preventive vaccine is found, the rate of new HIV infections in the United States is expected to remain at 50,000 plus annually. This may mean the new prevention campaigns, **without a vaccine, will not** significantly reduce new infections. Society has, in a sense, reduced new HIV infections to its lower limit.

Class Discussion: Is the last statement plausible—have we reached a point at which further expenditures will not significantly reduce the rate of infection—that all society can do now is wait on a preventive vaccine? What would be your solution given that we have actually reached this point and no vaccine is forthcoming?

SHAPE OF AIDS PANDEMIC: UNITED STATES

There has been a decline in new AIDS cases in every region of the United States. The decline began in 1996 and continues into year 2003.

Although the noticeable drop in new AIDS cases is a renewed cause for hope, the down side is the slowing progression to AIDS and to AIDS deaths (discussed next) means more HIV-infected

Shape of the HIV Epidemic, United States

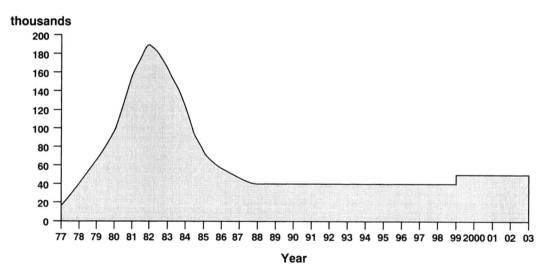

FIGURE 10-7   Estimated Rate of HIV Infection 1977 through 2003; United States. *(Source: Centers for Disease Control and Prevention)*

New HIV Infections

There are an estimated 950,000 people currently living with HIV in the United States with about 50,000 new HIV infections occurring in the United States annually since 1999.

By gender, 70% of new HIV infections each year occur among men, although women are also significantly affected.

By risk, men who have sex with men (MSM) represent the largest proportion of new infections, followed by men and women infected through heterosexual sex and injection drug use.

By race, more than half of the new HIV infections occur among blacks, though they represent 13% of the U.S. population. Hispanics, who make up about 12% of the U.S. population, are also disproportionately affected.

Estimates of annual new infections by gender, (N ≅ 50,000)

Estimates of annual new infections by risk, (N ≅ 50,000)

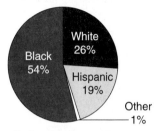

Estimates of annual new infections by race, (N ≅ 50,000)

To better understand how the HIV/AIDS epidemic is affecting men and women, it is critical we look at race and risk by gender.

Estimates of annual new infections in women, U.S., by race and risk

Estimates of annual new infections in men, U.S., by race and risk

FIGURE 10-8 A Glance at the HIV Epidemic in America. *(Source: Centers for Desease Control and Prevention updated)*

people with better health are available to spread HIV. According to the CDC, beginning in 2003 there were about 370,000 adult/adolescent people and 4000 children **reported** to be **living** with AIDS in the United States. The **estimated** number of people currently living with HIV is 950,000. The slowing of AIDS diagnosis makes tracking the epidemic harder. The ability to monitor the epidemic based on HIV infections does not, at the moment, compare with the CDC's ability to track the pandemic through the reporting of AIDS cases.

ESTIMATES OF DEATHS AND YEARS OF POTENTIAL LIFE LOST DUE TO AIDS IN THE UNITED STATES

"All my friends are dead." This expression is unique in a lifetime and is symbolic of reaching old age—except in a time of war. Too many young people worldwide have said it over the past 22 years because of AIDS.

Deaths Due to AIDS

Each year in the United States there are about 2,300,000 deaths. AIDS has, from 1991 through 1995, caused at least 40,000 of these deaths each year, and accounted for about 1.8% of all deaths for each of those years. That is, two people of each 100 who died, died of AIDS.

THE GOOD NEWS is that between the end of 1995 and the end of 1996, AIDS deaths dropped in the United States for the first time since the pandemic began—25% nationwide (about 12,600 fewer deaths). Between 1996 and 1998 deaths had dropped by about 75% (Table 10-7). Similar data was reported from Europe. The sudden drop in expected deaths due to AIDS is believed to be associated with the use of combina-

---

Table 10-7 New HIV Infections and AIDS Deaths in the United States

Year	New HIV Infections	AIDS Deaths	Accumulative 5-Year Intervals
1977	19,000	—	—
1978	40,000	—	—
1979	60,000	—	—
1980	90,000	30 (before 1981)	30
1981	160,000	128	
1982	190,000	463	
1983	160,000	1508	
1984	120,000	3505	
1985	70,000	6972	12,576
1986	60,000	12,110	
1987	50,000	16,412	
1988	40,000	21,119	
1989	40,000	27,791	
1990	40,000	31,538	121,546
1991	40,000	35,616	
1992	40,000	41,094	
1993	40,000	45,381	
1994	40,000	49,869	
1995	40,000	50,610	344,116
1996	40,000	37,794	
1997	40,000	21,922	
1998	40,000	17,949	
1999	50,000	17,172	
2000	50,000	15,245	454,198
2001	50,000	14,000	
2002	50,000	14,000	
2003	50,000	13,500	

Cumulative Deaths from AIDS in the United States from 1977 Through 2001. Data for years 2002 through 2003 are estimated. Worldwide, ending 2003 about 26 million people will have died of AIDS. AIDS deaths dropped by 75% from 1995 through year 2000. A similar or greater drop in AIDS deaths occurred in Europe over the same time period. It took from 1981 to about 1988, about 7 years, to reach the first 100,000 AIDS cases. Over the next 12 years there were an additional 700,000 AIDS cases.

tion drug therapy. (See Chapter 4 for more detail on the use of combination drug therapy.) Because of this enormous change in the natural history of AIDS, mortality no longer provides an accurate picture of the extent of the epidemic.

AIDS As a Cause of Death in the United States and Worldwide Beginning Year 2003

United States

♦ AIDS is no longer listed as one of the 15 leading causes of death for all ages.

♦ AIDS is the fifth leading cause of death among people ages 25 to 44.

♦ AIDS is the leading cause of death of black American men ages 25 to 44.

♦ AIDS is currently the fourth leading cause of death among all U.S. women ages 25 to 44, and the second cause of death among black women ages 25 to 44.

♦ AIDS is the seventh leading cause of death among children ages 1 to 14.

♦ In some cities in the northeastern United States, AIDS is the leading cause of death among children ages 2 to 5.

♦ In the United States between four and five people per hour become HIV-infected 365 days a year (40,000) and **every hour** about two people die (15,000). **Before 1996 one person died every 13 minutes.**

♦ Annually, from 1999 through 2002, there have been about 15,000 AIDS deaths and 50,000 new HIV infections. Thus, the number of HIV positive people has increased each year by about 35,000.

♦ Of those living with HIV infections, about 950,000 beginning 2003, 41% are white, 38% are black and 20% are Hispanic. Men make up 79% and women 21%.

♦ Through year 2010, an estimated 590,000 people will have died of AIDS.

Worldwide 2003 (See Figures 10-9, 10-10, and 10-11).

♦ Worldwide, 570 people become HIV-infected every hour, 365 days a year (5 million) and **every hour 342 people die** (3 million).

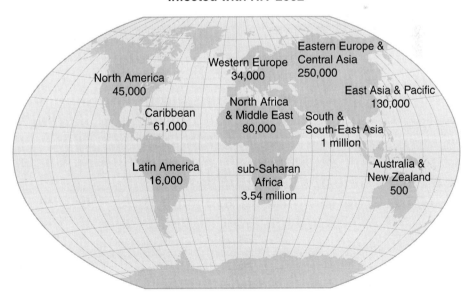

Global Estimates of Adults and Children Newly Infected with HIV 2002

Eastern Europe & Central Asia 250,000

Western Europe 34,000

North America 45,000

East Asia & Pacific 130,000

Caribbean 61,000

North Africa & Middle East 80,000

South & South-East Asia 1 million

Latin America 16,000

sub-Saharan Africa 3.54 million

Australia & New Zealand 500

Estimates are for the entire globe.
Total: 5 million

FIGURE 10-9 End of Year 2002 Estimate for New HIV Infections. The number of new HIV infections for 2001 was 5 million. *(UNAIDS, 2001 updated)*

- Ending year 2003, about 70 million people will have been HIV-infected, about 95% in developing countries.

- Nine out of ten HIV positive people are unaware they are infected.

- Ending year 2003, about 26 million people will have died of AIDS.

- 80% of those dying from AIDS are between ages 20 and 50. These are the people who enforce laws, harvest food, work the factories, heal the sick, keep students, and raise children.

- Ending year 2010 about 55 million people will have died of AIDS. Ending 2020 about 80 million people will have died of AIDS.

- If nothing changes, there will be an estimated 75 million to 100 million new HIV infections by 2020.

- It is estimated that new HIV infections will peak in year 2060.

Year End Estimates: Adult/Children Living with HIV Infection

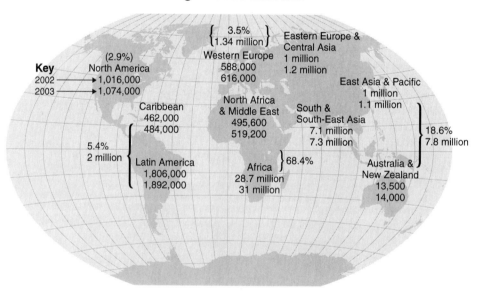

*Totals are estimates for the entire globe, %s for year 2002.

Total: 2002 — 42 million
2003 — 44 million

FIGURE 10-10   End-of-Year 2002 and 2003 Estimates of People Living with HIV Infection. Of the 42 million alive ending 2002, 96.4% are adult/adolescent, 50% are men, 46.4% women, and 3.6% are under age 15. *(UNAIDS, updated) Currently the Asia-Pacific region is experiencing over 1 million new HIV infections a year!*

Population and HIV Infection Rates in Selected African Countries

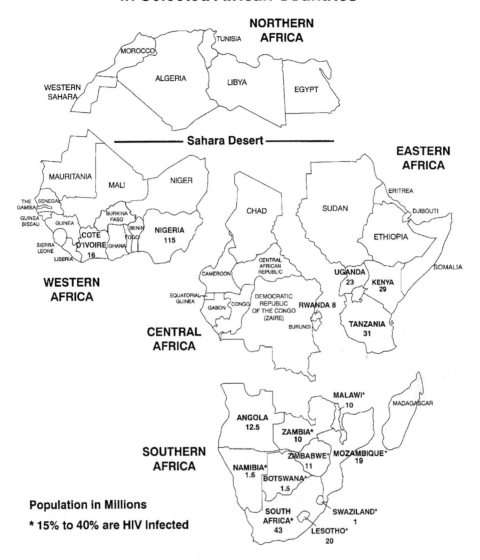

FIGURE 10-11 Map of Africa. Population of Africa = 800 million. Population of sub-Saharan Africa = 657 million. Prevalence of HIV infections and AIDS cases is highest in Southern Africa. South Africa with 43 million people has 4.9 million HIV-infected people, the highest incidence of HIV infection in the world. In seven African countries over 20% of the age 15-to 19-year-old population is HIV-infected, from 20% in South Africa to about 40% among adults in Botswana. The lifetime risk of dying from AIDS for a boy who is currently 15 is 65% in South Africa and near 90% in Botswana. Karen Stanecki of the U.S. Census Bureau reported that in KwaZulu Natal, a province of South Africa, HIV infection has reached 46%. In Francistown, Bostswana, HIV infection among adults is at 42%. Stanecki projected that AIDS deaths will peak in sub-Saharan Africa in 2020 at 6.5 million deaths/year; South Africa in 2010 at 940,000/year; Haiti in 2017 at 39,000/year; Thailand in 2000 at 66,000/year; Myanmar (Burma) in 2015 at 97,000/year; Brazil in 2002 at 623,000/year. *(Map courtesy of Centers for Disease Control and Prevention)*

Former Surgeon General C. Everett Koop has said on a number of occasions that **"AIDS is virtually 100% fatal."** Looking back over the number of AIDS cases diagnosed and comparing them to the number of AIDS patients who have died would indicate that a diagnosis of AIDS is a death sentence. Table 10-7 presents a sobering look at the numbers of AIDS patients who have died in America since those first CDC reported cases in 1981. People with HIV disease/AIDS were, through 1995, dying at the rate of about 3000 a month. **Over 95% of those diagnosed with AIDS in 1981 have now died.** And about 60% of AIDS cases diagnosed up through 1999 have died.

AIDS Deaths Postponed

Many of the deaths that would have occurred in the United States in 1996 through 2002 are being **POSTPONED** through the use of combination cocktail drug therapy and in particular the use of at least **one protease inhibitor** within the drug cocktail.

Six years of declining AIDS deaths means more Americans are living with HIV disease, which also means there are that many more people capable of spreading HIV.

The majority of AIDS deaths have occurred among homosexual/bisexual men (59%) and among women and heterosexual men who were injection drug users (21%). Most (75%) of AIDS deaths have occurred among people 25 to 44 years of age and about 24% occurred in those over age 45. In 1992, HIV disease/AIDS became the number one cause of death among black and Hispanic men ages 25 to 44 and second among black women ages 25 to 44 (*MMWR*, 1994b). Between January 1993 and December 1995 AIDS was the leading cause of death in all Americans aged 25 to 44 (*MMWR*, 1995a). For 1996 it dropped to second. In 2000, AIDS dropped to the 18th leading cause of death in the United States.

It now appears that for the age group 25–44, AIDS is the leading cause of death among black American men, third for Hispanics and sixth for whites. After rapidly increasing in the 1980s, the annual rate of death from AIDS peaked in 1995 at about 50,000 deaths, decreased through 1997, and from 1998 through 2002 ranged from 14,500 to 16,000 a year. According to the CDC, people now dying from AIDS increasingly consist of females, blacks and residents of the South.

According to the CDC, deaths from HIV disease/AIDS are currently underreported by 10% to 15%. Although most deaths occurred among whites, proportional rates have been highest for blacks and Hispanics.

The HIV/AIDS pandemic has taken on different forms in various parts of the world. In some areas, HIV infection has spread rapidly to the general population; in others, the spread has remained among higher-risk subpopulations, including sex workers and their customers, men who have sex with men, and injection drug users. Worldwide, the adult prevalence rate is 1.07% of the population, and 47% of infections occur among women. AIDS is the fourth leading cause of death worldwide and the leading cause of death in sub-Saharan Africa. According to estimates, about 26 million adults and children will have died of HIV/AIDS ending 2003. There are over 5000 AIDS deaths each day in Africa and that number is expected to rise to 13,000 a day by year 2005. Because the number of people infected with HIV continues to expand, the annual number of deaths worldwide can be expected to increase. Since 1999, one in five HIV related deaths were among children and over half the adults who died of HIV-related causes were women. Without effective measures to prevent its spread, experts estimate that AIDS could take 100 million lives by 2010 and exceed 200 million by 2020. These estimates worry epidemiologists because with so many people with compromised immune systems, where and when will a new virus or bacterium evolve to take advantage of this huge pool of endangered people before moving into healthy people?

UNITED STATES—WHO IS DYING OF AIDS?

The American AIDS epidemic once seen as a disease of middle-class gay white men has become a killer of minorities and the poor including African-American and Hispanic homo-sexual men, injection drug users, and innercity women.

Year 2001 and 2002 government statistics show that minorities account for about 7 in 10 new AIDS cases.

In proportion, since 1985, the rate of death was higher for women than for men (*MMWR*, 1996d). **Through the year 1990, over 120,000 people died from AIDS. By the end of 2003, about 495,000 people will have died from AIDS.** To place the death rate due to AIDS in perspective, each day in America in 2002, about 6000 people died from assorted causes while about 40 died each day from AIDS. Worldwide, an estimated 3 million people died of AIDS in 2001 and in 2002. Of these deaths, 46% were women and about 7% were children. Worldwide ending year 2003, of an estimated 75 million HIV-infected persons, about 44 million will be living with HIV disease. The rate of increase in new AIDS cases has slowed, but the number of new cases exceeds the number who die of AIDS by over 60% annually.

Prevalence and Impact of HIV/AIDS

However, if the impact of the disease is measured—by deaths, AIDS cases, or monetary losses—it is just beginning. The worldwide impact during the 1990s was 5 to 10 times that of the 1980s. As the pandemic continues, the United States will find itself progressively more involved with prevention/treatment programs and with the political changes that HIV/AIDS will bring about in countries with a high incidence of HIV/AIDS.

LIFE EXPECTANCY

In 1995, the Metropolitan Life Insurance Company published data that shows that life expectancy reached its peak in the United States in 1992 at 75.8 years. For the years 1993 and 1994 it dropped to 75.5 years. The forecast is that continued loss due to AIDS will further erode life expectancy.

A mortality analysis of homosexual males indicates that gay men in Vancouver, British Columbia, have a life expectancy 8 to 20 years shorter than nongay men in the same area (Hog et al., 1997). The researchers note that if the trend continues, "We estimate that nearly half of gay and bisexual men currently aged 20 years will not reach their 65th birthday." The study collected vital statistics from 1987 to 1992 and assessed mortality rates based on 3%, 6%, and 9% prevalence rates of homosexual and bisexual men. "Under even the most liberal assumptions, gay and bisexual men in this urban center are now experiencing a life expectancy similar to that experienced by all men in Canada in the year **1871.**"

CONNECTED BUT SEPARATE

Although all nations on Earth are connected in so many ways, there remains a separation of the **haves and have-nots**—the developed and developing nations.

Beginning year 2001 the developing nations have lost 6 million people to AIDS, tuberculosis and malaria, and 14 million people to communicable diseases annually. The practice of prevention and availability of medicines are paramount but neither is currently an option.

Worlds Apart

Beginning 2002, the **joint United Nations Program on HIV/AIDS (UNAIDS)** reported that each day, an estimated 14,000 men, women, and children in developing countries become infected with HIV. Forty-five percent of these infections occur in people ages 10 to 24. They are being infected at a rate of about 10 per minute, 600/hour, 14,400/day or 5 million/year. By the year 2020, there will be over 40 million orphans under the age of 15 in the 23 countries most affected by HIV. Most of these children will have lost their parents to AIDS. In contrast, in the industrialized world, new infections spread at the rate of 500 per day, less than one every 30 minutes. This disparity between rich and poor nations has increased dramatically over the course of the pandemic. In 1980, roughly twice as many adults were infected in sub-Saharan Africa as in North America; beginning 2003, **29 times** as many were infected. Altogether, UNAIDS estimates that about 95% of the world's current 42 million living HIV-infected people are in developing countries.

Africa, the HIV/AIDS Time Bomb: It Is Ticking Out of Control

Africa, with about 10% of the world's population, now accounts for about 90% of all new HIV infections. Beginning 2003, about 83% of all AIDS deaths have occurred in Africa. The United Nations in 2002 reported that in Africa's 25 worst affected countries, 7 million agricultural workers have died from AIDS since 1985 and 16 million more could die by 2020. Also, unless there is some immediate relief, by 2006 most Africans will not live to see their 48th birthday. Stefano Vella, president of the International AIDS Society, said in 2002, "This pandemic is not stabilizing, it is just beginning, it's just a baby beginning to grow." As a comparison, Vella said that if the United States had in proportion the same HIV infection rate as Botswana, between 35%–40%, there would be 40 million HIV-infected in America. Africa has been living with a biological terrorist for the past 22 years with no end in sight.

Deepening the Misery

To add to the HIV/AIDS problem in Africa, in May of 2002, reports out of Southern Africa, where as many as 20 million people are afflicted by hunger or malnutrition, reveal that this region of Africa is experiencing the worst food shortage in nearly 60 years, and HIV/AIDS is deepening the misery. Hunger is accelerating the onset of AIDS-related illnesses and death among household breadwinners. As a result, the AIDS epidemic is compounding the food problems by leaving the elderly and children to care for the sick, plant and harvest the crops, and take odd jobs for extra income. Seven countries facing the devastating drought have HIV prevalence rates over 20%: Botswana (40%), Lesotho (31%), Namibia (23%), South Africa (20%), Swaziland (34%), Zambia (22%), and Zimbabwe (34%).

By any and every measure, AIDS is a plague of biblical proportion. It is claiming more lives in Africa than in all the wars waging on the continent combined. AIDS is now the leading cause of death among all people of all ages in Africa and the progression of this pandemic has outpaced all projections (Figure 10-11). For example, in 1991, the World Health Organization predicted that by 1999 there would be 9 million infected and nearly 5 million deaths in Africa due to AIDS. Ending 2003, the numbers are about 29 million infected and 23.5 million deaths. Nearly all those currently HIV-infected in Africa will die around year 2010! **It is estimated that there are 11,000 new HIV infections each day in Africa.** From 1998 through 2002, AIDS killed, on average, 2.4 million annually, or over 6000 per day. With such overwhelming numbers, it is important to re-member that the data is about people not numbers, and not facts and figures, but faces and families (see Figures 10-12 and 10-13).

Of all reported AIDS cases, 91% are estimated to have been heterosexually acquired. Infections through blood transfusions and perinatal transmission from mother to child have also contributed to the spread of HIV across the continent. Tuberculosis (TB) is the most common opportunistic infection among AIDS patients in Africa. The contribution of the factors that facilitate transmission—high prevalence of STD, low rate of male circumcision, the unequal status of women, migration, poverty, and patterns of social mixing—differs by country. The HIV/AIDS pandemic in Africa is like an explosion in slow motion, a slowly moving chain reaction—no sound, no blinding flash, no intense heat, no mushroom cloud, no buildings destroyed—just one silent death after another with no end in sight. Whole generations of people are in jeopardy with so little hope to go around in the developing nations.

Survival after HIV Infection Compared to Survival in Developed Nations

Dilys Morgan and colleagues (2002) reported that survival in Africa after HIV infection prior to drug treatment is not very different than what occurs in developed or industrialized countries like the United States. The median survival from seroconversion was 9.8 years, which shows that HIV infection is not a more rapidly progressive disease in Africans. Once AIDS developed, the median survival was only 9.2 months, which is similar to that reported early in the epidemic in industrialized countries although much shorter than survival in these countries now. The majority of HIV-infected persons who die of AIDS most often have very low T4 or CD4+ cell counts at the time of death.

AFRICA IS DYING THROUGH DARWINIAN PERVERSION

The February 2001 issue of *Time* magazine labels AIDS in Africa a "Darwinian perversion" that is wiping out not the frailest but the fittest of its human species—farmers, miners, laborers, truck drivers, doctors, nurses, teachers, administrators, parliamentarians—while leaving societies "saturated

FIGURE 10-12 The Long Journey Home. Friends chant while carrying the body of their friend to his mother's home in Haiti. It is many miles up through the mountains to a small rural village where he grew up. He left home at the age of 15 to find work. He is now returned home for burial at age 28.*(Photo by Mike Stocker/South Florida Sun-Sentinel)*

FIGURE 10-13 Charles is 3 years old. He is HIV positive and has tuberculosis. He was admitted to Grace Children's Hospital in Port-au-Prince in January 2001 suffering from seizures, chronic fever, skin lesions, loss of appetite, and weight loss. His mother died of AIDS. *(Photo by Mike Stocker/South Florida Sun-Sentinel)*

with orphans" without the capacity to care for them. Richard Holbrooke, the former U.S. ambassador to the United Nations compares Africa's AIDS crisis to the Black Death or bubonic plague that annihilated a quarter of Europe in the 14th century. A 2001 feature in *The New York Times* warned that the worst is yet to come: "Someday, we may look back on the year 2001 with nostalgia for a time when AIDS was merely a health catastrophe . . . As they lose their most productive citizens, (African) nations themselves face collapse." Ignorance is the crucial reason the epidemic has run out of control. Surveys say many Africans are becoming aware that there is an incurable sexually transmitted disease called AIDS, but they don't think the risk applies to them. Their vague knowledge does not translate into changes in their sexual behavior. It's easy to understand why so many don't yet sense the danger when few talk openly about the disease. Africans are so beset by a roster of perils, famine, war, the violence of desperation or ethnic hatred, the regular illnesses of poverty, the dangers inside

mines or on the roads, that the delayed risk of AIDS ranks low.

UNAIDS, 2000

"**HIV will kill at least a third of the young men and women of countries where it has its firmest hold, and in some places up to two-thirds. Despite millennia of epidemics, war and famine, never before in history have death rates of this magnitude been seen among young adults of both sexes and from all walks of life.**" If death rates continue, even for a few more years, AIDS will kill more humans on the African continent than the 50 million who died on every front and in death camps in World War II.

Life Expectancy

AIDS already has sharply reduced life expectancy in many southern African countries. For instance, in Botswana, where more than one-third of adults are infected with HIV, life expectancy is now 39 in-

---

POINT OF VIEW 10.2

HIV STALKING AFRICA

A professor at South Africa's Pretoria University explained how HIV stalks the people of her country. "It is presumed if you get AIDS you have done something wrong. We have no language to talk candidly about sex, so we have no civil languages to talk about AIDS. As a result, the consequences of the silence march on: infection soars, stigma hardens, denial hastens death, and the chasm between knowledge and behavior widens." Because HIV is spread through sexual intercourse, migrant truck drivers and prostitutes commonly spread the virus.

Botswana, a country about the size of Texas, with a population of about 1.6 million, has the world's highest rates of HIV infection. In Francistown, where international highways and trade routes converge, at least 43% of adults are HIV positive. Prostitutes often trade sex for the transport of fruit, toilet paper and toys to families. In Gaborone, the capital of Botswana, 44% of those between ages 15 and 49 are HIV infected. Among women ages 25 to 30, about 50% are infected. Throughout the country there's premari-

tal sex, sex as recreation, obligatory sex and its abusive counterpart, coercive sex, transactional sex, sex as a gift, sugar-daddy sex, extramarital sex, and multiple partners. Men rarely agree to use condoms and women often engage in dry sex to please their partners, both practices significantly increasing the risk of contracting or transmitting HIV. The question asked but not answered is: How did HIV infection become so advanced in one of the most democratic, wealthiest, best educated and least corrupt nations in Africa?

Children orphaned by AIDS add another complex dimension to Africa's epidemic because communities are becoming saturated with them. "Most orphans drop out of school, suffer malnutrition, ostracism, psychic distress . . . girls fall into prostitution and older boys migrate illegally to South Africa, leaving the younger ones to go on the streets." The death toll from AIDS in Africa threatens to wreak the region's frail economies, break down civil societies, and incite political instability.

---

stead of 71, as it would have been without the disease. It is projected that by 2010, life expectancy will be 29 in Botswana, 30 in Swaziland, 33 in Namibia and Zimbabwe, and 36 in South Africa, Malawi, and Rwanda. Without AIDS, it would have been around 70 in many of those countries (Figure 10-14). More people died of AIDS each year from 1999 through 2002 in Africa than in all the wars on the continent during those years, including conflicts in Angola, Congo-Brazzaville, Sierra Leone, Somalia, Sudan, Ethiopia, and Eritrea. About one in 30 people are HIV-infected. Beginning year 2003, 90% of all African children with perinatal infection and 95% of all African AIDS orphans reside in sub-Saharan Africa.

Sub-Saharan Africa

The sheer number of Africans infected by this epidemic in this region is overwhelming. Ending 2003, there was an estimated 29 million people living in sub-Saharan Africa that have been infected with HIV and about 23 million people have died, about a quarter of them children. Beginning 2003, 70% of all people living with HIV live here as well as 90% of all cases of mother to child HIV transmission cases. In Rwanda, it is estimated that 80% of women are HIV positive resulting from rape by Rwandan soldiers during the genocide of a million Tutsi and Hutu. Overall, 55% of all new HIV infections in sub-Saharan Africa occur in women. In Botswana, Namibia, Swaziland, and Zimbabwe, current estimates show that between 20% and 30% of people aged 15 to 49 are living with HIV. In Zimbabwe, 30% to 50% of all pregnant women are now found to be infected and at least one-third of these women will pass the infection on to their babies. South Africa, which escaped much of the epidemic in the 1980s, is now being hit particularly hard.

South Africa

Nearly 5 million South Africans, roughly one in nine people and one in four adults are living with HIV/AIDS—and dying from it. Estimates are that ending 2010, about 7 million South Africans will have died from AIDS.

One in seven new infections on the African continent is occurring in South Africa, about 2000 infections per day. Ten percent or 200 are babies.

Military

In South Africa, according to *Johannesburg Mail and Guardian* newspaper, up to 70% of the South African National Defense Force may be infected with HIV. In one unit in KwaZulu Natal, 90% of troops are infected. Some military units near Pietermaritzburg and on the South African Mozambique border also had HIV infection rates higher than 70%. South Africa's military infection rate is similar to neighboring countries. In Malawi, 75% of the military is HIV positive, and in Mozambique, 80% have tested positive. Forces in the Democratic Republic of the Congo and Angola also have high rates of HIV infection.

WORKFORCE—SOUTH AFRICA: SOME EXAMPLES

In April 2002, NMG-Levy, Agence France-Presse reported that by 2005 about 30% of South Africa's labor force will be HIV positive. The pandemic is taking dramatic toll on the most productive members of the population, those in their 20s, 30s, and 40s.

Mining

AngloGold, a gold mining company in South Africa, reported that about 30% of its 44,000 employees are already HIV positive.

Agriculture

The International Labor Organization stated that by 2010 over 30% of the farmers in South Africa would be HIV positive.

Nurses

An estimated 20% or 35,000 South African nurses are HIV positive. A Netcare group nursing manager recently told delegates that half of first-year students at one of the province's four nursing colleges are HIV positive. At another of the colleges, 70% of students are attending a local HIV clinic. At another, 21% of the students have volunteered information that they are HIV positive. In addition, 200 nurses a month are going abroad. The nursing manager said, "In our organization we are losing registered nurses. We are sitting with nurses who are dying now, and the students are even worse off."

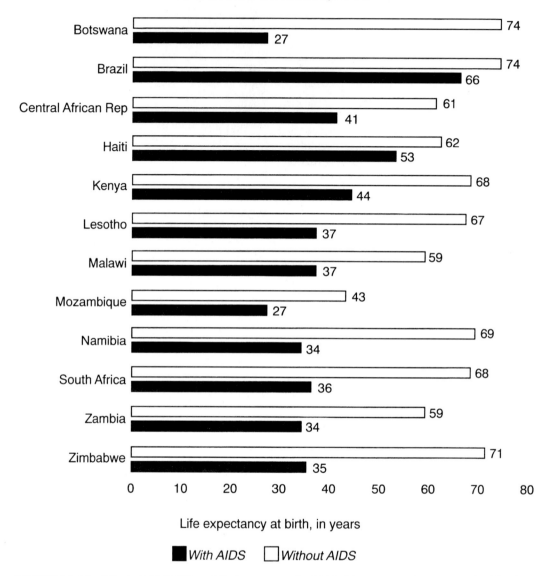

Projected Impact on Life Expectancy in Selected Countries, 2010

Country	Without AIDS	With AIDS
Botswana	74	27
Brazil	74	66
Central African Rep	61	41
Haiti	62	53
Kenya	68	44
Lesotho	67	37
Malawi	59	37
Mozambique	43	27
Namibia	69	34
South Africa	68	36
Zambia	59	34
Zimbabwe	71	35

Life expectancy at birth, in years

■ With AIDS   □ Without AIDS

FIGURE 10-14 Effect of HIV/AIDS on Life Expectancy. By 2010, life expectancies in many highly affected countries could drop below 30, reversing steady gains over the last century. According to a report by the U.S. Census Bureau presented at the 2002 XIV International AIDS Conference, AIDS will cause a drop in life expectancy in 51 countries over the next 20 years. The report also states that five African nations (Botswana, South Africa, Mozambique, Lesotho, and Swaziland) will experience more deaths than births by 2010, meaning populations will begin declining. The bureau predicts that life expectancy will drop to just 27 years in Botswana and Mozambique in the next eight years, while Swaziland will have an estimated life expectancy of 33 years, and Zimbabwe, Zambia, and Namibia will have an expected life span of 34 years. Without AIDS, the bureau said the life expectancy in Africa would have been approximately 70 years by 2010. *(Adapted from Henry J. Kaiser Foundation Facts Sheet, July 2002.)*

EDUCATION: TEACHERS AND STUDENTS—SOUTH AFRICA AND SOME COUNTRIES IN SOUTHERN AFRICA

As many teachers are dying every year of HIV/AIDS as qualify to teach, school districts exhausting their annual budgets within two months on transporting deceased teachers to their homes, widespread closure of schools because HIV/AIDS has stripped them of their teachers. These nightmare scenarios afflict Kenya, Zambia, Botswana, Uganda, the Central African Republic, and South Africa. The devastating impact of HIV/AIDS on teachers and learners was a repeated concern at a national policy conference on teacher training and development convened by the Department of Education in Midrand, Gauteng. The conference also heard that there has been an incredible 85% decrease in the number of students in pre-service teacher education programs between 1994 and 2002. These alarming trends are being identified at a time when the need for effective and widespread teacher training has never been greater. The country is poised to implement Curriculum 2005, the radically new teaching and learning methodology that has been on the drawing board since the mid-1990s. Nearly 400,000 in-service teachers have to be trained in the new curriculum by 2004. Where will they come from?

Nelson Mandela, the former president of South Africa, said in September 2000 that in South Africa, 10 teachers die every month from AIDS and one student dies of AIDS each week in each of the country's 74 colleges and universities—roughly 120 teachers and 3600 students a year. About one in eight teachers are HIV positive. In Durban Westville University in South Africa, about 25% of students are HIV positive.

Kenya lost 1000 teachers to AIDS in 1996, 1200 in 1997, 1500 in 1998, and over 2000 in 1999. The death rate is now up to 6205 teachers in 2002 or 17 a day of about 170/month, and the trend continues. Also, one in five secondary students and one in five college students are HIV positive in Kenya.

Zambia and Swaziland are losing about 130 teachers/month. Two teachers die for one graduated. So the teachers are not being replaced. The pool of uneducated becomes larger as does the number of students in the classrooms that continue. In Tanzania, it is estimated that over the next seven years, between 15,000 and 30,000 teachers will die of AIDS (2010). To date, in sub-Saharan Africa, some 2 million students lost their teachers to AIDS over the past several years. Many schools have closed because of teacher shortage.

In part of Malawi, Uganda, Botswana, and Zambia, over 30% of teachers are HIV positive. In the Central African Republic, 85% of teachers who died between 1996 and 1998 were HIV positive and died approximately 10 years before they were due to retire.

Burying the Dead

AIDS is the leading cause of death in South Africa. In 2002, over 40% of all adult deaths were due to AIDS.

In Soweto, South Africa, as in many South African cities and towns, burying those dying from AIDS has become a daily chore, They used to bury the dead on Saturdays. Too many are dying. "There are so many funerals, it is chaos. We don't know which funeral to attend. On some days we attend three funerals. Which neighbor or which family members' funeral should we attend? We must choose."

As AIDS continues to claim the country's young, it has transformed black neighborhoods into open-air funeral parlors and neighbors into widows, orphans, and grieving relatives.

OTHER TIME BOMBS: INDIA, CHINA, AND RUSSIA

The time bombs for the future are the world's most populous nations, China and India, each of which have over 1 billion citizens. HIV is now spreading rapidly in those countries, and because of their huge populations, even a fraction of the infection seen in Africa would be devastating.

India

If by 2010 just 2% of the Indian population is HIV-infected, that would be 20 million people. UNAIDS reports that about 7 to 8 million Indians are already infected and the virus is spreading rapidly in that country, primarily through heterosexual activities and injection drug use. During the June 5, 2001,

VARIOUS ASPECTS OF DEATH IN SUB-SAHARAN AFRICA

BURIAL CHANGES BECAUSE OF TOO MANY AIDS DEATHS IN ZAMBIA

AIDS has changed the way people live. Now it is changing the way they are buried. As the AIDS toll rises, Zambia's local government authorities complain that burial ground is being filled up almost as soon as it is designated and predict a serious shortage soon. Zambians are being encouraged to look at cremation as a burial option. This has elicited serious debate. Zambians are by nature a very superstitious people who fear changes in cultural practices. University of Zambia's Department of History Professor Yizenge Chondoka says to shift peoples' thinking from burial to cremation will be hard. There are certain rites that can only be performed at graveyards to complete the burial process and ensure that the spirit of those buried is at peace. He asks, "If we begin to cremate, where will these rites be performed?" There is a psychological process that people need to go through to accept cremation. Otherwise, any misfortune that befalls a family will be attributed to the dead person whose spirit is wandering because it has not gone through the burials rites and is not settled on some place. Chondoka says Zambians have shrines at burial sites where they consult the spirits of the dead in times of need. "If we begin to cremate and throw or keep ashes in small clusters in our houses, where will the shrines be put up?" Gertrude Chamabantu, a marriage counselor, says as a Christian nation, the dead should be buried with the proper funeral rites just as Jesus was buried. Lusaka has three designated cemeteries (besides unofficial ones), which can take about 10,000 graves, but these are already full and people are now squeezing their dead on what used to be thoroughfares. Chandoka says Zambia has adequate land for graveyards. However, because the sites in the immediate vicinity have been filled up, people will travel further to get to the graveyards.

Then there is the problem of economics, a teacher at the Zambian School of Education asks, "Do we really want valuable land to be taken up by graves?" AIDS is the leading cause of death in Africa. Beginning 2003, about 26 million people worldwide have died of AIDS. About 95% or 24.7 million of those deaths have occurred in Africa. About 6800 Africans die daily from AIDS. Death in Africa is a very public affair.

Funerals are big social events at which grief is expressed openly and lavishly. Families take large spaces in newspapers to announce the death of a loved one, complete with a picture, lists of achievements, and names of children. Now, about half of the faces staring out of the public death notices are young. They have died of AIDS. But in contrast to the public rites of death, this increasingly frequent cause goes whispered or unmentioned. AIDS is a taboo subject in Africa. She said, "At the rate we are dying (from AIDS), three quarters of Zambia will be a graveyard. There must be another way of disposing of our dead."

THE FUNERAL INDUSTRY—SOUTH AFRICA

Rising death rates in South Africa due to HIV/AIDS have led to the creation of a makeshift funeral industry. Many fly-by-night undertakers who are unlicensed and operate out of storefronts, compete to make funeral arrangements and leave bodies to decompose while they search for the cheapest means of disposal, creating a health hazard and raising costs to the government. The problem is greatest in Durban, capital of the hard hit KwaZulu-Natal province. Morgues and cemeteries have run out of room and the unlicensed undertakers are tempted to cut corners by mishandling bodies—burying them in mass graves or abandoning them in mortuaries. The government has not regulated the new undertakers (who are mainly black) because they were previously disadvantaged, but established funeral directors (mostly white and Indian) complain that the new undertakers would be subject to the same regulations. The newcomers said they are subcontractors for licensed morticians—they sell coffins and transport the body for burial while a licensed mortician washes, dresses, and stores the body. Sometimes licensed morticians front for the newcomers by picking up bodies at morgues for a fee, a violation of health regulations. This corpse shell game often results in bodies being moved several times or left to decompose. As AIDS death rise, the problem will only worsen. Currently, AIDS related deaths account for nearly a third of the country's 500 daily deaths and 40% of the deaths in KwaZulu-Natal. Deaths in South Africa could reach 16,000 a day by 2005, according to insurance experts. But talk of the rising death rate is all but taboo among government officials who, taking their cue from President Thabo Mbeki, barely acknowledge the extent of the HIV/AIDS epidemic or the rising death toll. Because of the stigma surrounding HIV/AIDS many families do not claim bodies, leaving the government to dispose of them at a cost of $150 each. The government has rejected the idea of cremating the bodies because African tradition stipulates that a person cannot enter the spirit world if his or her body is not buried intact. Because morgues and cemeteries are out of space, a black market has grown up in stolen burial equipment. Crooked morgue workers sell corpses to favored undertakers, or to the highest bidder, sometimes even before bereaved families arrive to claim a body—leaving the relatives no choice but to pay the undertaker who collected the remains. Rival hearse drivers carry pistols and exchange death threats. Most ominous of all, government hospitals are being left with more and more unclaimed bodies—mostly AIDS victims—to bury at unbudgeted public expense. Undertakers who bid for this work can be tempted to cut corners by mishandling bodies. This growing demand for mandatory pauper burials has already led to scandal: bodies allegedly dumped in mass graves or left unburied in mortuaries for months at a time. What to do with bodies in Africa is becoming a massive problem!

THE CASKET/BURIAL PLOT INDUSTRY— ZIMBABWE

Griffin Shea reported on the demand for caskets and burial plots in Zimbabwe in 2001. Deep in the shadow of Harare's office high rises, Luck Street is mostly islands of pavement in a river of mud and potholes. Despite its name, this side street in Zimbabwe's capital is where the city's least fortunate residents make their most-lasting purchases, a casket or coffin. With an economy in free fall and more than 3000 people dying of AIDS every week, coffin-making has become one of the country's few reliable sources of income. In outlying townships, vendors line up

caskets for sale next to tables of fruits and vegetables on the dusty roadside. But if you're on a budget—and almost everyone in Zimbabwe is— Luck Street is where you go for a bargain. At Sunshine Funeral Service, a darkened room behind a motorcycle repair shop, the owner and salesperson shows off his company's entire line of caskets, from a pressed-wood model that sells for about $15 to polished hardwood with shiny brass handles, $130. The owner said, "Last year, there were more people dying than in previous years. It is good business. People are dying." One thing that AIDS hasn't changed is the important place the funeral rites hold as part of the life cycle. Traditionalists say that the soul can take as long as a year to leave the body and join its ancestors in the spirit world—perhaps the reason for the traditional coffin burial. It is said that if people are not buried properly and given complete funeral rites by a medium, their souls will haunt their living relatives. After death, a number of rituals must be performed in order to assist the spirit. As funerals become an increasingly common part of life, Zimbabweans might have to find ways of blending their customs with modern realities. For about 30 cents per mile, the enterprising owners of Sunshine Funeral will send corpses back to their hometowns for burial, because most people prefer to be buried where they grew up. But skyrocketing inflation rates and a chronic fuel shortage have made that difficult for many urban dwellers, who are forced to buy a plot in cramped city cemeteries. According to Harare's director of cemeteries, eight of the city's 10 cemeteries are full. So the city is clearing five square miles of land to expand one of its cemeteries on the outskirts, where most of the graves will be dusty plots in the bare earth. The city does not maintain the gravesite. The effect will be something like Arlington National Cemetery without the grass or trees—acres of land covered with grave plots. The new space should give Harare enough room to keep burying its dead for the next few years. But with five square miles expected to fill quickly, Sunshine Funeral Services won't have to worry about closing its doors anytime soon.

twentieth anniversary of AIDS, a physician from India said on the *Jim Lehrer News Hour*, that he believes the real number of HIV-infected in India is between 8 million and 12 million.

The World Bank estimates that by 2006 there will be over 37 million HIV infected in India. The first case of AIDS was described in India in 1986. India is a vast heterogeneous country. Eighty percent of the people live in the countryside where many have never heard of HIV or AIDS. Some local authorities even challenge the existence of HIV or AIDS. Although it is believed that 83% of HIV infections occur through heterosexual intercourse with an infected partner, it is estimated that these will be between 4 million and 7 million HIV infections among female sex workers (prostitutes), their clients, and their families by year 2006.

Peter Piot, the Executive Director of UNAIDS, said in February 2002, "In the next few years, the number of HIV positive people in India could surpass the number of HIV positive South Africans if India does not step up prevention efforts. India currently has 3.8 million HIV-positive residents compared with 4.7 million HIV-positive South Africans. However, in India, HIV-positive adults account for only 0.7% of the national population, whereas South Africa's HIV-positive residents account for 20% of the population." Piot estimated that in 10 years, tens of millions of Indians could have HIV. Piot said he is particularly concerned about the epidemic in the Western state of Maharashtra where 2% of the adult population is HIV positive, and in the northeast where 30% to 40% of injection drug users have the virus. Also, the large migrant populations in Uttar Pradesh and Bihar make those states extremely vulnerable to the HIV/AIDS epidemic. The Indian government has launched a national program to combat the spread of HIV, but it is hindered by social and cultural beliefs. There's still a perception that HIV is something for the very poor, homosexual men, and drug users. The shame, stigma, and discrimination associated with AIDS make it very hard to have open discussions and deliver explicit messages about HIV/AIDS.

China

In August 2001, the deputy health minister held a first-ever news conference on the HIV/AIDS problem in China. A 2001 United Nations report estimated that over 1 million Chinese had HIV at the start of 2001, and that if current trends continue there could be 20 million by the end of 2010.

The first AIDS case was in an IDU discovered in the Yunnan province near the Burmese border in 1985. Since then HIV has spread rapidly among IDUs across China. Currently about 70% of China's IDU are HIV positive. Eighty percent of reported AIDS cases are among IDU and prostitutes. There are at least eight HIV subtypes and several HIV recombinants now circulating in China. China's central government has recently published a five-year plan to mobilize all parts of their society in HIV/AIDS prevention control. But, in June 2002, a United Nations report delivered scathing words about China's massive AIDS epidemic, stating that the country's efforts to stem the disease have had an "infinitesimally small impact." Titled "HIV/AIDS: China's Titanic Peril," the 89-page report portrays a government that has acknowledged the disease's spread but failed to contain or treat it on a large scale. Officials at some of the eight UN agencies that jointly issued the report stressed it wasn't an attack on the government, and praised increasing efforts by officials and the state media to address the scourge of HIV, the virus that causes AIDS. But, it is clearly a warning to a government that appears immobilized by the disease, even as a wealth of statistics confirm its rapid spread.

Russia

HIV quietly crept into Russia in 1987 through sex between gay men—a practice that was then illegal, making the disease an unspeakable taboo. But even as the numbers grew rapidly in the mid-1990s, primarily through intravenous drug use, few people paid attention. In his January 2002 address to the nation, Russian President Vladimir Putin spoke about the nation's overall health crisis but made no specific mention of HIV or AIDS. Peter Piot, the Executive Director of the United Nations AIDS Programs (UNAIDS) said in April 2002 that "Russia now has the fastest growing epidemic in the world, and I believe that the situation in Russia and the CIS (group of 12 ex-Soviet republics) is rapidly getting out of control." In year 2000 there were an estimated 80,000 HIV infected. Ending 2001 there were 250,000. According to the United Nations the actual number of HIV infected in Russia is about 800,000, while Russia's director of anti-AIDS Center, Vadim Pokrovsky, has suggested about a million Russians are HIV infected. If the current rate of infection continues, estimates are that over 5 million Russians will be infected by 2007. By 2015 between 5 million and 10 million will have died of AIDS. The major route of HIV transmission in Russia is through IDU. The age group most affected, as it is globally, is between ages 15 and 30. Half are under age 20. A major problem for Russia is that with this pandemic affecting the younger generations, Russia's shrinking population of 144 million people will continue to fall. Russia is faced by African-style depopulation, but in Africa its high birth rate moderates the effect of a large loss of life and will allow for population recovery.

SUMMARY

In 1981, the CDC reported the first case of AIDS in the United States, and, from that time onward, has constantly tracked the prevalence of AIDS cases in different geographical areas and within different behavioral risk groups. In all behavioral risk groups, the common denominator is the exchange of body fluids, in particular blood or semen. The heterosexual population at large is considered to be at low risk for HIV infection in the United States. By 1993, all states and the District of Columbia, Puerto Rico, and the Virgin Islands have reported AIDS cases in people who have had heterosexual contact with an at-risk partner.

A major problem exists in attempting to determine the number of HIV-infected people. Several different approaches have been used by the CDC to estimate the total number of HIV infections. These estimates can be evaluated by examining their compatibility with available prevalence data.

With respect to race and ethnicity, the cumulative incidence of AIDS cases is disproportionately higher in blacks and Hispanics than in whites. The ratio of black to white case incidence is 3.2:1 and the Hispanic to white ratio 2.8:1. This racial/ethnic disproportion is also observed in HIV-positive blood donors and in applicants for military service. Even among homosexual and bisexual men and IDUs, where race/ethnicity-specific data are available, blacks appear to have higher seroprevalence rates than whites.

With regard to prostitution, in a large multicenter study of female prostitutes, black and Hispanic prostitutes had a higher rate of HIV infection than white and other prostitutes. This disproportion existed for both prostitutes who used injection drugs and for those who did not acknowledge injection drug use.

The risk of new HIV infections in hemophiliacs and in people who receive blood transfusions has declined dramatically from 1985 because of the screening of donated blood and heat treatment of clotting factor concentrates. Evidence also indicates an appreciable decline in the incidence of new infections in homosexual men. However, the risk of new infections appears to remain high in IDUs and in their heterosexual partners. In several metropolitan cities, the prevalence of HIV infection in IDUs has been increasing.

Studies conducted by the CDC along with the American College Health Association revealed that in 1989, two college students per 1000 were HIV-infected.

There are some 5.3 million health care workers in the United States. Even though they are supposed to adhere to Universal Protection Guidelines set down by the CDC for their protection, a significant number are exposed to the AIDS virus annually. A relatively small number of those infected have progressed to AIDS.

Estimating the number of HIV-infected people in the United States continues to be a numbers game. Various agencies and private industries have, for different reasons, attempted to determine the number of HIV-infected people. The numbers from the different groups vary widely. However, the 1986 CDC estimated numbers of 1 to 1.5 million HIV-infected people may be too high. However, the number of new AIDS cases occurring each year are within 10% to 20% of the CDC estimated figures.

Beginning year 2003, with some 950,000 people HIV-infected in the United States and with 50,000 new infections occurring each year from 1999 through the year 2003, the face of AIDS in America is changing. **It's a younger and older face**

than it used to be. It's more likely to be a face of color than it used to be. More people with HIV disease and AIDS are from areas outside major cities. Overall, the number of new AIDS cases appears to be leveling. But the HIV epidemic should be viewed as many different epidemics in different stages that vary according to age, race, gender, and locality. Although gay and bisexual men continue to make up the largest portion of AIDS cases, the epidemic is increasing more rapidly among people who become infected through heterosexual contact and through sharing syringes to inject drugs. Every year women are composing a larger portion of AIDS cases, many who did not realize they were at risk. (See Chapter 11 for specifics on HIV/AIDS in women, children, and teenagers.)

RESOURCES

PEOPLE WITH HEMOPHILIA

Committee of Ten Thousand. (COTT) 800-488-2688 Hemophilia and AIDS/HIV Network for the Dissemination of Information (HANDI)

c/o the National Hemophilia Foundation.
800-424-2634; en espaÒol, ext. 3754

INJECTION DRUG USERS

Harm Reduction Coalition
2W. 27th St., 9th Fl., NYC, NY 10001; 212-213-6376

We the People
425 South Broad Street, Philadelphia, PA 19147; 215-545-6868; www.critpath.org/wtp

TRANSGENDER

International Foundation for Gender Education

Transgender hotline, referrals. 781-899-2212; e-mail ifge@ifge.org

PEOPLE OF COLOR

National Asian/Pacific Islander Consortium on AIDS and STDs
c/o Asian/Pacific Islander American Health Forum.
116 New Montgomery St. Ste.531, San Francisco, CA 94105; 415-512-3408; e-mail etta@apiahf.org

National Black Leadership Commission AIDS
105 E. 22nd St. Ste. 711, NYC, NY 10010;

212-614-0023; e-mail kimblca@aol.com

Latino Commission on AIDS
80 Fifth Ave., Ste. 1501, NYC, NY 10011;
212-675-2838

National Minority AIDS Council
1931 13th St. NW, Washington, DC,
20009; 202-438-6622

National Native American AIDS Prevention Center
134 Linden St., Oakland, CA 94607; 510-444-2051;
www.nnaapc.org

LESBIANS

Lesbian AIDS Project
A division of GMHC. 212-367-1355 or 212-367-1363

PRISONERS

American Civil Liberties Union National Prison Project
1875 Connecticut Ave. NW, Ste. 410, Washington, DC
20009; 202-234-4830

AIDS In Prison Project
www.aidsinfonyc.org/aip/index.html

Prisoner's Rights Project of the Legal AID Society
15 Park Row, 23rd Fl., NYC, NY 10038; 212-577-3530

REVIEW QUESTIONS

(Answers to the Review Questions are on page 489.)

1. How did the CDC estimate the numbers of HIV-infected people in the United States? In what year was this done? In retrospect, how accurate are their estimates?

2. Why are people placed in potential HIV risk groups?

3. True or False: The time it takes for HIV-infected people to become AIDS patients is different for each ethnic group, risk group, and exposure route. Explain.

4. What percentage of all U.S. HIV-infected IDUs are in the New York–New Jersey region?

5. What percentage of newborns from HIV-infected mothers are HIV-infected?

6. Eventually, what percentage of HIV-infected children will result solely from HIV-infected mothers?

7. What is the rate of college students currently HIV-infected? Is this more or less than the rate for military personnel? Explain.

8. Compare the college student rate of HIV infection with the rate of HIV infection for the general U.S. population.

9. What is the risk of a health care worker converting to seropositivity after exposure to HIV-contaminated blood?

10. What single job-related event causes the greatest risk of HIV infection among health care workers?

11. What percentage of the total number of AIDS cases in the United States represents health care workers?

12. Are health care workers more apt to become infected with the hepatitis B virus or the AIDS virus?

13. In mid-1989, the government's General Accounting Office said _____ cases of AIDS will have occurred in the United States by the end of 1991. How many did the CDC predict?

14. Do you think people of the United States openly and truthfully discuss their sexual habits with survey personnel? What does the text say?

15. Worldwide, how many AIDS patients are estimated to die by the end of 2003? In the United States?

16. Data on AIDS deaths indicated that of AIDS patients diagnosed between 1981 through 2002, in the United States,_____% had died.

Prevalence of HIV Infection and AIDS Cases Among Women, Children, and Teenagers in the United States

---

♦ A global estimate of HIV-positive women is presented.

♦ In proportion there are significantly more black and Hispanic women with AIDS than white women.

♦ Injection drug use is the major route of HIV infection for women.

♦ From 1994 through early year 2003 at least 38% of women infected in the United States contracted HIV from men through sexual intercourse.

♦ Injection drug use and prostitution are strongly associated with HIV infection.

♦ AIDS is the leading cause of death for women ages 25 to 34.

♦ First 100,000 AIDS cases in women in the United States were documented in December 1997.

♦ About 23% of all HIV-infected adult/adolescents in the United States are women.

♦ About 30% of all new HIV infections in the United States are in women.

♦ Women make up about 20% of all U.S. AIDS cases.

♦ Black American women make up 13% of the female population but made up about 65% of new AIDS cases in 2000 through 2002.

♦ In the United States, about 70% of new AIDS cases among women now occur among those aged 30 to 49, 18% among those aged 20 to 29, and 12% among women over age 50.

♦ Women make up about 36% of worldwide AIDS cases.

♦ Women make up about 41% of worldwide HIV positives.

♦ Of 3 million adult/adolescent AIDS deaths worldwide in 2001, 1.1 million were women.

♦ Pediatric means **under** age 13 in the United States and **under** age 15 in Canada and most underdeveloped nations.

♦ About 99% of new pediatric AIDS cases received the virus from their HIV-infected mothers.

♦ In proportion there are significantly more black and Hispanic pediatric AIDS cases than for whites.

♦ Perinatal HIV infection without anti-HIV drug intervention in the United States is about 25%; with drug intervention it is about 8%. With drugs and Cesarean section it's about 2%.

♦ Not all newborns that test HIV positive are HIV-infected.

♦ About 800,000 children under age 15 became HIV infected in 2002.

♦ By year 2015, there will be an estimated 44 million HIV/AIDS-related orphans under age 15 in 23 underdeveloped countries.

♦ Seven of 10 people are sexually active by age 19.

♦ Eighty-six percent of all sexually transmitted diseases occur in the 15 to 29 age group.

♦ The total number of HIV-infected teenagers is unknown.

♦ Black and Hispanic teenagers account for a disproportionate number of AIDS cases compared to whites.

♦ Teenagers are being exposed to quality HIV prevention but they choose to ignore it.

♦ Sex thrills but AIDS kills.

♦ Worldwide people ages 13 to 19 account for at least 50% of all new HIV infections.

♦ Worldwide women account for 58% of AIDS cases among people ages 13 to 19.

WOMEN: AIDS AND HIV INFECTIONS WORLDWIDE

The Gender Dimension of HIV/AIDS

Women over age 15 make up about 41% of the 44 million people worldwide living with HIV/AIDS ending year 2003. The heightened vulnerability that gender inequality has created is now evident across the world, with approximately 47% of all new adult infections occurring in women. In sub-Saharan Africa, 55% of the HIV-positive adults are women. In parts of Latin America and the Caribbean, the proportion has reached as high as 45% and this figure is on the rise. This alarming development must be recognized by concerned parties as an absolutely central consideration in the design of strategies to halt the spread of the disease worldwide.

Figures from UNAIDS show that the risk of infection is increasing for women everywhere—in developed and developing countries alike. For example, in France, women's share of reported AIDS cases increased from 12% in 1985 to 20% in 1995. In Spain, female AIDS cases rose from 7% to 19% of all AIDS cases during the same period. In Brazil the proportion of AIDS cases in women rose from 1% in 1984 to 25% in 1995. In the United States,

women represented 7% of AIDS cases in 1985 but 24% of new AIDS cases in 2002. Worldwide almost half of AIDS cases are women.

Through 1997, women, children, and teenagers seemed to be on the periphery of the HIV/AIDS pandemic. However, they have now become the center of this pandemic.

Worldwide ending year 2003, there will be an estimated 36 million AIDS cases out of 70 million people infected with HIV. About 11 million (30%) of these AIDS cases are **women.** Of the total HIV-infected, 41 million are men and 29 million are women (Figure 11-1).

In sub-Saharan Africa, the **ratio of women to men** infected with HIV/AIDS is currently 6:5. In Rakai and Masaka, rural districts of Uganda, a 1994 national report indicated that of 1300 young women aged 15 to 25, 70% were HIV-infected. When compared with HIV-infected young men of the same villages and age group, there was a female-to-male ratio of 6:1. In Rwanda and Tanzania, young women under age 25 accounted for 20% of female AIDS cases and men under 25 for less than 9% of male cases. The **male-to-female ratio** of AIDS cases among Ethiopian teenagers is 1:3; in Zimbabwe, it is 1:5. In Brazil, the **ratio of male-to-female** infection in Sao Paulo changed

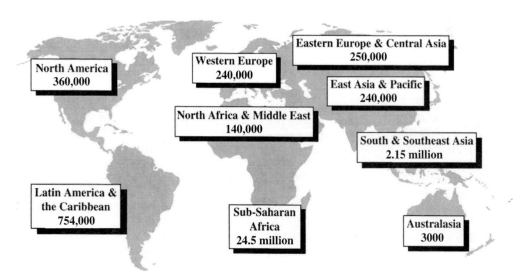

North America 360,000

Western Europe 240,000

Eastern Europe & Central Asia 250,000

East Asia & Pacific 240,000

North Africa & Middle East 140,000

South & Southeast Asia 2.15 million

Latin America & the Caribbean 754,000

Sub-Saharan Africa 24.5 million

Australasia 3000

Global Total: 29 Million HIV Positive Women

FIGURE 11-1 Estimate of HIV-Positive Women Worldwide Ending Year 2003. Ending 1993, women made up an estimated 8 million HIV cases. Ending year 2003 about 41% of all HIV positives worldwide were women! About 10 million women will have died.

from 42:1 in 1985 to 2:1 in 1995. In Northern Thailand, HIV prevalence among women coming to prenatal clinics reached 8% in 1993, and 72% of sex workers there are HIV-infected. In the United States, women as a percentage of HIV/AIDS cases rose to 8% from 1981 to 1987, to 20% in 1996 through 2002. Beginning year 2000, about 80% of HIV transmission worldwide was associated with heterosexual (vaginal) intercourse. Women are biologically more vulnerable to HIV infection than men because HIV in semen is in higher concentration than in vaginal and cervical secretions and because the vaginal area has a much larger mucosal area for exposure to HIV than the penis.

Transmission of HIV from male to female is 2 to 10 times more effective than from female to male (*World Health Organization*, 1994). Paradoxically, since time immemorial women have been blamed for the spread of sexually transmitted diseases. Among certain peoples in Thailand and Uganda, STDs are known as **"women's diseases."** In Swahili, the language of much of east Africa, the word for STD means, literally, **"disease of woman."** Also, it is not coincidental that the countries in which HIV is now spreading fastest heterosexually are generally those in which women's status is low.

The World Health Organization reported that globally, during 2002 there were 3 million AIDS deaths; 43.3% or **1.3 million of these deaths were women.** That is **over** two female deaths per minute! Four women become HIV-infected every minute!

UPDATE 2002 In June 2002, just prior to the XIV International AIDS Conference, a major report by UNICEF presented data on young women living with HIV/AIDS, compared to men, in 11 African countries. Their data is as follows: In Botswana, the percentage of young women living with HIV is 45% while the comparable figure for young men is 19%; in Lesotho, young women 51%, young men 23%; in South Africa, the numbers are 31% as compared to 13%; in Swaziland, 47% to 18%; in Zambia, 25% to 10%; in Zimbabwe, 40% to 15%; in Namibia, 29% to 8%; in Malawi, 18% to 8%; in Cameroon, 15% to 6%; in Central African Republic, 16% to 7%; in Rwanda, 13% to 6%. The pattern is comparable for almost all African countries.

UNAIDS also published a major report in the first week of July about the prevalence of HIV in-fection among women attending antenatal (before birth) care clinics in nine urban and 11 rural clinics. The prevalence in the urban clinics were: for Botswana, 56%; Lesotho, 42%; Malawi, 28%; Namibia, 31%; South Africa, 36%; Swaziland, 32%; Tanzania, 23%; Zambia, 31%; and Zimbabwe, 33%. The percentages outside major urban areas were: Botswana, 51%; Kenya, 31%; Lesotho, 26%; Malawi, 36%; Mozambique, 32%; Namibia, 32%; South Africa, 30%; Swaziland, 41%; Tanzania, 32%; Zambia, 31%; Zimbabwe, 71%.

These data help tell the story of why there are over 12 million AIDS orphans in Africa.

WOMEN: HIV-POSITIVE AND AIDS CASES—UNITED STATES

Women most at risk are ethnic minorities and the economically disadvantaged. Among sexually active teenagers, college students, and health care workers nationwide, nearly 60% of the heterosexual spread of HIV is among women (Pfeiffer, 1991).

In 1982, it was thought that all female AIDS cases were associated with injection drug usage. It soon became apparent that some of these women had become infected through heterosexual contact with HIV-infected males. Additional AIDS cases from heterosexual transmission appeared in 1983, and the percentage of female cases in the heterosexual category has continued to increase. The trend in heterosexual vaginal transmission may serve as a marker for future trends in HIV transmission.

HIV/AIDS in women is a national tragedy, but in addition, women are the major source of infection in infants. From 1993 through 2002, over 97% of HIV-infected children, aged 0 to 4 years, got the virus from their mothers.

At the end of 1988, women made up 6964 or 9% of the total adult AIDS cases in the United States. By the end of 2002, women accounted for over 150,000 AIDS cases (Table 11-1). **About 80% of all female AIDS cases have been reported in the eight years between 1993 and the beginning of year 2002.** They have been reported from all 50 states and territories. About 67% of these females are between the ages of 13 and 39 (HIV/AIDS Surveillance 1997 updated). Between 1989 and the beginning of year 2003, female AIDS cases were and continue to be twice as frequent among black women than among white, and almost three

AFRICA: POVERTY AND RITUALS LEAD TO THE SPREAD OF HIV

A woman from Zimbabwe explained her use of dry sex to please her man, but it is not by choice. She used herbs from the Mugugudhu tree. After grinding the stem and leaf, she mixed a pinch of the powder with water, wrapped it in a bit of nylon stocking, and inserted it into her vagina for 10 to 15 minutes. The herbs swell the soft tissues of the vagina and dry it out. That makes sex very painful. But she adds, "Our African husbands enjoy sex with a dry vagina."

Many African women concur that dry sex hurts, but it is common throughout southern Africa where the AIDS pandemic is out of control. Researchers who conducted a study in Zimbabwe had trouble finding a control group of women who did not engage in some form of the practice. Some women dry out their vaginas with *mutendo wegudo*—soil with baboon urine—that they obtain from traditional healers, while others use detergents, salt, cotton, or shredded newspaper. Research shows that dry sex causes vaginal lacerations and suppresses the vagina's natural bacteria, both of which increase the likelihood of HIV infection. Some AIDS workers believe the extra friction makes condoms tear more easily.

Africa contains thousands of cultures, some of which have strict sexual codes. But common to many sub-Saharan societies are the gender roles represented by dry sex: Women are unable to negotiate sex and so must risk infection to please the man. There are very few female checks and balances on male behavior. This stark inequality is part of the reason why HIV is spreading in countries with strict sexual codes, such as in Africa.

Lack of Authority

African women lack authority. Zimbabwe's Supreme Court ruled in 1999 that women have no more status of rights in the family than that of a "junior male"—usually an adolescent. In most sub-Saharan traditional cultures men pay for their wives, which gives them license to dominate the relationship. The very concept of marital rape doesn't exist in most of Africa and even the **aunties,** traditional marriage counselors for many young African wives, tell women that they cannot refuse sex with their husbands. Once a man has paid *lobola*—the word for dowry in several southern African languages, they are not forcing their wife to have sex. It's their right to have sex when they choose.

Many cultures especially in eastern and southern Africa provide home guardianship/widow inheritance. When a husband dies, one of his brothers or cousins marries the widow. This tradition guarantees that the children will remain in the late husband's clan and it also ensures that the widow and her children are provided for. When the guardian takes the widow, sexual intercourse is believed to cleanse her of the devils of death. A woman who refuses to take a guardian brings down *chira*—ill fortune on the entire clan. If her husband died of AIDS she might very well pass on the virus to her guardian. A Luo public health worker with the Red Cross said, "We have homes where all the males have died of AIDS because of this widow inheritance."

Poverty

The greatest inequality for women is poverty. Poverty is not a uniquely African phenomenon. Of the world's 1.3 billion people living in abject poverty, **70% are women**—and most of them face the same basic problems as African women. In developing countries women are trapped in their reproductive roles. In numerous studies on HIV, women from Latin America, Asia, and Africa report that they dare not insist on safer sex, or object to painful sex for fear of being abandoned by their men. In a 19-country study, the International Center for Research on Women found that the lower a woman's status, the greater her chance of becoming HIV-infected.

---

times higher in black women than in Hispanic women (Figure 11-2).

In the United States, ending 2003, about three quarters of the estimated 163,000 women living with AIDS are Black American or Hispanic, although they make up less than 25% of females nationwide.

Among the most alarming HIV/AIDS statistics to emerge is that of HIV transmission through heterosexual sexual contact. Of new HIV infections in women, acquired through heterosexual contact, in 2002 in the United States about 40% are women. Of AIDS cases that occur in women aged 13 to 24, about 76% are due to heterosexual contact.

Table 11-1 Reported AIDS Cases for Women, United States

Year	Number		Total
1981 (From June)	6		
1982	47		
1983	144		
1984	285		
1985	534		
1986	980		
1987	1701		
1988	3263		
1989	3639		
1990	4890		Through 1990
1991	5732	% Increase 1992–1994 151[b]	(15,489)
1992	6571		
1993	16,824[a]		
1994	14,379		
1995	14,100		Through 1995
1996	13,820		(73,095)
1997	11,651		
1998	10,500		
1999	10,800		
2000	11,000		Through 2000
2001	11,117		(130,989)
2002	11,300		
2003	11,225		Through 2003
Men	731,711		(estimated)
Total:[d]	895,000[c]		(163,289)

[a]The large increase in women's AIDS cases for 1993, over previous years was due to the January 1, 1993, implementation of the new definition of AIDS. Ending 2003, about 300,000 women will be living with HIV infection. Of these about 85,000 will be living with AIDS.

[b]Reported male AIDS cases for 1993 were up 113%, in women, 128% (Hirschhorn, 1995).

[c]Total AIDS cases include 9465 pediatric.

[d]Ending year 2003.

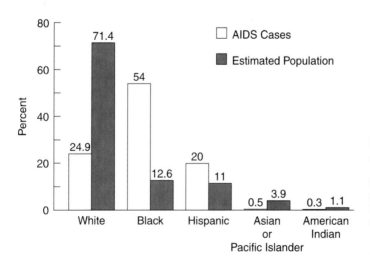

FIGURE 11-2 Incidence of AIDS Cases Among Women of Different Ethnic Groups, United States. Worldwide, every minute, four women become HIV-infected, and every minute, two women die of AIDS. *(Source: Global summary of HIV/AIDS Epidemic, 2001)*

PROFILE: WOMEN WITH HIV/AIDS IN THE UNITED STATES

Beginning year 2003, there were about 142 million American women in the United States.

The majority of women with AIDS in the United States reside in the Northeast and the South, are unemployed, and 83% live in households with income less than $10,000 per year. Only 14% are currently married, compared to 50% of all women in the United States, aged 15 to 44 years. Twenty-three percent (23%) of HIV-infected women live alone, 2% live in various facilities, and 1% are homeless. Approximately 50% have at least one child less than the age of 15 years. Similar to other population groups with AIDS in the United States, the majority of women with AIDS are from minority racial and ethnic groups, with 61% of all AIDS cases diagnosed in African-Americans, 19% in Latinos, and 18% in Caucasians (HIV/AIDS Surveillance 1998 updated).

Number of Women HIV-Infected and With AIDS

Between 1991 and 1995, the number of women diagnosed as having AIDS increased by 63%, more than any other group of persons reported as having AIDS, regardless of race or mode of exposure to HIV. Ending year 2002, about 300,000 women were living with HIV infection and of these about 76,000 women had AIDS (Wortley, et al., 1997 updated).

AIDS in Older Women

Entering year 2003, 7.6% or about 11,000 AIDS cases occurred in women aged 55 and older: White 3900, Black 5060, Hispanic 1870, all others 130.

Two Typical Senior HIV/AIDS Anecdotes

A soft-spoken, 63-year-old, self-described "churchy" woman from rural South Dakota, whose been living with HIV since her late 50s said, "I got very sick. I kept going to the doctor and he kept giving me antibiotics, and he would just kind of hit-and-run. He thought it was menopause, arthritis, high blood pressure, possibly a heart problem. Suddenly I found myself in the emergency room after two years of misdiagnosed infections, monthly visits to my primary care doctor, and an allergic reaction to daily doses of penicillin. That's where I was tested for HIV. When the doctor came into my room, I pulled on his sleeve and told him to sit down a minute. He said, 'What you have is really nasty, and you don't want to know.'"

In a second case, a 66-year-old woman said, "He was 10 years older than I was and he said, 'I've never worn a condom in my life and I'm not going to start now.'" Most older men say that. Older women won't insist that the man wear a condom. They don't ask where he's been. Older women especially don't pry. They can no longer have children, so why bother with condoms? Usually they tend not to be very assertive until they get HIV or an STD. Most seniors are first diagnosed with HIV in the hospital after they've already progressed to AIDS.

These two stories are typical of HIV-positive older women. The majority become infected through sexual contact with a husband or boyfriend. After months and sometimes years of being sick, they're tested for HIV as a last resort. Health care providers routinely fail these women by not readily screening them for HIV and other sexually transmitted diseases. They also neglect to ask about their sexual and drug-using behaviors. Ailments that accompany HIV often masquerade as signs of aging, throwing physicians even further off track. Fevers, night sweats, tuberculosis, chronic fungal infections, shingles, decreased vision, Pheumocystis carinii pneumonia, and cervical cancer can signal HIV, AIDS, or aging.

Figure 11-3 presents the cumulative **source** of U.S. female AIDS cases through 2002. In 2002, of the 38,000 persons reported with AIDS, 9000 (24%) occurred among women. The number of women AIDS cases increased steadily through 1993 and then began to decline. The decline is attributed to the use of prevention and antiretroviral drugs.

The median age of women reported with AIDS in 1998 was 35 years, and women aged 25 to 44 years accounted for 85% of female AIDS cases. Beginning year 2003, women aged 50 years and older accounted for 9% of all female AIDS cases. Most of these women became infected through heterosexual sexual activities (Schable et al., 1996 updated).

MARIA'S STORY

Maria is a Hispanic immigrant and former obstetrician in her home country who sees herself as having been victimized twice: once by her American husband, who infected her with HIV, and a second time by the legal system that bars her not only from U.S. residency (owing to her HIV status), but also from receiving her husband's benefits as a veteran. She nursed her husband for two years before he died of AIDS, only to learn that he had infected her. Upon applying for his veteran's benefits, she discovered that six months before her marriage, he had married another woman, who he also infected. The marriage licenses had been issued in the same building and same office. The first marriage invalidated her claim for widow's benefits, leaving her virtually penniless. Because of her HIV status, she has faced discrimination in housing and employment. Her salvation has been New York's ADAP program, which provides medications and medical care of HIV-positive people. As difficult as it has been in the United States, returning to her country would be far worse. Speaking through an interpreter, she said, "If I return to my country it would be sure death." Her family has rejected her, and medications and services are unavailable to those in her country without the means to pay for them. She has devoted herself to educating other Latina women to prevent them from spreading infection. Despite fears of deportation, she is determined to speak out about the plight of undocumented immigrants. "We need help for the sake of human rights. We live in limbo."

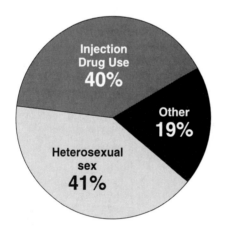

FIGURE 11-3 Cumulative Major Sources of HIV Infections in United States Women. *(Source: U.S. Centers for Disease Control and Prevention, Surveillance Report Year-mid 2002)*

Beginning year 2003, the Northeast region accounted for the largest percentage of AIDS cases reported among women (44%), followed by the South (36%), West (9%), Midwest (7%), and Puerto Rico and U.S. territories (4%). In the Northeast, 1.4% of women with AIDS resided outside metropolitan areas compared with 10.2% of women who resided outside metropolitan areas in the South. **Of all AIDS cases among women, 61% were reported from five states: New York** (26%), **Florida (13%), New Jersey (10%), California (7%), and Texas (5%).**

Of all new female AIDS cases, over 40% are associated with heterosexual transmission. The second most frequent cause was injection drug use at 40%. The AIDS rate for Hispanic women was eight times higher than for white women. The AIDS rate for black women was three times higher than for Hispanic women and 23 times higher than for white women.

[An excellent resource on HIV/AIDS in women can be obtained from the National Prevention Information Network, 1-800-458-5231 (formerly called the National AIDS Clearinghouse) and the Women's Information Service and Exchange (WISE), 125 Fifth St., N.E., Atlanta, Georgia 30308, (800) 326-3861.]

As the frequency of HIV/AIDS increases in women, the question of whether AIDS will explode in the heterosexual community of the United States becomes more a question of **when will the number of female AIDS cases equal male cases.** For the first time, in 1997 American women made up over 20% (22%) of AIDS cases for the year. In 1998 and 1999, 23% and in 2002, 26%. Worldwide, women accounted for 25% of all HIV-infected adults in 1990. Ending year 2003 that percentage will have risen to about 41%. The World Health Organization predicts that by the year 2005, women will constitute the majority of HIV-infected adults.

Transmission Categories

Heterosexual contact now makes up about 50% of all new adult/adolescent female HIV infections in the United States. Injection drug use is at 25% followed by blood transfusions and use of blood products at 4% and 1% of cases undetermined.

Artificial Insemination

To date there are six cases of transmission through **artificial insemination reported** in the United States, and six other cases are known to have occurred (Joseph, 1993 updated). Four of eight Australian women who received semen from a single infected donor became infected. HIV-contaminated semen had been injected into the uterus through a catheter. For other cases of men infecting women see Box 8.6.

Prostitutes

The term **prostitute** is used here in preference to the more recently coined **"sex worker."** No single term can adequately encompass the range of sex for money/drugs/friendship/accommodation transactions that undoubtedly occurs worldwide. How-ever, the term prostitute is at least relatively clear in referring to those who are directly involved in trading sex for money or drugs. In the United States, prostitutes represent a diverse group of people with various lifestyles. About 31% of female IDUs admit to engaging in prostitution. They need money to support their drug habit, pay rent, and eat. Cities with large numbers of IDUs subsequently have large numbers of prostitutes. Evidence is overwhelming—IDU, prostitution, and HIV infection are strongly associated.

ANECDOTE

I was referred to an eye doctor who is a specialist in retinal detachment in HIV/AIDS patients. After looking at my chart, the first thing he said to me was "Sex or drugs?" I knew he was trying to pigeonhole me. But I said, "Excuse me?" and he repeated, "Sex or drugs?" I told him, "I don't do drugs anymore and sex with you, I don't think so!"

Commentary: Women with HIV/AIDS have to deal with a lot of attitude from people, including health care providers.

POINT OF INFORMATION 11.3

HIV INFECTION AMONG WOMEN

There are over 6 million women ages 18 to 40 in the United States who are unmarried and having sexual relationships. Those most at risk for HIV infection are: **(1)** those who have multiple sexual partners (defined as having more than four different partners/year), and **(2)** those women who do not insist on the use of a condom.

Three of the nation's top five metropolitan areas with the highest incidence of AIDS in women are located in Florida within a 70-mile radius of each other (West Palm Beach, Ft. Lauderdale, and Miami). This area is an epicenter of HIV infection for Florida women. The other areas of highest incidence of AIDS in women are Puerto Rico, followed by New Jersey, New York, the District of Columbia, Florida, Connecticut, Maryland, Delaware, Massachusetts, Rhode Island, Georgia, and South Carolina. In Florida's Palm Beach County the rate is 24%; in Broward and Dade Counties, 18%. The epidemiologist for the state of Florida stated that what is happening in Florida is happening in innercities nationwide. What may distinguish the AIDS epidemic in women is that it hinges on the low self-esteem and lack of personal power experienced by women in many walks of life.

Most of Florida's women with AIDS are poor and receive their medical care through the public health system. Among women in South Florida, HIV transmission is associated with crack cocaine. Pam Whittington, director of the Boynton Community Life Center, a family support facility in southern Palm Beach County, said, "If you have 10 women on crack, probably eight of them are HIV-infected."

Crack cocaine is cheap and readily available. Its use contributes to anonymous, high-risk sex with multiple partners. Those who cannot afford crack exchange sex for it. In isolated communities of crack users, there is a high degree of sharing sex partners, many of whom are HIV positive.

In a multicity study, HIV antibody was detected in 13% of 1378 female prostitutes; 80% of the infected prostitutes reported using injection drugs (Darrow et al., 1989). For prostitutes **without** histories of injection drug use, HIV seroprevalence was 5%; HIV infection in this group was greater among blacks and Hispanics and among those who had had more than 200 paying sex partners. The point is that **non-injection-drug-using prostitutes in the United States play a small role in HIV transmission.** This is believed to be because of the low incidence of HIV infection among their male clients and on the insistence by many prostitutes that their clients use condoms (Felman, 1990). **In Africa, Asia, and other underdeveloped nations where the "Customer is King", prostitution plays a major role in HIV transmission.**

Women Who Have Sex With Women (Lesbians)

Research on female-to-female transmission remains inconclusive. But the large numbers of HIV-positive women and women with AIDS should alert women who have sex with women that they cannot assume their partners are uninfected because they are lesbians. It has been reported that 80% of lesbian women have had sex with men during their lifetime. Also, certain sexual behaviors common among lesbians probably put them at risk for transmitting and receiving HIV through vaginal fluid, menstrual blood, sex toys, and cuts in the vagina, mouth, and on the hands.

The evidence is clear: HIV infection is present among lesbians, and lesbians engage in behaviors that put them at risk for HIV infection, in some cases, at higher risk than most others in society. Whether or not lesbians put their female sexual partners at risk is less clear. In fact, there is a great deal of controversy about this question. Some HIV/AIDS investigators believe the risk of sexual transmission increases as the number of HIV-positive lesbians increases. Others believe that lesbians are not getting infected through lesbian sex, but only through unsafe behaviors like IDU. Female-to-female transmission has been reported

---

POINT OF VIEW 11.1

WOMEN + SEXUAL PARTNERS + DECEPTION = AIDS

Across the world, women in support groups or with a close friend have been telling their stories of **trusting** their sexual partners and ending up with AIDS. Their trust was violated—their lives forfeited. Here are but a few examples of the thousands of similar cases worldwide.

1. She is 48 years old with curly red hair and bags beneath her eyes. She slouches slightly in the office chair, stretching out her feet. From her eye shadow to her sneakers, everything is blue. Married to one husband for 28 years, she has children and grandchildren. She also has AIDS. She did not use drugs or have multiple sexual partners. **She did have sex with her husband without a condom!**

2. One 23-year old had a boyfriend with hemophilia; he never used condoms and never mentioned HIV, even though he had already infected another woman.

3. A divorced man with two children did not tell his 46-year-old girlfriend he had AIDS, even when he was hospitalized with an AIDS-related infection.

4. A seven-year live-in partner of a woman denied infecting her, even though he tested positive for HIV; she did not know he was having sex outside their relationship.

5. Because she had **only two boyfriends,** because "we were perfectly ordinary," they did not use condoms.

6. This woman with a baby did not know "my man was shooting up drugs and sharing needles." Not until he died of AIDS.

7. She **never** dreamed her partner had used a needle. When the doctor said she had AIDS, she replied, **"You have made a mistake. I cannot have AIDS. How could I have that?"**

All these women discovered their HIV status only after they became seriously ill with infections they should not have had. Heterosexual transmission is rising dramatically. A seldom mentioned fact is: A large percentage of infected women are married or in committed relationships.

---

in one case and suggested in another (Curran et al., 1988; Chu et al., 1994).

The July 1997 CDC **Facts** sheet reported on 1648 women who had sex with other women. Twenty percent (333) said they had sex **only** with other women but 97% of these (323) had other risks—mostly injection drug use. A separate study on over 1 million female blood donors found no HIV-infected women whose **only** risk was sex with women!

George Lemp and colleagues (1995) reported on HIV infection in 498 lesbian and bisexual women. Six were HIV-positive, but there was **NO** evidence of women-to-women transmission! The Women's AIDS Network (1988) of San Francisco states in their publication *Lesbians and AIDS* that if there is a possibility that either woman is carrying the virus, she should not allow her menstrual blood, vaginal secretions, urine, feces, or breast milk to enter her partner's body through the mouth, rectum, vagina, or broken skin.

Special Concerns of HIV/AIDS Women

First, HIV/AIDS has a profound impact on women, both as an illness and as a social and economic challenge. Women play a crucial role in preventing infection by insisting on safer sexual practices and caring for people with HIV disease and people with AIDS. The stigma attached to HIV/AIDS can subject women to discrimination, social rejection, and other violations of their rights. A study by Solley Zierler and colleagues (2000) estimates that about 21% of HIV-infected American women were assaulted by a partner or another relation after becoming HIV positive. The percentage of women receiving physical harm after receiving an HIV diagnosis in a developing nation is at least twice that found in America. In South Africa, for example, Gugu Dlamini was stoned to death by her neighbors after she revealed that she was HIV positive on World AIDS Day, 1999.

Women need to know that they can protect themselves against HIV infection. Women have a traditionally passive role in sexual decision making in many countries. They need knowledge about HIV and AIDS, self-confidence, the skills necessary to insist that partners use safer sex methods, and practice good medical care.

Efforts to influence women to practice safer sex must also be joined by efforts to address men and their responsibility in practicing safer sex.

Second, women become pregnant. Women who are ill and discover they are pregnant need information about both the potential impact of pregnancy on their own health and maternal–fetal HIV transmission.

Third, women have the role of mothering. From this role come two important consequences. **First,** when a woman becomes ill with HIV disease or AIDS, her role as caretaker of the child or children or other adults in the household is immediately affected. The family is severely disrupted and each family member has to make adjustments. **Second,** the mother must cope with her own life-threatening illness while she also deals with the impact of the disease on her family. Demographic studies show that many HIV-infected or AIDS women have young children; and these women are often the sole support of these children.

Fourth, a woman's illness may be complicated further by incarceration and the threat of foster care proceedings. If the mother is healthy enough to care for her child, she must still cope with the complex issues of medical and home care, school access, friends, and family stress.

Fifth, worldwide, women make up about 36% of AIDS cases and 80% of these women are mothers of children. An estimated 10 million women will have died of AIDS ending the year 2003, and about 29 million will have become HIV-infected. Yet, little is known about the HIV disease process in women and what is the appropriate standard for their clinical care. Initially, what became known about HIV disease was derived from studies on men, who for the most part differ from women in race, income, and risk behavior. And what female-derived information there is on HIV disease in women came mostly from studies on pregnant women that have focused primarily on perinatal issues. In 1986, only 3% of participants of federally funded HIV/AIDS clinical trials were women. By 2003, this figure was over 30%.

To date, too little is known about the pharmacokinetics of HIV/AIDS drugs in women, nor is it clear whether gender influences specific illnesses. For example, does HIV infection increase cervical and vaginal disease and pelvic inflammatory disease? Why are certain opportunistic diseases more aggressive and damaging to females? How are the drugs used to treat opportunistic infections metabolized in women?

Biology and the Clinical Course of AIDS Among Men and Women

According to Birgit van Benthem and colleagues (2002), sex differences with respect to response to HIV infection do exist. CD4 cell counts are higher in women than in men throughout infection and viral loads are lower initially in women than in men, although this difference eventually disappears. Despite these disparities, women have not been found to have a more rapid clinical progression to AIDS than men.

According to Arlene Bardeguez (1995) and other similar reports (Cohen, 1995; Garcia, 1995), biology does not influence the prevalence of AIDS-defining illnesses, with the exception of invasive carcinoma of the cervix and possibly Kaposi's sarcoma. Access to HIV-related care and therapies is the dominant factor influencing the prevalence of AIDS-defining illnesses among women. Injection drug use in HIV-infected women leads to a higher incidence of certain diseases, particularly esophageal candidiasis, herpes simplex virus, and cytomegalovirus. Once an initial diagnosis of AIDS has been made, several major AIDS-defining illnesses appear more frequently in women: toxoplasmosis, herpes genital ulcerations, and esophageal candidiasis.

The currently proposed female-specific markers of **HIV disease** include **cervical dysplasia** and **neoplasia** (tumor), **vulvovaginal candidiasis,** and **pelvic inflammatory disease** (PID). HIV-infected women will have a higher incidence of cervical abnormalities on routine screening.

The 14 most common AIDS-defining illnesses in HIV-infected women are listed in Table 11-2. **No biology-related differences in the survival of HIV-positive persons have been documented when equal access to medical care is considered.** The shorter observed survival of women in some studies is thought to occur because of the lack of access to physicians who are knowledgeable about HIV-related care and therapies. Shannon Hader and colleagues (2001) found no evidence between women and men infected with the virus in terms of natural history, progression, survival, and HIV-associated illnesses. Drug use, high-risk sexual behaviors, depression, and unmet social needs among infected women contributed to their underuse of HIV resources. Also in 2001, Timothy and colleagues reported that although viral loads were lower in women than men, the rates of progression to AIDS were similar.

In July 2000, a document entitled **"Guide to the Clinical Care of Women with HIV: 2000 Preliminary Edition"** was posted on the Web (hab.hrsa.gov/womencare.htm). The Ryan White CARE Act program of the Health Resources and Services Administration made this resource available to clinicians caring for women living with HIV/AIDS.

Female HIV/AIDS Deaths

Women's deaths in the United States rose from 18 cases in 1981 to about 80,000 beginning year 2003. That is, about 50% of all women with AIDS have died. AIDS is the leading cause of

Table 11-2 Frequency of AIDS-Defining Illnesses in HIV-Positive Women and Men

	Women (%)	Men (%)
Pneumocystis carinii pneumonia	34	36
Wasting syndrome	9	8
Esophageal candidiasis	20	12
HIV-associated encephalopathy	3	4
Herpes simplex infection	4	2
Toxoplasmosis of the brain	4	3
Mycobacterium-avium intracellulare complex	7	6
Extrapulmonary cryptococcosis	3	4
Cytomegalovirus infection	2	3
Cytomegalovirus retinitis	3	4
Extrapulmonary tuberculosis	3	2
Cryptosporidosis	2	3
Lymphoma (brain)	.3	.4
Kaposi's sarcoma	1.3	13

From *Morbidity/Mortality Weekly Report,* 1999.

death for all women between the ages of 25 and 34, the fourth leading cause of death for all women between the ages of 25 and 44, and the eighth leading cause of death in white women. It is the second leading cause of death for black women and the third leading cause of death for Hispanic women between the ages of 25 and 44 (MMWR, 1996b updated).

Identifying and Preventing HIV Infection

Currently, women make up 55% of adult/adolescent HIV infections in sub-Saharan Africa, 30% in Southeast Asia, and 20% in Europe and the United States.

Identification of HIV-Positive Women— At age 26, a woman and her physicians were baffled when she began suffering from a variety of strange medical conditions: fevers, throat sores, unexplained vaginal bleeding, and fatigue. **It took a variety of doctors and seven years to find out what was wrong. She tested HIV-positive!**

This woman's difficulty in getting diagnosed points out the extent to which women still are invisible when it comes to AIDS. After more than 21 years into the epidemic, the message still hasn't reached primary care physicians: Their female patients may be at risk. This young woman said, **"I went into doctors' offices and all they saw was a white, middle-class woman, not someone at risk for HIV."**

Early identification of women with HIV infection is a pressing problem. Risk-based screening at a Johns Hopkins perinatal clinic showed that 43% of HIV-positive women were not identified as at risk on the basis of such screening, with infection being found in 20 (9.5%) of 211 women admitting to at risk behaviors and in 15 (1.6%) of 949 who were not at risk according to their response to screening questions (Garcia, 1995).

Prevention: United States— To prevent HIV infection, women have been told to reduce their number of sexual partners, to be monogamous, and to protect themselves by using condoms. **But these goals, generally speaking, do not fit the realities of women's lives or may not be under their control.**

Women do not wear the condom. (A female condom is now available but not yet in heavy demand. See Chapter 9.) For women to protect themselves from HIV infection, they must not only rely on their own skills, attitudes, and behaviors regarding condom use, but also on their ability to convince their partner to use a condom. Gender, culture, and power may be barriers to maintaining safer sex practices.

Women who have more than one sexual partner in their lifetime often practice serial monogamy, remaining with one partner at a time. People living as couples reduce the number of their sexual partners. Still, in many phases of life, sex is practiced with new partners in new relationships. American women, on average, are single for many years before their first marriage; they might be single again after a divorce; they might marry again; and, in later phases especially, they might be widowed. **For some women, multiple partners throughout life**

BOX 11.1

ONE WOMAN'S COMMENTS ON HER HIV DISEASE TREATMENTS

"I was fired from my job when they found out I was HIV-positive. The boss said, You have a modern problem—and this is an old-fashioned business."

This woman, in 1995, was 29 years of age and HIV positive since age 22. When her T4 cell count dropped to 250, her M.D. put her on zidovudine (ZDV, also called AZT). She was not given any literature or verbal explanation of how this drug would affect her. In 12 months she became anemic; she could not sleep or hold down food, and her menstrual cycle became erratic. Without explanation, she next received two other HIV replication inhibitors, ddI and ddC.

The side effects were very bad: consistent premenstrual symptoms; mood swings; increased cravings for certain foods, alcohol, or drugs; breast tenderness; and bloating. But, there was no literature for her to read and her M.D. said, "I knew how the drugs affected men, but I knew nothing of what to expect when I gave these drugs to women." "I stopped taking these drugs—they were killing me faster than the virus! I have severe yeast infections, shingles, sinus infections, and a host of other infections. My M.D. is dealing with me like I'm some kind of experiment."

---

is an economic necessity, urging them to reduce the number of partners is meaningless unless the economic situation for these women is improved (Ehrhardt, 1992). In addition, public health strategies, not necessarily targeted to women, can also play an important role for women. Syringe exchange and drug treatment are important strategies because almost half of all HIV infections in women are due to injection drug use. Because women are now more likely to be infected by men through heterosexual contact, programs that specifically target men, especially IDUs, will have a beneficial impact on women's programs.

Prevention: Africa

Although they are exceptionally vulnerable to the epidemic, millions of young African women are dangerously uninformed about HIV/AIDS. According to UNICEF, in 2001, more than 70% of adolescent girls (aged 15–19) in Somalia and more than 40% in Guinea Bissau and Sierra Leone have never heard of HIV or AIDS. In countries such as Kenya and the United Republic of Tanzania, more than 40% of adolescent girls harbor serious misconceptions about how the virus is transmitted. One of the targets fixed at the UN General Assembly Special Session on HIV/AIDS in June 2001 was to ensure that at least 90% of young men and women should, by 2005, have the information, education, and services they need in order to defend themselves against HIV infection. As in other regions of the world, most countries

in sub-Saharan Africa are a considerable way from fulfilling that pledge. The vast majority of African women living with HIV do not know they have been infected. One study found that 50% of adult Tanzanian women know where they could be tested for HIV, yet only 66% of these have been tested. In Zimbabwe, only 11% of adult women have been tested for the virus. Moreover, many people who agree to be tested prefer not to return and learn the outcome of those tests. An additional problem is that in many African countries where pregnant women agree to undergo HIV testing, most have no access to drug therapy to prevent mother-to-child transmission of HIV. Over half of the HIV-infected women who were surveyed by Kenya's Population Council in 2001 said they had not disclosed their HIV status to their partners because they feared it would expose them to violence or abandonment. Not only are voluntary counseling and testing services in short supply across the region, but stigma and discrimination continue to discourage people from discovering or disclosing their HIV status.

Childbearing Women

The extent of HIV infection among pregnant women is often used as an indicator of HIV penetration into the population at large. By this yardstick, several Asian countries have serious epidemics. In some of India's HIV/AIDS surveillance sites, more than 2% of pregnant women are infected, with some sites as high as 6%. Myanmar recorded preva-

---

POINT OF INFORMATION 11.4

PREGNANT WOMEN AND KNOWLEDGE OF HIV TRANSMISSION

A report in the January 2001 issue of *Obstetrics and Gynecology* indicates that while most women in the United States are aware that HIV-infected pregnant women can transmit their infection to their infants, some are not so sure how the virus is actually passed on. Emmanuel Walter of Duke University Medical Center found that almost 40% of the 1400 pregnant women surveyed were not certain if an HIV-positive woman could transmit the virus to her baby via breastfeeding. About 33% thought that babies born to a woman with HIV would definitely become infected, and 49% were not aware that there are drugs than can help reduce the risk of newborns contracting HIV. It was

noted, however, that about 90% of the women questioned had been offered an HIV test during their pregnancy, with most agreeing to the test, and 60% said that routine HIV testing of all pregnant women should be required by law. Current data suggests that the rate of transmission is 2% or less when the maternal viral load is reduced to undetectable levels by highly active combination antiretroviral therapy or when zidovudine prophylaxis is combined with elective cesarean section. Since 1994, the number of cases of pediatric AIDS reported in the United States has declined by 86% among infants under the age of 1 year and 78% among children 1 to 5 years old.

---

lence rates of up to 5% among pregnant women in some areas in the country. In Thailand, HIV infection prevalence among pregnant women peaked at 2% nationally.

Worldwide each year, an estimated 2.3 million children are exposed to HIV before or during their birth and in 2000, 2001, and 2002 about 800,000 each year were born HIV positive. Of the 4 million women who become pregnant each year in the United States, 6000 to 7000 are estimated to be HIV-infected. These pregnancies now result in about 200 HIV-infected children annually.

Women, in general, have two children before they find out they are infected (Thomas, 1989 updated). The birth of an infected child may serve as a **miner's canary**—the first indication of HIV infection in the mother.

Pregnancy and HIV Disease— Early findings in pregnant women indicated that those with T4 or CD4+ cell counts of less than **300/µL** of blood were more likely to experience HIV-associated illness during pregnancy. Pregnant HIV-infected women exhibit a greater T4 cell count decline during pregnancy than do women without HIV infection. T4 cell counts in the HIV-infected do not return to prepregnancy levels. However, the overall declines in HIV-infected women likely represent declines that would have occurred in the absence of pregnancy and suggest that pregnancy does not accelerate disease progression (Newell et al., 1997; Bessinger et al., 1998).

Over the last 10 years, HIV-positive pregnant women have been attracting more attention from the medical establishment, **first,** because there are better medications for the HIV-positive mother and fetus, and **second,** because of the relatively high incidence of HIV births.

Class Discussion: Nationwide, approximately 2 of 1000 pregnant women are HIV-infected, an incidence much higher than that of fetal neural tube defects, for which pregnant women are screened routinely. Should all pregnancies be screened for HIV?

Reproductive Rights— These are central to a woman's right to control her body. The choices of becoming pregnant or terminating the pregnancy are continually disputed.

However, as more women become HIV-infected and give birth to HIV-infected children, childbearing may come under the surveillance of the state. Women of childbearing age may be among the first groups to undergo mandatory testing as part of an attempt to control the birth of HIV-infected newborns.

Reproductive rights take on new meaning with HIV-infected pregnancies. The state has traditionally expressed an interest in protecting the rights of the fetus. This interest was transcended **in the 1973 *Roe v. Wade* decision when the Supreme Court recognized a woman's right to choose an abortion.** The court ruled that a woman's right to privacy must prevail against the state's interest in protecting the future life of the fetus. (See Chapter 7 for recent information on preventing HIV infection of the fetus.)

INTERNET

Among the hundreds of websites containing information on HIV, there are key addresses that provide comprehensive information, including links to a vast array of other resources. The key sites listed here include special areas focused on **women and HIV.**

American Medical Association home page: http://www.ama_assn.org

This site is an avenue for accessing several valuable resources, including the JAMA HIV/AIDS Information Center (. . . /special/hiv/hiv-home.htm), JAMA HIV/AIDS best of the Net (. . . /special/hiv/bestnet/nethome.htm), and Online CME, which includes a series of Clinical Care Options for HIV. The last selection includes a female case study, "The Seropositive Patient: Initial Encounter," and a module on HIV and women.

Centers for Disease Control and Prevention (CDC) Home Page: http://www.cdc.gov

This site offers broad coverage of disease, health, risk, and prevention topics. Available publications include the MMWR and surveillance reports, as well as health statistics and slides. Of note is slide series L264 on women and HIV (. . . /nchstp/hiv_aids/graphics/women.htm).

HIV Insite: Gateway to AIDS Knowledge: http://hivinsite.ucsf.edu

This is a comprehensive site provided by the University of California, San Francisco AIDS Program at San Francisco General Hospital and the UCSF Center for AIDS Prevention.

BOX 11.2

RUTH'S POEM

This poem was written by a mother living with HIV, to her daughter.

Here I am, a few years on
It was hard enough explaining where
  Daddy had gone.
She knows there's something wrong with me
How can I explain about HIV?
I see the sadness, the fear in her eyes
Each time I have to be hospitalised,
And I see the way she looks at me
Each time I take my AZT.
"I thought these pills were to make you well,
so why are you still sick then? Go on mum,
  tell.
Quick mum, here, be sick in this basin."
I can see within her tiny mind racing.
"I'll help you mum, watch you don't fall."
And she treats me like a china doll.
Then the moment for something, I was very
  scared,
The question that I had not prepared.
"Why do I get a jag mum, why do I get
  blood taken?"

The moment of truth now, there can be no
  faking.
"Well, it's the doctors special way of
  knowing
that inside you there's no bugs growing;
tiny bugs that can make you unwell."
I had no choice but the truth to tell.
"You don't have these bugs darling, so
  there's no need to worry."
"But you have, mummy," she says in a hurry.
"Yes, my lamb, in me these bugs grow."
"When you die mummy, where will I go?"
I don't know the answer to that question,
Instead I make this stupid suggestion.
"Shall we go to the fridge and get some ice
  cream?"
Then we had a cuddle and I said, "I'm here."
I wish I could take away all her fear.
Her blood just now may not be infected,
But by HIV she's most definitely affected.
I don't fear dying any more,
Just for a special little girl who's only four.

  With Permission
  "© AVERT 2000"

Sister Connect: *Hotline for women with* HIV
  800-747-1108
Women Alive: *Treatment newsletter on the Web*
  800-554-4876;
  www.thebody.com/wa/
  wapage.html
WORLD: *Newsletter by and for HIV positive
  women.* P.O. Box 11535, Oakland,
  CA 94611

Resources for Children Whose PARENTS Have HIV/AIDS

There are workbooks tailored to the specific family situation (for example, one mother was losing her hair because of chemotherapy, so there are pictures of **mommy with and without her hair** in the workbook. Looking at pictures helps the child to accustom to the hair loss. Eventually, mommy without hair wasn't so scary.) Coloring pages, word searches, lots of fun things for parent and child to work through together. There are also a number of good children's books available such as "My Daddy Has AIDS," written by a

man in Dubuque, Iowa, for early elementary-age children.

Beth Wehrman
John Lewis Coffee Shop/AIDS Prevention Partnership
1202 W. Third St., P.O. Box 3733
Davenport, Iowa 52808
(319) 336-4517
email: bwehr@ix.netcom.com

Should You Tell Your Children You Are HIV Positive?
By Laura Damson, C.S.W.
BODY POSITIVE October 1997, Volume XI, Number 3
http://www.thebody.com/bp/oct97/tell.html

How to tell a 10-year old his mom has AIDS
Question/Answer by Michael Shernoff, *The Body*
http://www.thebody.com/shernoff/answers/quest 41.html

Ruth's Poem (Box 11.2)
This poem was written by a mother living with HIV, to her daughter.

Avert UK.
http://www.avert.org/poem.html

HIV-INFECTED WOMEN: DIFFICULT CHOICES DURING PREGNANCY

She was 19 years old, a nursing student, pregnant, and HIV positive. She spent $4\frac{1}{2}$ months of pregnancy in constant fear for herself and for her baby. She waited, her health began to falter, then she decided to have an abortion.

Several studies have reported that HIV-positive women who perceived their risk of infecting their fetus to be greater than 50% were more likely to abort than those who perceived a lower risk. HIV-positive women who chose to continue their pregnancy cited the desire to have a child, strong religious beliefs, and family pressure (Selwyn et al., 1989).

For women who are HIV positive, pregnancy poses difficult choices. First, pregnancy may mask the presence of HIV disease symptoms and having a child poses other questions such as: Can the mother cope with a normal or infected child? and Who will care for the child if the mother becomes too ill or dies? Such questions bring up a moral issue for

Class Discussion: Do couples have a right to have children when one of the partners is known to be HIV positive? If the woman is HIV positive? If both are HIV positive? Is there any stage of HIV disease/AIDS when you think a woman should lose the right to become pregnant? (See Chapter 7 for the four stages of HIV disease).

Listening to the Children
By Julian Meldrum
Body Positive UK Issue 224, June, 1998
http://www.bodypositive.org.uk/homepage. html

No specifics, but has some useful points for discussion.

A safe place for families, by Anette Goldstein *Canadian AIDS News*, Fall, 1997 (vol. X, no. 1) http://www.cpha.ca/cpha.docs/canews/X1/family. html

The Twin State Women's Network (TSWN) that serves women and families in Vermont and New Hampshire who are infected/affected by HIV and/or chronic hepatitis. Women and children's information can be reached at www.dartmouth. edu/~hivnet/women&children.htmld/index.html.

There are good books out now, and even a video about how parents can tell their children they have HIV or AIDS. The video is entitled **"Don't Shut Me Out."** It is available for $20 by sending a check to The Center for Special Studies, B-24, New York Hospital, 525 East 68th St., NY 10021.

PEDIATRIC HIV-POSITIVE AND AIDS CASES—UNITED STATES

The Pediatric HIV Conundrum

One of the biggest puzzles in understanding mother-to-child transmission of HIV is why the majority of babies born to HIV-infected women remain uninfected in utero, at birth and—perhaps most remarkably—during breastfeeding. It's even more remarkable in view of studies suggesting that cell-free viral load in breast milk can vary from undetectable to more than 200,000 copies per ml, meaning that a breastfeeding infant may ingest up to millions of viral copies each day. This apparent resistance puts infants in the category of exposed, seronegative individuals who can repel or effectively control HIV despite repeated exposures. Katharine Lazuriaga and Sarah Rowland-Jones have both documented cases of infants apparently clearing a transient HIV infection. It is these immune defenses that vaccine researchers seek to boost, or mimic, with a neonatal vaccine. But there is little hard data on just what they are and how this apparent protection works.

Pediatric AIDS in the United States affects two age groups: **(1)** infants and young children who became infected through perinatal (vertical) transmission, and **(2)** school-age children, the majority of whom acquired HIV through blood transfusions (mostly hemophiliacs).

Beginning year 2003, about 9400 pediatric AIDS cases were **reported** and about 5000 (55%) died from AIDS. Pediatric AIDS cases represent about 1.1% of the total number of AIDS cases to date. **It is estimated that for each pediatric AIDS case reported there are three to four other HIV-infected children.** Thus, an estimated 20,000 to

28,000 children in the United States have HIV (Luzuriaga et al., 1996; Rodriguez et al., 1996). Of the pediatric AIDS cases, 3% were/are hemophilic children who received HIV-contaminated blood transfusions or blood products (pooled and concentrated blood factor VIII injections). About 5% of pediatric AIDS cases occurred in nonhemophilic children who were transfused with HIV-contaminated blood. From 1995 on, virtually all HIV-infected newborns contracted HIV vertically. The Pediatric AIDS Foundation reported in April of 1995 that hospital costs for each HIV-infected newborn were $35,000 per year (*Nations Health Report*, 1995). In a study from Children's Hospital of Wisconsin, the cost of care for children with HIV was estimated at $418,863 per patient (*AIDS Clinical Care*, 1996:8, 23). Worldwide year 2002, about 2.9 million children are living with HIV disease and about 5.2 million have died from AIDS (Figures 11-4 and 11-5).

Reporting HIV-Infected Children

Beginning 2003, 35 states and the Virgin Islands reported **HIV-infected children.** They reported a total of 2256 HIV-positive children. **Of the 35 reporting states, only two are states that have a high incidence of pediatric HIV, New Jersey and Texas.** Nine states, New York (34%), Florida (13%), New Jersey (6%), California (5%), Texas (5%), Pennsylvania (5%), Maryland (3%), Illinois (2%), and Georgia (3%) have 73% of **all reported** pediatric AIDS cases. AIDS infection is now the **sixth** leading cause of death in children between the ages of 1 and 14.

Ethnic Prevalence of Pediatric AIDS Cases

Children of color make up 14% of all children in the United States but account for 57% of pediatric AIDS cases. Whites make up 70% of children and account for 18% of pediatric AIDS cases. Hispan-

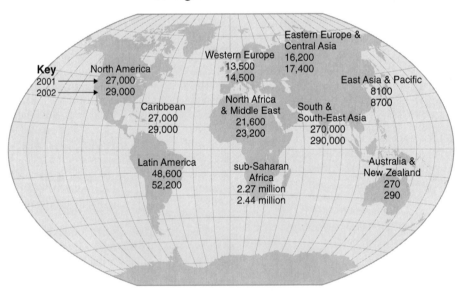

Year End Estimates: Children Living With HIV Infection

Totals are estimates for the entire globe.
Total: 2001- 2.7 million
2002- 2.9 million

FIGURE 11-4 Year 2001 and 2002 Global Estimates of Children Living with HIV Infection. Note that sub-Saharan Africa and South and Southeast Asia have the highest burden of HIV-infected children. *(Courtesy of UNAIDS updated)*

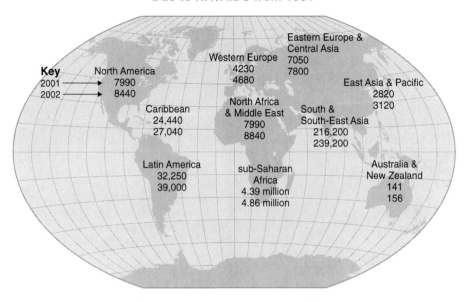

**Estimated Deaths in Children (<15 years)
Due to HIV/AIDS from 1981**

Key
2001 ⟶
2002 ⟶

North America
7990
8440

Western Europe
4230
4680

Eastern Europe &
Central Asia
7050
7800

East Asia & Pacific
2820
3120

Caribbean
24,440
27,040

North Africa
& Middle East
7990
8840

South &
South-East Asia
216,200
239,200

Latin America
32,250
39,000

sub-Saharan
Africa
4.39 million
4.86 million

Australia &
New Zealand
141
156

Totals are estimates for the entire globe.
**Total: 2001- 4.7 million
2002- 5.2 million**

FIGURE 11-5 Year 2001 and 2002 Global Estimates of AIDS Deaths in Children. Note the greatest number of children's deaths are occurring in sub-Saharan Africa and in South and Southeast Asia (*Courtesy of UNAIDS 2001 updated*). As tragic as the above data appear, these data on children dying of AIDS must be kept in perspective. Each year, inadequate drinking water and sanitation, indoor air pollution, accidents, injuries, and poisonings are just a few of the more preventable causes of 3 million deaths per year of children under age 5 and an estimated 12 million under age 15—about 20 times the number of children under age 15 who died from AIDS in 2002.

ics make up 12% of children and account for 23% of pediatric AIDS cases.

ORPHANED CHILDREN DUE TO HIV INFECTION AND AIDS

The word orphan is an English word that does not have an exact translation in many languages. The concept of orphan is a social construct, so the meaning assigned to it varies from one society to another. In the United States and Africa, typically the term is understood to mean a child who has lost either or both parents. UNAIDS reports orphans as children who have lost their mothers or both parents. They limit their estimates to chil-

dren below age 15. The UN Convention on the Rights of the Child defines children as being below age 18, unless the age of majority (adulthood) is reached under national law. Who is a child and who is an adult is defined differently in different countries and among different cultures. This further complicates the meaning of the word orphan because orphans are generally considered to be children.

Beginning year 2003, of the 14 million AIDS related orphans, 95% live or have lived in Africa. The problem of AIDS-related orphans will become much greater over the next 10 to 15 years.

AIDS orphans present a chilling illustration of the far-reaching effects of the AIDS pandemic.

His mother was young, single, and HIV positive. When she went to the hospital to give birth, she checked in under a false name and address and then slipped out of the hospital leaving her baby who was only a few hours old. Today the boy is 3 years old. No one has yet to offer him a home.

An increasing number of HIV-infected children are being left in hospitals because their HIV-infected mothers and fathers are unable to care for them and no one else wants them. The hospital becomes their home. James Hegarty and colleagues (1988) reported that for 37 children at Harlem Hospital Center, one-third of the total inpatient days and over 20% of the cost was for social rather than medical services. By year end of 2002, there were an estimated 35,000 AIDS-related orphan children in New York City.

As HIV continues to spread across the nation and HIV-infected women continue to become pregnant, the question is: **What will happen to their HIV-infected babies**? For one young woman who passed the HIV to her baby two years ago, the decision has been made. The baby has AIDS and is in foster care. The mother is very ill. The courts are now deciding whether her six other children should also be put in foster care.

Unless the course of the epidemic changes drastically, through the year 2003, the cumulative number of U.S. children, teens, and young adults left motherless due to AIDS will exceed 145,000. Over 70,000 children under age 15 have already lost their mother or both parents to AIDS. The great majority of these children, uninfected by the virus—will begin to affect already burdened social services in major American cities. Things will get immediately worse in such places, where children already spend years going from foster home to foster home and caseworkers are overwhelmed by long lists of families needing everything from housing to medical care. Using the same projections, as many as 98,000 young people 18 and under will become motherless and in some cases be called upon to care for younger family members.

The Silent Legacy

Orphans are often referred to as the silent legacy of AIDS. It is expected that about a third of the children orphaned in America will be from New York City, which has the nation's largest number of AIDS cases. Other cities expected to be hit hard are Miami, Los Angeles, Washington, Newark, and San Juan, Puerto Rico. Most of these orphans will be the children of poor black or Hispanic women whose families are already dealing with stresses like drug addiction, inadequate housing, and health care. Relatives who might in other circumstances be called upon to care for the children often shun them because of the stigma attached to AIDS.

HIV-infected women who abandon their babies are often already sick themselves and face an early death. Few can bear the thought of watching their children struggle through a short life should they have passed the virus during pregnancy. Though the majority of infected mothers do not abandon their offspring, such babies are becoming an increasingly common feature of the AIDS pandemic almost everywhere. And they are part of a larger problem that is turning out to be one of the most serious social consequences of the pandemic—**THE PHENOMENON OF AIDS ORPHANS.**

Sub-Saharan Africa

The HIV/AIDS orphan crisis is one of the greatest humanitarian and development challenges facing the global community. The orphan epidemic is still in its infancy. In the years and decades ahead, the impacts of HIV/AIDS on children, their families, and their communities will grow far worse—expanding to dimensions difficult to imagine at present. To date, over 90% of all children infected through mother-to-child transmission have been in sub-Saharan Africa. During 1995 through 2002, on average 600,000 children were born with HIV infection annually (about 1600 per day); of these children, in 2002 87% were in sub-Saharan Africa, 11% in Southeast Asia, 2% in Latin America and the Caribbean. HIV incidence among children in sub-Saharan Africa, Southeast Asia, and the Caribbean is higher than HIV incidence among children in all other regions of the world. HIV/AIDS prevalence among children is almost 35 times higher in the developing world than in the industrialized world. It has been estimated that 38% of the children in Southern and East African countries could be orphaned because of parental HIV/AIDS cases by 2010.

By the year 2015, there will be 44 million orphans under the age of 15 (one in three under age 5) in the 23 countries (30 million of these

NKOSI JOHNSON 1989–2001

Nkosi Johnson died on February 4th, at home in Johannesburg, South Africa. He was 12 years old. But he left his mark on the world by telling his story of how the others reacted to his infection. Nkosi Johnson is to Africa what Ryan White (see Chapter 13, Figure 13-1) means to America. Both young heroes of the HIV/AIDS pandemic, experienced similar discrimination because they were diagnosed with AIDS. Doctors gave Nkosi nine months to live when he was 2 years old. His foster mother took him in because his HIV-positive mother could not support him. In 1997, he took on parents at the Melville Primary School who did not want him admitted. He won. He completed grade four at the school in 2000. At the age of seven, he was labeled South Africa's longest surviving child living with HIV. Nkosi's collapse in December 2000, left him semi-comatose. He died in February 2001. Nkosi will be remembered internationally for his brave speech at the Durban 2000 AIDS Conference in South Africa. He will be remembered as an AIDS activist. Nkosi challenged the South African government's policies on AIDS and brought together millions of South Africans in the fight against the disease. Nkosi is a hero in South Africa. He will be remembered as someone who has broken the silence about AIDS, and especially about the experience of children with HIV. He has left behind a history of fighting stigma and discrimination.

orphans will live in 19 countries in sub-Saharan Africa) most affected by HIV. Most of these children will have lost their parents to AIDS.

The vast majority of the children orphaned by the AIDS pandemic, will be in sub-Saharan Africa, where formerly the extended family could always be relied upon to take on the dependents of those who died. But today the continent's age-old, traditional social security system—which has proved itself resilient to so many social changes—is buckling under due to the unprecedented strain caused by the increasing number of AIDS cases.

Mother to Child Transmission (MTCT) or Vertical HIV Transmission

Vertical transmission means that HIV passes directly from the infected mother into the fetus or infant.

Stigma— Stigma is particularly strong surrounding mother-to-child transmission. The very phrase "mother-to-child" itself may be stigmatizing as it puts all the responsibility of transmission on the mother and none on the father of the child. Stigma stops women coming forward to get themselves tested. It reduces their choices when it comes to health care and family life once they are diagnosed as HIV positive and has a negative effect on their quality of life. Equally troubling is the lack of sympathy or respect given to pregnant women with HIV, especially in the developing nations where they are open to blame, ridicule, and rejection. For example, in rural Zambia a man stated, "If a pregnant woman is sick and has a sick and premature baby who dies before 3 months, then we know she is affected [infected with HIV] and turn away from her. This is our [HIV] test!"

Timing of HIV Transmission— Worldwide, over the past two years, 1.6 million HIV-infected children were born. Over 95% of these children were born in underdeveloped countries.

The exact time of HIV transmission to the fetus during pregnancy is unknown. It has been shown to occur as early as the fifteenth week of gestation, at or near the time of delivery and through breast-feeding.

Breast-feeding by mothers with HIV infection established **before** pregnancy increases the risk of vertical transmission by 14%. When a mother develops primary HIV infection while breast-feeding, the risk of transmission rises to 29%. In general, it is believed that 50% of HIV-positive babies are infected during the last two months of pregnancy and about 50% are infected during the birthing process or through the early months of breast-feeding (Miotti et al., 1999).

A working definition of the timing of maternal HIV transmission has been established to differentiate infants infected **in utero (in the uterus)** from those infected near the time of or **during delivery** (perinatally). In utero infection occurs in approximately 20% of HIV-infected infants. Children who are infected in utero have a more rapid progression to AIDS and generally become symptomatic during the first year of life. Those infected perinatally have no detectable HIV at birth but demonstrate HIV in the blood by 4 to 6 months of age. These children constitute the majority of HIV-infected

infants and have a slower progression to AIDS, about 8% per year (Diaz et al., 1996).

Breast-feeding: Global Summary

♦ Where no drugs or other methods of prevention are administered and the baby is breast-fed by its HIV-positive mother, the risk of infection is about 30–35%.

- Where no drugs are administered and the baby is not breast-fed by its HIV-positive mother, the risk of infection is about 20%.

- Where a one-month course of AZT (zidovudine) is administered and the baby is not breast-fed, the risk of infection is about 10%.

- Where a one-month course of AZT is administered and the baby is breast-fed by its HIV-positive mother for up to six months, the risk of infection is about 18% at that age.

- Where two antiretrovirals, AZT and 3TC (lamivudine) are administered at the time of labor, and to mother and baby for one week following delivery, the risk of infection at six weeks of life, with breast-feeding, is around 11%. If the drugs are given from the 36th week of pregnancy, continued in labor, and given for a week after delivery, the risk of infection at six weeks of life, when the baby is breast-fed is about 9% (Background Brief UNAIDS, 1999).

Rate of Transmission— The worldwide rate of HIV transmission from mother, **without drug therapy,** to child varies geographically. In Africa, maternal transmission is as high as 50%, producing about 1600 infected babies **a day.** In Europe and the United States, without the use of antiretroviral drugs the overall rate is 25% to 30% producing less than 500 infected babies **a year.** The U.S. Public Health Service and 16 other national health organizations have recommended that HIV testing be offered to all women at risk prior to or at the time of pregnancy. Through year 2002, only six states, Arkansas, Connecticut, Florida, Michigan, New York, and Tennessee require health care providers to HIV-test every pregnant woman as early as possible in her pregnancy unless she refuses. The rate of vertical HIV transmission in New York state has decreased dramatically from 25% to 3.5% since the implementation of its 1996 law requiring (a) HIV counseling and offer of an HIV test to all pregnant women, and (b) infant HIV testing and maternal notification. Because of this law, over 99% of HIV-infected New York women and their children have been linked to counseling and medical care.

Newborns: HIV Positive

Because newborns who test HIV positive may not be HIV-infected, infected mothers in developed nations are advised not to breast-feed their chil- **dren.** The reason a newborn can test positive and not be infected is because the mother's HIV antibodies can enter the fetus during pregnancy (gestation). Because of the presence of maternal HIV antibody, the newborn may appear to be infected but is not. The HIV antibody will be lost with time and the child will revert to **seronegativity** (no HIV antibody in the serum). Mothers in underdeveloped nations have been advised to breast-feed because of the lack of available health care and nutrition. On average, an estimated 350,000 newborns worldwide became HIV-infected through **breast-feedings** each year between 1997 and the beginning of 2003.

UPDATE 2002 In June of 2002, President George W. Bush has committed $500 million in overseas aid to support HIV testing for pregnant women and treatment to prevent HIV transmission to their babies. President Bush explained that this money would be made available for the next 16 months, focused on 12 countries in Africa and others in the Caribbean "where the problem is most severe and where our help can make the greatest amount of difference." President Bush said, "We have a three-part strategy. First, in places with stronger health care systems, we will provide voluntary testing, prevention, counseling, and a comprehensive therapy of antiretroviral medications for both mother and child, beginning before the delivery, and continuing after delivery. This combination has proven extremely effective in preventing transmission of the HIV virus. Second, in places with weaker health care systems, we'll provide testing and counseling, and we will support programs that administer a single dose of nevirapine to the mother at the time of delivery, and at least one dose to the infant shortly after birth. This therapy reduces the chances of infection by nearly 50%. Third, and most importantly, we will make a major effort to improve the health care delivery systems in targeted countries. This will allow more women and babies to receive comprehensive therapy. It will allow for better and longer treatment and care of all AIDS victims. And it will lead to better health care, in general, for all the country's citizens. This major commitment of my government to prevent mother-to-child HIV transmission is the first of this scale by any government, anywhere. In time, we will gain valuable experience, improve treatment methods, and sharpen our training strategies. Health care systems in targeted countries will get better. And this will make even more progress possible. And as we see what works, we will make more funding available."

Perinatal Transmission— Many factors that influence perinatal HIV transmission are not known; but, influencing factors do exist because one mother gave birth to an HIV-infected child followed by an uninfected child who was followed by an infected child (Dickinson, 1988)!

There are multiple factors involved in HIV transmission risk, including maternal immunity and viral load, placental conditions, route of delivery, duration of membrane rupture, and fetal factors (birth order, gestational age). This knowledge has led to trials of various interventions, such as drug therapy to reduce viral load (the number of HIV RNA strands present in the mother's blood at the time of birth) and cesarean section to reduce HIV exposure during delivery.

Viral RNA Load Associated With Perinatal HIV Transmission— Although the close association between stage of HIV infection in a pregnant woman and likelihood of perinatal transmission has been established, there are no precise numerical criteria for pregnancies at **high** and **low** risk of transmission. Viral load measurements are now helping to quantitate this risk.

Separate studies in 1996 and 1997 on pregnancy and viral loads showed that mothers who did not transmit HIV to their children had a low plasma HIV RNA level (less than 30,000 copies/mL) while mothers with plasma HIV RNA levels above 30,000 copies/mL transmitted HIV, especially mothers who had over 50,000 copies of plasma HIV RNA per milliliter at delivery. An RNA copy number of 50,000 has scientists calling it a breakpoint for defining a high-risk pregnancy for HIV transmission.

Breast-feeding, Drug Therapy and HIV Transmission

Without question, one of the most significant accomplishments of the HIV/AIDS era has been the dramatic reduction in transmission of HIV between mother and child. In America, from 1992 until the present time, perinatal transmission has declined over 80% and it is now possible, using combination anti-HIV drug therapy, to achieve

Groups (ACTG) of pregnant women to date, has lowered the incidence of HIV-infected newborns from HIV-infected mothers (Figure 11-6).

Summary of Results of ACTG Protocol 076— Enrolled women were assigned randomly to receive a regimen of either ZDV or placebo. There was a 60% reduction of HIV transmission into newborns within the ZDV group! Based on what has been recently learned about perinatal transmission and viral load, ZDV may be reducing HIV transmission by reducing viral load. ZDV did not appear to delay the diagnosis of HIV infection.

In short, the use of ZDV is known to reduce perinatal HIV transmission. But it is not 100%, because 8% of ZDV-treated pregnancies will still deliver HIV-infected infants. And that is if therapy is given to all HIV-positive pregnant women! (See Chapter 8 for more information on HIV transmission and zidovudine therapy.)

Entering year 2003, a number of ACTG participants have received a variety of combination drug therapy, which includes the use of protease inhibitors. Perhaps the best news to date is the work of Laurent Mandelbrot and colleagues (1998) presented at the 12th World AIDS Conference. **The French study reported that of women who took zidovudine and had a cesarean section delivery, and did not breast-feed, mother-to-newborn HIV transmission occurred less than 1% of the time.** A study by the National Institute of Child and Human Development in Washington combined the findings of that study with several others in Europe and North America and found that Cesarean sections when combined with zidovudine treatment, cut the transmission to about 2%.

In 1999, researchers at Makerere University in Kampala, Uganda, and Johns Hopkins University in Baltimore gave HIV-infected women a single dose of **nevirapine** (a non-nucleoside reverse transcriptase inhibitor) during labor and another dose to their infants within three days of birth. The infection rate dropped from 25% to 13%. At a cost of about $4, the nevirapine regimen is some 70 times cheaper than AZT given during the last month of pregnancy. And nevirapine can be stored at room temperature. If adopted widely in developing countries, the treatment could prevent prenatal HIV transmission in up to 400,000

FIGURE 11-6 Drops of Danger. This woman nurses her 4-month-old son. She, her husband, and three other children have been diagnosed with AIDS. She did not know she could pass HIV to her newborn via breast-feeding. She said that her husband was her only sexual partner. After her health began to decline and she tested HIV positive, her husband refused to be tested and he abandoned the family for another woman. *(Photo by Hilda M. Perez/South Florida* Sun-Sentinel*)*

transmission rates as low as 1%–2%, compared to 25%–30% a decade ago.

In 1999, two studies that were perhaps the first, demonstrated the relationship of viral load and mother-to-child breast-feeding HIV transmission. The higher the maternal viral load the greater the chance for HIV transmission via breast-feeding (Katzenstein et al., 1999; Plaegaer et al., 1999).

Nucleoside Reverse Transcriptase Inhibitor Monotherapy that Appears to Reduce HIV Transmission During Pregnancy— For many HIV investigators, the hard search for drugs to combat HIV replication has paid off. The use of **zidovudine** (ZDV), in all AIDS Clinical Trials newborns per year. Year 2001 French data showed that using AZT and **lamivudine** (a nucleoside reverse transcriptase inhibitor) reduced HIV transmission to 1.6%.

The best news is that Mary Culnane and colleagues (1999), Patricia Garcia and colleagues (2001), and Ruth Tuomala and colleagues (2002) found **no** significant differences in growth, cognitive development, or immunologic function in children age 5 exposed to zidovudine and other FDA approved antiretroviral drugs excluding tenofovir during pregnancy (in utero) and during their first six weeks of life.

Class Discussion: Present factual, medical, and economic reasons for and against the use of a C-section on 100 women to prevent one HIV transmission. Also discuss the fact that neither a C-section nor abandonment of breast-feeding is practical for women in poor countries.

States and Territories Most Affected by Pediatric Cases

There is evidence that HIV was present in female IDUs as early as 1977 because their babies developed AIDS (Thomas, 1988). As the number of HIV-infected women of childbearing age rises, so does the number of HIV-infected babies.

In the United States pediatric AIDS is most widespread among blacks, Hispanics, and the poor of the innercities (Figure 11-7). Beginning year 2003, New York continues to have the highest incidence of pediatric AIDS cases followed by Florida, New Jersey, California, Puerto Rico, and

Texas. Combined, these cases accounted for 66% of all AIDS cases reported among children.

Risk Exposure for Mothers of HIV-Infected Newborns

Risk exposures for HIV infection among the mothers of children with perinatally acquired AIDS included injecting drug use (40%), sexual contact with a partner with or at risk for HIV/AIDS (35%), and receipt of contaminated blood or blood products (2%). No risk was specified for 13% of cases. Ten metropolitan areas account for more than 50% of all pediatric AIDS cases: New York City, Miami, Chicago, Los Angeles, San Juan, Washington, DC, Philadelphia, Newark, New Jersey, Baltimore, and Ft. Lauderdale report the largest numbers. The epidemic is also spreading into smaller communities. Beginning 1999, pediatric AIDS cases have been reported in all 50 states.

AIDS Cases among Children Declining

The findings reported in "AIDS Among Children—United States, 1996" present a documented decline in the incidence of pediatric AIDS. From 1993 through year 2000, the estimated **annual** number of pediatric AIDS cases declined over 80% from 1017 in 1992 to less than 200 beginning year 2003.

There are many reasons to believe that with continued HIV counseling of HIV-positive pregnant women and use of AIDS drug cocktails that lower viral loads, fewer children will become

FIGURE 11-7 Josh, Age 3, Has Advanced-Stage AIDS. His older brother died from AIDS. Their mother died of AIDS, leaving them as AIDS orphans. *(Photo by Hilda M. Perez/South Florida Sun-Sentinel)*

DISTURBING THOUGHTS

Much has been said over the past year, by politicians and the press, about getting cheap antiretroviral drugs into developing countries in order to extend lives and reduce the transmission of HIV from the HIV-infected mother into her infant. However, Karen Beckerman of San Francisco General Hospital (2002) says that treatment programs that use antiretrovirals to prevent mother-to-child transmission are likely to succeed only in creating a generation of orphans and ruining the treatment chances of mothers. Beckerman raised the question "Is it justifiable to visit the antiretroviral mistakes of the industrialized world on regions that have been devastated by the HIV epidemic but are at least antiretrovirally naïve?" She states that active deployment of AZT/3TC during delivery for millions of pregnancies may prevent hundreds of thousands of pediatric infections per year. However, these same women and their infected children exposed to short-course zidovudine plus lamivudine or single-dose nevirapine will be at substantial risk of treatment failure when antiretroviral therapy becomes available. Instead of inducing resistance to AIDS drug therapies, prophylaxis against mother-to-child transmission must be linked to preventing the creation of orphans.

On average, about 600,000 HIV-infected babies have been born each year over the past five years. But, save these children for what? To become orphans by the millions who then become street urchins who are poorly fed, undisciplined, unsheltered, and uncared for? These children form gangs and add to the growing crime wave in all orphan-populated cities. About 30% of these orphans are HIV positive and require care they cannot get. They are left in already crowded hospitals and homes that offer little more than a place to die. Regardless of the town, city, or country's economic plight, the growing mass of orphans tends to further decrease the economy

and care available to healthy adults and school-age children. It is not universally agreed that saving an infant born to an HIV-infected mother is a sensible use of public funds in poor countries. It has been written that President Mbeki of South Africa follows this reasoning. He believes the cost of drugs and care would ruin the economy of South Africa. He is not alone in his beliefs. The infant will be born into extremely difficult circumstances. Death is predicted at least for its mother and probably for its father. Should public dollars be invested in preventing infant deaths—an investment that will translate into a rising tide of orphans? In hard-hit countries such as Zimbabwe, Botswana, Malawi, Namibia, Swaziland, and South Africa, it is predicted that by 2005, one in three children younger than 15 years will be orphaned. Currently, about 40% of South Africa's population of 42 million people are under the age of 15. A report from the 2002 14th International AIDS Conference from UNAIDS states that 50% of South African new mothers could die because of HIV, and that mortality among 15- to 34-year-olds will be 17 times higher because of AIDS.

The U.S. Census Bureau reported at these meetings that ending 2005 there will be 20 million AIDS-related orphans (up from 14 million ending 2003) worldwide; by 2010 there will be 25 million. A Swiss-based association, Francois-Xavier Bagnoud, predicted that ending 2010 there would be about 100 million AIDS-related orphans.

Class Discussion: Take a stand, for or against saving the lives of some 42 million orphans who will populate the underdeveloped nations by year 2015. Support your presentation with facts, not just emotions. Answer the question, "Is the social cost of so many young people being raised without parental or adult guidance too high to tolerate?"

infected and this will translate into a continued decrease in children with AIDS.

This possibility was inconceivable to many clinicians, families, and patients not too long ago. The rapid decline has many physicians suggesting that a goal of eliminating perinatal transmission may be attainable in the United States. However, Patricia Fleming of the CDC, told those in atten-

dance at her presentation at the 2002 14th International AIDS Conference, that it would be difficult to get the numbers much lower because the treatment isn't always effective. An estimated 130 HIV-positive babies still would have been born even if all the pregnant women had received treatment. The number of infected babies is likely to grow in the future because of the rise in new infections among women. Fleming said, "The simple fact is that the best way to prevent new infections in babies is to prevent infections in women."

To counter the good news (the 80% drop in babies born with HIV) Roland Foster, Congressional aide and member of the oversight committee on Foreign Federal HIV/AIDS programs said, "The truth is the CDC has no idea how many babies are being born with HIV, and its plan, which relies on voluntary rather than routine HIV screening, has fallen short. Nearly half of pregnant women are still not being tested for HIV."

Although many children have benefited from the present achievements, there are many more in the developing world awaiting the translation of progress into practice.

Conflicting Reports on Breastfeeding, Drug Therapy—Whether and Which Drugs Should be Used Leads to Confusion

In reviewing the recent literature on breastfeeding, a variety of conflicting data has been reported by the respected authorities in this field of HIV/AIDS research. For example, it is not understood how AZT, nevirapine or other drugs lowers the vertical HIV transmission rate, yet the following statements have been made:

1. If you give AZT or nevirapine to 100% of pregnant women, the mother should not breastfeed for fear of HIV transmission.

2. If you give AZT or nevirapine, there is no way that safe and healthy formula or water to make formula is available or obtainable in most developing nations where vertical transmission rates are highest.

3. If you don't breastfeed, the babies will die of other diseases because they will lose the immunological benefits against these diseases that breastfeeding provides.

4. More babies will die because they are not breastfed than will die from the small percentage that become HIV infected perinatally.

5. Prenatal care, immediate delivery as soon as the water breaks, clean birth canal, treatment of infections, etc., will reduce to a minimum the chance of perinatal transmission.

6. The key is the maternal HIV viral load, not AZT or nevirapine. Even with antiviral drugs, if the viral load is high, the mother will transmit. If the viral load is low, the mother will not transmit.

7. Treat all pregnant women with antiretroviral drugs regardless of viral load or T4 or CD4+ counts.

8. The risk of transmission of HIV through breastfeeding is not high. UNAIDS estimate the additional risk of transmission of HIV through breastfeeding, over and above that occurring during pregnancy and birth, to be about 15%. This means that if 100 HIV-infected mothers breastfeed their babies, 85 of them will not be infected through breastfeeding.

9. A study published in 1999 and followed up in 2001 found that exclusive breastfeeding (with the addition of no other foods and liquids) leads to no additional risk of transmission of the virus than when there is no breastfeeding at all. And a review by the WHO Collaborative Study Team in 2000 noted that babies in developing countries who were not breastfed were placed at a much higher overall risk of death from other infections.

10. On a scale of competing risks, a baby born in sub-Saharan Africa has a much greater chance of survival if breastfed even by an HIV-infected mother than if breastfeeding is withheld.

11. The issue of HIV and breastfeeding cannot be separated from the global reality of increasing malnutrition and mortality rates among children in many sub-Saharan African countries. That breastfeeding with all its benefits should also pose a significant risk of HIV transmission is one of the ultimate public health paradoxes and will likely continue to be a major challenge for the prevention of HIV infections in infants living in resource-poor settings.

12. Perhaps the most sobering comment concerning breastfeeding and the use of therapy is the "active use of drugs for millions of pregnancies may prevent hundreds of thousands of pediatric infections per year. However, these same women and their infected children exposed to short course zidovudine plus lamivudine or single-dose nevirapine will be at substantial risk of treatment failure when antiretroviral therapy becomes available."

"Instead of inducing resistance to antiretroviral drugs, prophylaxis against mother-to-child transmission must be linked to preventing the creation of orphans. We know that 3% to 4% of HIV-infected sub-Saharan mothers die within a year of delivery. Within 2 years, 11% of HIV-infected breastfeeding mothers die. Their babies are unlikely to survive infancy. An older child who survives the death of mother will join the rapidly growing global ranks of orphans under 15 years of age, predicted to reach 44 million by 2010. With or without antiretroviral prophylaxis, most of these children will not be HIV infected. They will face extraordinary risk of inadequate nutrition, housing, and health care, in addition to servitude, harshness, abuse, and acquisition of HIV infection themselves. By 2020, sub-Saharan teenagers will outnumber adults rendering already politically unstable regions potentially explosive. However, although support for home care, community programs, and government services are routinely mentioned as effective responses to the global orphan tragedy, strategies to prevent the creation of orphans—that is, saving the lives of parents—are rarely discussed. This is particularly disturbing in view of the developed world's experience that treatment of maternal HIV disease results in transmission rates far lower than transmission prophylaxis alone" (Karen Beckerman, 2002, *Lancet* 359:1168–1169).

Life Span of Untreated HIV-Infected Newborns in sub-Saharan Africa

According to Taha Taha and colleagues of Johns Hopkins University (2000) over 50% of HIV-infected newborns die within 12 months. Eighty-nine percent of HIV-infected children alive at 6 months died by age 3 years. In comparison,

---

BOX 11.4

JOHANNESBURG, SOUTH AFRICA

There is a major crisis in this city. There are so many HIV/AIDS-associated orphans that the city cannot handle the problem. In one case, in response to the problem, a Baptist minister built a steel delivery box into a wall on her Johannesburg church. Unwanted infants can be safely left there by their mothers rather than left to die in dustbins or drains. Thirteen babies were deposited at this "Door of Hope" in the first three months. Some social workers criticized the project, suggesting it encourages abandonment. But the minister disputes the charge, and has called on the government's Children Protection Unit to drop its threat of prosecuting mothers caught leaving a baby in the box.

---

the authors note that in a European study, only 18% of HIV-infected children died by age 3 years, and a U.S. study found that 75% lived to age 5 years.

CONTACTS FOR INFORMATION ON USE OF ANTIRETROVIRAL DRUGS DURING PREGNANCY

For a copy of newest "US Public Health Service Recommendations for Use of Antiretroviral Drugs in Pregnant Women Infected with HIV-1 for Maternal Health and Reduction of Perinatal HIV-1 Transmission in the United States," contact: **CDC National Prevention Information Network**, 800-458-5231, http://www.cdcnac.org or **HIV/AIDS Treatment Information Service**, 800-448-0440, http://www.hivatis.org.

Pediatric AIDS Resources

American College of Obstetrician and Gynecologists— Website: www.acog.org

♦ Important News For Pregnant Women tear pad: Information for patients on routine pregnancy tests, including HIV (both English and Spanish versions). Printed on tear pads for easy use by providers or counselors.

AIDS Alliance— Website: www.aidsalliance.org

♦ Pregnant Women and HIV Counseling and Testing Recommendations: Brochure of AIDS Alliance's recommendations to providers and policy makers regarding prenatal HIV testing.

National Pediatric and Family HIV Resource Center— Website: www.pedhivaids.org

♦ HIV Infection and Pregnancy: This PowerPoint slide set is an educational curriculum for healthcare providers.
♦ Labcoat Pocket Laminated Cards on HIV Antiretroviral Therapy in Pregnancy, 2001: Easily accessible recommendations for antiretroviral therapy to prevent transmission during pregnancy and for infants exposed to HIV. Lists toll free numbers and websites of national resources.

Association for Maternal-Child Health Programs— Website: www.amchp.org

---

GLOBAL HIV INFECTIONS
IN YOUNG ADULTS

Over the summer of 1999, especially in the United States, young people ages 10 to 24 flocked to theaters to experience the **Dark Side of the Force**. Many thousands saw the STAR WARS movie repeatedly. But the real **Dark Side** of their lives is the threat of HIV infection and the **Force** should be their education to prevent their infection. About half of all new HIV infections in the United States and worldwide are occurring in this age group. Hopefully, reading this section will encourage the young to stay on the **Light Side with the Force**.

In April of 1998 the Joint United Nations Program on HIV/AIDS (UNAIDS) released a report showing that five young people aged 10 to 24 are now infected with HIV every minute, one every 12 seconds, and drew attention to the fact that Eastern Europe has emerged as a particular trouble spot for young people and HIV.

The UNAIDS report was released to mark the launch of a year-long initiative, **"Force for Change: World AIDS Campaign With Young People,"** which aims to promote the participation of young people, and strengthen support for young people in their effort to fight AIDS. This report found that overall, children and especially young people still carry the heaviest burden of new infections. Among the key findings of the report (updated) are:

♦ More than half of all new HIV infections acquired after infancy occur among young people.

♦ Of the 44 million persons living with HIV/AIDS ending year 2003, at least a third are young people.

♦ Every day, 7500 young people worldwide acquire the virus. This translates into 2.7 million infections each year in this group (ages 10 to 24).

♦ In the worst affected countries, HIV is spreading fastest among young people below the age of 24 years—at the peak of fertility. And in places where the virus is spread predominantly through heterosexual intercourse—notably sub-Saharan Africa—young women outnumber young men among those becoming infected. Studies sponsored by UNAIDS show that in western Kenya about one girl in four between the ages of 15 and 19 is living with HIV compared with one in 25 boys in the same age group. In Zambia, in this age range, 16 times as many girls as boys are infected. In rural Uganda among 20- to 24-year olds,

there are six young women who are HIV positive for every infected young man.

♦ **Overall, young people ages 14 to 24 account for at least 50% of all those who now become HIV-infected.**

Young People and HIV/AIDS

Young people are central to any discussion of HIV/AIDS because there are so many! There are about 1.2 billion people aged from 15–24 in the world. They make up 20% of the global population. Young people are and will continue to be the sector of the population most affected by HIV/AIDS. As today's children grow up, the proportion of 15- to 24-year olds will continue to increase, particularly in developing countries where more than 80% of the world's young people live. At present rates, about 8000 young people aged 15–24 are infected every day or 2.9 million a year—About six young people every minute!

MTV Youth Poll— In 2000, less than 25% of young people surveyed in 16 countries across Asia, Europe, and the Americas consider themselves well informed about HIV/AIDS. Among the 16- to 24-year olds surveyed by the worldwide television network, 60% are concerned about becoming infected by HIV but just 24% said they know a lot about the disease. Some 25% of poll respondents believed only promiscuous people contracted AIDS and 17% said it was improbable they would ever be exposed to the virus. (This means that 83% do not consider themselves to be at risk!) Seventy-nine percent of the poll respondents said they relied mostly on television as their news source for information about HIV/AIDS.

Additional Information on Young People and Their Knowledge About HIV/AIDS—2000

Young people in the Pacific and East Asia are unprepared to handle HIV/AIDS. A survey of 10,000 youth ages 9 to 17 conducted by UNICEF shows that children in 17 Asia-Pacific countries have an alarming ignorance about HIV/AIDS. UNICEF said the survey was a representative sample of 300 million children in the region and indicated that 33 million youth "lacked basic knowledge about the disease." The survey found that 60% of 9- to

13-year olds and 25% of the 14 to 17 age groups knew "absolutely nothing" about, or "only the name" of HIV/AIDS. In addition, while 68% of the older age group knew that unprotected sex was a method of contracting HIV, only 41% knew about condoms. The results of this survey should serve as a wake-up call to the governments and societies in this region on how much more needs to be done to educate young people about HIV/AIDS.

United States—South Carolina 2000

A study of 1000 teenagers and adults in South Carolina reveals a significant lack of information regarding basic knowledge, awareness of community services, and perception of personal risk for HIV and AIDS. The researchers reported their findings at the 128th annual American Public Health Association meeting in Boston. They found that 14% of the teens believed there was a vaccine for HIV while 36.6% of the teens and 20% of the adults said the virus is transmitted through blood donation. Also, nearly 50% of teens and adults did not think there were HIV or AIDS patients living in their communities.

Why the High HIV-Infection Rates Among Young People?

To some extent, the high infection rates reflect the preponderance of young people in the world. The global population is young. Between 1960 and 1990, when **the world population grew by 75%,** the proportion of young people **increased by 99%.** Of the world's young people, 85% live in developing countries, and this is where over 90% of the pandemic is now concentrated. But population percentages tell only part of the story. There are special reasons why young people are exposed to infection. Remember, that above all **HIV is a sexually transmitted virus.** Adolescence and youth are times of discovery, emerging feelings of independence, and the exploration of new behavior and relationships. It is also a time of examination, rebellion, and change. By definition adolescence is about taking risks and experimentation. Sexual behavior, an important part of this, can involve risks; the same is true of experimentation with drugs. At the time, young people get mixed messages. They

are often faced with double standards calling for virginity in girls but early and active sexual behavior in boys. They have been told **"Just say NO"** since the early 1980s, yet abuse continues, perhaps because they are confronted with hundreds of millions of dollars worth of media images of sex, smoking, and drinking as glamorous and risk-free. They are told to be abstinent, but exposed to a barrage of advertisements using sex to sell goods. Compounding the challenge, in the name of morality, culture, or religion, young people are often denied their right to education about the heath risks of sexual behavior, and to important tools and services for protection. Among the world's young people, some are more exposed to HIV than others. Those living in what UNICEF terms, "especially difficult circumstances" include young people who are out of school, who live on the streets, who share needles with other injecting drug users, engage in commercial sex, or are sexually and physically abused. Young men who have sex with men are disadvantaged by the lack of information and services available to them and directed to their needs.

TEENAGERS: HIV-POSITIVE AND AIDS CASES—UNITED STATES

Teenagers often say, **"I KNOW HOW TO BE SAFE,"** but the statistics on teenage pregnancy, smoking, drinking of alcohol, drug use, and in particular, injection drug use, sexual behavior, and the use of contraceptives indicates otherwise. **Studies on teenage risk-taking continue to show that about half of teens are NOT WORRIED ABOUT BECOMING INFECTED WITH HIV AND THAT RELATIVELY FEW TEENAGERS HAVE CHANGED THEIR SEXUAL BEHAVIORS**

BECAUSE OF THEIR CONCERNS ABOUT THE HIV PANDEMIC.

Teenagers/Young Women at Greatest Risk

In the United States, 25% of all new HIV infections are estimated to occur in young people between the ages of 13 and 20. And at least 50% occur in people under age 25. While more research needs to be done on this topic, several factors associated with teenagers and young women are clear: **(1)** they tend to be partnered with **older men** who have had more sexual partners and have a greater chance of being infected with HIV and other sexually transmitted diseases (STDs); **(2)** their risk of HIV infection is greater because of their immature cervix and relatively low vaginal mucous production presents less of a barrier to HIV; and **(3)** many lack the education, social status, economic resources, and power in sexual partner relationships to make informed choices.

Safer Sex: Sex Thrills but AIDS Kills

There was a time when safer sex meant not getting caught by your parents. With time, sexually transmitted diseases and in particular HIV/AIDS have changed the meaning of safer sex. Today, over half of teenagers (aged 13 to 19) in the United States have had sex by the time they reach 16, and 7 in 10 are sexually active by 19. Many enter the sexual arena unprepared for the responsibility of their actions (Table 11-3). About 1 million teenage women become pregnant, outside of marriage, each year.

Whether or not society openly discusses it, teens are having sex. Many women—and most men—have their first sexual relations prior to marriage, usually during their teens, and most often those first encounters are unprotected. Research in family planning has revealed that the quality of reproductive health information is generally low among adolescents. This is a reflection in part of the lack of social acceptance of providing sex education and contraceptive services to teens in many countries. In the developing world, contraceptive services are often available only to married women, and in some situations, only to women who have already borne one or more children.

The guiding philosophy in dealing with sexuality in many cultures is **"If you don't talk about sex they won't do it."** This logic, however, is critically flawed. Teenagers are sexual beings at varying stages of self-awareness and understanding. Many teenagers continue to engage in sexual intercourse despite lack of access to any accurate information about sex and, in most cases, engage in "unsafe sex." **Safer sex requires an ability to distinguish between risky and nonrisky sexual activities and the emotional security to choose safer sex.**

Teens, Sexual Partners, and Sexually Transmitted Diseases

In a nationwide survey, 19% of high school students have had four or more sex partners by their junior year and 29% had four or more by their senior year (*MMWR*, 1992). Teenagers are experiencing skyrocketing rates of sexually transmitted diseases (STDs). **Every 10 seconds a teenager somewhere in the United States is infected with an STD.** (That's equal to 3 million teenagers aged 13 to 19 years.) People under age 25 account for 66% of all new STDs every year. One in four teens will contract an STD before finishing high school. In California, for example, 15- to 19-year olds have the highest rates of gonorrhea and chlamydia of any age group in the state. Experts fear that if these diseases are being transmitted, then HIV is too (California Department of Health Services, 1995).

Table 11-3 Sexually Active Teenagers by High School Year and Age (%)

High School Year	Age Group	Female	Male	Combined
9th Grade	14–15	31.9	48.7	40.3
10th Grade	15–16	42.9	52.5	47.7
11th Grade	16–17	52.7	62.6	57.7
12th Grade	17–19	66.6	76.3	71.5

Source: CDC HIV/AIDS Surveillance Report, November 1991:1–18.

WARNINGS DON'T WORK!

They heard endless warnings about the dangers of intravenous drug use, about the wisdom of using condoms. Many even knew older relatives, neighbors, and friends who had died because of AIDS. But somehow, it didn't add up. Not me, they said. Couldn't happen to me. And so a 16-year-old girl became infected with HIV because she had unprotected sex with a friend. A 14-year-old boy never took his condom out of its wrapper, and now he is HIV positive. A 16-year-old girl trusted her boyfriend, a drug user. She shouldn't have. Risky sexual behavior is nothing new among young people. But medical professionals find it disturbing that the risk-taking continues despite extensive educational campaigns. Black American youths are paying an especially high price. That is a major change from the early 1980s when gay white men made up the majority of young people infected with HIV. For many young people, HIV has become just one of the many problems in their lives, like if they are going to get a good meal, who they are going to live with, whether they are going to school.

HIV-INFECTED CHILDREN: LIVING LONGER—PAYING A PRICE

AIDS, in America, is the seventh leading cause of death in 15- to 24-year-old people.

Adolescents infected with HIV since birth are a new population in the ever-changing HIV/AIDS pandemic. Data from the CDC shows that before 1996, HIV-infected children lived to an average age of 9. After 1996, with the use of antiretroviral drugs, the average age has risen to 14 and continues to climb.

Six years ago, an estimated three children died each week of AIDS at Detroit's Children's Hospital. Today, that rate has dropped to about one child per year. But as the children's life expectancy increases, so do the number of complex social issues they must face, especially during adolescence. One mother of an HIV-positive child said she dreads the issue of dating because it's going to be emotionally crippling. "Unless current attitudes about those infected with HIV change, my daughter will not be very popular and that will hurt. It will just crush her." (Recommended reading, see Parker, 2000.) Her daughter is one of Michigan's 123 children under age 13 living with HIV. They have had their car tires flattened and parents of classmates forbade their children from playing with her. In response to these issues and new issues such as dating, Children's Hospital has hired social workers and psychologists to hold support groups for these children, bringing them together to help them understand they aren't alone. This is a growing problem nationwide.

In April of 1992, the *MacNeil/Lehrer Report* estimated that 40,000 to 80,000 teenagers will become HIV-infected during the 1990s. According to recent CDC estimates, it happened. Yet AIDS cases are relatively rare among **13- to 19-year olds.** This is because of the 9- to 15-year time average from HIV infection to AIDS diagnosis. In 1981, there was **one** reported teenage AIDS case, by 1991 there were **789** reported AIDS cases. Beginning 2003, there were an estimated 5000 (0.6% of the total AIDS cases). From 1991 to 2003 the number of AIDS cases in 13- to 19-year olds increased by 83%.

HIV/AIDS WON'T AFFECT US!

In 1996, it was estimated that at least two teenagers per hour were becoming HIV-infected (8760 per year) and this will increase markedly through the year 2003 (Office of National AIDS Policy 1996). Regardless of available information on prevention, meaning that **teenagers do know** how HIV is transmitted, there has been a continuing increase in HIV infections within the preteen and early teen population! They continue to engage in sexual intercourse **without condoms!**

FEDERAL PUBLIC HEALTH POLICY SUPPORTS ABSTINENCE-ONLY PROGRAM: SEX EDUCATION

IN ONE LESSON—NO SEX!

Jenny, a cartoon teenage virgin, is about to give in to her boyfriend and climb into the backseat of his car. Suddenly, the emergency brake gives out and his car rolls until it teeters from a cliff off lover's lane. Their lives hang in the balance. That is when Windy, the good witch in high-tops, leaps to the rescue. "Paul loves me," Jenny protests. Windy asks, "Oh. Is that why he asked you to do something that could mess up your life forever?" Using her time machine, Windy shows Jenny how she would have awakened pregnant. **Had the car's brake not failed her boyfriend's condom would have.** The cartoon, shown to sixth-graders at Burbank Elementary School, is one weapon in an arsenal of films, celebrity rallies, and school classes pushing a message of chastity in classrooms around the nation. Currently, only 18 states and the District of Columbia require schools to provide sex education!

Will it work? Years of heated debate on the failure versus benefits of **sexual abstinence-only** education continues. However, in August of 1996, with the passage of the **Welfare Reform Act** the United States Congress allocated $50 million annually for five years to states that would institute abstinence-only educational programs (no discussion of contraception). To qualify, states have to match $4 of federal money with $3 of state money. Thus the yearly total for abstinence-only education is $87 million. This legislation specifically requires funded programs to teach the social, psychological, and health gains to be realized by abstaining from sex; that abstaining from sexual activity outside marriage is the expected standard for all school-age adolescents; that a mutually faithful monogamous relationship in the context of marriage is the expected standard of human sexual activity; and that **abstaining from sexual activity is the only certain way to avoid pregnancy, STDs, and other associated health problems.**

Clearly there are numerous health, economic, and social benefits in delaying sexual onset in teenagers like disease prevention, but scientists say they can **not** identify a long-term advantage to abstinence programs relative to safer sex programs. Perhaps young people should receive two messages: one, promoting abstinence and the delay of sexual activity, the other, warning against high-risk behaviors and teaching teens how to protect themselves. These messages are not contradictory, but they are complex. "Don't drink, but if you drink, don't drive" is a similar complex message that has saved many people from death on highways. Prevention scientists offer significant evidence that safer-sex interventions work. But there is no clear and compelling evidence that abstinence-only programs work (DiClemente, 1998). The work of John Jemmott and colleagues (1998) and Douglas Kirby and colleagues (1998) demonstrate that for those adolescents that were sexually experienced at the beginning of their study, there was **no difference** in the proportion of the adolescents in the abstinence program relative to those in a safer-sex program with regard to having sexual intercourse. For those **not** sexually experienced, abstinence education was effective for a short time (three months). After 12 months the adolescents in the two groups were each as likely to become sexually active and were similar in their pregnancy and sexually transmitted disease rates. At press time, two states, California and New Hampshire, decided against the program and returned the federal money.

Abstinence Catching on in Africa

Kenya—where 2.3 million out of 30 million people are HIV infected, where 700 people die each day from AIDS, President Daniel Arap Moi has urged Kenyans to abstain from sex for at least two years to try to curb the spread of AIDS. The government announced plans to import 300 million condoms.

Swaziland—where 25% of its people are HIV positive, King Mswati III declared a five-year sex ban on women under age 18 in order to help stop the spread of HIV. Any man breaking this rule will be liable to pay about $160 or an animal, such as a cow. The tradition of preserving maidens' chastity, known as Imabali YeMaswati or Flower of the Nation, will be policed by traditional chiefs who still rule over much of Swazi society to preserve virginity among girls and combat AIDS. Under the rite, the girls wear woolen "do not touch me" tassels or different colors depending on their ages.

Women in relationships and older than 19 years would be expected to wear red with black tassels, and those still virgins will wear blue with yellow.

Irony—King Mswati, eight weeks after his declaration, broke his sex ban rule. He married a 17-year-old woman as his 8th wife. He was fined one cow.

Teenagers' Perception of Abstinence

The 2001 Alan Guttmacher Institute survey revealed that those aged 15 to 19 considered oral sex to be a substitute for sex. They believe that oral sex is risk free! In addition to this survey are the data from other public health care workers who have found that young people believe that neither anal nor oral sex places them at risk and that these activities maintain their virginity! In defense of these young people it can be said that health educators themselves are no more clear. A 2000 survey found that nearly a third believed that oral sex was abstinence behavior. And why not? In 1998, President Clinton, in testimony about an affair with a White House intern said, with great sincerity, that he had not had "sexual relations" but had engaged only in oral sex!

Update 2002—In April 2002 the Congress allocated an additional $33 million for use in abstinence-only programs. In 2003, the annual total is now $135 million.

Update May 2002—An interim report written by independent researchers, (Mathematica Policy Research, under contract to the Department of Heath and Human Services), stated that there is still no evidence that abstinence-only programs prevent teen sex, pregnancy, or disease. Despite claims by advocates, no reliable evidence exists on whether the programs work. Most studies of abstinence education programs have methodological flaws that prevent them from generating reliable estimates of program impacts.

Class Discussion: Is it good science, poor politics, or poor science and good politics, or some other combination of events that made it logical for the federal government to earmark tax dollars specifically for abstinence-only educational programs? Do you sense a religious involvement in the government policy? Explain.

Two groups, teenage (adolescent) gay men and teenage women infected via heterosexual sex, account for about 75% of teenage HIV infections. Race is an important factor with regard to who becomes infected. Sixty-one percent of AIDS cases that occur in people ages 20 to 24, occur in blacks and Latinos, but they were HIV-infected in their teens (Collins et al., 1997)!

How Large is the Teenage and Young Adult Population?

In the United States there are about 28 million teenagers between the ages of 13 and 19 (70% white, 15% black, 15% Hispanic). This number is expected to increase to 43 million over the next 24 years (Sells et al., 1996). There are 18 million people ages 20 to 24, and about 22 million between the ages of 25 and 29. That's 68 million people between the ages of 13 and 29. Over 86 percent of all STDs occur in this age group. It has been estimated that 34% of all heterosexual adults with AIDS were infected with HIV as teenagers.

Estimate of HIV-Infected and AIDS Cases Among Teenagers and Young Adults

The total number of HIV-infected teenagers is unknown. **Federal health agencies estimate that teenagers make up about 20% or 190,000 of the HIV-infected population.** They are a silent pool for eventual cases of AIDS. About 20% of the total number of AIDS cases in the United States, or 1 in 5 occur in people ages 20 to 29 (about 170,000 beginning 2003). Most of these people, given the 9- to 15-year period before being diagnosed with AIDS, were infected as teenagers! About 50% of HIV-infected teenagers come from six locations: New York, New Jersey, Texas, California, Florida, and Puerto Rico. The overall male-to-female ratio of AIDS cases in the United States is now about 7:1, but among 13- to 19-year olds, the ratio in 1997 became about 1:1.

HIV SPREADING RAPIDLY AMONG TEENAGE GAY MALES

Combined results of the first two national surveys of young gay and bisexual men showed that 7% in the surveys were HIV-infected (HEALTH, 1996 updated). Researchers interviewed 5273 men ages 15 to 22 in six urban counties: Miami's Dade County, Dallas County, and Los Angeles, San Francisco, Santa Clara, and Alameda counties in California. Results of the interviews demonstrated that 5% of the young men ages 15 to 19 and 9% of those ages 20 to 22 were HIV-infected. Four percent of whites, 7% of Hispanics, and 11% of blacks were infected. And, 38% reported unprotected anal sex within the previous six months. These 1996/1999 data, when compared to those data of a similar 1994/1995 survey, were about the same! Education and prevention control measures do not appear to be changing teenage gay sexual behaviors with regard to preventing HIV infection.

In New York City, teenagers account for 29% of all New York AIDS cases. Sixty percent of new HIV infections in women now occur during their adolescent years. **About 500,000 people in the United States under the age of 29 are HIV positive.**

Teenagers and Incidence of AIDS Cases by Gender and Color

Updating the CDC report with 4219 cumulative adolescent/teenager (ages 13 to 19) AIDS cases through June 2001 likely means there will be about 4250 AIDS cases beginning 2003. Overall, it is estimated that there are 12,000 AIDS cases in people under age 20. Over half were diagnosed before age 5.

Teenagers of color account for 47%, whites 32%, and Hispanics 19% of reported teen AIDS cases. Among males, white teenagers account for 41% of reported teen AIDS cases, followed by blacks (36%) and Hispanics (21%). Among females, black teenagers account for 66%, white

---

POINT OF VIEW 11.3

THOUGHTS AND COMMENTS FROM A GENERATION AT RISK

"If you're going to educate kids about AIDS, you have to educate them about drugs as well. If you're a youth, you're going to experiment with drugs, especially if you live in a metropolitan area. Even though you get stupid with drugs, you still think about things you don't want to do, but you do it anyhow."—**16-year-old HIV-positive youth from San Francisco**

"We grow up hating ourselves like society teaches us to. If someone had been 'out' about their sexuality. If the teachers hadn't been afraid to stop the 'fag' and 'dyke' jokes. If my human sexuality class had even mentioned homosexuality. If the school counselors would have been open to a discussion of gay and lesbian issues. If any of those possibilities had existed, perhaps I would not have grown up hating what I was. And, just perhaps, I wouldn't have attempted suicide."—**Kyallee, 19**

"People say HIV is this or that group's problem, not mine. But for HIV, it's a matter of risk behaviors, not risk groups. Because if you say it's a risk group thing, I don't identify with that group, so I'm not at risk. That makes people feel invincible to HIV."—**HIV-positive youth**

"I was infected with HIV by my first partner when I was 16 years old. Now at 20 I have this virus that's taking my life because everything I heard when I was younger was sugar-coated. We need more complete information than what we are being given. Even the pamphlets concerning HIV/AIDS prevention are too basic and bland. We need to know real stuff."—**Ryan, age 20**

"We, the young people of this country, need a place where we can go to ask our questions, where we won't be teased or ridiculed. We need a place where we can ask about our mixed up feelings, about sex, and about AIDS."—**15-year-old high school student from Concord, NH**

"If I could talk to the President, or a Senator, or anyone in the Federal Government who can make a difference, I'd tell them to take a look, learn a lesson from the youth that are currently dealing with the disease. Listen to them, hear their stories and then see that they have a future. If they don't have that future, then we don't have an America."—**Allan, San Francisco**

(Adapted from a *Report to the President,* March 1996)

CAN LIFE GET WORSE THAN BEING YOUNG, HOMELESS, AND DYING OF AIDS?

Regardless of cause, to have AIDS and nowhere to go, no one to help, to have no one who cares about you means that one has hit the bottom rung of life. **Many young people are there now!** There are 15,000 to 20,000 young homeless people just in New York City. About 40% of them sell themselves in order to survive. Too many are becoming HIV-infected because of the demands of their lifestyle. A few examples should make the point.

Case 1. In the 10th grade he was kicked out of his home—over time he meandered to San Francisco's tenderloin area. He began working as a street prostitute and injecting drugs. **He wanted to become HIV-infected.** He said he actually cried when he tested HIV negative. At age 19 he tested positive. This time he cried because he now recognized the mistakes he made along the way. He had no money, no job skills, and no friends. Once, near death he said he had an epiphany (a sudden perception—the essential nature of a thing). He went to a clinic, received job training, gave up drugs, got a job and said, "I really want to live!"

Case 2. Her history begins in a North Carolina group home. She left and drifted to Georgia where she believes she became infected from a man who gave her $300 to have unprotected sex. She said she was a night child—she went to night clubs and adult bookstores to pick up her tricks. By her 21st birthday she said she was ready to jump off the Golden Gate Bridge—if she could find it. After finding help at a clinic she is now preparing to take her GED (graduate equivalence degree).

Case 3. He was raped by the son of his foster parents. His life was spent in a series of Milwaukee foster homes. He became HIV positive at age 13. He found his way to San Francisco. He said "I felt I would be accepted there, it's a city that understood AIDS and the people that have it." He goes to a clinic that services 3000 other young homeless people. He believes he has been sentenced to death. He has not been able to become comfortable with his HIV status. (Adapted from Russell Sabin, *San Francisco Chronicle*, Oct. 18, 1998.)

---

for 17%, and Hispanic for 17%. **Teenage females, unlike their adult counterparts, are more likely to become infected with HIV through sexual exposure than through injection drug use.** A program that followed a large group of HIV-infected adolescents found that although 85% of females contracted HIV infection through heterosexual intercourse, very few were aware that their male partners had HIV infection at the time of their exposure (Futterman et al., 1992).

Categories of Teenage HIV Infection

From 1996 through 2002, the breakdown for HIV infection among teenagers was estimated as follows: males who have sex with males account for about 29%, patients with hemophilia and other coagulation disorders account for about 31%, heterosexual contact represents about 14%, injection drug use about 17%, and non-hemophilia-related transfusions and organ donations about 9%.

YOUNG PEOPLE AND HIV/AIDS WORLDWIDE AND IN AFRICA

The Most Vulnerable

Worldwide, HIV-infected young people ages 15 to 24 are at the center of the HIV/AIDS pandemic. According to the Bloomberg School of Public Health at Johns Hopkins University report, "Youth and HIV/AIDS: Can We Avoid Catastrophe?" (2001), although 15- to 24-year-olds make up 20% of the world population, they account for over half of the 70 million HIV infections, ending year 2003. Ending 2003, of the 44 million people living with HIV/AIDS, about 19 million or about 43% are people ages 15 to 24 (Figure 11-8). Young women are especially vulnerable and account for about 65% or about 12 million of these HIV infected youth. Of the estimated 19 million HIV-infected young people, 77% live in sub-Saharan Africa as do 90% of the world's orphans. UNAIDS estimates that over half the population of sub-Saharan Africa is under age

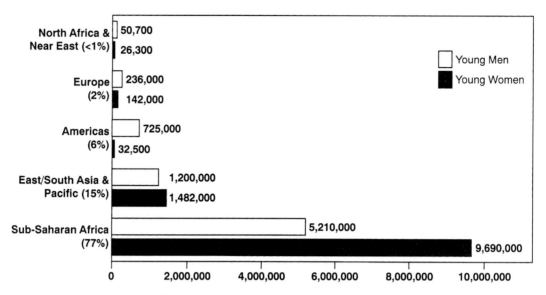

FIGURE 11-8 Estimated Worldwide Young People Ages 15 To 24 Living with HIV/AIDS by Region and Gender Ending Year 2003 Total 19 Million *(Source: UNICEF Updated).*

18. About 15% of the 19 million youth living with HIV infection reside in East/South Asia and the Pacific region of the world. Twenty-two years into this pandemic and millions of young people still know little, if anything, about HIV/AIDS. According to UNICEF, in 2002, over 50% of young people (aged 15–24) in more than a dozen countries, including Bolivia, Botswana, Cote d'Ivoire, the Dominican Republic, Ukraine, Uzbekistan, and Vietnam, have never heard of AIDS or harbor serious misconceptions about how HIV is transmitted. There were 5 million new HIV infections in 2001 and in 2002, 42% or about 2.1 million infections occurred in people ages 15 to 24 at the rate of almost 5800 infections per day (Figure 11-9).

In July 2002, the Henry J. Kaiser Foundation reported that ending 2010 there will be 21.5 million people ages 15 to 24 worldwide living with HIV/AIDS (New report on Global Impact of HIV/AIDS on Youth, amandam@kff.org).

Africa

Between 50% and 85% of all 15-year olds in some African countries with AIDS will eventually die of the disease prior to reaching age 50!

AIDS deaths totaled 3 million in 2002, with about 26 million dead since the epidemic was recognized 22 years ago. But the disease's largest impact will be on African youth. Currently, about 11 million young adults ages 13 to 24 are infected. AIDS' spread among African youth, propelled largely by heterosexual sex, is most pronounced among **teenage girls who have a rate of infection five times that of young boys.** Although men's infection rates increase as they age, young women are particularly vulnerable to HIV because they are likely to have sex with older men and much more likely to be infected during vaginal intercourse with an infected partner. **The result of such a large number of HIV infected young people will be a population imbalance unheard of even after massive wars.** The world has never before experienced death rates of this magnitude among young adults of both sexes across all social strata. UNAIDS Director Peter Piot said, "We are only at the beginning of the actual impact on societies of AIDS. The demographic effects will only be getting worse in the coming years, even if by some miracle HIV infection suddenly stopped."

David Rogers, vice chairman of the National Commission on AIDS (which dissolved in 1993), said, "We have let issues of taste and morality interfere with the delivery of potentially life-saving information to young people."

Class Discussion: Do you think he is correct? What is the down side of his statement?

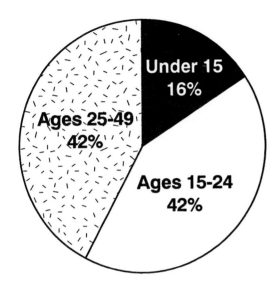

N = 5 million

FIGURE 11-9 Worldwide New HIV Infections by Age Group. UNAIDS estimates that there were 5 million new HIV infections each year since 1999 for a total of 25 million new infections ending year 2003. The percentages for each age group in the figure are averaged percents for years 2001, 2002, and 2003. *(Source: UNAIDS Updated)*

Runaway Teenagers

Each year since 1993, an estimated 3 million adolescents dropped out of high school. Youth dropouts have higher frequencies of behaviors that put them at risk for HIV/STDs, and are less accessible to prevention efforts. Many teenagers run away from home.

The Homeless

An estimated 1 to 2 million runaway teenagers are homeless each year. These youth may engage in behaviors such as injection drug use, having multiple sexual partners, exchange of sex for money or drugs, and unprotected sexual intercourse that place them at risk for HIV infection. HIV seroprevalence studies among homeless youth have shown rates that are higher than adolescents in other settings (Rotheram-Borus et al., 1991).

In nine of 16 STD testing sites, HIV seroprevalence rates among homeless youth were higher than the median rates of youth attending STD clinics within the same city. These studies can only hint at how far HIV has infiltrated specific groups of teenagers.

If you are a teenager or know of one who needs help or has HIV/AIDS questions, call: **NATIONAL TEENAGERS AIDS HOTLINE** 1-800-234-8336.

Adolescent AIDS Program: Montefiore Medical Center, 111 E. 210th St., Bronx, NY 10467; (718) 882-0023

AIDS Community Alliance: Works with HIV positive and HIV-affected individuals. 44 North Queens St., Lancaster, PA 17603; (717) 394-3380

Bay Area Young Positive: Youth-run, offers counseling, resources, newsletter. 518 Waller St., San Francisco, CA 94117; (414) 487-1616; e-mail: **BAYPOZ@aol.com.**

SUMMARY

AIDS surveillance and HIV seroprevalence studies indicate that a significant proportion of HIV infection among women in the United States is acquired through heterosexual contact. Because more men than women are HIV carriers, a woman is more likely than a man to have an infected heterosexual partner. The predominance of heterosexually acquired HIV infection in women of reproductive age has important implications for vertical HIV transmission to their offspring: Nearly 30% of children with AIDS were infected by mothers who acquired infection through heterosexual contact. One of the greatest tragedies of the AIDS pandemic is orphaned children. They are left in hospitals because (1) their parents have died of AIDS or cannot care for them, or (2) no one wants them. AIDS at present is relatively rare among 13- to 19-year olds, but 20% of AIDS cases, due to a 9- to 15-year period before AIDS diagnosis, had to begin with HIV-infected teenagers.

INTERNET

1. **The Coalition for Positive Sexuality (CPS) Website (http://www.positive.org/cps)**, which provides information and advice on sexuality, is produced by and targets adolescents. The Coalition is a grassroots volunteer group based in Chicago. Their self-described mission is: "to give teens the information they need to take care of themselves and in doing so, affirm their decisions about sex, sexuality, and reproductive control; second, to facilitate dialogue, in and out of the public schools, on condom availability and sex education." Included among the topics is information about safe sex, birth control, STDs, pregnancy, and being gay. Homosexual relations are discussed in the same manner as heterosexual relationships.

2. Although CPS is aimed at youth in general, **Oasis (http://www.oasismag.com)** targets and is written primarily by gay youth. Most of the columns written by contributors, who range in age from 14 to 22, read a lot like personal high school journals, an approach that undoubtedly makes readers feel comfortable—like hearing from a friend. A monthly advice column on sexual health is written by a physician and an epidemiologist, who are based in the San Francisco area.

OTHER USEFUL SOURCES

National Network Run Away Youth Service: 202-783-7949

Am Institute for Teen AIDS Prevention: 817-237-0230

Teen AIDS Student Coalition on AIDS, Washington, DC: 202-986-4310

Positive Pediatrics/AIDS: 518-798-8940

Teen AIDS **CDC**: 1-800-342-2437

REVIEW QUESTIONS

(Answers to the Review Questions are on page 489.)

1. Ending year 2003, how many women are expected to be HIV positive worldwide?

2. Globally, what percent of **new** HIV infections occur in women?

3. What are the major routes of HIV transmission into women?

4. What is the most likely way a female prostitute in the United States becomes HIV-infected?

5. During the year 2002, how many women worldwide will have become HIV positive and how many will have died from AIDS?

6. AIDS is now the _____ cause of death for all women between ages _____ and _____. It is the _____ leading cause of death in _____ women between the ages of _____ and _____ and the _____ cause of death for black women ages _____ to _____.

7. Beginning year 2003, how many HIV-infected women are of childbearing age in the United States?

8. Beginning year 2003, how many states have not reported a pediatric AIDS case?

9. Since 1995, what percentage per year of HIV-infected newborns received HIV from their mothers?

10. List three major factors that are associated with perinatal HIV transmission.

11. Where do most of the orphaned AIDS children come from? Why are they called AIDS orphans?

12. What percentage of teenagers have had sexual intercourse by the age of 16?

13. Currently, _____ teens per hour are being HIV-infected in the United States? Worldwide _____ per hour?

14. How many teenagers are there between the ages of 13 and 19 in the United States?

15. What two groups of teenagers in the United States (adolescents) account for the most HIV infections _____, _____? What is the percentage _____?

16. What percentage of all new HIV infections in the United States occur between ages 13 and 20?

17. About how many people in the United States under the age of 29 are estimated to be HIV positive?

18. Is race an important factor with regard to who becomes HIV-infected _____? What race or races have the largest number of HIV-infected young adults _____?

19. Of the 44 million people living with HIV disease ending 2003, how many are young adults _____?

20. What is the National Teenagers' AIDS Hotline telephone number?

Testing for Human Immunodeficiency Virus

CHAPTER CONCEPTS

- ELISA means enzyme linked immunosorbent assay; it is a screening test for HIV infection.
- Western blot is a confirmatory HIV test.
- The ELISA test has been used to screen all blood supplies in the United States since March 1985.
- HIV screening tests can produce both false positives and false negatives.
- A positive ELISA test only predicts that a confirmatory test will also be positive.
- False-positive readings result from a test's lack of specificity.
- There is a relationship between the incidence of HIV in the population being tested and the number of false positives reported. The higher the incidence, the fewer the false positives.
- Levels of test sensitivity and specificity must be determined.
- Several new screening and confirmatory HIV tests are now available.
- June 27 is national HIV Testing Day.
- Screening of nation's blood supply is improved.
- Saliva and urine HIV tests are FDA approved.
- The polymerase chain reaction test is the most sensitive HIV RNA test currently available.
- Other HIV RNA tests available are Amplicor and the branched-DNA test.
- Rapid HIV test kits used in other countries now to be used in the United States.
- AIDS cases have been reported in all 50 states.
- Forty-four states have some form of HIV reporting system.
- Competency and informed consent are necessary for most HIV testing.
- Mandatory HIV testing does not mean people can be forced to undergo testing.
- HIV testing, for the most part, is on a voluntary basis.
- Compulsory HIV testing is used in the military, prisons, and in certain federal agencies.
- Forty-one states offer anonymous HIV testing.
- FDA approves two home HIV Test Kits.
- U.S. Public Health Service guidelines for annual prenatal HIV counseling and voluntary HIV testing of all pregnant American women.
- New York is the first state to legislate mandatory HIV testing and disclosure of newborn HIV status to mother and physicians.
- American Medical Association endorses mandatory HIV testing of all pregnant women and newborns.

Let's begin this chapter by asking, **WHY DOES TESTING MATTER? ANSWER:** The most basic epidemiology holds that early knowledge of where a virus is moving—into which populations—is essential to slowing its spread. Even if a disease cannot be cured, knowing who the infected people are may help prevent the transmission of the disease to other people.

Beginning year 2003, of the estimated **42 million** living HIV-infected people worldwide, at least **half** became infected **before age 25.** About 10% know they are HIV positive. HIV testing is not readily available in many places in developing nations. Where HIV testing is available, testing is seen as an important part of prevention and care. This chapter presents HIV testing information and some of the important problems connected with **whom, how,** and **where** to test.

HIV antibody testing has been with us since 1985. Testing technology has evolved considerably over the years, with a variety of new and improved tests coming into use, both in research and daily practice. Because determining one's HIV status is the first step in treatment decisions, it is important to understand the tests being used today, including their limitations.

DETERMINING THE PRESENCE OF ANTIBODY PRODUCED WHEN HIV IS PRESENT

HIV-antibody testing is a readily available, inexpensive, reliable, and accurate method to identify whether a person is infected with HIV. **HIV antibodies are found in the blood and in other body fluids.** When properly performed, HIV-antibody testing is highly sensitive and specific.

Currently there are at least nine tests that detect HIV antibodies, antigens, or the nucleic acid of HIV in a person's body fluids. They are the: enzyme linked immunosorbent assay (ELISA), Western Blot, Polymerase Chain Reaction (PCR), saliva and urine tests, Aplicor, branched DNA test, immunofluorescent antibody assay, rapid HIV test kits, and at-home HIV test kits. They are discussed in the following pages.

REQUESTS FOR HIV TESTING

Public HIV/AIDS clinics in the United States are becoming overwhelmed with requests for HIV testing. Most of the requests are repeats. Beginning year 2003 the CDC estimated that about 60% of the 950,000 living HIV-infected persons in the United States have been tested. The majority of those people **at risk** who have **not** been tested includes most **hardcore IDUs and sexual partners of IDUs** and people who are image sensitive. Currently, about 50 million blood and plasma samples are HIV tested annually worldwide. In the United States about 25 million blood and plasma samples are HIV tested annually.

In the developing world, where the greatest number of HIV-infected people are concentrated, the picture is very different. About 90% of the infected people do not know they are infected! HIV

SIDEBAR 12.1

ANNUAL NATIONAL HIV TESTING DAY

National HIV testing day began June 27, 1995. It was initiated by the **National Association of People Living with Aids** in conjunction with the **CDC.** June 27, 2003, is the ninth anniversary. The purpose of the annual **HIV Testing Day Campaign** is to encourage those at risk for HIV to take personal control and responsibility for their own health. It is estimated that about 300,000 Americans are unaware they are HIV-infected. In 2002 over 11,000 national, state, and local organizations participated in the campaign.

---

testing is done mostly for purposes of surveillance, which involves very small population samples and is done anonymously. **Few people have any hope of treatment, so they feel little incentive to get tested.** But even those who would want to know may not be able to find out. In many countries, there are no voluntary testing and counseling facilities; people have no acceptable way of learning if they are HIV-infected. An ongoing study at a rural hospital in South Africa suggests that only 2% of people who are HIV positive know their status. The situation in urban Kenya is equally poor. Of 63 randomly chosen women who tested HIV positive in one study, only one was aware that she was infected.

REASONS FOR HIV TESTING

HIV testing is done to monitor the pandemic; to determine how many people are infected, how many are being infected in a given time period (incidence), and their location. Testing is used to determine the impact of prevention efforts to slow the spread of HIV, to prompt behavior change and to provide entry into clinical care. Also, if necessary, to provide a starting point for partner notification and education, and to protect the nation's blood supply.

Take the Test: Take Control

There is an immediate need to change perception about being HIV positive so that people feel good about taking the test to protect themselves and others, rather than the discrimination that now exists against those who have taken the test.

HIV TESTING OF WOMEN IN AFRICA

About 90% of Africans living with HIV do not know they have acquired the virus. One study has found that 50% of adult Tanzanian women know where they could be tested for HIV, yet only 6% have been tested. In Zimbabwe, only 11% of adult women have been tested for the virus. Moreover, many people who agree to be tested prefer not to return and discover the outcome of those tests. But, in Abidjan, Cote d'Ivoire, 80% of pregnant women who agree to undergo a HIV test do return to collect their results. However, of those who discover they are living with the virus, fewer than 50% return to receive drug treatment for the prevention of mother-to-child transmission of the virus. In addition, more than half of the women who know they have acquired HIV and who were surveyed by Kenya's Population Council in 2001 said they had not disclosed their HIV status to their partners because they feared it would expose them to violence or abandonment. According to UNICEF, African women are dangerously ignorant about HIV/AIDS. More than 70% of adolescent girls (aged 15–19) in Somalia and more than 40% in Guinea Bissau and Sierra Leone, for instance, have never heard of AIDS. In countries such as Kenya and the united Republic of Tanzania, more than 40% of adolescent girls harbor serious misconceptions about how the virus is transmitted. One of the targets fixed at the UN General Assembly Special Session on HIV/AIDS in June 2001 was to ensure that at least 90% of young men and women should, by 2005, have the information, education, and services they need to defend themselves against HIV infection. As in other regions of the world, most countries in sub-Saharan Africa are a considerable way from fulfilling that pledge. There are too few counseling and testing centers available. Testing at this time **is not** in their future.

AVOIDING HIV TESTING

In August 2001 the CDC released the results of a 10-year survey of 19,000 AIDS patients in 12 states who were asked, "When did you first learn you were HIV-infected?" Forty percent who learned of their HIV infection had AIDS at the time or developed AIDS within 12 months of their HIV positive test. In a second 2001 report on 434 high-risk HIV-positive people, researchers at Kaiser Permanente found that 40% of these people demonstrated signs and symptoms of HIV infection for over a year before being tested.

The Need for Routine HIV Testing

After 22 years of educating people about HIV/AIDS, the majority of adults/adolescents in the United States have never been tested for HIV. Unless people are tested in greater numbers, it may be impossible to break the cycle of HIV transmission in America. The failure of educational programs to stem the rates of 40,000 to 50,000 new HIV infections annually may need to be replaced by new policies on HIV testing. Joseph Inungu, a Central Michigan health science professor is recommending an HIV test as part of the routine tests performed on office patients. Inungu analyzed data on people ages 18 to 80 who participated in a national Health Interview Survey conducted by the National Center for Health Statistics. He found the groups least likely to be tested for HIV were men, people over the age of 50 or between age 18 and 19, people with a low level of education, people in rural areas, and people in the Northeast or Midwest. While adolescent groups are among the fastest growing population of HIV/AIDS sufferers, few are tested for HIV unless they come to a physician for a sexually transmitted disease. Older populations—over the age of 50—have tended to feel they were not at risk but have actually seen increases in the numbers of cases of HIV. The groups that were most likely to get tested included non-Hispanic blacks, people with higher educational levels, and people who were separated, divorced, or widowed.

IMMUNODIAGNOSTIC TECHNIQUES FOR DETECTING ANTIBODIES TO HIV

Refinements in the field of immunological testing, serology, and the study of antigen–antibody reactions have produced test names that reflect the component parts of the test being used. In most cases, tests are based on the detection of antibodies present in the serum, in this case antibodies to HIV. One immunological test uses antibodies, which if present in the person's serum, form a complex with a given antigen. An enzyme is then connected to the antibody. The presence of the antibody can be determined by adding a reagent that will form a colored solution if antibody to HIV is present. This is called the **enzyme linked immunosorbent assay** (ELISA, el-i-sa). The ELISA test was first used in 1983 to detect antibodies against HIV.

Because the ELISA test detects the presence of antibodies made against HIV, it is called an **indirect test.** This test suggests that HIV is or was present. The Western Blot test, presented next, is also an indirect test for the same reason. Indirect tests stand in contrast to those tests that directly test for the presence of HIV's nucleic acid—a **direct test.** These tests say that HIV is currently present in the system. They are presented after the indirect tests presented next.

ELISA HIV ANTIBODY TEST

A Fable for the HIV/AIDS Era

It was a medieval mystery. Somehow, needles were finding their way into some of the kingdom's haystacks. Cows were eating the needles: not a good thing. The king sent out a proclamation offering a sack of gold to the first person able to find a needle in a haystack. After 20 days, the contestants were still trying to locate the needles hidden among 10 haystacks placed in the palace courtyard. The king was despondent. From his tower he could see thousands of haystacks in fields across the kingdom. "This is terrible," he said. "Either our cows go hungry while we look for the needles, or we let them eat the hay along with some needles. Either way it's not good for the cows. We need a way to tell which haystacks have the needles; then we can feed our cows the good hay while we figure out how to get the needles out of the bad haystacks." He was a logical king. In 1981 the needle had no name but its presence was known. The search for this needle—like those in the haystacks—was intense and even after the needle was found to be HIV, investigators had to find a way to distinguish between those who carried and did not carry HIV—which haystacks carried the needles. Because HIV was in human blood it was essential to protect the nations' blood supply, thereby preventing people from receiving contaminated blood and blood products. But, like the good king, it took time to find the means to find the needle in the blood supply—HIV.

It was not until 1985—nearly four years after the first cases of AIDS were announced—that an antibody test was developed that could indicate whether a person was infected with HIV. Even after this discovery, the fact that there were no effective treatments for those who tested HIV positive, coupled with the widespread perception of stigma associated with HIV infection left many questioning the value of HIV testing. That equation shifted markedly with the availability of potent combination therapy, which significantly delays the progression of HIV disease in many people. There is now widespread consensus among public health officials and community leaders regarding the importance of HIV testing and counseling in order to link individuals who test positive with medical care and to counsel them on how to reduce the risk of further transmission.

The initial application of the ELISA test outside the research laboratory was used primarily in large-scale screening of the nation's blood supply. ELISA **testing of the existing blood supply and all newly donated blood began in the United States in March 1985.** Very quickly, however, testing also became seen as an important aspect of HIV prevention. In recent years, the discovery of treatments for HIV and associated opportunistic infections has further increased the benefits of early detection. Today, HIV testing is seen as an integral part of both the nation's prevention and treatment efforts.

The ELISA test is used as a screening test because of its low cost, standardized procedures, high reproducibility, and rapid results.

The ELISA test is now semi-automated. It uses an antigen derived from HIV cultivated in human cell lines. One such line is the human leukemia cell line **H9.** Whole viruses isolated from H9 **are disrupted** into subunit antigens for use. The subunits of HIV are then bound to a solid support system.

Two different solid support systems are used in the seven ELISA screening test kits licensed in the United States. Some attach the antigens onto small glass beads (Figure 12-1), while others fix the antigens onto the sides and bottoms of small wells (microwells) in a glass or plastic microtiter plate. The serum to be tested is separated from the blood and is diluted and applied to the HIV-coated solid support systems (Figure 12-2). The

---

BOX 12.1

AN ASSUMPTION OF AIDS WITHOUT THE HIV TEST: IT SHATTERS LIVES

Case 1

San Francisco—For six years, a 53-year-old gay male lived in the world of AIDS. He stopped working, suffered the painful side effects of experimental drugs, and waited to die.

Now his doctors say he never had the disease.

His health shattered by AIDS treatment, his livelihood lost, he filed a $2 million claim against Kaiser Permanente health maintenance organization. He claims he underwent sustained treatment for full-fledged AIDS without receiving an HIV test.

His attorney said, "For six years he thought that the most he had was six months to live. So every day he'd wake up and think 'Is this the last day of my life?'"

To begin, this male says he checked into a San Jose hospital affiliated with Kaiser in 1986 with respiratory problems and doctors told him he had pneumocystic pneumonia, considered a sure sign of AIDS at the time.

He underwent tests but **was not** given one to determine the presence of HIV, the virus associated with AIDS.

In 1986, he began taking the drug zidovudine in high doses, which gave him a chronic headache, high blood pressure, and peripheral neuropathy—permanent pins and needles pains from his calves to his feet. He is battling an addiction to Darvon and other prescription drugs.

Under doctors' orders, he quit his job as a skin care technician and lives on government welfare and disability benefits of $600 a month.

(Associated Press, 1992)

Case 2

In 1980, she had received a blood transfusion during surgery at a hospital in this Southeast Georgia town. During a checkup for a thyroid problem, a decade later, at a clinic in Hialeah, Fla., her blood was taken for testing.

On November 13, 1990, her telephone rang. She was asked to come down to the local health clinic where she was told she had AIDS. They were not sure how long she had to live. She was

45 years old. Her three sons were then teenagers; their father had died.

She kept the television on continually in a usually unsuccessful effort to block out the thought of AIDS.

The nights were the worst.

"I'd go to bed every night thinking about dying. What color do you want the casket to be? What dress do you want to be buried in? How are your kids going to take it? How will people treat them? I was afraid to go to sleep."

In 1992, her doctor put her on didanosine, (ddl), which brought on side effects that included vomiting and fatigue.

"I had put my kids through hell. They were scared for me."

When she joined a local hospice group for AIDS patients, counselors heard her story and noted that her T cell counts had remained consistently high. At their suggestion, she was retested.

In November 1992, nearly two years to the day she was told she was HIV positive, another call came. She was greeted at the clinic with these words: **"Guess what? Your HIV test came out negative!"**

She sued the Florida Department of Health and Rehabilitative Services—the agency that performed the test—and the clinic and doctor who treated her.

A jury awarded her $600,000 for pain and suffering but cleared the clinic and said the bulk must be paid by the agency.

Case 3

Every day, four times each day, for six years Mark swallowed his antiretroviral drugs. Mark was told by a "fine physician" that he was HIV positive in July of 1990. Regardless of the drugs, Mark felt sick and suffered further physical effects and depression. For reasons not given, Mark moved from Chicago to Ohio. His new physician was puzzled that Mark did not demonstrate signs or symptoms of HIV infection. His tests on Mark came back **HIV negative.** On investigation, the Chicago clinic could not produce any documents showing that Mark was ever HIV tested!

ELISA test takes from 2.5 to 4 hours to perform (Carlson et al., 1989) and costs between about $8 in state-sponsored virology laboratories and about $60 to $75 in private laboratories.

In accordance with FDA recommendations, effective June 1992, blood collection centers in the United States began HIV-2 testing on all donated blood and blood components. The CDC does not

THE MIAMI HERALD AND CHICAGO TRIBUNE, 1985

Miami Herald

In September 1985, the **Metro Commissions** of Dade County Florida voted to require **all** food service workers in Dade County be HIV tested. The commissioners' motivation is not in question. Aware of how the AIDS panic has hurt restaurant patronage in several other cities, they properly wanted to calm fears and protect food service jobs. Inadvertently, though, the Metro commissioners may have sent the wrong signal. Medical experts say that AIDS is not spread by the kinds of contact that food handlers have with a restaurant's patrons or with their food. By ignoring this advice, commissioners implicitly seem to be questioning it. This may heighten the public's fears, not calm them. That is especially evident when one notes the test's inability to do what is expected of it. Richard Morgan, Dade's health director, says that testing all 80,000 of Dade's food service workers would take a year. So even if AIDS were spread through food—which it is not—the test would be of dubious value. A food service worker might test clean one day, become infected the next, continue working, and escape detection for months. Moreover, the high worker turnover in this seasonal business means that large numbers of these costly tests would continue to be given indefinitely. Thus the costs would not necessarily diminish much, after all current workers had been tested. The AIDS-test requirement is part of a broader health-care ordinance that commissioners tentatively approved.

Chicago Tribune

In early 1985 Chicago's Health Commissioner protested federal guidelines requiring that blood donors be informed if their blood was HIV positive. In response the following article appeared on April 10, 1985: "Chicago Health Commissioner Lonnie Edwards is wrong to protest federal guidelines requiring that blood donors be informed if tests show that their blood contains antibodies to the virus linked to AIDS (acquired immune deficiency syndrome). The new test for AIDS antibodies is being phased into use in the nation's blood banks, after its approval early in March by the Department of Health and Human Services. Blood found to have AIDS antibodies will be discarded. By late April, all blood banks in the Chicago area will be doing such screening. But the antibody test is still controversial. It cannot show whether a blood donor currently has AIDS. A positive result only indicates that a person has been exposed at some time and in some way to the virus believed to cause the usually fatal disease—not that he is immune to it or that he will eventually become ill and die of it. Another problem is that the test is not totally accurate; both false negatives and false positives can occur. Some homosexual groups oppose the use of the AIDS screening test on the grounds it could violate individual privacy or that a third party might obtain test results and use them to discriminate against donors. But the presence of HIV in the nation's blood supply is becoming a serious problem. Dozens of recipients of blood or blood-based products have already died of AIDS presumably acquired from blood donors. In a few instances, these victims have passed the disease on to their spouses and young children.

---

recommend routine testing for HIV-2 other than at blood collection centers (*MMWR*, 1992).

Understanding the ELISA Test

The ELISA test determines if a person's serum contains antibodies to one or more HIV antigens. Although there are some minor differences among the FDA-licensed kits, test procedures are similar.

Problems with the ELISA Test

Any HIV screening test must be able to distinguish those individuals who are infected from those who are not. **The underlying assumption of an ELISA test is that all HIV-infected people will produce detectable HIV antibodies.** There are, however, problems with this assumption. **First,** although rare, there are documented cases of individuals who remain antibody negative but are able to spread HIV. These individuals do not produce antibodies to HIV! **Second,** the HIV-infected population in general does not produce detectable antibodies for six weeks to one or more years after HIV infection. This is called the **window period. Most often, HIV antibody is detectable within 6 to 18 weeks.** Thus, HIV-infected people can test HIV-negative. **This is**

Solid Supports

A. Bound HIV Antigens

Microbeads

B. A Microtiter Well from a Microwell Plate

Bound HIV antigens

Blood/Serum dispensed into each receptacle

1 Bead is placed in each tube

Microwell Plate

Solid-phase antibody complex

Antibody

1 hour incubation (HIV antibodies if present complex with HIV antigen)

Removal of excess serum or blood

Wash

Add anti-human Immunoglobin G linked to horseradish peroxidase-conjugate solution

2 hour incubation (conjugate attaches to antigen-antibody on solid phase)

Withdraw excess solution

Wash

Add substrate (o-phenylenediamine or azinobenzthiazolium)

Color develops

Substrate reacts with peroxidase to produce a yellow-orange color in those tubes or microwells containing HIV antibodies. The intensity of the color is proportional to the amount of antibody present in the serum.

FIGURE 12-1 The ELISA Test. **A.** Microbeads with attached antigen in test tubes. **B.** Antigens bound to walls and bottom of microtiter wells. **C.** Microbeads are 7 mm in diameter. The test takes between 2.5 and 4 hours to perform.

C.

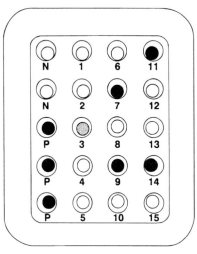

D.

E.

FIGURE 12-1 *(Continued)* **D.** Microwell plates showing positive (yellow) and negative (clear) test results. The microtiter dispenser handles eight microwells at a time. (**C.** and **D.**: *Photographs courtesy of the author*) **E.** Specimens positive for HIV antibody have a deeper color in this microwell tray. Serum specimens from 15 patients were tested for antibodies to HIV. Two negative and three positive control specimens are provided in the first column. In wells 7, 9, 11, and 14, the dark yellow color change, matching the color in the three positive control wells, indicates that the specimens are positive. Well 3 shows a weakly reactive result. The remaining specimens showed no color change and were interpreted as negative for HIV antibodies. *(Adapted from Fang et al., 1989)*

a false negative result. In some HIV-infected persons, the virus ties up the available antibody as their disease progresses. Testing at this time may also produce false negative results.

An Unusual Case— At the VA Medical Center in Salt Lake City in 1997, a man tested **HIV negative 35 times over a four-year period.** Because his wife was HIV positive and because he demonstrated symptoms of HIV disease, p24 and PCR assays were performed—he was HIV positive. [p24 antigen (see Point of Information 12.2) and the PCR test are explained later in this chapter.] This case is unusual because (**1**) he is falsely negative almost four years beyond the window period; (**2**) the strain of HIV is typical of that found in the United States; and (**3**) the strain of HIV is closely related to the strain infecting his wife (Reimer et al., 1997). This may be one of the rare non-HIV antibody-producing people reported.

False positive reactions may also occur. This means that the person's serum does not contain antibodies to HIV but the test results indicate that it does. Christine Johnson (2000) has compiled a list of 66 conditions taken from HIV/AIDS scientific literature that can cause false positive results.

People may test **false positive** who have an underlying liver disease, have received a blood transfusion or gamma globulin within six weeks of the test, have had several children, have had rheumatological diseases, malaria, alcoholic hepatitis, autoimmune disorders, various cancers, acute cytomegalovirus infection, or DNA viral infections; are injection drug users; or have received vaccines for influenza or hepatitis B (Fang et al., 1989; MacKenzie et al., 1992). In each case, the person may have antibodies that will cross-react with the HIV antigens giving a false positive reaction. Other reasons for false positives are laboratory errors and mistakes made in reagent preparations for use in the test kits.

Why is the ELISA Test Sensitivity and Specificity Set High?

Because the original purpose of the ELISA test was to screen blood, the sensitivity (ability to detect

A.

C.

B.

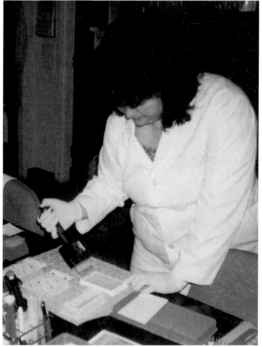

D.

FIGURE 12-2 Semi-Automated ELISA Test. **A.** Serum samples are individually machine diluted with a special solution 1 to 400 to achieve a balance between the amount of antibody to the amount of antigen. Antibodies, if present in the individual sera, attach to the HIV antigens in each well. **B.** Excess serum is withdrawn from each sample and the beads are washed. The antihuman immunoglobulin-horseradish enzyme conjugate is added to each prepared sample. **C.** The samples are incubated. **D.** Each sample receives the chromogen or substrate (o-phenylenediamine or azinobenzthiazolium). A yellow-orange color appears in samples that contain antibodies to HIV. *(Courtesy of Florida Department of Health, Retrovirology Unit, Jacksonville)* low-level color formation; see Figure 12-1) of the test was purposely set high. It was reasoned that it was better to have some false positives and throw away good blood rather than to take in any HIV-contaminated blood. Thus the ELISA test is a **positive predictive value** test. It only predicts that the serum tested will continue to test positive when a test with greater specificity, called a **confirmatory test,** is done.

In 1985, during the first month of donor screening, 1% of all blood tested HIV-antibody positive. On ELISA retesting of these samples, only 0.17% (17/10,000) were HIV-antibody positive. On subjecting these samples to a confirmatory test, only 0.038% (4/10,000) were actually HIV positive. These early tests produced about 24 false positives for every true positive result. The main reason for such a high false positive rate or **lack of specificity** was that something other than HIV produced an antibody or other substance that reacted with HIV antigen causing the HIV test to appear positive.

Although high sensitivity tests eliminate HIV-contaminated blood from the blood supply, there is a downside to high sensitivity testing when proper procedure is **not** used. People told that they have tested positive have become emotionally distraught. Former Senator Lawton Chiles of Florida, at an AIDS conference in 1987, told of a tragic example from the early days of blood screening in Florida. Of 22 blood donors who were told they were HIV positive by the ELISA test, seven committed suicide.

There continue to be false positive reactions among blood donors and low-level risk populations because of a **low prevalence** of HIV infection in such populations. The American Red Cross Blood Services laboratories report that using current ELISA methodology, a specificity of 99.8% can be achieved (*MMWR,* 1988a).

Positive Predictive Value— The positive predictive value of the ELISA test indicates the percentage of true positives among total positives in a given population. To determine a positive predictive value:

Number of true positives ÷ Number of true positives + false positives) × 100%

There is also a negative predictive test. A negative predictive value refers to the percentage of individuals who test truly negative; they **do not** have HIV. It is determined by:

Number of true negatives ÷ (Number of true negatives + false negatives) × 100%

To safeguard against false-positive tests, the CDC recommends that serum that tests positive be retested twice (in duplicate). If both tests are negative, the serum is considered HIV-antibody negative and further tests will only be done should signs or symptoms of HIV infection occur (Figure 12-3). If one or both of the tests is positive, the serum is subjected to a confirmatory test, usually a Western blot (WB) (Figure 12-4). At blood banks, if the initial ELISA test is positive, the blood is discarded. If an individual's serum subjected to a confirmatory test is positive, the person is considered to be HIV-infected.

Although confirmatory tests can be used to determine true-positive results, they are too labor intensive and expensive to be used in screening a large population. Thus the positive predictive value of an ELISA test is an important first step in large-scale screening. Recall, however, that **the predictive value depends on the prevalence of HIV infection in the population tested.** The higher the prevalence of HIV infection in a given population, the more likely a positive ELISA test is to be a true positive; and conversely, the lower the prevalence of infection, the less likely a positive ELISA test is to be a true positive.

Levels of Sensitivity and Specificity in Testing for HIV— A test's **sensitivity** is its capacity to identify **all** specimens that **have** HIV antibodies in them. A test's **specificity** is its capacity to identify **all** specimens that **do not have** HIV antibodies in them.

Sensitivity is determined as follows:

Number of true positives ÷ (Number of true positives + the false negatives) × 100%

If 100 persons are actually HIV-infected and the test identifies only 90 of them as such, then we can say that the test has 90% sensitivity.

Specificity is determined as follows:

Number of true negatives ÷ (Number of true negatives + false positives) × 100%

Assume that, in a group of 500 people being tested for HIV antibodies, 100 individuals are actually not infected. If test results show that only 90 out of the 100 are identified as not having the virus, then the test has 90% specificity.

FIGURE 12-3 Incoming Specimens. About 900 to 1000 blood specimens are received each day and are prepared for testing. From those samples, those testing negative are reported out in 8 to 10 hours. Positive samples are reported out in 3 to 4 days.*(Courtesy of Florida Department of Health, Retrovirology Unit, Jacksonville)*

FIGURE 12-4 Western Blot Strips. Each WB strip contains nine separate antigenic proteins of HIV. Human serum or blood is applied directly to the strips. See text for details on reactions. Because false positives can sometimes occur with the ELISA test, additional testing is needed to evaluate specimens that are repeatedly reactive by ELISA. The Western blot is more specific but less sensitive than the ELISA and is recommended for blood banks and organ donor centers. Its clinical usefulness in trials to aid in evaluating specimens that are questionably positive by other methods has been proven. It is not a screening test because it lacks a high level of sensitivity. *(Courtesy of Roche Biomedical Laboratories, AIDS Testing Brochure)*

WESTERN BLOT ASSAY

The gold standard for determining a true positive HIV-antibody test is still the **Western blot** (WB). This test is a method in which individual HIV proteins are used to react with HIV antibody in a person's serum. It should be understood that the WB test is not a **true gold standard** because it is not 100% certain, but it can come close to 100% if properly used.

Human leukemia cells, in which HIV is being cultured, are lysed or broken open, and the mixture of cell components and HIV components (proteins) are separated from each other. The

— BOX 12.2 —

PRETEST PATIENT INFORMATION

It is important that you read and understand the following information before having the HIV-antibody test.

This test is not a test for AIDS, but a positive result does mean that there is a high probability an HIV-infected person will eventually develop AIDS.

Only anonymous test results remain absolutely confidential.

What Does the Test Reveal?

The test reveals whether a person has been exposed to HIV. The test detects the presence of HIV antibodies, an indication that infection has occurred. It does not detect the virus itself nor does it indicate the level of viral infection, **only that one has been infected.**

It is important to find out whether you are HIV positive or negative so that you can prevent spreading the virus to others and seek early medical intervention.

What Tests Will Be Done?

Wherever the test is done, the procedures are similar. A blood sample is taken from the arm and analyzed in a laboratory using the *ELISA* test. If the first ELISA test is positive, the laboratory will run a second ELISA test on the same blood sample. If positive, another test, called Western blot, is run on the same blood sample to confirm the ELISA result.

What Do the Test Results Mean?

See Table 12-1.

Table 12-1 The Meaning of Antibody Test Results

A Positive Results	B Negative Results
If you test positive, it does mean: 1. Your blood sample has been tested more than once and the tests indicate that it contained antibodies to HIV. 2. You have been infected with HIV and your body has produced antibodies. **If you test positive, it does not mean:** 1. That you have AIDS. 2. That you necessarily will get AIDS, but the probability is high. You can reduce your chance of progressing to AIDS by avoiding further contact with the virus and living a healthy lifestyle. 3. That you are immune to the virus. **Therefore, if you test positive, you should do the following:** 1. Protect yourself from any further infection. 2. Protect others from the virus by following AIDS precautions in sex, drug use, and general hygiene. 3. Consider seeing a physician for a complete evaluation and advice on health maintenance. 4. Avoid drugs and heavy alcohol use, maintain good nutrition, and avoid fatigue and stress. Such action may improve your chances of staying healthy.	**If you test negative, it does mean:** 1. No antibodies to HIV have been found in your serum at the time of the test. **Two possible explanations for a negative test result exist:** 1. You have not been infected with HIV. 2. You have been infected with HIV but have not yet produced antibodies. Research indicates that most people will produce antibodies within 6 to 18 weeks after infection. Some people will not produce antibodies for at least 3 years. A very small number of people may never produce antibodies. **If you test negative, it does not mean:** 1. That you have nothing to worry about. You may become infected; be careful. 2. That you are immune to HIV. 3. That you have not been infected with the virus. You may have been infected and not yet produced antibodies.

(Adapted from the San Francisco AIDS Foundation)

BOX 12.2 *(continued)*

Positive Result—A positive result suggests that a person has HIV antibodies and may have been infected with the virus at some time. People with a positive result should assume that they have the virus and could therefore transmit it:

♦ by sex (anal, vaginal, or oral) where body fluids, especially semen or blood, get inside the partner's body;

♦ by sharing injection drug "works" (needles, syringes, etc.);

♦ by donating blood, sperm, or body organs; or

♦ to an unborn baby during pregnancy or to a newborn by breast-feeding.

Negative Result—If it has been four to six months since the last possible exposure to HIV, then a negative result suggests that a person is probably not infected with the virus. However, **false negatives** can occur. For example, if the test was too soon after HIV exposure, the body may not have had time to produce HIV antibodies. **Collectively, studies show that 50% of HIV-infected persons seroconvert (demonstrate measurable HIV antibodies) by three months after HIV infection and 90% seroconvert by six months. a small percentage seroconverted at one year or later. Most important, a negative result does not mean that you are protected from getting the virus in the future—your future depends on your behavior.**

Inconclusive Result—A small percentage of results are inconclusive. This means that the result is neither positive nor negative. This may be due to a number of factors that have nothing to

do with HIV infection, or it can occur early in an infection when there are not enough HIV antibodies present to give a positive result. If this happens, another blood sample will be taken at a later time for a retest.

How Accurate or Error-Free is the Test Result?

The result is accurate. However, as with any laboratory test, there can be false positives and false negatives.

False Positive—A small percentage of all people tested may be told they have the HIV antibody when they do not. This can be due to laboratory error or certain medical conditions that have nothing to do with HIV infection.

False Negative—Some people are told that they are not HIV-infected when, in fact, they are. This can happen when the test is taken too soon after being infected—the body has not had time to produce HIV antibodies. This is called the **window period.**

Should the Test Be Performed?

Whether to have the test done is a personal decision. However, knowing your antibody status can help you address some very difficult questions. For example, if the test is negative, what lifestyle changes should be made to minimize risk of HIV infection? If the test is positive, how can others be protected from infection? What can be done to improve your chances of staying healthy?

(Source: Roche Biomedical Laboratories, Inc.)

---

viral proteins are placed on a polyacrylamide gel, which then gets an electrical charge. The electrical current separates the viral proteins within the gel.

POINT OF INFORMATION 12.1

HIV TESTING OF TEENAGERS

Laws regarding the counseling and testing of persons younger than 18 years of age generally give minors the ability to be tested for STDs without parental consent or knowledge, but not all states classify HIV as an STD! Through 2002, at least 16 states had such laws specific to HIV. One in four (25%) of sexually experienced teenagers aged 15 to 17 have been tested for HIV.

SIDE ISSUES 12.2

A FALSE POSITIVE HIV REPORT

In January 2002, a man in Oklahoma City was awarded $1.4 million because he was wrongfully told he was HIV positive. At age 40 he received the news from a Health Maintenance Clinic. During the following four years, he became depressed, despondent, abused alcohol, and attempted suicide twice. Thinking he was HIV positive, he had unprotected sex with known HIV positive partners. Reviewing his file to determine when he became infected he learned that his test four years earlier was HIV negative. He filed suite for negligence and won.

IMPROVED ELISA TESTING, BLOOD DONOR INTERVIEWS, SCREENING FOR P24 ANTI-GEN, AND NUCLEIC ACID TESTING LOWERS HIV IN NATION'S BLOOD SUPPLY

The increased sensitivity of current HIV-antibody ELISA tests, improved donor interviewing about behaviors associated with risk for HIV infection, and deferral of donors who test positive for HIV, hepatitis, human T-cell leukemia virus type 1 (HTLV-1), or syphilis have considerably improved the safety of the U.S. blood supply. In 1993, approximately six per 100,000 blood donations collected by the American Red Cross tested positive for HIV antibody. In addition, an estimated one in 450,000 to one in 660,000 donations per year (18–27 donations) were infectious for HIV but were not detected by current screening tests.

In February 2002, a Texas man became the first person to get HIV from a blood transfusion in the United States since new screening tests began in 1999. The infected blood given to the Texas man came from a heterosexual donor who didn't think he was at risk for HIV. The man donated his blood four times during 2000. At the time of his last donation, tests showed that his blood carried HIV. This prompted intensive testing of samples from his previous donations—including the blood given to the Texas man.

Screening for p24 Antigen—In August 1995, the FDA mandated that all blood and plasma collection centers screen all blood for p24 antigen. The FDA recommended p24 screening as an additional safety measure because recent studies indicated that p24 screening reduces the infectious window period (the FDA approved Coulter p24 antigen blood test detects HIV as early as 16 days after infection). Among the 12 million plus annual blood donations in the United States, p24-antigen screening is expected to detect four to six infectious donations that would not be identified by other screening tests. FDA regards donor screening for p24 antigen as an interim measure pending the availability of technology that would further reduce the risk for HIV transmission from blood donated during the infectious window period (*MMWR*, 1996 updated).

Nucleic Acid Testing—Beginning the spring of 1999, the American Red Cross and 16 member laboratories of the America's Blood Centers began testing donor blood for the human immunodeficiency virus (HIV) type-1 and the hepatitis C virus with a new research testing method known as **nucleic acid amplification testing** (NAT). This testing is conducted under well-defined Investigational New Drug (IND) research protocols approved by the Food and Drug Administration (FDA). Currently there are four molecular techniques available to detect the presence of infectious microorganisms in donor blood by amplifying the nucleic acid sequences specific to the microorganisms. Use of these techniques provides a much higher level of sensitivity and specificity than routine testing methods currently provide. Despite the current screening of donor blood for the detection of antigens to HIV and hepatitis B (HBV) and antibodies to HIV and hepatitis C (HCV), there still remains a residual risk of posttransfusion infection from HIV or hepatitis viruses acquired from donors donating blood in the early window period of infection. The power of NAT is its ability to detect the presence of infection by directly testing for viral nucleic acids rather than by indirectly testing for the presence of antibodies. The efficacy of such screening depends on the prevalence of the infection in the population and the duration of the window period. In most Western countries, HCV shows a higher prevalence and longer window period (80 days) than HBV (56 days) and HIV (16 days).

This explains why NAT detection of HCV is the primary focus of implementation of this approach to blood screening. The use of NAT could theoretically close the window period of HIV from the current 16 days to approximately 10 days as well as the window period of HCV from the current 70 to 80 days to approximately 10 to 30 days. This would reduce the risk of transfusion-transmitted HCV from approximately one in 100,000 units transfused to one in 500,000 to 1,000,000 units transfused.

Pitfalls to the Use of NAT

There are some serious drawbacks to the use of NAT. For example, a cost-effective, automated system does not yet exist to perform the test on individual donor blood samples. The requirement of specially trained lab technicians, space constraints, a minimum 12 hours required to perform NAT and the cost of a NAT test kit, which is currently 10 times higher than the ELISA test kit, will be difficult to overcome. Also, as NAT currently exists there is a 1% chance of obtaining false negative results. Regardless, NAT testing continues at Red Cross Blood collection centers.

Conclusion

In order to pursue its stated policy of seeking innovative means to increase the safety of the blood supply and to allow compliance with the European requirements, the FDA, in September 2001, licenced the first NAT for use in the screening of blood plasma donors for HIV and cytomegalovirus. FDA approval of NAT for broad scale commercial use came in February 2002.

   UPDATE FDA Issues Emergency Guidelines Regarding HIV, Hepatitis C Testing of Donated Blood To speed the transportation of blood products to areas affected by terrorist attacks in New York City on Sept. 11, 2001 the FDA released

new emergency guidelines allowing donated blood to be shipped to crisis areas before HIV and hepatitis C testing is complete. An FDA statement says that due to the "recognized need for rapid and high volume blood collections under non-routine circumstances," some blood may have to be shipped before all testing is complete. The agency normally requires all blood donations be tested for such diseases before the blood is shipped. The emergency guidelines state that if the blood products are shipped before FDA testing has been completed, the product must be labeled "For Emergency Use Only" and must list the tests that have not yet been completed. The blood must indicate if screenings for HIV-1, HIV-2, and hepatitis C are not complete. The tests for the viruses should be completed "as soon as possible" and "appropriate actions taken in the event of a reactive screening test result."

This is called gel electrophoresis. The smallest HIV proteins will move quickly through the gel, separating from the next larger size, and so on.

   Each different protein will arrive at a separate position on the gel. After proteins of similar molecular weight collect at a given site, they form a band; these bands are identified based on the distance they have run in the gel. Because each band is a protein produced as a product of a different HIV gene, the gel band patterns give a picture of the HIV genes that were functioning and the location of each gene's products on the gel (Figure 12-4 and Table 12-2). The protein or antigen bands within the gel are "blotted," that is, transferred directly, band for band and position for position, onto strips of nitrocellulose paper (Figure 12-4).

   Once the antigen bands have been formed, serum believed to carry HIV antibodies is placed directly on them. That is, a test serum is added directly to antigen bands located on the nitrocellulose strip. If antibodies are present in the serum, they will form an antigen–antibody complex directly on the antigen band areas. After the strip is washed, the HIV antibody–antigen bands are visualized by adding enzyme-conjugated antihuman immunoglobulin G to the strip. Then the substrate or color agent is added. If antibody has complexed with any of the banded HIV proteins on the nitrocellulose strip, a color reaction will occur at the band site(s) (Figure 12-4). Positive

test strips are then compared to two control test strips, one that has been reacted with known positive serum and one that has been reacted with known negative serum.

   In contrast to the ELISA test, which indicates only the presence or absence of HIV antibodies, the WB strip qualitatively identifies which of the HIV antigens the antibodies are directed against. **The greatest disadvantage of the WB test is that reagents, testing methods, and test-interpretation criteria are not standardized.** The National Institutes of Health (NIH), the American Red Cross, DuPont company, the Association of State and Territorial Health Officers (ASTHO), and the Department of Defense (DoD) each define a positive WB differently.

   It can be concluded from the criteria set up by different organizations to define a positive result that although the WB may be the gold standard of confirmatory testing, there is **no** agreement on what constitutes a positive WB test (Miike, 1987).

   The WB procedure is labor intensive, takes longer to run (12 to 24 hours), and is therefore more costly than the ELISA test. **The WB is less sensitive than the ELISA but more specific.**

   Because the WB lacks the sensitivity of the ELISA test, it is not used as a screening test. Despite the high specificity of the WB, false positives do occur, but they occur less frequently than with

Table 12-2 Description of Major Gene Products of HIV Capable of Inducing Antibody Response

Gene Product[a]	Description
p17/18[b]	GAG[c] protein
p24/25	GAG protein
p31/32	Endonuclease component of POL[d] translate
gp41	Transmembrane ENV[e] glyco-protein
p51/52/53	Reverse transcriptase component of POL translate
p55	Precursor of GAG proteins cleaved to p18 and p24
p64/65 p66	Reverse transcriptase component of POL translate
gp110/120 gp120	Outer ENV glycoprotein
gp160	Precursor of ENV glyco-protein

[a]Number refers to molecular weight of the protein in kilodaltons; measurement of molecular weight may vary slightly in different laboratories.

[b]Where two bands on acrylamide gel are too close for easy identification, they are presented as such, p51/53, etc.

[c]GAG = core.

[d]POL = polymerase.

[e]ENV = envelope.

(Adapted from *MMWR*, 1988a)

ELISA tests because the WB is only run on serum, blood, oral fluid, and urine already **suspected** of containing HIV antibodies.

Indeterminate WB

Western blots may also turn out to be **indeterminate** in HIV infections. Meaning, a person can be infected, but the blot is not conclusive—it looks positive but it may not be or is too poor to tell. The indeterminate WB results can occur either during the window period for HIV seroconversion, or during end-stage HIV disease. Indeterminate WBs have **occurred in uninfected individuals because of cross-reacting autoantibodies** related to recent immunization, prior blood transfusion, organ transplantation, autoimmune disorders, malignancy, infection with other retroviruses (for example, HIV-2), or pregnancy. Some patients have a persistent pattern of indeterminate reactivity that remains stable over several years in the absence of true HIV infection.

In general, most persons with an initial indeterminate Western blot result who are infected with HIV will develop detectable HIV antibody within one month. Thus, clients with an initial indeterminate Western blot result should be retested for HIV infection after one month. According to CDC (*MMWR*, 2001), persons with continued indeterminate Western blot results after one month are unlikely to be HIV infected and should be counseled as though they are not infected unless recent HIV exposure is suspected.

Relative Costs of ELISA and Western Blot Tests

The cost incurred to identify each true positive HIV individual in a population with a 10% prevalence for HIV infection is presented in Table 12-3. Cost estimates are for tests performed on a contractual basis, that is, for screening large numbers of people versus testing of individuals. Note that the difference is quite significant.

Table 12-3 Incurred Costs To Identify True Positive HIV-Antibody-Containing Sera in a Population With a 10% Prevalence of HIV-Antibody-Infected People

Price of testing under negotiated contracts:
    Low estimate: $4.41 per specimen tested
    High estimate: $7 for each ELISA, $60 for each Western blot
    Price for individual testing: $47.50 for each ELISA, $121 for each Western blot

Best case:
    Number of true positives: 9920
    Number of ELISAs performed: 100,000
    Number of Western blots performed: 9960 + 1900 = 10,860
    Low estimate: $4.41 × 100,000 divided by 9920 = $44
    High estimate: $7 × 100,000 plus $60 × 10,860 divided by 9920 = $136.25
    Individual testing: $47.50 × 100,000 plus $121 × 10,860 divided by 9920 = $611.30

(Adapted from Miike, 1987; adjustment reflects charges through 2002)

NEW ELISA TESTING PROCEDURES REVEAL EARLY VS. LATE HIV INFECTION

STARHS—A Sensitive/Less Sensitive HIV Test

The best data for understanding recent changes in HIV transmission are measurements of the number of new infections in a defined time period (incidence of infection). But this has been difficult because ELISA testing simply gave a positive or negative response to the presence of HIV antibody without regard to the actual time of infection. However, in mid-1998 (Jensen et al.) through 1999 (McFarland et al.) a new testing strategy provided a means to detect new or early HIV infections versus older HIV infections. The new testing technique is called **STARHS** (the **Serologic Testing Algorithm for Recent HIV Seroconversions**). The test uses two different ELISAs to test a single blood sample to tell if an infection is old or new. By more accurately pinpointing the time of infection, STARHS may help patients identify when and from whom infection took place. Because people can live symptom-free with HIV for over a decade, there was no way previously to tell when they might have become infected. But the new technology changes that. For example, while it's hard for many sexually active people to recall the names and addresses of all their partners, spanning years of activity, it is typically a simple matter to make a list for the past four months. Armed with this new information, public health authorities can track down individuals who appear to be spreading HIV, and—for the first time—interrupt the chain of transmission on a large-scale basis.

HOW IT WORKS

The standard ELISA blood test is **very sensitive** and measures the presence of antibodies against HIV. The very sensitive or **highly tuned ELISA**

tests can pick up even minute numbers of antibodies present in the first days of infection before the immune system has mounted a full response to the virus. Conversely, a less sensitive diluted or **detuned ELISA does the reverse.** It detects only the presence of antibodies at higher levels that typically appear three to six months after infection. By administering both the standard and detuned ELISA tests at the same time, technicians can tell an individual's stage of infection. In brief, if someone tests positive on the sensitive test and negative on the **detuned** test, they likely have a recent infection. Positive results on both tests indicate the infection is more than four to six months old.

EARLY FINDINGS

Beginning year 2000, use of the sensitive/less sensitive ELISA testing in a San Francisco HIV/AIDS clinic revealed the following: (a) about 20% of clients are in the early phase of infection. This says that 20% sought testing within less than four months of getting infected. (b) Out of several thousand tested, not one single woman has come up positive. (c) One individual came up positive even though his only sexual activity was oral. The researchers have confirmed he acquired his HIV **orally.** (d) None of the Bay Area's IV-drug users have turned up positive for recent infection, except those who are gay. The researchers believe these men acquired HIV not from needles, but from sex. (e) All the newly acquired HIV infections have been in gay men, mostly white, in their thirties. A map of where those men live today matches—almost to the block—a 1984 map of San Francisco AIDS cases compiled by epidemiologist Andrew Moss from University of California, San Francisco.

OTHER SCREENING AND CONFIRMATORY TESTS

There are a variety of HIV-antibody and HIV-antigen detection tests now on the market and others are on their way. A few of these tests have been singled out because they are currently in use or because of their potential to make a contribution in the field of HIV antibody–antigen testing methodology.

Immunofluorescent Antibody Assay

The **immunofluorescent antibody assay** uses a known preparation of antibodies labeled with a fluorescent dye such as fluorescein isothiocyanate (FITC) to detect antigen or antibody. In the direct fluorescent antibody test, fluorescent antibodies detect specific antigens in cultures or smears. In the indirect fluorescent antibody test, specific antibody from serum is bound to antigen on a glass slide.

The indirect procedure is modified for use in detecting antibodies to HIV. Cells that are HIV-infected will have HIV antigens on their cell membranes and will later fluoresce when the antihuman fluorescent conjugate is added.

A diluted sample of a person's serum is placed on a slide prepared with HIV antigens and incubated to allow antibody–antigen reaction if there are HIV antibodies in the serum. The slides are then rinsed to get rid of excess serum and other materials. Fluorescent antihuman antibody is then placed on the slide and incubation allows antihuman HIV antibody complexing to occur. The slide is again rinsed and dried. Fluorescence, if any, is observed using a special fluorescence microscope. The indirect fluorescent antibody (IFA) test is now used in many laboratories as a screening procedure. In as much as the sensitivity and specificity of the IFA test are similar to the Western blot, this method has been proposed as an alternative confirmatory test for positive ELISA results. The IFA method is relatively simple and is one of the quickest tests available.

In late 1992, the FDA approved Fluorognost for marketing, the first assay for HIV-IFA confirmation and screening.

The assay allows doctors to do in-office tests for antibodies to HIV in human serum or plasma. As opposed to the Western blot test, the current standard confirmation test, Fluorognost posts almost no indeterminate test results. In addition, the test takes only 90 minutes to complete, while the Western blot takes from 12 to 24 hours to process. This FDA-approved test allows smaller health care facilities, emergency rooms, and doctors' offices to conduct in-office HIV screening and confirmation with accuracy, ease, and low overhead.

Polymerase Chain Reaction

Interactions between HIV and its host cell extend across a wide spectrum, from latent to productive infection. The virus can persist in cells as unintegrated DNA, as integrated DNA with alternative states of viral gene expression, or as a defective DNA molecule. Determining the fraction of cells in the blood that are latently or productively infected is important for the understanding of viral pathogenesis and in the design and testing of effective therapies. Determining the number of infected cells in a heterogeneous cell population and the proportion of those cells that are carrying the virus but not producing new viruses requires the identification of the proviral DNA and viral mRNA in single cells.

The polymerase chain reaction (PCR) is a technique by which any DNA fragment from a single cell can be exponentially multiplied to an amount large enough to be measured (Figure 12-5). This technique indirectly measures **viral load** and thus enables an assessment of viral load and viral expression in different parts of the body of HIV-infected patients. Thus PCR could be an ideal diagnostic test for HIV infection, since it directly amplifies proviral HIV DNA and does not require antibody formation by the host. It is already used in settings where antibody production is unpredictable or difficult to interpret, such as in acute HIV infection or in the perinatal/postnatal period. For HIV testing, the technique used is to copy a segment of proviral DNA found in cells such as T4 lymphocytes and macrophages that carry the

---

POINT OF VIEW 12.1

SOME RELATIVE DRAWBACKS TO THE CURRENT HIV SCREENING TEST— ELISA/WESTERN BLOT

Regardless of the high sensitivity and high specificity or overall test performance, there are a few test-related problems. For example, although only 24 hours are required to complete the ELISA/Western blot testing procedures, most labs batch specimens for processing, causing a one- to two-week wait for definitive results. One study has shown that 40% of those tested never returned for their test results. Perhaps because of concern about maintaining anonymity or other factors, many individuals with HIV are not tested until they develop symptoms. Up to one-third of patients receive their HIV diagnosis within two months of an AIDS diagnosis.

Cost and time investment of the two-step process (pre- and posttest counseling) have also impeded testing. Even when tested without charge at a publicly funded clinic, clients must take time out of work or caring for children for waiting time, counseling, or travel. The true cost of this process has been estimated at $41 per test. And, individuals tested in private offices may incur not only the cost of the test by commercial or hospital labs, but also the physician's office fee (Sax et al., 1997).

Polymerase Chain Reaction

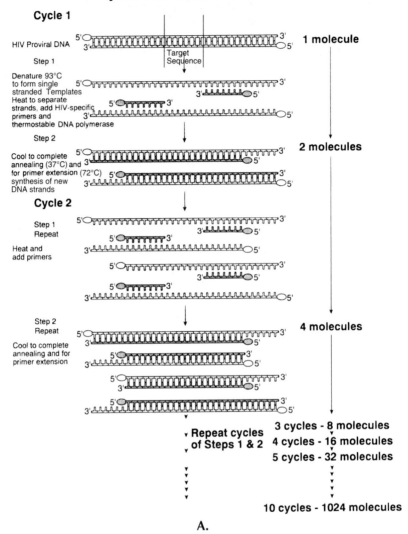

Cycle 1

HIV Proviral DNA — 5' ... 3' / 3' ... 5' — **1 molecule**

Step 1 — Target Sequence

Denature 93°C to form single stranded Templates Heat to separate strands, add HIV-specific primers and thermostable DNA polymerase

Step 2

Cool to complete annealing (37°C) and for primer extension (72°C) synthesis of new DNA strands — **2 molecules**

Cycle 2

Step 1 Repeat

Heat and add primers

Step 2 Repeat

Cool to complete annealing and for primer extension — **4 molecules**

▾ **Repeat cycles** ▾ **of Steps 1 & 2**

3 cycles - 8 molecules
4 cycles - 16 molecules
5 cycles - 32 molecules

10 cycles - 1024 molecules

A.

FIGURE 12-5   A. Polymerase Chain Reaction. A source of DNA containing the sequence to be amplified is mixed with two primers, nucleotide triphosphates and the DNA polymerase Taq 1 (Taq 1 is a DNA polymerase derived from the bacterium *Thermus aquaticus*). The primers are synthetic oligonucleotides of *known sequence*. Therefore, the boundaries of the DNA sequence to be copied are already known. *Cycle 1*: Primers are added in excess (1 million-fold). Using DNA polymerase, the primers are extended by DNA synthesis. The first cycle takes about five minutes. *Cycle 2*: The product from cycle 1 is denatured, reannealed, and primer extension occurs once again. This cycle takes place as many as 50 times so that the primer-extended sequence increases thousands of times. The original DNA sequence can be amplified exponentially according to the formula 2^n, where *n* is the number of cycles. In theory, 25 PCR cycles would result in a 34 million-fold amplification. However, since the efficiency of each cycle is less than 100%, the actual amplification after 25 cycles is about 1 to 3 million-fold. The size of the amplified region is generally 100 to 400 base pairs, although stretches of up to 2,000 bases can be efficiently amplified. In HIV-infected cells, the DNA template is a specified region within the provirus (Keller et al., 1988).

B.

FIGURE 12-5 *(continued)* **B.** Photograph of a thermocycler—the machine used to run the PCR. *(Photograph courtesy of the author)*

virus. **The PCR is so sensitive that it can detect and amplify as few as six molecules of proviral DNA in 150,000 cells or one molecule of viral DNA in 10 μL of blood.**

Finding these few molecules of DNA to copy and amplify is, as the saying goes, like finding a needle in a haystack. The needle in this case is the proviral DNA molecule. It is only a miniscule fraction of the total DNA content of a given cell and far less when mixed in with the DNA of over one million cells as used in some HIV PCRs.

One of the first uses of the PCR in HIV/AIDS research was to show that HIV was present in people who were suspected of being infected but did not produce HIV antibodies. The HIV provirus was detectable in their cells. The PCR's most recent use has been in the detection of HIV provirus in newborns of HIV-infected mothers (Rogers et al., 1989).

In 1993, researchers reported that, in HIV-infected persons, 4% to 15% of peripheral blood lymphocytes were infected with HIV. The percentage of these cells that contained HIV mRNA, an indicator of viral replication, ranged from less than 1% to 8%. The data indicate that, in HIV-positive individuals, a significant proportion of peripheral blood lymphocytes are infected with HIV, but that the virus is in a latent state in the majority of these cells.

Now that there are some good anti-HIV therapies available to help slow the onset of AIDS, the diagnosis of individuals who carry the provirus is critical because they may benefit from early treatment. The PCR test will become even more important with the advent of an HIV vaccine. Vaccinated people will become HIV-antibody positive. The PCR test will be used to identify those who are truly HIV-infected.

RAPID HIV TESTING

A rapid test for detecting antibody to HIV is defined as a screening test that reveals the presence or absence of antibodies for human HIV during the length of the patient's visit to the clinic, which is usually between 10 and 30 minutes. In the United States, 10% to 20% of pregnant women do not know their HIV status at the time of delivery. In Africa and Asian countries, it is estimated that over 90% of pregnant women do not know their HIV status at delivery. But the HIV status of pregnant women is essential to prevent mother-to-child HIV transmission.

Rapid HIV test results are also necessary for deciding whether to initiate treatment for health care workers after accidental exposures to patient body fluids and there is a need for rapid HIV tests to assist with diagnosis and appropriate treatment of persons who may have opportunistic infections due to AIDS in urban emergency departments, which have been shown to have high rates of undiagnosed HIV infection among their patient populations. In short, the value of rapid HIV tests in public health has been well established.

There are over 30 different rapid HIV tests currently marketed worldwide. Six rapid tests were recently evaluated in the United States for their sensitivity and specificity in detecting human HIV. The Single Use Diagnosis System (SUDS) is the only one approved by the FDA through mid 2002. Additional SUDS tests are in different stages of development; they differ mainly in the peptide or recombinant antigen used to bind the HIV antibodies present in the patient's serum. The FDA-licensed rapid SUDS HIV antibody test has a sensitivity of 99.9% and a specificity of 99.6%. The sensitivity and specificity of the SUDS rapid HIV test are comparable to those of the ELISA. The benefits of rapid testing are greatest for clinics that serve a population with a high prevalence of HIV but have experienced low rates of patients who return to learn their HIV test results. Facilities that serve clients who have low risk for HIV infection and who come from communities with low HIV prevalence will experience a higher proportion of false positive tests.

The **HEMA-STRIP** and **SERO-STRIP** are used to test for HIV antibody in over 20 countries. Those and other rapid HIV tests used outside the United States require no additional equipment. These **one-step** assays have all reagents contained in a tube-like device that has a strip containing antigens. Whole blood, oral fluid, or serum is placed at the tip of the device and or membrane allowed to diffuse along the strip or membrane impregnated with reagents where reaction with the antibody occurs. These tests can be completed in less than 10 minutes, require no addition of reagents, and contain a built-in quality control reagent. These assays offer attractive features and may be the tests of the future in America.

What Is the Difference between a Rapid HIV Test and an Enzyme Immunoassay (EIA)?

The rapid HIV test is easier to use and produces results more quickly than the EIA does. The sensitivity and specificity of the rapid HIV test are just as good as those of the EIA. Persons whose rapid HIV tests are **negative** can be given a **definitive** negative result without a return visit. Persons whose tests are **positive** can be counseled about the likelihood of their infection and to return for confirmation testing.

In the ELISA test, a diluted sample of a person's blood is placed into a microwell of a test plate (Figure 12-1) that is coated with HIV antigen and the test sample is allowed to come to equilibrium in the microwell. It takes some time for the antibody to diffuse out and complex or attach to antigen in the microwell. In a rapid test, the test sample can be more highly concentrated. When the test sample is placed on a rapid test membrane, it spreads out across the membrane and immediately penetrates the membrane, which contains HIV antigen. Antibody/antigen complexing begins immediately. As such, the antibodies complexed to HIV antigen are taken out of solution as the test sample runs through the

---

POINT OF INFORMATION 12.4

CAUTION REGARDING RAPID TESTS

New York health officials are dealing with a state regulation adopted in 1999 that requires the screening within 48 hours of women who present for labor and whose HIV status is not known. If the women refuse the test, their babies are tested at birth. However, the rapid Single Use Diagnostic Systems (SUDS) HIV test used is not always accurate or used correctly. Preliminary data from the first four months after the regulation went into effect show that 32 women were identified as HIV positive with a rapid HIV test. A confirmatory test later showed that 17 of those women did not have HIV and 13 of their babies had already been started on preventive antiretroviral therapy. A study conducted at a Bronx hospital in the summer of 1999 found that two out of three SUDS positive tests were false positives. In addition, one study by the New York City Department of Health revealed a 45% false positive rate with SUDS, while another showed that it missed HIV-2 infection. The New York Health Department does not require the use of SUDS, only that hospitals have results within 48 hours. The CDC is currently studying other rapid screening tests that are thought to be about as reliable as the ELISA and Western blot tests.

WHY ONLY ONE FDA-APPROVED RAPID HIV TEST IN THE UNITED STATES?

Why are rapid HIV tests that are available in Japan, France, and Thailand unobtainable in the United States? The answer seems to lie with big companies that make the conventional HIV tests. Because of a web of patents and intellectual property agreements, these corporations have been keeping rapid testing out of the U.S. market. The problem stems not from testing for HIV-1, the most common HIV infection in the world, but with patents that cover testing for HIV-2, and AIDS-causing virus most prevalent in West Africa. Although HIV-2 infections have been reported in areas with large immigrant populations such as New York, overall, infections with the HIV-2 are rare in the United States. When a test for HIV-2 became available in 1990, the

CDC recommended that HIV blood screening tests should be able to detect both types of HIV. Although the FDA requires that blood screening tests check for HIV-2, the agency does not ask the same of tests used to diagnose HIV in individuals. Yet producers of HIV diagnostic assays have voluntarily adopted the standards such that an HIV test should be able to test for all forms of HIV prevalent in the world. In 2001, the FDA gave a clear signal that diagnostic products that test for HIV-1 alone would receive a favorable review, given sufficient research outcomes. Reportedly, this has unlocked the gates and several rapid test makers have submitted applications. It's possible that an approval could come in early 2003.

---

membrane. Thus, the rapid test allows for immediate screening of a test sample for HIV antibody. If antibody to HIV is present the test is positive. If no antibody/antigen complex is found the test is negative. This is quick and efficient versus an ELISA HIV test which, because of having to wait for diffusion equilibrium, takes hours to complete and requires more expensive equipment and personnel to accomplish. In short, the rapid test provides a large surface area with a high concentration of HIV antigen covering the membrane surface. When varying concentrations of HIV antibody pass over and through the membrane they attach to the antigen, providing a rapid positive reaction within minutes.

In March 1998, the CDC changed its policy on the use of rapid HIV screening tests in the United States. Based on its studies, about 750,000 out of **2.5 million** people annually **do not** return to anonymous test centers to find out their **ELISA** test results. The CDC now feels that early disclosure of results (10 minutes rather than two weeks) will cut down on the number of people who do not return for their results. Therefore, the CDC has recommended that physicians use the SUDS test, and the FDA will most likely approve other rapid test kits in early 2002 (*MMWR*, 1998b updated).

Saliva and Urine Tests

By the end of 1994, there were at least nine **serum** HIV-antibody **screening** tests and four confirmato-

ry tests available in the marketplace. Because HIV antibodies are present in body fluids other than blood (for example, urine and saliva), HIV-antibody assays have been developed for their use. **Collecting samples of urine and saliva is noninvasive, easier, less dangerous, and less expensive.** Such tests are particularly useful in developing nations where there is a shortage of refrigeration and sterile equipment (Constantine, 1993; Frerichs et al., 1994).

At least one HIV saliva test, **OraSure** (Figure 12-6), had received FDA approval for use in the United States in late 1994. But the FDA withheld permission to market OraSure until June of 1996. Previously, people whose OraSure had tested positive had to give a blood sample to confirm the results. Now both the initial and confirming (Western blot) tests can be performed with the OraSure pad. OraSure is comparable to blood tests in cost and speed, but the FDA says it is slightly less accurate than blood tests. Although the OraSure kit performs well, at this point its niche in the clinical lab is not entirely clear. The manufacturer suggests it may be useful for needle-phobic patients and in mass screening programs in which phlebotomy (drawing blood) is not readily available. A home version now being developed for marketing here should have a wide appeal (Gallo et al., 1997). Entering year 2000, one urine test, **Sentinel,** (Seradyn) a screen HIV test, was FDA approved on August 6, 1996. In May of 1998, the FDA approved a **urine Western blot** test. Now the confirmatory test can be done in urine. It is **less** sensitive and specific than blood

FIGURE 12-6 HIV-antibody testing and OraSure technology. OraSure is a simple lollipop-like device that is an easy-to-use oral HIV-antibody testing technology now available to consumers through health professionals. The product does not require the use of needles or blood and is about as effective as traditional HIV blood tests. A specially treated pad attached to the handle is placed by the patient between the lower cheek and gum for two minutes. The pad is then placed in a vial with preservative and sent to a clinical laboratory for testing for the presence of HIV antibodies, the same way blood samples are tested. *(Photograph courtesy of Epitope, Inc.)*

testing. **The test is available only to professional laboratories** (Sax et al., 1997 updated, 1999).

HIV Gene Probes

Gene probes or genetic probes are an idea borrowed from methodologies used in recombinant DNA research. The idea is to isolate a DNA segment, make many copies of it, and label these copies with a radioisotope or other tag compound. If the DNA sequence copied is contained in any of the HIV genes, the labeled copies of this DNA sequence can be used to hybridize or attach to DNA of cells that contain HIV DNA. This method of DNA probe analysis eliminates the need of searching for HIV gene products or antibodies to these products to prove that a person is HIV-infected.

At least two HIV-specific probes are on the market. One uses a radioactive sulfur label on the DNA for detection (^{35}S). This probe hybridizes to about 50% of the entire HIV genome and most specifically hybridizes to the HIV polymerase region. A second probe, also using ^{35}S, is an **RNA probe.** It is being used to detect HIV RNA in pe-

ripheral blood or tissue samples. **RNA probe hybridization allows detection of one HIV-infected cell out of 400,000 uninfected cells.** Specifically, the assay detects the presence of HIV in whole white blood cells as soon as the virus begins to replicate. The ^{35}S-labeled probes enter the white blood cells and combine with HIV; the procedure does not require DNA extraction and results are obtained in just over one day (Kramer et al., 1989).

Passive Hemagglutination Assay

There continues to be an urgent need for an inexpensive, accurate assay for anti-HIV screening in the developing world. Scheffel's results (1990) indicate that the **passive hemagglutination assay (PHA)** is a good candidate. The assay is simple to perform and requires no expensive equipment or precision pipettes. The reagents appear very stable even in adverse conditions. However, the assay requires a minimum of three hours before a reading can be made.

The accuracy of the assay is reportedly excellent, with 100% sensitivity on some 890 HIV-positive serum samples and sensitivity equal to or better than the second-generation ELISA.

VIRAL LOAD: MEASURING HIV RNA

Recent studies have shown that a very rapid turnover of HIV RNA occurs in the plasma of infected patients, with approximately 30% of the total virus population in the plasma being replenished daily. Continual viral replication and rapid T4 or CD4+ cell turnover play a central role in the pathogenesis of HIV infection. **High plasma HIV RNA levels have been shown to be a strong predictor of rapid progression to AIDS after HIV seroconversion, independent of T4 cell count.** These findings have led to increased interest in quantitating HIV RNA in patients for prognostic purposes. HIV RNA viral load measurements are used in the management of HIV-infected patients, both in predicting rate of progression and monitoring response to antiretroviral therapy (see Chapters 4, 7, and 11 for additional information on HIV RNA load). Until June of 1996, reliable measures of HIV RNA were available only in research laboratories. And, the quantitation of HIV from a clinical specimen required very expensive, labor-intensive, and

BLOOD VS. URINE: OUTCOME OF HIV TEST MAY DIFFER (DISCORDANT RESULTS)

In December 1998, **Clinical Reference Laboratory (CRL),** one of the country's leading clinical reference laboratories, announced the results of the largest study to date showing a significant proportion of individuals—approximately one of every 1000—within the low-risk population test **positive** for HIV antibodies **in their urine** and **negative in their blood.** The results suggest that people being tested for HIV antibody should have both their blood and urine screened. The presence of antibody against HIV in the urine indicates, at the very least, a prior exposure to the virus. Scientists believe that the reason some persons show antibodies in their urine, but not in their blood is based on their ability to compartmentalize the virus; the virus is contained to specific body tissues.

In June 2001, the FDA approved Calypte's urine-specific Western Blot test. The approval eliminates costly duplicative testing, as well as the wasteful practice of providing kit controls for both urine and serum in the same kit. Calypte's urine test product has a longer shelf life than the chemicals used in serum HIV test kits, making this test more appealing to the international market.

difficult-to-reproduce culture techniques. Recently, however, quantitation of HIV viral load in plasma specimens has been accomplished with a variety of techniques that measure HIV RNA and are less expensive and easier to perform. Currently, three commercial assays are available: (**1**) FDA Approved Amplicor HIV Monitor Test, which couples reverse transcription to quantitative polymerase chain reaction (PCR) (Roche Molecular Systems); (**2**) Bayer Quantiplex HIV RNA assay, a branched DNA (bDNA) technology; and (**3**) Nucleic Acid Sequence-Based Amplification (NASBA) (Organon) (Technika). Because in June of 1996 the FDA approved Amplicors' first generation test and in March 1999 the **ULTRASENSITIVE** test, they are briefly reviewed. In addition, the branched-DNA test will also be presented because it is near FDA approval.

Amplicor HIV Monitor Test

This multistep test includes specimen preparation, reverse transcription and PCR, and nonradioactive detection. Plasma samples (200μL) are treated to lyse the viral particles and release RNA; isopropanol is then added to precipitate the RNA. This first step renders the sample noninfectious and safe for laboratory workers.

The new Amplicor HIV Monitor Ultra-Sensitive Test has a three-log dynamic range; its lower limit of sensitivity is about 50 copies of HIV RNA/mL. The assay is reproducible and 5-fold differences in HIV RNA copy number are easily discernible. Using stored samples for comparison, it is possible to detect the high levels of HIV RNA that occur in acute infection and the suppressed levels of circulating virus that follow seroconversion.

Branched-DNA Testing

Another new assay for measuring HIV levels directly, developed by Chiron, uses a branched-DNA (bDNA) technology to amplify a signal to indicate the presence of HIV RNA. The bDNA assay was first designed in 1989 (Horn et al., 1989) and improved upon for use in HIV detection by Urdea (1993) and Dewar (1994).

Using the bDNA assay, nucleic acids can be detected **directly in clinical samples** by means of signal amplification. Signal amplification of HIV RNA occurs when branched oligode-oxyribonucleotides (bDNAs) hybridize to the target HIV RNA and incorporate many alkaline phosphate molecules onto the target HIV RNA. The complex of HIV RNA plus bDNA plus alkaline phosphate is then exposed to dioxetane, which is then triggered by an enzyme to luminesce (give off a light that can be detected with a measuring device, a luminometer) (see Figure 12-7). The luminescence means that HIV RNA is present and the brighter the light (or signal) the more HIV RNA is present in the test sample. The current assay, Chiron's Quantiflex 340 can measure down to 40 copies of HIV RNA/ml of sample.

DETECTION OF HIV INFECTION IN NEWBORNS

Early detection of HIV infection in newborns and children is important because it may prevent

FIGURE 12-7 Branched-DNA Assay for HIV RNA Quantification. Schematic outline of bDNA assay. HIV is concentrated from 1-mL aliquots of patient's plasma. Pellet is then resuspended in mixture of proteinase K, lithium lauryl sulfate, and target probes. Extract is added to wells of 96-well microplate, incubated overnight at 53° C, and washed. bDNA amplifier is then added, incubated at 53° C, and washed, followed by addition of alkaline phosphatase probes, another wash, and addition of the chemiluminescent substrate. *(Adapted from Dewar et al., 1994)*

unwarranted toxicity from the use of antiretroviral agents in children who are not infected, and it can allay the fears of parents with potentially afflicted but uninfected newborns. However, early diagnosis of HIV infection in children born to HIV-positive women is difficult owing to the presence of maternal IgG antibody in the newborn that may persist until the child is about two years old. Thus serological detection of HIV infection in neonates is complicated by the presence of immune complexes, consisting of passively transferred maternal antibodies and HIV antigens. Steven Miles and colleagues (1993) have used a rapid assay designed to disrupt these immune complexes in order to permit the detection of a specific HIV antigen. Their preliminary work correctly identified p24 antigen in the blood of 29

out of 29 children. These children tested HIV positive, but when the maternal antibodies were treated to separate the p24 antigen present (the antigen would be present because the virus was present), they found p24 antigen. Children who were HIV positive but lacked the presence of the p24 antigen were falsely positive—they contained only the mother's HIV antibodies. Although this technique is simple to perform and accurate when compared to other methods of HIV detection in newborns, additional testing of this technique is required before its adoption. If a mother is known to be HIV-infected, cells from the newborn can be subjected to HIV blood culture or polymerase chain reaction tests. These two techniques, although very accurate, are not yet ready for the screening of all newborns. They can detect the presence of HIV in the first few days of life.

FDA APPROVES TWO HOME HIV ANTIBODY TEST KITS

On May 14, 1996, the FDA, which for years opposed home-based HIV testing kits because of the lack of face-to-face counseling, reversed its stance by saying the benefits of early detection of HIV infection outweigh any risks posed by the test. FDA Commissioner David Kessler said, "We are confident that this new home system can provide accurate results while assuring patient anonymity and appropriate counseling."

The FDA approved the home test **because** in a 1994 study by the Federal Centers for Disease Control and Prevention of people at increased risk of infection, like injection drug users and sexually active homosexual men, 42% indicated that they would use a home test.

Test Kit Operation

A person who buys the kit uses an enclosed lancet to prick his or her finger and places three drops of blood on a test card with an identification number. The card is mailed to a laboratory for HIV testing, and samples that test positive are retested to ensure reliability. People who use the home system do not submit names, addresses, or phone numbers with the specimen sent in on filter paper. Therefore, **the HIV test results are anonymous.** To get results, the individual calls three days later and punches into the phone his or her identification number.

If the caller's test results are positive or inconclusive, he or she will be connected to a counselor who will explain the results, urge medical treatment, and, if necessary, make a referral to a local doctor or health clinic. If the person's results are negative, he or she will be connected to a recording that will note that it is possible to be infected with HIV and still test negative if the antibodies to HIV haven't yet developed. A counselor is available for anyone who tests negative and wants to discuss the results.

The FDA said that the kit is as reliable as tests conducted in doctors offices and clinics.

Test Kit Availability

The first FDA-approved HIV test kit, called Confide HIV Testing Service, was made available in June 1996. It was withdrawn from the marketplace in June 1997 due to poor sales. A second FDA-approved HIV home test kit went on sale nationwide in July 1996. This kit, called **Home Access Express-HIV Test** (Figure 12-8) (1-800-448-8378), lets people take a blood sample at home, mail it to a laboratory, and, three days to a month later, learn by phone their results. The two tests are very similar to each other with regard to use and performance.

Pro and Con of Home-Use HIV Test (Collection) Kits

Pro— Those who favor HIV home testing point to the discouraging statistics using current HIV testing methods stating that 80% of people in high-risk populations are unwilling to use standard testing services. They note frequent instances of substandard HIV testing even in physician's offices, with test results delivered in brief phone calls or left on telephone answering machines. Also offered **in support of home-based testing is that the existing system of testing is inefficient and wasteful because 98% of tests are HIV negative.** Thus, there is an enormous amount of money spent on HIV-negative results that should be spent elsewhere. With respect to the need for face-to-face counseling, they cite the success of suicide hotlines and crisis counseling services in support of using home telephone HIV counseling procedures.

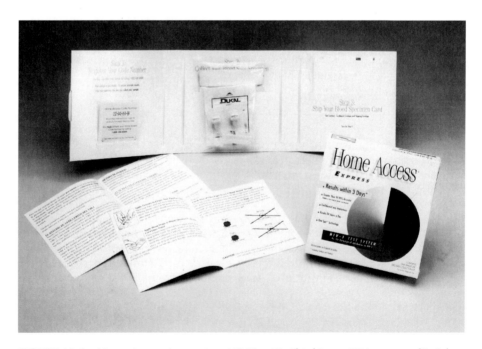

FIGURE 12-8   Home Access Anonymous HIV Test Kit. This kit was FDA-approved in July 1996 and provides access to professional counseling and medical/social service referrals 24 hours a day, 7 days a week. *(Photograph courtesy of Home Access Health Corp., Illinois)*

FEDERAL TRADE COMMISSION WARNS OF POOR HIV HOME TEST KITS

The FDA has not approved home-use HIV test kits, which allow consumers to purchase a test kit, collect a sample in private, and **interpret their own HIV test results** in a few minutes. The Federal Trade Commission has warned that some home-use HIV test kits, many of which are available on the internet and in the "gray" market (i.e., unauthorized imports), supply inaccurate results. These tests are different from FDA-approved home sample collection kits, which allow consumers to purchase test kits, collect a sample in private, send the sample to a laboratory for testing, and telephone for their HIV test result, counseling, and referral.

Beginning 2001, the U.S. Federal Trade Commission issued a warning about a dozen home HIV tests sold over the internet. In a con-

sumer alert, the agency cautioned, "Using one of these kits could give a person who might be infected with HIV the false impression that he or she is not infected." FTC tests showed that when a known HIV-infected sample was used, the tests indicated that the sample was not infected—**a false negative.** At least three HIV home test kits have already led to criminal prosecution. The FDA said the tests were **"medically useless"** and the distributors were fined or put in prison. The internet advertisements have falsely stated or suggested that the kits were cleared by various well-known health groups, the FDA and the WHO. However, the U.S. Food and Drug Administration has approved only The Home Access Express home HIV test kits.

Con— Those against the use of home testing say that this is just one more instance of the telephone substituting for face-to-face contact in medical practice. They suggest that **bad health news of this magnitude and complexity should be given in person.** They also point out that these test kits will probably be used mostly by affluent people who are well, but worried, while the poor, at-risk people continue to remain untested. In addition, there is the risk of the tests being used coercively by employers or the police. The potential for human rights violations are great.

Possible use of the tests by adolescents and young adults is especially controversial. Currently, there are no age restrictions on the purchase of home kits. Although the box states that the test is "recommended for persons 13 and over," anyone who can afford a kit can buy one. If adolescents use the tests, how can they be served effectively by telephone counselors? In addition, many advocates for youth have expressed concern about possible coercion of youth to be tested by parents, guardians, or older adults.

For a more thorough review of the issues on HIV home testing, read **"Testing for HIV at home: What are the issues?"** (Schopper et al., 1996).

Remarks— It remains to be seen just how many of the undiagnosed thousands of HIV-infected persons home-based kits manage to capture—and at what cost—and whether the sys-

tem will be more helpful than abused. **CLASS QUESTION: WHAT DO YOU THINK WILL HAPPEN? GIVE SOME EXAMPLES.**

REPORTING HIV INFECTIONS

In May of 1998 a report from the CDC advised all states not currently requiring name-based, laboratory reporting of positive HIV tests to implement **"integrated HIV and AIDS surveillance"** (*MMWR*, 1998a). The CDC now believes that surveillance AIDS data is not sufficient to track the AIDS pandemic in the United States. The CDC believes that HIV diagnosis and reporting will more accurately reflect trends and incidence of the national pandemic. **The issue now is not whether HIV infections should be reportable at the federal level, but rather how to proceed with the reporting!**

All 50 states and the District of Columbia require health care providers to report new cases of AIDS to their state health departments. Beginning year 2003, 44 states required some form of name reporting of HIV-infected people (Table 10-7). The 44 states that require HIV reporting have over 60% of the population and accounted for over 60% of reported AIDS cases through 2002. Based on the number of HIV infections reported to the CDC, over 300,000 people out of the estimated 950,000 HIV-infected in the United States do not know they are infected. Beginning 2003, only 12 states classified HIV/AIDS as a sexually transmitted disease. Sixteen states classify HIV/AIDS as a communicable disease and 23 states classify HIV/AIDS as a **separate** category of disease. Only 12 states authorized physicians to inform partners of HIV/AIDS patients (*Medical Tribune*, 1991 updated).

Does the United States Need a National System for HIV Reporting?

Lawrence O. Gostin of Georgetown University Law Center in Washington, DC, and colleagues state that the United States now needs a national system of HIV case reporting. Up to now, the AIDS surveillance system has ". . . formed the cornerstone of the nation's efforts to monitor and characterize the HIV pandemic." Because this system reports **advanced** cases of HIV infection, [AIDS] it only ". . . provides a snapshot of a decade-old epidemic." Gostin and colleagues believe that the compelling need for accurate monitoring of HIV infection and for effective medical and public health interventions **mandates a fundamental reevaluation of AIDS surveillance.** They argue that there is now a **new era** of more sophisticated treatments for HIV infection, that current treatment of HIV using reverse transcriptase inhibitors and protease inhibitors reduces mortality and delays progression of disease. Thus anti-HIV therapy has provided a **defining moment** in this pandemic and, unless our current HIV/AIDS surveillance system is revised to include reporting of all HIV infections, authorities will not have reliable information about the prevalence, incidence, and future directions of HIV infection. And they will not be able to provide therapy intervention when it will do the infected the most good.

WHO SHOULD BE TESTED FOR HIV INFECTION?

Testing for antibodies to HIV is an important first step in establishing a diagnosis of HIV infection. Testing every person may be counterproductive. Attempts to isolate or publicly identify people with HIV/AIDS can actually fuel the spread of HIV. People outside the tested group may feel invulnerable, and then fail to make necessary changes in their behavior.

The effects of stimulating a false sense of security are well illustrated in Germany where, in certain towns, prostitutes are required to be checked for certain STDs every week and are given health inspection cards. Many customers think these cards guarantee against disease and so refuse to use condoms.

The problem is not confined to Germany. **A European shipbroker whose work frequently takes him to southeast Asia, where he has a regular sex partner, said: "I tell her when I'm due to arrive and she has an HIV test just before. If she has an up-to-date health card I know I'm safe."**

In fact, a negative HIV test is no guarantee the tested person is **truly** HIV negative—he or she may be in the **window period.** The decision to test must be based on people's risk behaviors and/or symptoms. As to who **needs** to be HIV tested, a complete history and physical examination will give the best answer to this question. Decisions based on individual indications are often more appropriate than decisions based on one's classification (for example, all pregnant women or all single men between 20 and 49 years of age). Initial assessment for current or past behaviors (within the past 10 years) should include:

1. Persons with **risk behaviors** such as:
   a. Anal sexual activity, male or female
   b. Injection drug use
   c. Frequent casual heterosexual activity
   d. Encounters with prostitutes
   e. Previous treatment for sexually transmitted diseases (*Condyloma acuminata* (genital warts), herpes simplex virus, gonorrhea, syphilis, Chlamydia)
   f. Blood transfusions, especially before 1985
   g. Sexual activity with partners having any of the above
   h. Infants born to women involved in any of the above

2. Persons with symptoms such as:
   a. Fever, weight loss (unexplained)
   b. Night sweats
   c. Severe fatigue
   d. Recent infections, especially thrush and shingles (varicella-zoster)

3. Persons with **signs** (based on physical exam) such as:
   a. Weight loss
   b. Enlarged lymph nodes and/or tonsilar enlargement

c. Oral exam (candidiasis, oral hairy leukoplakia)

d. Skin lesions (Kaposi's sarcoma, varicella-zoster, psoriasis)

e. Hepatosplenomegaly (enlarged liver)

f. Mental status examination showing changes

4. Pregnant women who have demonstrated high-risk behavior.

5. Prisoners. A number of states (about 20 beginning 2003) now have legislation to HIV test all incoming and/or outgoing (released) inmates of state prisons (see Chapter 10). The rate of HIV infection in prison populations is about 2.1%. In New York, Florida, Texas, and California the rate is between 3% and 4%. The turn over rate in some state inmate populations is 50% per year. Many of these inmates become infected in prison, and are released to spread HIV in the general population.

Acceptance of HIV testing is reportedly lower when clients have been tested previously and are fearful of their ability to cope with their test results. Testing is more likely to be accepted when:

a. Clients perceive their own HIV risk and acknowledge behaviors placing them at increased risk

b. Testing is voluntary and routinely offered to clients rather than clients having to request it

c. Protections for client confidentiality are in place

d. Anonymous testing is available

e. Alternate HIV test technologies are offered to clients

f. Providers recommend testing as part of appropriate medical care

g. Providers and clients perceive HIV counseling and testing to be beneficial for early diagnosis and prevention purposes

6. Gay and bisexual men. Hoping to head off a new surge of infections, the government recommended for the first time, in May of 2002, that sexually active gay and bisexual men get tested at least once a year for HIV. Previous guidelines from federal health officials have been less specific, urging doctors to recommend HIV tests for patients whose behavior might put them at risk for infection.

Addressing Barriers to HIV Testing

Knowledge of HIV infection status can benefit the health of individual persons and the community. Thus, HIV testing should be as convenient as possible to promote client knowledge of HIV infection status. Efforts should be made to remove or lower barriers to HIV testing by ensuring that:

♦ Testing is accessible, available, and responsive to client and community needs and priorities;

♦ Anonymous and confidential HIV testing are available;

♦ The testing process considers the client's culture, language, sex, sexual orientation, age, and developmental level; and

♦ Confidentiality maintained. (In some places, like rural communities, **confidentiality** can't be assured, so people may decide not to get tested. The stigma that has existed since the beginning of the pandemic hasn't changed. Because the mechanics of transmission are so well understood, and society in general sees it as preventable, people have the attitude: "You know better, why did you get it?" Especially for women, the fear of being isolated in their communities can be very powerful. Many infected women have children they want to protect from school gossip. In addition, they aren't used to being part of a community that is ostracized, such as gay males and injection drug users.)

Acceptance of HIV testing is reportedly lower when clients have been tested previously and are fearful of their ability to cope with their test results. Testing is more likely to be accepted when:

♦ Clients perceive their own HIV risk and acknowledge behaviors placing them at increased risk;

♦ Testing is voluntary and routinely offered to clients rather than clients having to request it;

♦ Protections for client confidentiality are in place;

♦ Anonymous testing is available;

♦ Alternate HIV test technologies are offered to clients;

♦ Providers recommend testing as part of appropriate medical care; and

♦ Providers and clients perceive HIV counseling and testing to be beneficial for early diagnosis and prevention purposes.

WHY IS HIV TEST INFORMATION NECESSARY?

A recent CDC random-digit-dial telephone survey of Americans ages 18 to 65 revealed that **42% of those surveyed** said they had been HIV tested. Geographic differences were great. For example, 26% of people in South Dakota said they had been tested versus 60% in Washington, DC (*MMWR*, 1999). The CDC also reported that about 25 million Americans are HIV tested each year. Some 10,000 publicly funded counseling and testing programs conduct about 2.5 million of these tests annually.

Thirty percent of adults who seek HIV testing do so to find out their HIV status; 12% are tested because of hospitalization or surgery; 16% for application for insurance; and 7% to enter the military. Another 1% are referred by their doctor, the health department, or sexual partner, and 4% are tested for HIV for immigration reasons (Hooker, 1996).

Knowledge of HIV infection status allows infected persons and their infected partners to seek treatment with retroviral agents, prophylaxis against *Pneumocystis carinii* pneumonia, tuberculosis skin testing and tuberculosis prophylaxis (if appropriate), and other types of therapy and vaccines that may delay or prevent the opportunistic infections associated with HIV infection. Such measures have been shown to delay the onset of AIDS in infected persons and to prolong the lives of persons with AIDS. Counseling and testing may help some persons change high-risk sexual and drug-use behaviors thereby preventing HIV transmission to others.

IMMIGRATION INTO THE UNITED STATES

Having HIV can make it very difficult to immigrate into the United States. Everyone 15 years of age and older who applies for a "green card" has to take an HIV test. If you test HIV positive you cannot get a green card unless you get an HIV waiver. An HIV waiver is a special permission from the Immigration and Naturalization Service (INS) that allows an HIV-positive person to obtain permanent residency. A green card applicant who is the spouse, unmarried child, or parent of a U.S. citizen or legal permanent resident may be able to get a waiver if he or she meets the other requirements. Before you can get a waiver, you must show the INS that you are able to pay your medical expenses if you get sick. In other words, you must show that you will not need government benefits such as Medicare or free county services. You must also show that you are not a danger to the public health—that is, you must demonstrate knowledge of how HIV is spread and what you can do to minimize the chances of transmission.

Section 212(a)(1)(A)(I) of the Immigration and Nationality Act renders inadmissible any applicant for a visa or admission who is found, according to the regulations published by the secretary of health and human services (HHS), to have a communicable disease of public health significance, which includes HIV infection. However, in view of humanitarian and family unity concerns, the law also provides waivers to inadmissibility, which are discretionary and granted on a case-by-case basis. Two specific waiver policies have been implemented for applicants seeking admission as **nonimmigrants** (for a temporary period of time) who are inadmissible due to HIV infection:

Routine HIV Waiver Policy— Nonimmigrants may be granted a waiver for admission to

BLACK MINISTERS LEAD BY EXAMPLE

During June 4 and 5, 2000, at least 50 black ministers in Chicago were HIV tested. Jessie Jackson, who led the movement, said, "There's a certain taboo and even a certain shame to AIDS." Balm in Gilead, a national organization established 12 years ago to help African-American churches deal with AIDS began airing television commercials about how the clergy can help. While similar mass testing has taken place in At-lanta, this is the first movement in Chicago and the first time Jackson's Rainbow/PUSH coalition has been involved. In the United States, AIDS is the number one cause of death of African-American men and women 25 to 44 years old. Statistics show that in Chicago, two-thirds of all new AIDS cases from 1999 through 2001 were among black Americans, compared to 37% one decade before.

the United States for 30 days or less to attend conferences, receive medical treatment, visit close family members, or conduct business. The applicant must demonstrate that he or she is not currently afflicted with symptoms of the disease; there are sufficient assets, such as insurance, that would cover any medical care that might be required in the event of illness while in the United States; the proposed visit to the United States is for 30 days or less; and that the visit will not pose a danger to public health in the United States.

The Designated Event Policy— This policy facilitates the admission of HIV-positive persons to attend certain designated events, which are considered to be in the public interest, such as academic and educational conferences and international sports events. To initiate the process, HHS writes a letter to the Department of State (DOS) regarding a specific event. DOS recommends the event to the attorney general who designates the event and authorizes a blanket waiver. This blanket waiver allows HIV-positive applicants seeking admission to the United States specifically to participate in the designated event to be admitted for the duration of the event without being questioned about their HIV status.

If the INS discovers a noncitizen is HIV positive, he or she can be prevented from entering the country even if they have a green card. The INS does not require an HIV test to reenter. However, they are allowed to ask you if you have HIV. If you reenter the United States with AIDS-related materials such as pamphlets or medicine such as AZT in your luggage, or if you are clearly sick, the INS may ask you if you are HIV positive and detain you for medical examination. However, tourists and other nonimmigrants such as business people, temporary work-ers, or those seeking medical treatment are generally not asked to take an HIV test. There is no HIV test when applying for citizenship. Only persons applying for permanent residency are required to be tested by the INS. always consult with an immugration/naturalization attorney.

Illegal Immigrants and HIV

According to immigration authorities, an unknown number of the 7 million undocumented immigrants in the United States are infected with HIV and the secretive existence they live out of fear of deportation is adding to their health risks, according to medical experts. In the worst cases, immigrants are dying because they cannot access health care or they are spreading the disease because they do not know they are infected. Undocumented persons with HIV may be getting a patchwork of inconsistent care, turning to emergency rooms for treatment of opportunistic infections and then returning to the shadows, afraid that deportation to a homeland without medicines or health care is a certain death sentence.

Immigration and Entry into Foreign Countries

An increasing number of foreign countries require that foreigners be tested for HIV prior to entry. This is particularly true for students or long-term visitors. Information available from 185 countries beginning 2003 reveals that 61 countries require an HIV test prior to entry, on arrival, or on application for residency. Entering 2003, a total of 101 countries have entry or residence restrictions against HIV-infected people. There are 65 countries that have no restrictions. **Before traveling abroad, check with the embassy** of the country to be visited to learn entry requirements and specifically whether or not HIV testing is a requirement. If the foreign country indicates that U.S. test results are acceptable "under certain conditions," prospective travelers should inquire at the embassy of that country for details (which laboratories in the United States may perform tests and where to have results certified and authenticated) before departing the United States. For a copy of HIV Testing Requirements for Entry into Foreign Countries, send a self-addressed, stamped, business-size envelope to: Bureau of Consular Affairs, Room 5807, Department of State, Washington, DC 20520.

UPDATE 2001 Chengdu, China, the sprawling capital of China's Sichuan province, has become the first city in China to adopt legislation dealing directly with people infected with HIV. The Chengdu City AIDS Prevention and Management Regulations, which went into effect in May, prohibit AIDS patients and people who have tested positive for HIV from marrying. They order police to test people in high-risk groups, such as prostitutes and drug users, within five days of an arrest and require separate incarceration facilities for those who have tested positive. The regulations also mandate HIV tests for returning Chinese who have been abroad for more than a year, and they suggest that pregnant women with AIDS be persuaded to abort their fetuses if medicine that could prevent the transmission of the HIV to the child is unavailable. Another part of the law bans people with HIV or AIDS from working as kindergarten teachers or surgeons, among other professions. Violators are subject to large fines. On a national level, China, 15 years after its first recorded AIDS death, is still in a state of flux as to how to deal with a sharply increasing number of HIV infected and AIDS cases.

Vietnam

In Vietnam, the Ministry of Health issued a circular that contains seven lists of occupations banned to HIV/AIDS-positive people. For example, Medical Services: surgery, obstetrics, blood transfusion, dermatology, cancer, injection, acupuncture, biopsy, endoscopy, and other medical services in direct contact with patient's blood and biological fluids; Everyday Life services: haircutting, hair drying, hair perm and washing, manicuring, ear piercing, nostril piercing, massage, and vital point pressing; warming, drying, and sterilizing instruments for medical checkup and treatment; providing direct services in hotel rooms and lounges; working and dancing girls in ballrooms; and providing food or care to children in nurseries, kindergartens, early childhood classes, and service establishments.

An Example of How HIV-Infected Immigrants Impact the Host Country

A 2002 survey by the Times of London found that African immigrants accounted for 80% of new HIV cases reported in the United Kingdom in 2001. Africans also composed nearly 25% of the total number of people in the country living with HIV. According to the Times of London, many Africans who seek treatment at U.K. hospitals say they are on vacation, others are asylum seekers and are therefore entitled to free health care, and others had been recruited by the government to work in the United Kingdom as teachers or nurses. Their Human Rights Act gives overseas visitors with HIV the right to stay and be treated for the rest of their lives if treatment is not available at home. The influx has strained the National Health Care system, which is experiencing longer waiting lists for routine operations, insufficient money for medical drugs, and low pay for staff, according to the Times London and former member of Parliament Robert Kilroy-Silk, a U.K. talkshow host. Kilroy-Silk added that language barriers, which necessitate translators, are also driving up costs and slowing down care. He also said, "It's no wonder we have a Third World health service. It's because we've become the health service for the Third World." However, Jean-Emil Yebga, spokesperson for Blackliners, a support group for HIV-positive blacks, said most Africans in need of treatment do not receive it because they are afraid for their immigration status. So the impact of imported cases of HIV is even larger than expected.

Testing for HIV Infection

With about 42 million HIV-infected people living in almost all the countries of the world, and with about 950,000 of them living in the United States beginning year 2003, the question of HIV testing on either a voluntary or a mandatory basis cannot be ignored.

U.S. PUBLIC HEALTH SERVICE (USPHS) RECOMMENDATIONS FOR HIV COUNSELING AND VOLUNTARY TESTING FOR ALL PREGNANT WOMEN

Knowledge of HIV status is important for several reasons. **First,** women who know their serostatus can gain access to HIV-related care and therapies (such as *Pneumocystis carinii* pneumonia prophylaxis, TB screening, and antiretroviral therapy) during pregnancy and postpartum as needed. **Second,** HIV-infected women can be offered antiretroviral therapy to potentially block maternal–fetal transmission of HIV. **Third,** an obstetrician would postpone rupture of amniotic membranes and avoid scalp electrodes or other potentially invasive procedures, all of which may be cofactors for enhanced transmission of HIV. **Fourth,** antiretroviral drugs can be offered to infants of HIV-seropositive women who have recently delivered.

This report (*MMWR,* 2001) contains the recommendations of a 10-member USPHS task force on the use of zidovudine to reduce perinatal transmission of HIV. In summary, the recommendations are:

1. Health care providers should encourage all pregnant women to be tested for HIV infection, both for their own health and to reduce the risk for perinatal HIV transmission. Four million women become pregnant each year in the United States.

2. HIV testing of pregnant women and their infants should be voluntary. In voluntary testing, the reason for the test, how it is administered, and the person's right to privacy and confidentiality must be explained.

This allows the person the choice of taking or refusing the test and giving or not giving demographic data.

3. Three states require health care providers to counsel and offer HIV testing to women as early in pregnancy as possible so that informed and timely therapeutic and reproductive decisions can be made.

4. Uninfected pregnant women who continue to practice high-risk behaviors (such as IV-drug use and unprotected sexual contact with an HIV-infected or high-risk partner) should be encouraged to avoid further exposure to HIV and to be retested in the third trimester of pregnancy.

5. For women who are first identified as being HIV-infected during labor and delivery, health care providers should consider offering intrapartum and neonatal antiretroviral drugs.

In mid-1995 the CDC reported that routine HIV counseling and voluntary testing for all pregnant women has already proved effective in several communities nationwide. In one innercity hospital in Atlanta, for example, 96% of women chose to be tested after being provided HIV counseling.

According to the Pediatric AIDS Foundation, about $350 million a year could be saved by testing pregnant women for HIV. The average hospital bill for a baby born infected with HIV is $35,000 annually for the 8 to 10 years the child lives.

Benefits of HIV Testing— Testing for the presence of HIV antibodies or antigens as early as possible when HIV is suspected can provide substantial health benefits to the individual, for example, early combination anti-HIV drug therapy reduces viral load and extends the quality of life for the infected, and reduces the risk of transmitting the virus to others.

TESTING, COMPETENCY, AND INFORMED CONSENT

Competency is often used interchangeably with capacity; it refers to a person's ability to make an

A WEAK LINK IN HIV TESTING

The movement from a **positive** test result to treatment is a weak link in the overall care of the HIV-infected. Jeffrey Samet and colleagues (1998) reported that although a majority of patients (61%) sought medical care in the first year after their diagnosis, 39% delayed treatment for longer than one year, 32% for longer than two years, and 18% for longer than five years. Their report did not include those persons using home testing kits. It is believed that these people are even further removed from testing to medical care followup.

informed decision. For example, to consent to medical treatment, a person must be mentally capable of comprehending the risks and benefits of a proposed procedure and its alternatives. While a health care provider can assess competence, a legal finding of competency is often required based on the testimony of a mental health professional. Mental illness by itself does not indicate that a person is incompetent to make medical decisions. Various degrees of mental incapacity may occur with HIV infection, requiring an assessment of competency. AIDS dementia complex (ADC) occurs in approximately 70% of HIV-infected patients at some point in HIV disease/AIDS and may interfere with the patient's capacity to provide an informed consent.

Informed Consent

Informed consent is not just signing a form but is a process of education and the opportunity to have questions answered. The concept of informed consent includes the following components: full disclosure of information, patient competency, patient understanding, voluntariness, and decision making. The process of obtaining informed consent involves appropriate facts being provided to a competent patient who understands the information and voluntarily makes a choice to accept or refuse the recommended procedure or treatment.

When the concept of informed consent is applied clinically, complexities arise regarding both the content and the process. The concept contains ambiguous requisites such as "appropriate" facts, "full" disclosure, and "substantial" understanding. The process is affected by many variables including the communication skill and range of practice style of the physician; the maturity, intelligence, and coping strategies of the patient; and the interaction between the physician and the patient (Hartlaub et al., 1993).

Testing without Consent

Beginning 2003, at least 29 states had laws that allowed HIV testing without informed consent under certain conditions. The required conditions vary and include:

1. Patient or other authorized person is unable to give or withhold consent.
2. Test result will help determine treatment.

BOX 12.4

BOXER STRIPPED OF FEATHERWEIGHT TITLE AFTER POSITIVE HIV TEST

It took Ruben Palacio 12 years to win a world title. On the eve of his first defense, he became the first champion to test positive for HIV. The British Boxing Board of Control said, "We can't risk the life of another boxer by letting him fight. It's a kind of disease that can be spread via blood contact, and boxing is a sport where that is likely to happen."

Palacio is the first active world title holder known to have tested positive for the AIDS-causing virus. Esteban DeJesus, who held the WBC lightweight boxing title in the 1970s, contracted AIDS after his retirement and died in 1989.

HIV testing has been a routine part of the prefight medical examination in Britain for several years. In February 1990, African heavyweight champion Proud Kilimanjaro of Zimbabwe was barred from a fight with Britain's Lennox Lewis because he refused to give details of an HIV test to the British Boxing Board of Control.

His manager said, "This brings the HIV thing into perspective. Instead of going home with the largest paycheck of his life, he is going home with an HIV test result that means he will die."

In March of 1996 Tommy Morrison, a former U. S. heavyweight contender disclosed that he is HIV positive (see Figure 8-7). Beginning year 2003 at least nine states require professional fighters and kickboxers, licensed in those states, to be HIV-tested.

---

3. Patient is unable to give consent, and physician can document that a medical emergency exists and that the test is needed for diagnosis and treatment.
4. Test is needed to protect the health of other patients, health workers, emergency or law enforcement personnel.
5. Several states require posttest counseling.
6. In 27 states, teenagers must have signed parental consent to be HIV tested. In 23 states (Alabama, Arizona, California, Colorado, Connecticut, Delaware, Florida, Georgia, Hawaii, Illinois, Iowa, Michigan, Nebraska, Nevada, New Mexico, North Carolina, North Dakota, Ohio, Rhode Island, Tennessee, Utah, Washington, Wyoming) **minors can consent** to HIV testing and treatment.

Generally, HIV antibody testing without consent is legally considered **battery.** Legal liability for "unlawful touching" may result from performing an HIV antibody test without consent. Such a procedure may also constitute an illegal search.

Question: Are federal and state governments overly emphasizing personal privacy at the expense of prevention? (Defend your answer with examples/situations.)

Voluntary Named HIV Testing

In **voluntary named** HIV testing, the individual freely provides his or her name. In this type of testing, an individual voluntarily seeks to learn his or her HIV status and receives a result that is known both to the individual and the test provider/testing agency. An advantage to named testing is that health care providers can contact the person tested if he or she does not return for the testing result.

Voluntary Unnamed HIV Testing

HIV testing is voluntary, but the identity of the person being tested is not placed on the blood sample or the testing form. As a result, the only person who can link the test result with an individual is the person being tested. This form of testing may encourage people concerned about the HIV infection status to obtain testing as it eliminates risk of discrimination or stigmatization. However, it places the exclusive responsibility for seeking counseling, support, and preventive measures on the individual who is infected. **Unnamed testing permits reporting of test data to public health authorities without the risk of breaching confidentiality.** Many public health authorities currently prefer voluntary unnamed testing to named testing.

Testing that is voluntary may miss populations that disproportionately need to be reached. The people least likely to have the virus, it appears, are the most likely to say yes to a test, and the people most likely to be infected are the most likely to say no. In one study, infection rates were 5.3 times as high among people who refused HIV testing as among people who consented to it. In voluntary anonymous, the downside is that such testing reduces the probability that they will return for posttest counseling and linkage to follow up services and a substantial reduction in partner notifications (Moser, 1998).

Mandatory HIV Testing

HIV testing is **mandatory** if it is required to participate in a process or activity that is not itself required. For example, if an HIV test is required for travel to some foreign countries, or to donate blood, this is considered mandatory testing because, while the test is required, one is not required to travel or donate blood. In mandatory testing, care must be taken to ensure that people are not in fact **forced** to undergo testing. At least **in theory,** mandatory testing is a form of voluntary testing: People can decide not to participate in the process or activity for which testing is required. **In practice,** however, the degree of voluntary consent is in some cases questionable. For example, in a situation where employment is not possible unless one agrees to be tested and one needs that job, the **voluntary** nature of the test appears to have vanished (*AIDS, Health and Human Rights,* 1995).

Many people advocate mandatory HIV screening for everyone. They believe that this is the best way to stop the transmission of HIV. But others oppose such testing. For example, some Christian groups oppose mandatory testing because if pregnant women knew they were infected with HIV, this would increase abortion rates. Others oppose testing because of civil rights concerns and the fear that individuals identified as HIV positive would be subjected to social stigma.

Why Mandatory Testing?

Mandatory testing is for the protection of a certain group or the public at large. Although it is not anonymous, results are kept confidential on a need-to-know basis. Mandatory testing for HIV continues to be angrily debated primarily because of the possibility of error when running large numbers of test samples, inadvertent loss of confidentiality, and lack of overall benefit to those who are found to be HIV positive. Mandatory HIV testing is routine for blood donors, and military and Job Corps personnel.

Mandatory HIV Testing of Newborns and Disclosure of Test Results to Mothers and Physicians

Perhaps no call for mandatory HIV testing has caused as much recent controversy as those requiring all pregnant women or all newborns to be tested. On June 26, 1996, New York became the **first** state in the nation to mandate and disclose the HIV status of newborns to mothers and physicians. Governor George E. Pataki signed into law legislation known as the **"Baby AIDS" bill,** which authorizes the state health commissioner to establish a comprehensive program of HIV testing of newborns. The governor said, "This law extends our efforts to do everything we can to reduce the number of babies born with this devastating virus. This information can be used to help mothers make important health care decisions for themselves and their children. We will no longer allow infants to be used as statistical tools in some scientific study. Today, we recognize the HIV infant as a living, breathing human being whose right to medical treatment must be respected."

The passage of this bill was immediately followed by the American Medical Association announcement endorsing mandatory testing of all pregnant women and newborns for the AIDS virus. Entering year 2003 only the states of Connecticut, Arkansas, Tennessee, and New York require health care providers to HIV test **every** pregnant woman as early in her pregnancy as possible—**if she refuses the test** the baby is tested.

Compulsory HIV Testing

In compulsory testing, a person cannot refuse to be tested. Compulsory testing may be forced onto an individual, groups, communities, or even entire populations. A court may order an individual to be tested, or a government may decree or legislate that, for example, commercial sex workers, homosexuals, prisoners, hospital patients, or persons seeking immigration must be tested.

In Colorado, Florida, Georgia, Kentucky, Illinois, Michigan, Nevada, Rhode Island, Utah, and West Virginia, HIV **testing is compulsory for people convicted of prostitution.** However, many prostitutes are back on the streets before their test results are in. In many cases, the prostitutes could not be found for follow-up counseling. In Duval County, Florida, county judges agreed to impose a 30-day jail term for convicted prostitutes, a time period long enough to get their test results and provide counseling. Prostitutes have to sign the test results sheet. They are released as soon as they do.

Under Florida law, a prostitute who knows he or she is carrying HIV but continues to offer sexual favors can be jailed for one year.

In June 1999, the state of Oregon passed legislation that allows a judge to order a person accused of a crime to be tested for HIV. The person also would be tested for other communi-

cable diseases if he or she transmitted bodily fluids to a victim. The results would not become public records.

At least 45 states and the District of Columbia authorize HIV testing for charged or convicted sex offenders (Hooker, 1996 updated).

Fear of Mandatory Testing— If a massive mandatory screening test program was implemented, would it be possible to keep results confidential (See Box 12.5)? What would be done with the information? For example, would the state prevent an uninfected person from marrying an infected one? Officials fear that mandatory testing will drive many people who might have volunteered for anonymous testing underground and away from the health care system. These people will be lost to the counseling and education that would benefit them and others. The reason for going underground would be fear of discrimination and social ostracism if found to be HIV-infected.

A case can be made that a compulsory program could maintain strict confidentiality even with large numbers of people being tested. But, it would appear that the political powers and public in general are not ready for broad-scale compulsory screen testing in the United States.

Confidential, Anonymous, and Blinded Testing

Both confidential and anonymous testing involve the use of informed consent forms that are, to date, with exception of the U.S. military, Job Corps workers, and certain criminals, done on a voluntary basis. Blinded testing **does not,** because of procedure, require informed consent.

Confidential HIV Testing— The person's name and test results are recorded. A consent to HIV testing must be given freely and without coercion. The volunteer does not have to provide any information unless he or she wants to. Individuals to be tested in a state laboratory complete a HIV Antibody Form. The consent form explains in simple terms what the presence of HIV antibody does and does not signify. It explains the uncertain medical outcome and potential social and legal implications of a positive test result. The consent form assures confidentiality, but **warns that the result is part of the patient's medical record, to which others may have access under certain conditions.** Some centers provide com-

FLORIDA: HEALTH CARE WORKER LEAKS CONFIDENTIAL HIV INFORMATION

As of October 1, 1996, the state of Florida mandated there be at least one anonymous and confidential HIV counseling and testing site in each of its 67 counties. As of January 1, 1997, all persons testing HIV positive who request health services must give up their identity.

Penalties— Any person who violates the confidentiality of the new laws commits a misdemeanor of the first degree punishable by imprisonment not to exceed one year.

Update 1997— The state of Florida delayed the identification of HIV-positive people until they are more certain that the state can assure patient confidentiality. This concern resulted from a Pinellas County health care worker who left the office, in September 1996, with a computer disk containing the names of about 4000 HIV-infected people. The disk included names of people with AIDS and other personal information, including telephone numbers, addresses, date of birth, information about how they got AIDS, and other health information. The disk was sent to the *Tampa Tribune* and the *St. Petersburg Times* newspapers! **Florida began mandatory HIV reporting in July 1997.**

---

pletely anonymous testing; this option is available to the patient and his or her physician.

The following example demonstrates one of the problems with confidential testing: A young homosexual male with signs of oral thrush agreed to an HIV test. Later that day, he called and asked that his blood **not** be sent to the lab. He was a teacher in a parochial school and feared the results would be revealed. His sample was set aside, but the laboratory courier mistakenly took it for testing. The result was positive, yet no one could tell the patient. A malpractice attorney said to make certain all records of the test were deleted and to send the patient a letter urging him to return for a blood test. He never appeared (Wake, 1989).

Many national public health agencies and committees favor a confidential screening and counseling program that includes all individuals whose behavior places them at high risk of HIV exposure. These agencies recommend that the following eight groups seriously consider volunteering for periodic HIV antibody testing:

1. Homosexual and bisexual men
2. Present or past injection drug users
3. People with signs or symptoms of HIV infection
4. Male and female prostitutes
5. Sexual partners of people either known to be HIV-infected or at increased risk of HIV infection
6. Hemophiliacs who received blood clotting products prior to 1985
7. Newborn children of HIV-infected mothers
8. Immigrants from Haiti and Central Africa since 1977

The Public's Question— The situation surrounding confidentiality for patients infected with HIV is comparable to circumstances that dictate our reporting of sexually transmitted diseases and cancer. The reason for reporting these cases to the CDC is that valuable epidemiological data may be gathered. These data can then be used to document geographical location, prevalence, routes of transmission, and those groups of people that may be at highest risk for these diseases. **If these diseases are reportable for the ultimate benefit of individuals susceptible to sexually transmitted diseases and cancer, shouldn't HIV-positive people be reportable for the same reasons?** It is questions such as this that are bringing about a change in public opinion concerning confidential HIV testing and use of test results.

Anonymous HIV Testing— No name is ever given. This is also a form of voluntary testing. It differs from confidential testing only in that those who request anonymity receive a bar coded identification number. They provide no personal information and they come back at a predetermined time to find out if their test number is positive or negative. No followup occurs. Forty-one states have anonymous test sites providing over 2 million tests a year (Nash et al., 1998 updated). Things change when the individual seeks treatment: If one goes to a doctor and the doctor does a viral load test, he reports the person and their viral load test to the health department. There is no way to keep treatment for HIV anonymous.

Blinded HIV Testing— This occurs when blood or serum is available for HIV testing as a result of another medical procedure wherein the patient's blood has been drawn for analysis. In this case, the demographic data have been recorded and can be used for epidemiological studies even if the name of the individual is withheld and a bar code is used. In 1988, the CDC asked for a blinded study of all 1989 newborn blood samples taken in certain cities in 45 states for metabolic studies. The name and other demographics of each newborn were recorded on the label of each tube. After the metabolic tests were completed, the name was changed into a bar code and leftover blood was sent to a state HIV testing center.

New York began a study of this type in 1987. Since then, New York has blind-tested about 250,000 newborns. The statewide incidence rate for HIV-infected newborns was 0.7%, or seven per 1000. (Recent anti-HIV therapy before and following birth has cut the incidence by half.)

Class Discussion: Present reasons for and against blinded testing.

HIV Testing Consent and Counseling

Requirements for consent and counseling vary from state to state. Most, but not all, states require specific informed consent—sometimes in writing—for HIV testing. Approximately one-fifth of states require pre-test counseling, with many listing specifically what that counseling must include. The U.S. Department of Health and Human Services recommends that all HIV testing include counseling that covers the test itself, basic information about HIV and AIDS, how to avoid spreading the virus, the confidentiality of the results, the possible impact of the results on the per-

son being tested, and discussion of to whom results should be disclosed, such as sex or needle-sharing partners. Counselors should also be able to give referrals to medical and psychosocial support services. Counseling and consent procedures vary greatly, remain controversial and may continue to change. Even states that require informed consent may allow HIV testing without consent in special circumstances. For example, many permit involuntary testing of a patient when health workers have been exposed to the person's blood. Some test prisoners or people accused of sex crimes, and at least four states require mandatory testing of newborns, which indirectly reveals the mother's HIV status.

PERSON-TO-PERSON: DISCLOSURE OF HIV INFECTION

Disclosure is a general term referring to the act of informing persons or authorities of an individual's serostatus or to the fact that such information has been transmitted to a third party, with or without the individual's consent. The term disclosure may be used in the context of both reporting and partner notification. Disclosure outside the health system should not but does occur through reporting of cases of HIV infection and/or of AIDS informally, either intentionally or unintentionally. Disclosure to selected individuals is of course an explicit and integral part of partner notification (discussed in Chapter 9). The decision to disclose an HIV diagnosis is a complex issue for those infected. Although research has shown that suppressing difficult emotions and thoughts can be damaging to one's physical and emotional health, sharing an HIV diagnosis with others can also be stigmatizing and potentially damaging due to society's views of the illness. Negative emotional consequences of disclosure have shown to include rejection, abandonment, and isolation. Nevertheless, disclosure is an issue that all patients face because it is a prerequisite for proper health care and, in many cases, necessary for the receipt of appropriate emotional support from others.

Should I Tell? Michael Stein (1998) surveyed 129 patients, (89 men, 40 women) at two eastern urban hospitals, seeking their first primary care for HIV infection, that had sex in the past six months. They were asked if they had disclosed their HIV infection to their sex partners. **Forty percent said they did not inform their sexual partners.** And of these 40%, over half (58%) did **not** use a condom all the time. The survey subjects were mostly poor, often illegal drug users, and commonly lacked high school education, but researchers believe withholding HIV information is widespread. Among those surveyed, 46% were black, 23% were Hispanic and 27% were white. Whites and Hispanics were three times more likely to tell partners than blacks. Subjects with only one sexual partner were three times more likely to have told their partners than subjects with multiple partners. "The public health message is that if you are not absolutely sure of the HIV status of your partner, you should be having safer sex."

Reasons for Nondisclosure: risk of rejection, stigmatization, revealing sexual orientation, revealing IDU, and breach of privacy that could lead to loss of employment, housing, and insurance.

Class Discussion: Provide other reasons for nondisclosure.

BOX 12.6

CONFIDENTIALITY AND SEXUAL PARTNER BETRAYAL

This story took place in an HIV/AIDS clinic in the South. A husband and wife came into the clinic for an HIV test. They said the **only** reason for requesting the test was that they wanted to begin a family and hoped that nothing in their past would have led to either of them being HIV positive. The tests were completed.

The husband came in on a Monday; the wife came in that Friday.

Monday A.M.

Counselor: Mr. X, your test came back HIV positive.

Reactions and counseling were similar to those presented in this chapter. Then Mr. X said he wanted to be the one to tell his wife; **he insisted on it.** The counselor agreed, Mr. X left the clinic agreeing to come back for a follow-up counseling session.

Friday A.M.

Counselor: Mrs. X, your HIV test was negative.

Mrs. X: That's wonderful news. I can't wait to tell my husband. We've been waiting for my results. I want to get pregnant immediately.

Mrs. X received HIV-negative counseling and left the clinic very happy.

Clearly, the husband did not tell his wife the truth about his test results. A follow-up phone call to the husband went unanswered; so did a letter from the clinic. Several months later, Mrs. X called the counselor to tell her that she was pregnant!

Question: What do you think the counselor should do now?

1. Inform the woman about her husband.
2. Take no action.
3. Call the husband and discuss the situation.
4. Threaten the husband with legal action if he does not tell his wife.
5. Your position?

Discuss the moral, ethical, and legal responsibilities of each participant.

SUMMARY

HIV infection can be detected in three ways: first, by HIV-antibody or antigen testing prior to the signs and symptoms of AIDS; second, by detecting the presence of HIV nucleic acid; and third, by physical examination after symptoms occur.

The test most often used to screen donor blood at blood banks and individuals referred to testing centers is the ELISA test. ELISA (enzyme-linked immunosorbent assay) is a highly sensitive and specific test that determines the presence of HIV antibodies in a person's blood or serum. The ELISA test was first used in 1985 to reduce the number of HIV-infected blood units for blood transfusions.

Because the ELISA test is only a predictive test that gives the percentage chance that a person is truly positive or truly negative, serum from those who test positive is retested in duplicate. If still positive, the serum is then subjected to a Western blot (WB) test. The WB is a confirmatory test. If it is also positive, the person is said to be HIV-infected.

Other screening and confirmatory tests are available. The indirect immunofluorescent antibody assay (IFA) is relatively quick and easy to perform. Although it can be used as a screening test, it is generally used as a confirmatory test. The test is similar to the ELISA test except that the analysis is made by looking for a fluorescent color, indicating the presence of HIV antibodies, with a dark field light microscope.

Rapid HIV test kits require no special equipment and can be performed in less than 10 minutes. These tests are a major contribution in Third World countries that do not have the equipment or trained personnel to run ELISA and WB tests. The CDC recently (mid-1998) encouraged physicians to use such tests in the United States.

The polymerase chain reaction (PCR) is a process wherein a few molecules of HIV proviral DNA can be amplified into a sufficient mass of DNA to be detected by current testing methods. It can determine if newborns of HIV-infected mothers are truly HIV positive. The branched-DNA assay offers a means of detecting the presence of HIV RNA directly within the clinical sample.

Gene probes are also being used to detect small HIV proviral DNA sequences in cells of people who are HIV-infected but not yet making antibodies.

REVIEW QUESTIONS

(Answers to the Review Questions are on page 489.)

1. What is the acronym for the most commonly used HIV-antibody test and what does each letter stand for?

2. What basic immunological assumption is this test based on?

3. Does a single positive HIV antibody result mean the person is HIV-infected? Explain.

4. Is there a specific test for AIDS? Explain.

5. What is currently the most frequently used HIV confirmatory test in the United States?

6. What is the name of one additional confirmatory test in use in the United States?

7. How is HIV antibody detected in the ELISA test?

8. True or False: All newborns who are antibody positive are HIV-infected and all go on to develop AIDS. Explain.

9. What is the greatest shortcoming of the ELISA and WB tests?

10. What are the two major problems in interpreting ELISA test results?

11. What two factors may account for false positive and false negative results?

12. What is the relationship between false positive results and prevalence of HIV in the population?

13. In an HIV screening test, what is a positive predictive value? Why is it called a predictive value?

14. What is the current gold standard of confirmatory tests in the United States?

15. What is the major problem in using this test?

16. Why is the polymerase chain reaction (PCR) considered so useful in HIV testing? Name two situations when PCR can be significant in HIV testing.

17. True or False: Two home-use HIV antibody test kits are now available in the United States.

18. Using the ELISA test, when are HIV antibodies first detectable?

19. How early are HIV antigens detectable in human serum?

20. What are three benefits of early identification of HIV-infected people?

21. Name the four kinds of testing privacy available to people who want to take an HIV test.

22. What is the major difference between an anonymous and a blind HIV test?

23. Why would someone want an anonymous test?

24. True or False: The ELISA serological test is adequate to confirm HIV infection.

25. True or False: Pre- and post-HIV-antibody test counseling is recommended any time an HIV-antibody test is performed.

13
AIDS and Society: Knowledge, Attitudes, and Behavior

In the end, they will say, we died not at the hands of our enemies, but in the silence of our friends.

Martin Luther King

THE NEW MILLENNIUM AND HIV/AIDS

HIV/AIDS is becoming more of a global disaster with each passing year of the new millennium. This disaster will be with us for many years to come, perhaps lifetimes to come—like smallpox, the Bubonic Plague, cholera, and other diseases from ancient times. It does not appear that there are any new surprises that scientists are about to spring on this virus—but this virus continues to surprise our best scientists. HIV just keeps spinning its genetic building blocks looking for its next jackpot—how to overcome the next onslaught of antiretroviral drugs. Those jackpots keep coming up and the virus is winning the drug war. In developed nations, like America, too many people think the AIDS crisis is over—they have been fooled by erroneous television and press coverage. Globally in 2002, 3 million people died of AIDS and 5.3 million new infections occurred. But wait, estimated numbers of AIDS deaths and new infections for 2003 and 2004 are even higher!

AIDS in the new millennium is like a train heading toward a horrific wreck. As the train gains speed, the global rate of HIV infections increases. As T4 or CD4+ cells drop, the distance to the wreck becomes shorter; on impact millions more will have died of AIDS. Like the **Energizer bunny,** HIV infections keep on going and going and . . .

AIDS COALITION TO UNLEASH POWER: ACT UP

June of 2003 marked the 22nd anniversary of the first official report that a deadly new illness was showing up in young men. All those initially reported were gay men suffering from a previously unseen form of severe immune deficiency. In subsequent weeks and months, the illness that was initially known as Gay-Related Immune Deficiency (GRID) and eventually called AIDS began to reveal itself in additional reports, particularly through the discovery of groups of men exhibiting an otherwise rare form of cancer known as Kaposi's Sarcoma. This was the beginning and recognition of an unfolding global tragedy to come. To remember or recall the beginning of this pandemic in America is to recognize and honor the generation of people who fought so hard to build the organizations, tools, and the scientific and political support for confronting the newly recognized disease. The gay, lesbian, and transgender communities and their heterosexual supporters must be acknowledged for their immediate, aggressive, and humanitarian response to AIDS. Years before government was ready to accept its rightful role, these communities were caring for the sick, fighting for treatment and research, and making remarkable changes in personal and organizational behavior to curb the risk of AIDS. Their efforts and accomplishments are without precedent in modern medical history. In years past, an AIDS action group called ACT UP (AIDS to Unleash Power) under its mantra, "Silence = Death," urged people to get out there and raise hell because nobody else is doing anything about this disease. In order to promote prevention, they draped a 35-foot condom over Republican Jesse Helms' house, scattered the ashes of people who died of AIDS on the White House lawn, and tossed a coffin in front of a San Francisco hospital after an AIDS patient was denied a liver transplant. And these were some of the milder forms of protest. But it took these actions to get the attention of mainstream America and its politicians. Today's more recently infected people may not recognize the names of those who demonstrated in the streets, stopped meetings, defied government policies, and demanded adequate research funding and better medicines for this new disease, but they should know that without the efforts of these early warriors in the AIDS battle, the nationwide infrastructure of AIDS care, prevention and treatment education would be much less than it is. It is the successes achieved by gay empowered ACT UP that later empowered women and heterosexuals to demand action for better drugs and a government commitment to finding an HIV vaccine, and which served as model for international AIDS activism that has recently achieved great price reductions in HIV/AIDS drugs for their countries. ACT UP has also served as a model for people with other diseases, like female breast cancer, to form action groups to demand more from their government.

Whatever weakness and failings exist in the current structures, they do provide structures to build and improve upon. Those who have passed on have left a legacy that can serve as a guide in the future as the epidemic cuts its way through new groups around the world.

HIV/AIDS IS AN UNUSUAL DISEASE

AIDS, like other severe epidemics in America, has a powerful social force that has allowed it to become established and that has promoted its rapid spread. But this disease is unique in the sense that it seems to track the fault lines in our society and profits from the social flaws and weaknesses inherent in societies in transition. The spread of AIDS is determined by very powerful social and economic factors. (See Federal Response to AIDS—end of chapter).

The epidemic is not afflicting us because of chance or bad luck. HIV was destined to spread because of specific social and economic factors. HIV is mainly sexually transmitted and therefore closely associated with and intertwined in people's relationships. The forces in our society that promote lasting and loyal relationships, unity, social order, and stable family and community life inhibit epidemics. The forces inherent in a disordered social environment, in which there is a high degree of family and community instability, where individual and community stress is high, and where significant numbers of people are dislocated from their homes and families, serve to aid the spread of this disease. AIDS is a schizophrenic condition. It is a pandemic worldwide, but it has not yet fully emerged. It often promotes stigma and rejection at the very time when people need comfort, compassion, and support. Stigma and discrimination further serve to propagate the disease because in this climate individuals do not feel confident or free to disclose their status, often not even to their sexual partners or their spouses. The disease remains silent and spreads relentlessly. HIV is transmitted through our most creative and spiritual potential, our ability to create life. It is also passed in the breast milk of mothers to their newborn infants; the very food of life can sow seeds of death. These spiritual connections can trigger negative and harmful perceptions and thoughts, promoting the concept that this epidemic is God's punishment to the wicked and to the sexually immoral. These can easily be translated into negative actions, blame, and rejection, further serving to keep the epidemic hidden and invisible, and fostering continued denial of the problem and its spread. Unlike most other terminal or life-threatening diseases, this one affects mainly the young and middle-aged adults, the adults on whom we all depend; they drive the economy, they parent and teach the children, they care for the sick, and keep the planes and trains running on time.

AIDS IS HERE TO STAY

The past 22 years of the global AIDS pandemic have taught us that HIV disease is a **permanent part of life on planet Earth. HIV is simultaneously a virus and a phenomenon.** When it is viewed only as a virus, it is hard to see why HIV prevention is a problem. People normally want to avoid harming themselves and others. When viewed as a phenomenon, HIV points to the many personal and societal causes of disease transmission. It points to the difficulties people have in making their intentions match their behavior. It points to the inequalities in relationships, which help to spread HIV. It points to societies' reluctance to prepare young people to manage their intimate relations, to admit to sexual diversity, to responsibly manage complex health and social

problems such as drug abuse, and to provide access to health care. It points to the world's failure to care about improving living conditions in poor countries.

AIDS

Acquired Immune Deficiency Syndrome (AIDS) is an illness characterized, according to CDC criteria, as the presence of antibody to HIV and a T4 cell count of less than $200/\mu$ L of blood, or by the presence of HIV and certain opportunistic infections and diseases that affect both the body and brain.

AIDS was first described in the United States in 1981. Who would have thought then that 22 years later about 70 million people or about 1 in every 100 people on planet Earth would be infected with the virus that causes AIDS? And that this virus, regardless of the involvement of the world's governments, the best scientists, and the expenditure of about $275 billion just in America, continues to spread out of control in many nations of the world. There is no way at the present time to prevent the 5 to 6 million new HIV infections each year. No drugs offer a cure, and most of the 42 million living with HIV-infected cannot afford and will not receive those drugs that offer **some** temporary improved quality of life. An HIV-preventative vaccine **now** is wishful thinking. But, there is one commodity in plentiful supply—BLAME—**enough for everyone, everywhere.**

SIDEBAR 13.1

A MOTHER'S NIGHTMARE

Recently, at a bus stop, a woman saw a man walking toward her. The man was so thin she could see his face, leg, and arm bones. His eyes were sunken and sad. As he got closer, she recognized it was her son! Her only son! He was living in the streets, an injection drug user; he told her he was dying of AIDS. She was too stunned to be hurt, she just put her arms around him and let him cry.

There are some things mothers can fix—this wasn't one of them. But she set out trying to find him a place to live and a doctor to care for him. At age 35, her son is watching himself shrink into an old man. His mother, age 61, wonders how she will pay for his burial.

BLAME SOMEONE, DÉJÀ VU

The greater **hostility** and greatest **stigma** tends to be assigned to diseases in which individuals are seen as responsible for having the disease; in which the disease's course is fatal; in which fear of transmission is a major issue; and in which the disease leads to highly visible and frightening physical expressions. All these conditions are associated with HIV disease and AIDS. With AIDS more than any other disease in history, people have found verbal mechanisms for distancing themselves from thoughts of personal infection. Worldwide, from the onset of this pandemic, people have learned in a relatively short time to **categorize, rationalize, stigmatize,** and **persecutize** those with HIV disease and AIDS. AIDS statistics are published in categories to identify how many gay or bisexual men, injection drug users, persons with hemophilia, and so on, have developed AIDS. Also listed are the countries, states, and cities with the highest incidence of the disease, along with which racial and ethnic groups are highest among reported AIDS cases. **By focusing on categories of people, have we made it possible for society to rationalize that AIDS belongs to somebody else? Have we made the thought of HIV/AIDS somewhat impersonal? HAVE WE FOUND A WAY TO BLAME SOMEONE ELSE?**

Placing blame does not always require reason and tends to focus on people who are not considered normal by the majority. Thus, minorities and foreigners are often singled out to blame for something, sometimes anything. Epidemics of plague, smallpox, leprosy, syphilis, cholera, tuberculosis, and influenza have historically focused social blame onto specific groups of people for spreading the diseases by their "deviant" behavior. Blaming others leads to their stigmatization and persecution.

While the Black Death, an epidemic of Bubonic Plague, swept across Europe in the 14th century, blame was variously attached to Jews and witches, followed by the massacre and burning of the alleged culprits. In Massachusetts between 1692 and 1693, some 20 people were hanged or burned at the stake after being accused of having the powers of the devil. Eighty percent of those accused were women. When Hitler blamed Jews, communists, homosexuals, and other **undesirables** for the economic stagnation of Germany in the 1930s, the result was death camps and ultimately the second World War. Now there is a new plague—HIV/AIDS. **What blame comes packaged with this new disease?**

Jonathan Mann, former head of the World Health Organization's Global Program on AIDS, said in 1998 that there are really three HIV/AIDS epidemics, which are in fact phases in the invasion of a community by the AIDS virus.

First is the epidemic of silent infection by HIV, often completely unnoticed. **Second,** after a period of incubation/clinical latency that may last for years, is the epidemic of the disease itself, with an estimated total of 26 million AIDS deaths worldwide beginning 2003.

Third, and perhaps equally important as the disease itself, is the epidemic of social, cultural, economic, and political reaction to HIV/AIDS. **The willingness of each generation to place blame on others when believable explanations are not readily available simply recycles history. We have been there before; we have placed blame on others and it will continue.** With respect to the HIV/AIDS pandemic, blame has been disseminated among nations. There is no shortage of political, economic, social, or ethical issues associated with this **new** disease.

FEAR: PANIC AND HYSTERIA OVER THE SPREAD OF HIV/AIDS IN THE UNITED STATES

With the 1981 announcement by the U.S. Public Health Service and the CDC that there was a new disease, AIDS quickly became a symbol for our darkest fears. Responsible public officials gave out conflicting messages: **reassurance** on one hand and **alarm** on the other. **Public panic and hysteria began.**

People with HIV disease and AIDS are still abused, ridiculed, and maligned. Some people believe that AIDS is divine retribution for immoral lifestyles. People who have not indulged in high-risk lifestyles (for example, newborns and recipients of blood products) continue to be labeled as **innocent victims,** implying perhaps that other HIV-infected individuals are guilty of the behavior that led to their infection and therefore deserve their illness.

Families and communities continue to be divided on their beliefs and acceptance of HIV/AIDS patients. Federal and state agencies stand accused of a lack of commitment and compassion in the war against AIDS. The bottom line is that **value judgments** are associated with HIV/AIDS because the disease involves the most private areas of people's lives—**sex, pregnancy, drug use, and finances.**

The Fear Factor

Worldwide, the political, medical, and legal communities used the media or vice versa, to scare people about a new disease called AIDS. **The result has been to scare people into fearing other people rather than the disease.** For example, a 1990 survey of 1000 black American church members in five cities found that more than one-third of them believed the AIDS virus was produced in a germ warfare laboratory as a form of genocide against blacks.

Another third said they were **unsure** whether the virus was created to kill blacks. That left only one-third who disputed the theory.

These findings held firm even among educated individuals. Rumors that AIDS was created to kill blacks have circulated in the black community for years, and the belief is still endorsed by some black leaders.

A poster in the Swiss STOP AIDS Campaign focuses on how we think about people with AIDS:

> For the doctors, I am HIV-positive; for some neighbors, I am AIDS-contaminated; for my friends, I am Claude-Eric.

Soon after young homosexual men began dying in large numbers, a barrage of frightening rhetoric began filling the airwaves, television, the popular press, and even the most reputable scientific journals. The AIDS disaster was here. One health care administrator stated, **"We have not seen anything of this magnitude that we can't control except nuclear bombs."**

In 1986, Myron Essex of the Department of Cancer Biology at the Harvard School of Public Health noted,

> The Centers for Disease Control and Prevention (CDC) has been trying to inform the public without overly alarming them, but we outside the government are freer to speak. The fact is that the dire predictions of those who have cried doom

ever since AIDS appeared haven't been far off the mark . . . The effects of the virus are far wider than most people realize. It has shown up not just in blood and semen but in brain tissue, vaginal secretions, and even saliva and tears, although there's no evidence that it's transmitted by the last two.

In 1987, columnist Jack Anderson reported that the Central Intelligence Agency (CIA) concluded that in just a few years heterosexual AIDS cases would *outnumber* homosexual cases in the United States. Also in 1987, Otis Bowen, former secretary of health and human services, said AIDS would make the Black Death that wiped out one-third of Europe's population in the Middle Ages pale by comparison. In 1988, sex researchers William Masters, Virginia Johnson, and Robert Kolodny stated in their book, *New Directions in the AIDS Crisis: The Heterosexual Community,* that there was a possibility of HIV infection via casual transmission—from toilet seats, handling of contact lenses from an AIDS patient, eating a salad in a restaurant prepared by a person with AIDS, or from instruments in a physician's office used to examine AIDS patients.

In contrast to these reports is the 1988 article by Robert Gould in *Cosmopolitan* reassuring women that there is practically no risk of becoming HIV-infected through ordinary vaginal or oral sex even with an HIV-infected male. The vaginal secretions produced during sexual arousal keep the virus from penetrating the vaginal walls. His explanation was: **"Nature has arranged this so that sex will feel good and be good for you."**

Reaction Based on Fear

In December 1997, a male entered a bar and held a syringe full of blood against a female patron's throat. He said the blood contained HIV. He demanded money. He was caught and charged with robbery and attempted murder, pending the outcome of HIV tests of the blood from the syringe. **The man felt the fear of AIDS would be sufficient to rob the bar.**

In Taiwan, people with HIV have been hired to work as debt collectors. The widespread fear of HIV/AIDS is being used to force people to pay their debts. The HIV-infected need a job and the loan agency needed a clever way to get their money back. The loan agency believes it's a proper business agreement.

Fear of AIDS is understandable, given that AIDS is fatal and is communicable. AIDS appeared suddenly and spread quickly—it took a number of years to identify the virus that causes it and the mechanisms for spread. Yet, today the routes of transmission are well established and widely known, as are the precautionary measures that can be taken to prevent its spread. Early on, fear of AIDS took an unhealthy turn, anxieties are projected on to those who are hit the hardest by the disease, and the fear of AIDS became an irrational fear of people with AIDS.

ACTIONS OF COURAGE

There are far too many heroes of this pandemic to list here, and the heroes come from every walk of life and profession. So many have answered the call for help, compassion, and human kindness. But there are a few examples that might be considered either sufficiently different or unusual enough to mention. And although unusual, even these actions have been demonstrated by many.

First, in 1979, when gay pride was rising, a teenage male took a male friend to the prom in Sioux Falls, South Dakota. The national media were there to record the moment; the camera lights glared as he and his date danced; gay activists were elated. It was the first time a same-sex

couple had been allowed to attend an American prom. This male couple faded into obscurity—until January 1993. **His death from AIDS was reported to the CDC.**

The next examples of courage are about two courageous teenagers. He was a husky eighth-grader from Missouri who wore a peace symbol around his neck and was diagnosed with HIV in the summer of 1991. He recalled the day his mother called him into the house to give him the news. "I was getting ready to play baseball. I said, 'Does this mean I'm going to die?' She said, 'Not today.' I said, 'Can I go play baseball now?'"

He had problems with prejudice. For example, a few parents in neighboring towns didn't want their children to play against his baseball team. **"I quit the team because I didn't think it was fair for them to not get to play because of me."**

A 14-year-old girl in Detroit who goes by the nickname of Slim has very grown-up responsibilities at home.

"It's hard, but I won't show you or let you see my pain," she said. "I was always taught to be strong."

She's had to be. Her mother, a single parent, died of AIDS. Later she learned that her sisters were also infected.

One sister died in April of 1993 at age 9. Then in November, her 6-month-old sister died. Her third sister died.

Through it all, she has been responsible for giving medications and intravenous feedings to everybody, around the clock.

"I want people to know what's going on. But I don't want anyone's pity."

WHOM IS THE GENERAL PUBLIC TO BELIEVE?

Because of the complexity of HIV disease, a great deal of press coverage of AIDS issues reflects what scientists say to journalists. A journalist's responsibility is to check that the facts are accurate, but not necessarily to judge their overall merit. Why should a good story be spiked just because other scientists disagree with the data interpretation? **When scientists say contradictory things to the public, how can the public assess whom to believe?** Science has a duty to inform and educate the public, but it must neither frighten people unnecessarily nor give them unjustified expectations. Claims of **"AIDS cures"** in the popular press need to be based on much more than just test tube data. **Whatever the need to attract research funding, is five minutes of fame ever worth a day of fear or weeks of false hopes for many?** The popular press has provided HIV-infected persons with a roller coaster ride between hopelessness and fantasies of imminent cure.

As a result of journalistic promises, there was and still is a range of emotions that run from real hope of a cure to public panic and hysteria. In at least five states, children with AIDS were barred from attending local public schools. The case of 12-year-old Ryan White of Kokomo, Indiana, was made into a TV movie, *The Ryan White Story,* in 1989.

BOX 13.1

EXAMPLES OF UNCONTROLLED FEAR AND HOSTILITY

In September 1985, in Stamford, Connecticut, a murder suspect with AIDS is escorted into court by police wearing rubber gloves. Fourteen prospective jurors promptly asked to be removed from the case for fear of catching AIDS from being in the same room. In Atlanta, November 1985, a man develops a nosebleed while being driven to a jail in a squad car. After he tells police that he has AIDS he is rushed to the hospital and the car is quarantined for 21 days.

In 1986, a very ill AIDS patient on an airline flight spilled some urine from a drainage bag on the seats and carpet. After the patient deplaned, several rows of seats around the area were taped off; the contaminated area would be removed. Crew members and airline union leaders expressed outrage at the exposure of passengers and crew to this threat. The clean-up crew refused to remove the carpet, even using rubber gloves.

BUT WE HAVE LEARNED SINCE THEN, RIGHT? **WRONG!**

In April 1993, an American Airlines flight crew requested that all pillows and blankets be changed on a plane that carried a group described by an internal communication as "gay rights activists." A representative for American Airlines apologized saying that such action was completely and totally inappropriate and that American Airlines has a strict policy against discrimination of any individual or group. **But it happened.**

In June of 1995 a delegation of 50 gay and lesbian elected officials was met at the White House by uniformed Secret Service officers wearing rubber gloves. The officers were apparently concerned about the risk of infection from HIV.

CAN IT HAPPEN AGAIN? In September 1997 his sister told ambulance personnel that her sick brother had AIDS and had to go to a specific county hospital. They said they could **not** go outside their county line. She called a multi-county ambulance service. After arrival,

neither ambulance service personnel would go near her brother. Her young daughter held an oxygen mask on him while she drove him to the hospital. He died later that evening. The sister filed an AIDS discrimination suit against the ambulance services. (Case pending)

SURELY NOT IN 1998! In September 1998 a federal judge barred the eviction of an HIV-positive man who was to be evicted from public housing. The infected male is suing the manager of a federally subsidized housing complex. The manager is said to have told people that she did not want the complex contaminated with AIDS.

In Cleveland, **November 1998,** a black American sex worker was forced, as part of his plea bargain, to appear on an NBC-affiliated TV station WKYC to identify himself as a person living with HIV. The judge said her goal with the unusual sentencing was to protect the public. In **December 1998, Gugu Dlamini of South Africa was beaten to death the day after she revealed that she was HIV positive during a commemoration of World AIDS Day, December 1, 1998.** She was one of many unsung heroes of the daily struggle against HIV. Her death reminds us how stigmatizing the disease AIDS still is, and how much courage it takes for people with HIV to be open about their condition because fear still controls people's behavior.

In **Colonial Heights, Virginia, February 1999,** the 4th U.S. Circuit Court of Appeals found that although the Americans With Disabilities Act prohibits discrimination against people with AIDS, the law does not require **U.S.A. Bushidokan,** in Colonial Heights, to accept **Michael Montalvo,** then 14, for its Japanese-style sparring classes. Michael was 12 when he attempted to join the karate school. The owners barred him from class after learning about his HIV infection. The decision drew criticism from AIDS groups, which said it reflects fear rather than legitimate health concerns. An AIDS Action leader said,

---

BOX 13.1 *(continued)*

"Communities are right to become concerned about HIV, but cases like this detract from giving young people the information they need and give a false sense of how it is transmitted." The Montalvos, who have since **moved out of Virginia** because they believe public disclosure of Michael's infection led to discrimination, plan to appeal to the U.S. Supreme Court.

December 1999—Mercy Makhalemele of Kwamashu, South Africa, told her husband that she was HIV positive. He shoved her into a pot of boiling water, scalding her. But she still had to go to her job selling shoes. Her husband came to her job and told her to go home, get her things, and leave him. He could not live with someone with HIV. That was 10 A.M. By 3 P.M.

she was fired from her job. Adding to all this, her only child, age 2-and-a-half, was diagnosed with AIDS. She was unable to find treatment for her. Her child died thereafter.

February 2000—The *Los Angeles Times* reported on the death of **Israeli** pop star **Ofra Haza.** She died of AIDS. Her condition and death were a closely guarded family secret because of the stigma associated with an AIDS death in Israel.

The way people with HIV are treated is likely to continue to be based more on fear, prejudice, and judgmentalism than on the facts of science. Supreme Court rulings are not going to change that. What the courts do, however, is make it absolutely clear that such prejudicial behavior will not be legally tolerated.

In some localities, police officers and health care workers put rubber gloves on before apprehending a drug user or wear full cover protective suits when called to the scene of an accident. In other communities, church members, out of fear of HIV infection, have declined communion wine from the common cup.

Since the epic announcement in 1981, HIV/AIDS has refashioned America. HIV/AIDS is a disease molded to the times, one that has wedged apart the thinly concealed fault lines of American society by striking hardest at the outcasts—gay men, injection drug users, prostitutes, and impoverished whites, blacks, and Hispanics. **HIV/AIDS has brought forth uncomfortable questions about sex, sex education, homosexuality, the poor, and minorities.** The disease has inevitably polarized the people, accentuating both the best and worst worldwide. Many churches, schools, and communities have responded to the new disease with compassion and tolerance; others have displayed hate and reprisals of the worst kind.

As Camus wrote in *The Plague,* **"The first thing (the epidemic) brought . . . was exile." Anyone who carried the disease could inspire terror. They became pariahs in society.**

People with hate in their hearts torched the house of the Ray family and their three HIV-positive hemophilic children in Arcadia, Florida. Someone shot a bullet through the window of Ryan White's home to let the teenager know he should not attend the local high school. After he died,

his 6-foot, 8-inch gravestone was overturned four times and a car ran over his grave!

Early on, the federal government and its public health apparatus showed little interest in the HIV/AIDS epidemic. **Former president Ronald Reagan never once met with former Surgeon General C. Everett Koop to talk about AIDS despite Koop's pleas.** Koop said, "If AIDS had struck legionnaires or Boy Scouts, there's no question the response would have been very different."

By the time former president of the United States Ronald Reagan delivered his first speech on the AIDS crisis in 1987 over 40,000 men, women and children had been diagnosed with AIDS and over 28,000 Americans had died of AIDS. Recently released documents from the Reagan's administration show that the president's delay in addressing the AIDS issue was based on the perceived "political risk" in doing so. It took nine years and over 115,000 AIDS deaths before the U.S. Congress and former president George Bush enacted the nation's first comprehensive AIDS-care funding package— the Ryan White CARE Act (1990).

The primary purpose of the act is to provide emergency financial assistance to localities that are disproportionately affected by the human immunodeficiency virus epidemic. An eligible metropolitan area (EMA) is any metropolitan area for which there have been reported to the CDC a cumulative total of more than 2000 acquired immune deficiency syndrome (AIDS) cases for the most recent five years for which data are available. The amended act requires formula grants based on the estimated number of persons living with AIDS in the EMA. Estimates were derived by using methods specified in the act. The amount of funds received by each EMA (under Title I) or state (under Title II) is determined by the locality's proportion of the total estimated number of living persons with AIDS.

Misconceptions About AIDS Linger

Despite widespread reports that casual contact does not spread the virus, families have walked out of restaurants that employed gay waiters and hospital workers have quit rather than treat HIV/AIDS patients.

In 1989, a man was barred in Anderson, Indiana, from coaching his daughter's intramural basketball team because he had been diagnosed with AIDS. The 37-year-old father received the virus in a blood transfusion during open heart surgery in 1984.

POINT OF VIEW 13.1

A SOUTHERN UNIVERSITY STUDENT'S EXPERIENCE

A southern university student taking a senior semester course on HIV/AIDS in 1999, experienced firsthand the fear-related ignorance that still exists.

This student had accompanied her friend to the office of a physician in a nearby small town. While the student was in the waiting room, she was using the time to read the given class assignment in her textbook, **AIDS Update 1999**. People coming into the office would **look over** at the empty chairs on each side of her—then look at her and decide to sit elsewhere. Even as the office filled and fewer and fewer seats were available, no one chose to sit near her. She said, "People took one look at the book and chose another seat some distance from me." She said, **"So much for education on nontransmission of HIV by casual contact!"**

UPDATE—Since placing this event in this book, students in each of my HIV/AIDS courses through 2002 have experienced similar discrimination while reading their AIDS UPDATE book in a beauty salon, and in the office waiting rooms of a physician, veterinarian, optometrist, and a car wash.

Each example points out that regardless of education, the public still assumes the virus can be casually transmitted. **IT IS FEAR THAT IS BEING TRANSMITTED BY CASUAL CONTACT—NOT THE VIRUS.** How would you react if a good friend, classmate, or co-worker told you he or she was HIV positive? What if you found out that your child's schoolmate, a hemophiliac, had AIDS? What if you were told this child had emotional problems or a biting habit? What if your work put you in direct physical contact with people who might be HIV positive?

An AIDS diagnosis for one person resulted in his physician's refusal to treat him, his roommate left him, his friends no longer visited him, his attorney advised him to find another attorney, and his clergyman failed to support him. They were all afraid of **"catching" AIDS.** In another case, a mother whose young son has AIDS sent cupcakes to his classmates on his birthday. School officials would not permit the children to eat the cupcakes. The elementary school principal said **the school had a policy against homemade food because it could spread diseases such as AIDS.**

In Jacksonville, Florida Leanza Cornett (Miss America 1993) using her reign as a national platform to teach about AIDS, was told by public school officials not to use the word **condom** while addressing student groups. In Bradford County, Florida, she was told she could not mention the name of the disease (AIDS) in three elementary schools she planned to visit.

In Hinton, West Virginia, one woman was killed by three bullets and her body dumped along a remote road. Another was beaten to death, run over by a car, and left in the gutter. Each woman had AIDS and told people so. And each, authorities say, was killed because she had AIDS. Lawyers and advocates for AIDS patients say the similar slayings, two counties and six months apart, illustrate AIDS' arrival in the American countryside and the fear and ignorance it can unearth.

In Calcutta, India, October 2000, the body of a 45-year-old male who died of AIDS laid in the morgue of a hospital for 45 days because undertakers refused to take it for cremation. The "doms"—low-caste Hindus who take bodies for cremation—refused to remove the corpse after learning that he died from AIDS. Some of the doms threatened to stop work unless the body was removed immediately by someone else.

India accounts for 60% of HIV cases in Asia and 20% of the world's HIV infections. But AIDS awareness is still extremely limited and the HIV-infected are more often than not ostracized by their families and local communities. The fear and stigma associated with HIV/AIDS has no boundaries.

What Do We Know?— Beginning year 2003 and 22 years of the AIDS epidemic, it is clear that the scare headlines and tactics lack substance. From what has been learned about the biology of HIV, it appears that the virus is not casually nor easily spread but it has reached the magnitude of the great plagues and a vaccine has not yet been found!

AIDS Epidemic Parallels the Syphilis Epidemic in the United States— The social and medical history of the AIDS epidemic parallels the syphilis epidemic. It was feared that syphilis was casually transmitted via pens, pencils, toilet seats, toothbrushes, towels, bedding, medical procedures, and kissing. Immediate concern about casual transmission indicates the depth of human fears about disease and sexuality. Concerns about hygiene, contamination, contagion, pain, and death are expressions of anxieties that reveal much about contemporary society.

Fallout from AIDS: The Spector of Discrimination— The biggest difference between HIV/AIDS and other diseases is the larger amount of social discrimination. Society does not reject those with cancer, diabetes, heart disease, or **any** other health problems to the degree that it rejects people with HIV disease or AIDS.

The AIDS pandemic has taught people about risk behavioral groups, homosexuals in particular. In some, this has promoted tolerance and understanding; in others, it has reinforced feelings of hatred. Information on HIV disease and AIDS, how it is spread and how to prevent becoming infected has, over the past 20 years, become a part of TV talk shows, movies, TV advertisements, and newspaper and magazine articles.

Phil Donohue, host of a former popular TV show, said **"On *Donohue,* we're discussing body cavities and membranes and anal sex and vaginal lesions. We've discussed the consequences of a woman's swallowing her partner's semen. No way would we have brought that up five years ago. It's the kind of thing that makes a lot of people gag."**

The language, photography, and art work used by the media are explicit and have upset certain religious groups. They believe that open use of language about condoms, homosexuality, anal sex, oral sex, vaginal sex, and so on promotes promiscuity.

CLASS QUESTION: How can people learn to prevent HIV infection and AIDS without talking about sexual behavior and injection drug use? Does it seem at times as if opponents of sex education would rather have people suffer with AIDS than have them learn about sex?

Regardless of who is correct, few could have predicted in 1980 the casualness with which these topics are now presented in the media. If the AIDS pandemic has done nothing else, it surely has affected the nature of public discourse. In 1987, prior to the TV broadcast of the **National AIDS Awareness Test,** viewers were warned of objectionable material. By 1990, few if any such viewer warnings were given. It is as if to say that no one can afford to be ignorant of this information because it may save your life.

How Can Information Help?— There is great hope that information will lead the nation past its social prejudice and forward to compassion for those who are HIV-infected or have AIDS. More than any disease before, AIDS has proved that ignorance leads to fear and information can lead to compassion. **The need for compassion is great.**

Admiral James Watkins, chairman of the 1988 Presidential Commission on the HIV Epidemic, reported that "33% to 50% of physicians in some of our major hospitals would not touch an AIDS patient with a ten-foot pole."

A friend of a dying AIDS patient who was in the hospital with pneumocystic pneumonia went to visit him. As he was leaving, his dying friend said, **"Thank you for coming—thank you for touching me."** He said, "I can't even imagine being at a point in my life that I would be so grateful for someone touching me, that I would have to say thank you."

It would appear that although biotechnology has provided methods of HIV detection, new drugs, and hope for a vaccine, human emotional responses have not changed much from those demonstrated during previous epidemics like the plague, cholera, influenza, and syphilis.

—— BOX 13.2 ——

HOW SOME PEOPLE RESPONDED AFTER LEARNING THAT SOMEONE HAD AIDS

VIGNETTES ON COMMUNITY BEHAVIOR AND AIDS

In **Colorado Springs, Colorado,** Scott Allen's wife, Lydia, had contracted HIV from a blood transfusion hours before son Matthew was born. A second son Bryan was also born before Lydia learned of her HIV infection. Scott wasn't infected, but was **dismissed** as minister of education at First Christian Church in Colorado Springs when he sought his pastor's consolation. Matt was **kicked out** of the church's day care center and the family was told to find another church.

When the family moved to Dallas and moved in with Scott's father, Allen, and his wife, church after church refused to enroll Matt in Sunday school. **Allen, a former president of the Southern Baptist Convention** wrote in his book, *Burden of a Secret: A Story of Truth and Mercy in the Face of AIDS,* "Good churches. Great churches. Wonderful People. Churches pastored by fine men of God, many of whom I had mentored. **Nobody had room for a boy with AIDS."**

Bryan, an infant, died in 1986, Lydia died in 1992, and Matt died in 1995.

In **Ohio,** a man was erroneously diagnosed as being HIV-infected. Within 12 days of learning the test results, he lost his job, his home, and he almost lost his wife. **The error almost cost him his life:** He had planned to commit suicide on the very day he received notice that he had received the wrong test results!

In **Maryland,** a court of appeals upheld a lower court's ruling permitting courtroom personnel to wear gloves to prevent picking up the AIDS virus. The court did suggest that the gloves were unnecessary.

In **New York,** a minister said that he was in a religious "Catch-22": He wanted to show concern and compassion for AIDS patients, but there are definite biblical injunctions against homosexuality. "How," he asked, "can I support these people without supporting homosexuality?"

In **Florida** in 1987, Mrs. Ray, the mother of three hemophilic HIV-infected sons (Ricky, 14; Robert, 13; and Randy, 12) turned to her pastor for confidential counseling. He responded by expelling the family from the congregation and announcing that the boys were infected. As a result, the boys were not allowed to go to church, school, stores, or restaurants. Barbers refused to cut their hair. Some townspeople interviewed said they were terrified at having the boys in the community. They had to move to another town! The Rays sued the DeSoto County School District. They agreed to pay a $1.1 million out of court settlement in 1988. Ricky Ray died of AIDS on December 13, 1992, at age 15. Robert, age 15, was diagnosed with AIDS in 1990; Randy, age 14, was diagnosed with AIDS in May of 1993. Both are living at this writing.

In **Florida, Broward County** parents packed school meetings and teachers filed a class action grievance saying a student's presence endangered their health. District officials determined that the 17-year-old mentally handicapped boy with AIDS would be educated by a teacher in an isolated classroom in the school. The student received $3\frac{1}{2}$ years of isolated education. For the $1\frac{1}{2}$ years, maintenance people would not walk into the portable classroom. Instead, they would leave packages or supplies in the doorway. The teacher and an assistant got used to doing their own cleaning. The one student cost over $50,000 per year to educate.

In **Duval County, Florida** (1990), the foster parents of a 3-year-old AIDS child who was infected by his mother, were forced to leave their church because other parents insisted that the child not be allowed to attend the church nursery. The pastor went along with the majority. When presented with CDC findings that HIV is not casually transmitted, one parent scoffed, **"I called the CDC for information and they asked me what I was going to use it for." He then asked the congregation, "How can you believe anyone like that?"**

In **California,** a young man arrived home one evening to find that the locks had been changed. A few days later he discovered that everything he had ever touched had been thrown out—clothes, books, bed sheets, toothbrush, curtains, and carpeting. Even the wallpaper had been stripped from the walls and trashed. The day before, he had told his friends he had AIDS. "Overnight, I had no friends. I slept on park benches. I stole food. I passed bad checks. No one would come near me. I was told that I had 14 weeks to live."

In a second California incident, volunteer fire fighters refused to help a 1-year-old baby with AIDS at a monastery that cares for unwanted infants. The baby was reported to be choking. Although the fire department has agreed to respond to such calls in the future, one fire fighter quit, saying he was frightened because he had not been trained to deal with victims of acquired immune deficiency syndrome.

BOX 13.2 *(continued)*

In **New Jersey,** a bartender could not tell his parents or friends he had AIDS. It meant confessing that he was gay. He feared it might also mean the loss of family, friends, lovers, and insurance. He was expressing signs and symptoms and paying out of pocket for medical bills rather than file an insurance claim.

In **Charlotte, North Carolina,** in 1993, a bride wore an ankle-length chiffon dress, white above and flowered black below. She'll wear the dress again, at her husband's funeral. The groom was diagnosed with progressive multifocal leukoencephalopathy (PML), a relentless viral infection that attacks the nervous system and causes brain lesions. About 4% of people with AIDS contract the disease. No cure exists.

A legal marriage would make the groom ineligible for Medicare and Medicaid, which he can't afford to lose. So their wedding had to be symbolic and legally nonbinding.

Both wanted a wedding as a sign of commitment. He also wanted it for psychological support: It tells him that his wife will be there as things get worse.

PML has already begun to separate the newlyweds. He has developed speech problems. Sometimes he doesn't remember what he's doing.

From the wreckage, they have clutched love.

"Love is—period," she said. "We don't qualify it. We don't distinguish between heterosexual and homosexual. When love is there, the physical form it takes is just a detail."

In **Charleston, West Virginia,** in July of 1995, a 10-year postal mail carrier who refused to deliver mail to a couple with AIDS was indefinitely suspended with pay after an educational class failed to change his mind. The mailman said he was afraid of cutting himself on the home's metal mail slot and becoming infected from envelopes or stamps the couple had licked. Postal sources said the mailman was to be fired.

In **Texas,** a father with AIDS cried while praying that his three children would not be treated as cruelly. The man, in his mid-20s, was mugged because he looked too weak to fight, hit with rocks by people who found out he had AIDS, and in one incident a man broke a bottle over his head screaming that he was out to kill AIDS. During one beating, an attacker said, "After we kill you, we will kill your wife and children in case they have AIDS."

Almost daily, similar senseless acts of violence and cruelty occur across the United States as a response to AIDS. Such episodes of panic, hysteria, and prejudice are perpetuated by the very people society uses as role models: clergy, physicians, teachers, lawyers, dentists, and so on. Philosopher Jonathan Moreno said, **"Plagues and epidemics like AIDS bring out the best and worst of society. Face to face with disaster and death, people are stripped down to their basic human character, to good and evil. AIDS can be a litmus test of humanity."**

THE LIFE OF RYAN WHITE

In Kokomo, Indiana, Ryan White was socially unacceptable. He was not gay, a drug user, black, or Hispanic. He was a hemophiliac; he had AIDS. His fight to become socially acceptable, to attend school, and to have the freedom to leave his home for a walk without ridicule made Ryan a national hero (Figure 13-1).

FIGURE 13-1 Ryan White was diagnosed with AIDS in 1984 and died on April 8, 1990. This young male became another teenage AIDS tragedy. He gained the respect of millions across the United States before he died of an AIDS-related lung infection. *(Courtesy AP/Wide World Photos)*

BOX 13.2 *(continued)*

Ryan's short life was a profile in courage and understanding. Like many other people with AIDS, Ryan tried to change the public's misconception of how HIV is transmitted. Ryan suffered most from the indignities, lies, and meanness of his classmates and his classmates' parents in Kokomo, Indiana. They accused him of being a "fag," of spitting on them to infect them with the virus, and other fabrications. Ryan said he understood that this discrimination was a response of fear and ignorance. Ryan got the virus from blood and blood products essential to his survival. Ryan's wish was to be treated like any other boy, to attend school, to study, to play, to laugh, to cry, and to live each day as fully as possible. But AIDS was an integral part of his life. AIDS may not have compromised the quality of his life as much as the residents of his community did. One day, at age 16, as Ryan talked about AIDS to students in Nebraska, another boy asked Ryan how it felt knowing he was going to die. Showing the maturity that endeared him to all, Ryan replied "It's how you live your life that counts." Ryan White died, a hero of the AIDS pandemic, at 7:11 A.M. on April 8, 1990. He was 18 years old.

Gregory Herek and colleagues (1993) determined via telephone interviews that HIV/AIDS stigma is still pervasive in the United States. They interviewed 538 white adults and 607 African Americans. Nearly all respondents indicated some stigma. Regardless of race, men were more likely than women to support preventive policies such as quarantine and said they would *avoid* persons with AIDS.

AIDS EDUCATION AND BEHAVIOR

I said education was our **"basic weapon."** Actually it's our **only** weapon. We've got to educate everyone about the disease so that each person can take responsibility for seeing that it is spread no further.

C. Everett Koop
Former U.S. Surgeon General

For some, the occurrence of recently estimated 50,000 new HIV infections in the United States each year is evidence that HIV education and prevention efforts have failed. If HIV prevention programs are held to a standard of perfection and are expected to protect 100% of people from disease 100% of the time, the efforts are by definition doomed to failure. No intervention aimed at changing behaviors to promote health has been or can be 100% successful, whether for smoking, diet, exercise, or drinking and driving. For example, even though warnings regarding the health effects of smoking were issued in 1964, warning labels on cigarettes were not mandated until 1984, and smoking-related illness still remains a major cause of death.

Because some of the behaviors and activities that need to change in order to avert HIV infection are **pleasurable**, it should be no surprise if short-term interventions do not lead to immediate and permanent behavior changes. An important difference between HIV infection and other life-threatening diseases is that HIV can be contracted by a single episode of risk-taking behavior. **Once HIV-infected there is no second chance— no giving up the behavior, like drinking alcohol or smoking, that will make any difference;** HIV disease progresses to AIDS. The adverse effect of smoking, alcohol, or diet on health usually manifests after years of smoking thousands of cigarettes or after years of drinking or poor dietary choices.

After 22 years of experience with HIV, it has demonstrated that lasting changes in behavior needed to avoid infection can occur as a result of carefully tailored, targeted, credible, and persistent HIV risk-education efforts. Given experience in other health behavior change endeavors, no interventions are likely to reduce the incidence of HIV infection to zero; indeed, insisting on too high a standard for HIV risk-reduction programs may actually undermine their effectiveness. A number of social, cultural, and attitudinal barriers continue to prevent the implementation of promising HIV risk-reduction programs. The remote prospects for a successful prophylactic vaccine for HIV and the difficulty in finding long-lasting effective drug treatments have underscored the importance of sustained attention to HIV prevention and education.

The goals of educating people about HIV infection and AIDS are to promote compassion and social understanding and to prevent HIV transmission. To achieve these goals, accurate

This sounds so easy: Educate people and they will do the right thing. **Wrong.** Knowledge does not guarantee sufficient motivation to change sexual behavior or stop the biological urge to have sex. Education has not stopped teenage pregnancy, nor has the knowledge about cigarettes causing lung cancer stopped people from smoking.

Perhaps the reason education is not as effective as it could be is because the public receives its education by daily doses from the mass media. With so much going on in the world, people have become more or less dependent on the media for information essential to their well-being. Gordon Nary (1990) said, **"The public wants to know what's right or wrong in five three-second images or 25 words or less. It wants simple problems with simple solutions. It wants *Star Wars* with good and evil absolutely defined. The media often responds to these demands."**

Mathew Lefkowitz (1990) says that the word AIDS has been infused with an irrational fear that has nothing to do with the illness. He states that the word AIDS has been politicized in such a way that it can and has been used as a weapon. Lefkowitz relates the

information must be provided that makes people aware of their risk status. People at minimum risk can continue their safer sexual lifestyles. People at high risk should determine their HIV status, alter behaviors, and practice safer sex.

BOX 13.3

WHEN ONE WITH AIDS COMES FORTH

Father Paul made the decision to preach on AIDS because of a phone call he had received informing him that a former parishioner was coming to Jacksonville. "George has AIDS. He will be in Church on Sunday. With your permission, he will be receiving Communion."

Father Paul granted permission and welcomed George's attendance. He sensed, however, that some might not agree to have George in church or receive Communion. In his parish, a number of people refuse to believe that HIV is not transmitted by saliva from the lavitha (Communion cup).

By Sunday morning's sermon, over 60% of the congregation had learned of George.

Father Paul began his sermon, "Today's Gospel lesson, Luke 10:25–37, tells us the Parable of the Good Samaritan . . . The Parable challenges us to take stock of who our neighbors are who have needs that we can meet. . . . is it not also true that our neighbors are being harmed by AIDS? . . . Many Orthodox Christians are good about reaching out to the needy and indigent. But we are not so willing to reach out to those with AIDS."

Father Paul said that he would be dishonest if he did not admit having concerns about people receiving Communion after George. "I did not fear for myself, I feared for them, and especially for my two daughters who receive Communion regularly."

Father Paul reminded everyone about the faith of The Church. He addressed the question, "Can AIDS be contracted through casual contact and specifically from the Eucharistic Chalice?" He said, "Communion is the Body and Blood of our Lord. In the Gospel of John, chapter 6, Jesus speaks to us of His Body and Blood as being agents of life, NOT of sickness and death. Similarly, St. Ignatius of Antioch alludes to Communion as the 'medicine of immortality' which allows one to eternally abide with God. To believe, therefore, that one can contract sickness and AIDS from Holy Communion is blasphemy against the Holy Spirit. It is also to render everything that the Bible and the Church teaches about Communion meaningless."

As he spoke, he saw George near the back of the Church. Though only 47 years old, George looked 60. George was weak, abnormally thin, spoke with a rasp, and walked with a cane.

Before Sunday's Liturgy, Father Paul had discussed with George his pastoral concerns about the people's anxieties. Without asking, he proposed a solution, he would receive Communion last.

Father Paul introduced George to the congregation and announced that he would be receiving last.

At Communion time, several of the congregants assisted George to the front of the church. Then, the same individuals and several others lined up behind him.

About 10 people received Communion after George. Father Paul asked one why he did it. "Father, did you not tell us in your sermon that we had to be Good Samaritans? It would have been a very unloving and discriminatory act to allow George to go last."

George died several weeks later in New York City. The news was received with sadness.

George, thank you for coming to Jacksonville. God brought you to us to help us grow. May God remember you in his Kingdom.

(Adapted with permission from Father Paul Costopoulos, Jacksonville, Florida)

FREEDOM FOR COMPASSION: CHILDREN AND AIDS

Charlie the doll was pressed against the antique glass case. Jeff, a blue-eyed, blond-haired boy of 10, looked at him closely. "Someday Charlie will leave this cage," he pondered, "and someday he will be free."

A few visits later, Jeff devised a plan to buy Charlie. He began his task by seeking employment as a leaf raker, a car washer, and the best of panhandlers among friends. After a while his hope faded and his energy waned, but he did not despair. He had met adversity before; in fact, for most of his life. When Jeff was 4 years old, he had contracted AIDS.

The family of John Calvin Presbyterian Church met Jeff because other congregations had turned him away, telling his family that Jeff's illness was a punishment from God. Jeff planned his own memorial service, but five different congregations ignored him by making excuses that the songs he had chosen from the play, "Peter Pan," and the balloons he had requested would not be appropriate.

One Sunday morning as I was beginning my sermon, Jeff's mother wheeled him down the main

BOX 13.3 *(continued)*

aisle to a front pew. I wondered what would happen if this church rejected him, too? How would the other children treat him? Could this congregational family risk enough to love Jeff and his family in the same way in which God loved them? But my fears were relieved after church at the coffee fellowship. Parents introduced themselves to Jeff's mother and the children included Jeff within their circle of games. People earnestly gathered to accompany Jeff and his family on their special journey: members ran errands, provided transportation, and brought in food. This outpouring of help came at a crucial time: Jeff's mother had given up her own business to take care of Jeff, emotional pressures contributed to Jeff's parents' divorce, the family lost their home to bankruptcy court, and Jeff's brother and sister suffered from the prejudice of schoolmates and others.

A few weeks prior to Jeff's death, I bought Charlie the doll. As Jeff's fragile hands began to untie the shiny silver ribbon that secured the purple box, large tears began to trickle down his sunken cheeks. When he discovered what was inside, Jeff smiled and said, **"Now he's free . . . and someday I will be, too." Jeff's freedom arrived on March 2, 1988.**

Those of us who knew Jeff have gained freedom as well. Jeff, and others like him, have introduced us to a new appreciation of life. Through them we have been reminded of how fragile we are and of our precious responsibility to live each moment fully. Together we have discovered the gift that no person, no circumstance, no condition— even the AIDS virus—can take from us. We have discovered God's gift to us in Jesus Christ.

John Calvin Presbyterian Church is now a better-educated congregation. Jeff helped to teach us the importance of risking and reaching out. Our church has adopted a resolution stating that we are committed to minister intentionally with people with AIDS and their families. We provide office space to the Tampa AIDS Network, an advocacy, support, and fund-raising group serving the Tampa Bay area. A number of members and I are part of a growing coalition of volunteers serving on task forces, care-giving programs, and support groups.

In the midst of our congregation's activity we are still keenly aware of the continuing apathy, ignorance, and prejudice permeating much of the religious community. Many underestimate the possibility of this disease intruding into their lives and communities. Much work remains to be done with few to accomplish it.

Jeff's memorial service was just as he had planned it. The sanctuary of the church was filled with the nurses and doctors who had worked with him, the many hospice volunteers who had given him solace, his buddies from the Tampa AIDS Network who had held his hand, the many other friends he had made on his journey. Hundreds of brightly colored helium balloons were released into the sky at the end of the service. We celebrated Jeff's life—and ours as well. Our celebration continues as we minister with others who are traveling this very difficult path. Our strength and hope are renewed with each encounter, for we have been given the freedom for compassion.

Adapted from Rev. Jim Hedges, pastor of John Calvin Presbyterian Church, Tampa, Florida, in *Church and Society*, Vol. 79, No. 3(January/February 1989). Reprinted with permission.

parallel between today's use of the word AIDS with Eugene Ionosco's classic absurdist play *The Lesson*. In the play, a professor stabs a girl to death with the word *knife*—not with a knife but with the **word knife**. It appears that today the word *AIDS* is being used to stab those whom we fear; namely the HIV-infected. How long will it take the educational process to work? **THE VIRUS IS NOT AS MUCH OUR ENEMY AS WE ARE.** For example, in Washington, DC, 1995, because a national public radio commentator was furious at U. S. Senator Jesse Helms of South Carolina for having the audacity to suggest that the government spends too much money on AIDS research, he said, "I think he ought to be worried about what's going on in the good Lord's mind because if there is retributive justice, he'll get AIDS from a transfusion—or **one of his grandchildren will get it.**"

Perhaps zealots need to realize that the purpose of civil exchange is to arrive at wisdom through reasoned debate, not to verbally intimidate those who differ into silence. **Class Discussion: WHAT IS YOUR OPINION?**

Public AIDS Education Programs

Over the years billions of dollars have been spent by federal and state health departments to inform the public about cardiovascular risks, health risks associated with sexually transmitted diseases (STDs),

AFTER 20 YEARS, AMERICANS STILL SAY AIDS IS A TOP HEALTH CONCERN FOR THE NATION AND THE WORLD.

New Survey Finds Sense of Urgency and Personal Risk Highest Among Minorities and Young People

The Henry J. Kaiser Family Foundation's *National Survey of Americans on HIV/AIDS* is a nationally representative survey of adults 18 and older. The survey was designed by staff at the Foundation and Princeton Survey Research Associates (PSRA), and conducted by telephone by PSRA between August 14, 2000, and October 26, 2000. Interviews were conducted with 2683 adults including an oversample of African Americans and Latinos. Interviews were completed in both English and Spanish according to the preferences of the respondent.

AIDS Still Seen As Major Health Problem

When asked to name the most urgent health problem facing the United States in 1995, 44% said AIDS. In 2000, 26% said AIDS. Nearly half of Americans (49%) think HIV/AIDS, in general, is a more pressing problem for the nation today than it was a few years ago. More than one-third (37%) name HIV/AIDS as the most urgent international health problem, ranking it number one among all global health issues. More than four in ten Americans (43%) say they know someone who is either living with HIV/AIDS or has died of AIDS, and more than one in three (37%) say they are personally concerned about becoming infected. And 71% of parents are worried about their children becoming infected.

Desire for More Public and Private Action and Support for Broad Range of Policies

Two-thirds (66%) of Americans believe that the federal government is not doing enough to fight the epidemic in the United States, and more than half believe state and local governments (59%) and schools (51%) are not doing enough. Majorities also say that corporate America (56%) and parents (66%) should be doing more. Americans express strong support for federal spending on AIDS. More than half (55%) say the federal government should be spending more on AIDS, another 25% say spending is about right, and 5% say spending is too high. Most believe that prevention and education (86%), finding a vaccine (83%), and treatment and care (75%) should all be federal policy priorities. Support for some more controversial policies is also notable. Nearly all Americans (97%) want high school sex education to address HIV transmission and prevention, and 90% would include information about condoms. A majority of Americans (58%) also favor needle exchange programs, while 35% oppose them. Two-thirds (66%) of Americans support U.S. spending on AIDS in sub-Saharan Africa, while 29% oppose it. Most (81%) also think that drug companies should be willing to cut AIDS drug prices in developing countries. While the public supports federal spending on HIV/AIDS, AIDS policies will have to compete with other priorities for a seat at the budget table. Polls consistently show that other issues—such as education, health care, and Medicare; social security; and a tax cut—top the public's priority list for federal dollars.

African Americans, Latinos, and Young People Especially Concerned

The demographics of the epidemic in the United States are reflected in the heightened concerns expressed by those hardest hit. African Americans represent 12% of the U.S. population and Latinos 13%, but they represent 47% and 19% of reported AIDS cases respectively. Young people are also disproportionately affected: Americans under age 25 account for about half of all new HIV infections.

Information, Misinformation, and Discrimination

The survey findings show that after 20 years, most Americans know the basics about AIDS. Nearly all Americans are now aware that HIV can be transmitted through unprotected intercourse (99%), sharing intravenous needles (99%), and unprotected oral sex (91%). Eighty-six percent know there are drugs that can extend the lives of those living with HIV/AIDS, and 89% know that no cure has yet been found. However, some significant misconceptions and gaps in knowledge persist:

♦ One in five (22%) Americans believes that sharing a drinking glass can transmit HIV or is unsure about the risk of this activity.

♦ Sixteen percent believe that touching a toilet seat can or might transmit HIV.

♦ More than half (58%) do not know that having another sexually transmitted disease, such as herpes, increases their risk of HIV infection. Less than half (43%) are aware of available treatments to prevent mother-to-child transmission.

♦ Many want more information on specific AIDS-related topics. The two things Americans most want to know more about are how to talk with children about HIV/AIDS (44%) and information about HIV testing (26%).

The majority of Americans (84%) believe that people with HIV and AIDS still face some or a lot of prejudice and discrimination in the United States today, although fewer than one in five

(17%) thinks discrimination has increased in recent years. One-third (33%) of Americans are concerned that others would think less of them if it were known that they had been tested for HIV. Forty-three percent of Americans say they have been tested for HIV, representing a slight increase since 1995, when 37% said they had been tested. More than one in four Americans (28%) say they would be uncomfortable working with someone who has HIV/AIDS. Those who think HIV can or might be transmitted through toilet seats, drinking glasses, or kissing are much more likely to express such discomfort. (Source: The Henry Kaiser Family Foundation. The AIDS Epidemic at 20 Years: The View from America. A National Survey of Americans on HIV/AIDS.)

BOX 13.4

THE WAY WE ARE

The young man worked alongside a 35-year-old woman helping to teach the disabled to function. She was very attractive with a wonderful sense of humor. He watched her every movement—he was in love from a distance; she inspired him to new heights in his work and thoughts about his future. She understood his emotions so she was not surprised when, after work one evening, he offered dinner and a moonlight walk around the lake. During the walk, she could tell from the conversation that his young hormones were flowing—as were her own. In the awkwardness of saying goodnight she said, "I know you want me—I would like that very much." As his broad face glowed she said, **"I must share something with you. I have been diagnosed with AIDS but there are no outward signs yet."** The love that moments before surged through his body crashed down around him; he felt ill yet sympathetic—his urge for sex vanished. He could not bring himself to look at her as he said, "Please forgive me, I just can't." She nodded her understanding and explained following an auto accident in 1984 it was either a blood transfusion or death. **"I made the choice for life and whatever comes with it."** The young man cried as he walked home. He left the job the next morning.

BOX 13.5

ANECDOTE: FATHER AND SON EXCHANGE SEX INFORMATION

"Son, I think it's time we had a talk about sex."
"O.K., Dad, what do you want to know?"

---

specific state and federal legislation. Tobacco advertisements were outlawed on TV and drivers in some states who are not buckled up must pay a fine. But even with laws to support these educational programs, many adults have failed to change established behavior patterns. In the larger cities, educators must combat the fear that AIDS is a government conspiracy to eliminate society's "undesirables"—minorities, drug addicts, and homosexuals. They must overcome cultural and religious barriers that prevent people from using condoms to protect themselves.

Another problem is that educational programs are not preventing individuals from acquiring one or more STDs, using drugs, drinking to excess, driving drunk, failing to use seat belts or motorcycle helmets, and smoking. It might also be added that there have always been educational programs against crime, but in 1989 through 1999 more new jails were built in the United States than ever before. And this expanding jail-building program continues! In short, educational programs on TV, radio, in newspapers, and in the popular press have achieved only limited success in changing peoples' behavior.

It is not that education is unimportant; it is essential for those who will use it! That is the

smoking and lung cancer, chewing tobacco and oral cancer, drug addiction, alcohol consumption, and seat belt use to name just a few. In some cases these campaigns were eventually supported by

THE RED RIBBON

Frank Moore II, a Manhattan painter who was instrumental in launching the overlapping red ribbon as a symbol of AIDS awareness in 1991, died April 22, 2002, from AIDS-related complications at the age of 48. Moore, who said that his paintings represented a journal of his long battle with HIV, was a board member of Visual AIDS, a Manhattan-based group that raises money to fund artists with HIV/AIDS and helps maintain the art of people with the disease. The red ribbon became an international symbol of AIDS awareness and has been used in other colors by groups to represent different causes.

The color red was chosen because the disease was a blood-borne disease. The shape of the ribbon was meant to signify the connectedness of all of us with or without the disease, but who wanted to make a statement of visible support for those who were infected or had AIDS.

THE EVENT

We were sitting in a small Italian restaurant. I had just come back to town from a presentation on AIDS. The jacket I wore still had the red ribbon on the lapel. As we enjoyed our meal, I noticed a woman at the next table who appeared to be glaring at me and making statements to her companion. At one point her voice became loud enough for us to hear her say, "I am sick and tired of those people trying to push the lifestyle of homosexuals down our throats" as she was looking right at me. She then said, "That red ribbon is a sign of a sick person trying to make all of us sick too. That ribbon and all that it stands for ruins my day." With that she and her companion left the restaurant.

That outburst left my family and me embarrassed and confused. My children deserved an explanation. I don't think I have ever explained the idea of the red ribbon to anyone before. Like so many things we observe in life, after a while they become understood by each in his or her own way. This woman expressed her way rather forcefully. To my children I said that the ribbon is a symbol to call attention to a social problem that needs a solution. I went on to say, "Do you recall the song 'Tie A Yellow Ribbon Round the Old Oak Tree' in 1973 and what that meant? And, do you recall the ribbons tied around trees, on car antennas, mailboxes and so on while our 56 service men were held captive in Iran in 1980 and again for our captives in the 1991 Persian Gulf War? Remember the first lady Nancy Reagan's campaign using red ribbons for 'Just say no to drugs' and more recently the pink ribbons for women against breast cancer and most recently the purple ribbons for stopping violence in our schools? These are all symbolic gestures to show support for those enduring suffering and pain. All of the ribbons then and now serve to connect people emotionally, to help unite people in a common cause, to help people feel less isolated in a crisis."

I explained to my children that the problem with the red ribbon now is similar to what occurred over the long time period our soldiers were in captivity—people begin to wear the ribbon as an accessory.

The Author

catch. Although education must be available for those who will use it, too few, relatively speaking, are using the available education for their maximum benefit. In general, people, especially young adults, **do not do what they know. They sometimes do what they see, but most often do what they feel.** In short, knowledge in itself may be necessary but it is insufficient for behavioral change. A variety of studies have failed to show a consistent link between knowledge and preventive behaviors (Fisher, 1992; Phillips, 1993).

Costs Related to Prevention— The assertion that spending more money on educational programs will ensure disease prevention for the masses, as the examples given suggest, may not be the case. In particular, peoples' behaviors regarding the prevention of HIV infection do not appear to be changing significantly despite the billions of dollars used to produce, distribute, and promote HIV/AIDS education. The major educational thrust is directed at how not to become HIV-infected. Most of this information is being given out to people from age 13 and up.

The problem with AIDS education is that communicating the information is relatively easy but changing behavior, particularly addictive and/or pleasurable behavior, is quite difficult.

FIGURE 13-2 Dawn Beckhols at age 23, about the time of her infection. She believed that she became infected via one sexual encounter while on vacation. Dawn died of AIDS on July 13, 1997, at age 33. *(Photo courtesy of L. Schwitters)*

numbers of future HIV infections in the United States will occur in individuals who did not know the virus was transmitted through sexual contact and IV drug use. Yet new infections over the past 4 years occurred at an incidence of about 50,000/year.

Evidence accumulated between 1983 and 1987 indicates that homosexual and bisexual males modified their sexual behavior and this resulted in a drop in AIDS cases among them. There is also evidence that some IDUs have begun wearing condoms. But recent evidence suggests that some of these people are being drawn back to their former practice of unprotected sex and needle sharing. The disease is showing signs of a resurgence in the gay community as health workers struggle to get their message to a new generation and to older gays who seem to have lost the motivation to protect themselves.

In 1982, there were 18 new HIV infections for every 100 uninfected gay men in San Francisco. That rate dropped to 1 per 100 in 1987 but rose to 2 per 100 in 1993. For gay men younger than 25, it is 4 per 100.

Although humans are capable of dramatic behavioral changes, it is not known what really initiates the change or how to speed up the process.

Public School AIDS Education: Just Say Know

Some information relevant to AIDS education can be learned from educational programs that have been designed to reduce pregnancy and the spread of STDs among teenagers. However, data from a variety of high school sex education classes offered across the country indicate that teenagers are learning the essential facts but they are not practicing what they learn. **They do not do what they know.**

Risky sexual behavior is widespread among teenagers and has resulted in high rates of STDs. Over 25% of the 15 million STD cases per year occur among teenagers. One teenager is infected with an STD every 10 seconds in the United States. One in six teens has been infected with an STD. Over 50% of sexually active teenagers (11 million) report having had two or more sexual partners; and fewer than half say they used a condom the first time they had intercourse (Kirby, 1988).

Most cigarette abusers know that smoking causes lung cancer and would like to quit or have tried to quit. Likewise, many alcoholics have tried to quit. But both cigarettes and alcohol are pleasurable to those who use them. The mass media have provided near saturation coverage of key AIDS issues and **it is very unlikely that significant**

EXAMPLES OF ADULT REACTIONS TO HIV/AIDS VS. THE COURTS

Case 1—In September 1998, a mother in the state of Maine, who feared powerful AIDS drugs would kill her HIV-infected 4-year-old son rather than extend his life won the right Monday to refuse treatment for the boy. A state judge refused to give custody of her son to the state Department of Human Services, which had argued his mother was jeopardizing his health. The mother said that she saw her 3-year-old daughter go through an agonizing death while on the drug AZT, and she did not want her son to suffer the same way. The mother is infected with HIV and has stopped taking medication as well. She passed the virus on to her son at birth. She has two older children who do not have the virus. The judge found that there was insufficient evidence that the boy's health was in jeopardy from being denied medical treatment. He also found that evidence suggested the combination of drugs was still experimental and carried the risk of side effects while not guaranteeing a positive outcome.

UPDATE AUGUST 2001 According to an Associated press report in the *Los Angeles Times,* the 7-year-old boy is healthy and happy despite a chronic ear infection.

Case 2—In April 1999, a juvenile court judge in the state of Oregon **refused** to give up state custody of an infant born to an **HIV-positive woman** who wants to breast-feed. **The judge said,** "The parents may choose to run that risk with the child, but the court may second-guess that decision." The 4-month-old boy will be allowed to live with his family, but a caseworker from Oregon's Office for Services to Children will visit periodically to ensure that the order is being fulfilled. The mother's case rested on the contention that HIV does not cause AIDS and cannot be transmitted through breast milk, however, witnesses for the state testified that breast milk from an infected mother has a very high risk of virus transmission.

In April 2000, the wife and husband lost an appeal. The child remains under state control—**no breast-feeding permitted!**

Class Discussion: What do you think, can this work for the child?

Teenage Perceptions About AIDS and HIV Infection in the United States— A recent survey by *People* magazine indicated that 96% of high school students and 99% of college students knew that HIV is spreading through the heterosexual population; but the majority of these students stated that they continued to practice unsafe sex. Combined data from surveys performed in 1988–1989 indicate that among sexually active teenagers, only 25% used a condom. Peter Jennings stated in a February, 1991, AIDS Update TV program that 26% of American teenagers practice anal intercourse. Data such as these have prompted a number of medical and research people to express concern for the next generation. If HIV becomes widespread among today's teenagers, there is a real danger of losing tomorrow's adults. Available data suggest that teenagers have not appreciably changed their sexual behaviors in response to HIV/AIDS information presented in their schools or from other sources.

Teenagers at high risk include some 200,000 who become prostitutes each year and others who become IDUs. About 1% of high school seniors have used heroin and many from junior high on up have tried cocaine (Kirby, 1988). A large number of children from age 10 and up consume alcohol. **Is it possible that too much hope is being placed on education to prevent the spread of HIV?** Teenagers must be convinced that they are vulnerable to HIV infection and death. Until then, it only happens to someone else. The World Health Organization estimates that worldwide, beginning 2003, there were between 12 and 14 million HIV-infected teenagers.

Teenagers, like adults, must be convinced of their risk of infection but not with scare tactics. Behavior modification as a result of a scare is short lived. However the information is given, it must be internalized if it is to be of long-term benefit.

College Students— Everyone must know and act on the fact that a wrong decision about having sexual intercourse can take away the future. For example, a young college student had a three-year nonsexual friendship with a local bartender. She was bright, well educated, and acutely aware of AIDS. After drinks one evening, as their friendship progressed toward sexual intercourse, she asked him if he was "straight" (a true heterosexual) and he said yes. **But he was a bisexual! It was a single sexual encounter.** She graduated and left town. She found out that the bartender died of AIDS three years later. She did not think much of it until she was diagnosed with AIDS five years after their affair. **This young, talented, bright, and personable girl lost her future.** This brings home the point that it is difficult to change something as complex as personal sexual behavior regardless of knowledge. It also brings up at least one other important point in personal relationships: **telling the truth.**

Nothing but the Truth?

During the 1988 Psychological Association Convention, the following facts were presented with respect to telling the truth or lying in order to have sex. The data came from a survey of 482 sexually experienced southern California college students:

1. 35% of the men and 10% of the women said they had lied in order to have sex.
2. 47% of the men and 60% of the women reported they had been told a lie in order to have sex.
3. 20% of the men and 4% of the women said they would say they had a negative HIV test in order to have sex.
4. 42% of the men and 33% of the women said they would never admit a one-time sexual affair to their long-term partner.

Although these data come from a 1988 study, data on telling the truth, when it comes to acquiring sex, is most likely the same today.

Researchers at the French National Research Institute reported in 2002 that men and teenage boys are far less likely than females to tell their main sexual partners they have been diagnosed with HIV or other sexually transmitted disease (STD). Researchers found that 14% of men diagnosed with an STD in the past five years had not told their main partners, compared with just 2% of women. Similarly, 51% of boys who had been diagnosed with an STD had not talked about it with their partner at the time, in contrast to 9% of girls. In a 2002 online poll Gay.com/PlanetOut.com Network wanted to know what people thought about the fact that a San Francisco court awarded $5 million in damages to a man who claims he was infected with HIV from his ex-lover, a former city health commissioner, who lied about his HIV status. When asked, "Should lying about one's HIV status to a sexual partner be a crime?" more than two-thirds—69%—respondents said yes, 8% said no. Another 20% answered, "only if someone is infected as a result."

Adult Perceptions About HIV Infection and AIDS in the United States— A 1996 survey by the **Kaiser Foundation: Survey on Americans and AIDS/HIV** found that with respect to having confidence in AIDS sources, 6% **did not** believe the public health officials, 9% **did not** believe the U.S. surgeon general, 11% **did not** believe the newspapers, 16% **did not** believe Magic Johnson, 17% **did not** believe church/religious organizations, 25% **did not** believe the media and 34% **did not** believe the U.S. government. Thirty-three percent of people **did not** know there are drugs and other treatments for HIV disease or AIDS and 29% **did not** know there were ways to **prevent** or reduce the spread of AIDS. Less than 5% could name a single person that they thought was a **national leader** on AIDS.

The Workplace— If a person is **not** working near or beside someone who is HIV positive, they will be relatively soon! But they may not know it because a person's right to privacy prevails over an employee's right to know.

Recently, 2000 adult employees were phone interviewed during a national survey concerning their attitudes about AIDS. The survey (Hooker, 1996) revealed that:

♦ AIDS is the **chief health concern** among 20% of U. S. employees (cancer was the primary concern of 32%; heart disease of 7%).

THE RIGHT TO PRIVACY

Arthur Ashe (Figure I-1) died of AIDS in February of 1993; he was *forced* to go public about having AIDS. Did that affect his life? Yes. He had to alter a lifestyle he was trying to live with his family. He could no longer live a normal day with his family.

The immediate defense from the press, which forced Arthur Ashe to go public, is that it serves the public interest to identify prominent people with AIDS. The news media says that it increases awareness—and therefore, theoretically, action—to fight back against AIDS. **DO YOU AGREE?**

Organizations can write and broadcast about HIV/AIDS any time, about anybody they want to. **IS THIS MORALLY RIGHT?**

Some defenders of the news media say that a public figure cannot have it both ways—cannot deliberately keep himself in the limelight with sports equipment endorsements and so forth, and then turn around and say, "I want to be a private person." **But what is public and what is private?**

As Ellen Hume asks, "Is there no moment of a public figure's life that is not open to prurient exposure? Does being a political officeholder or, as in Ashe's case, a sports champion, mean that the public owns all of your life, including your life in the bedroom, the doctor's office, the church confessional or the psychiatrist's couch?" **WHAT IS YOUR REPLY TO HER?**

Ms. Hume asks, "Should journalists end their scrutiny of public figures?" She thinks not. But she says, **"Not every revelation serves the public interest.** No American president and few athletes, astronauts, journalists or other heroes could have survived this Spanish Inquisition. Isn't it time for the press to develop a more sophisticated sense of priorities and ethics to go along with its extraordinary new power?" **WHAT IS YOUR REPLY?**

ual employee who is diagnosed with HIV. The probability of sickness and death obviously affects the individual and his or her ability to continue to contribute to the organization's activities and goals.

Employees' fear of AIDS can create a widespread loss of teamwork and productivity, and create an environment that is inhumane and insensitive toward the infected employee.

As the incidence of HIV and AIDS increases, the impact on organizations will obviously increase as well. While there are important logical and moral reasons for ensuring that infected people are not discriminated against, there are also practical reasons for addressing the employee HIV/AIDS problem.

An educated workforce, aware of the facts regarding diagnosis, testing, treatment, and transmission of HIV, can have a positive impact on the overall health of all employees. People are more inclined to openly acknowledge their HIV status and to seek treatment when assured of a supportive workplace environment. This increases productivity.

Whether additional public education will change these attitudes over time is unknown. See the surgeon general's brochure, "Understanding AIDS" (Figure 13-3).

A recent Georgia Tech survey found that workers who received educational brochures or pamphlets about the disease were more likely to have negative feelings toward HIV-infected co-workers than employees who received no information. The results suggest companies should be more concerned about the kind of messages workers receive. By focusing only on practices that can transmit the disease, many educational materials neglect to deal with the social, emotional, and humanitarian aspects of the problem. Education may be the key, but we need to look closely at what kind of education that should be.

American Perceptions about HIV/AIDS in Developing Nations Based on the Henry J. Kaiser Telephone Toll of 1,042 Randomly Selected Adults in 2002

- 74% supported President Bush's proposal to spend $500 million over three years to stop mother-to-child HIV transmission.
- 31% said the United States was not spending enough on HIV/AIDS in developing countries.

- 67% of employees predicted that their co-workers would be uncomfortable working with someone with HIV or AIDS.
- 32% thought an HIV-positive employee would be fired or put on disability at the first sign of illness.
- 24% said that an HIV-positive employee should be fired or put on disability at the first sign of illness.
- 75% of employees said they wanted their employers to offer a formal AIDS education program.

AIDS can have a variety of impacts in the workplace. The obvious one, of course, is on the individ-

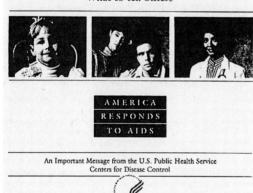

What You Should Know About AIDS

Facts about the disease
How to protect yourself and your family
What to tell others

AMERICA
RESPONDS
TO AIDS

An Important Message from the U.S. Public Health Service
Centers for Disease Control

FIGURE 13-3 Understanding AIDS. This public health pamphlet contains eight pages of HIV/AIDS information. It was sent to 107 million homes in the United States in 1988, at a cost of $22 million. Fifty-one percent of those who received the pamphlet did not read it! *(Courtesy CDC, Atlanta)*

♦ 80% said that HIV/AIDS in other countries would affect the quality of life in America.

♦ 51% said that America has no more obligation to fund HIV/AIDS in other countries than other wealthy countries.

♦ 47% said additional funding for HIV/AIDS in Africa would not lead to meaningful progress.

♦ 80% said that Africans were unwilling to change their unsafe sexual practices to prevent HIV infection.

♦ 75% said the African government was not doing enough to help fight HIV/AIDS.

♦ 51% said HIV/AIDS prevention and treatment is a high priority for U.S. spending on health care in Africa.

♦ 67% said that the worst is yet to come for Africa.

The survey also found that many Americans think the HIV/AIDS crisis in the United States is over. Only 17% identified HIV/AIDS as the country's most urgent health problem.

♦ 15% of white Americans believe a cure for AIDS exists.

♦ 25% of Black Americans believe a cure exists.

♦ 18% of Latinos believe there is a cure.

♦ 46% of Americans are "not at all concerned about contracting HIV."

THE CHARACTER OF SOCIETY

Key HIV/AIDS Related Laws Enacted through 2002

The following laws were enacted specifically to protect those living with HIV.

The Americans with Disabilities Act of 1990 (Public Law 101–336) prohibits discrimination against any qualified individual with a disability—including people living with HIV/AIDS—in employment, public services, telecommunications, and public accommodations.

The Ryan White Comprehensive AIDS Resources Emergency (CARE) Act of 1990 (Public Law 101–381) authorizes funds to "improve the quality and availability of care for individuals and families with HIV diseases." The CARE Act provides funding to cities, states, and other public and private non-profit entities to develop, coordinate, and operate systems of care. Congress has twice reauthorized the Act, which is currently authorized through September 2005.

The Housing Opportunities for People With AIDS (HOPWA) Act of 1991 (Public Law 101–625) provides housing assistance to low-income people living with AIDS. Funds are allocated to states and cities.

The National Institute of Health Revitalization Act of 1993 (Public Law 103–43) provides authority for a permanent, independent Office of AIDS Research at NIH and requires the director of that office to "act as the primary Federal official with responsibility for overseeing all AIDS research conducted or supported by NIH."

The Ricky Ray Hemophilia Relief Fund Act of 1998 (Public Law 105–369) mandates a single payment of $100,000 to any individual infected with HIV if the individual has any blood-clotting disorder and was treated with blood-clotting agents between July 1, 1982, and December 31, 1987.

The Ticket to Work/Work Incentives Improvement Act of 1999 (Public Law 106–170) enables states to create new Medicaid buy-in programs for working individuals with disabilities and authorizes state demonstration programs to provide Medicaid to workers with potentially severe disabilities, including HIV/AIDS, who are not yet disabled.

The Global AIDS and Tuberculosis Relief Act of 2000 (Public Law 106–264) authorizes funds for U.S. participation in the global response to HIV/AIDS, TB, and malaria.

Rumors of Destruction

Today, friends are asked on street corners, at social gatherings, or over telephones: "Did you hear that he/she has AIDS?" Or: "Do you believe that he/she might be infected? You never know with the life they lead!" Some of the famous people **rumored** to have HIV/AIDS are Madonna, Elizabeth Taylor, Burt Reynolds, and Richard Pryor.

Rumors ruin lives. People suddenly subtly lose services; the lawn boy quits, no reason given. Quietly, job applications are turned down or car and homeowner insurance policies are canceled, and so on. In one case, after rumors of HIV infection spread in a small town, a man, if he was served in local bars at all, received his drinks in plastic cups. A health club refunded his membership dues. His apartment manager asked him to leave and when his toilet backed up the maintenance man came in wearing a hat over a World War II gas mask, deep water fishing boots, a raincoat, and rubber gloves. In frustration, he had an HIV test. The results were negative and he gave copies of the test to every "joint" in town, his physician, dentist, theater manager, grocery store manager . . . **He felt this approach was better than running. Do you agree?**

In another case in Brantly County, Georgia, population 11,077, the 22-year-old mother of a 2-year-old son was the subject of a rumor that she was HIV-infected. The rumor also stated that she had had intercourse with 200 men in the past year. To convince the townspeople, she took the HIV test and was not HIV-infected. This young woman had to circulate the results of her blood test around town, but it was still not enough to stop the rumor. A newspaper in nearby Waycross quoted an unnamed source saying that this woman was HIV positive. **The rumor goes on!**

There was the case of a compassionate person who opened a home for helping AIDS patients. Rumor quickly spread that the entire neighborhood was in danger, especially after the mail carrier refused to deliver mail and was ordered to wear rubber gloves and return to the post office for disinfection! To help the neighborhood understand AIDS and stop unfounded fears, a seminar was held at the AIDS home, **but no one would enter the house.**

A young person with AIDS reluctantly returned home—it meant revealing that he was gay to his family—and to the community. He said to his parents, **"I have good news and bad. The bad is that I'm gay. The good is I have AIDS. I won't be around long enough to interfere with anyone."** Once the word got out, a catering service refused to do the annual family Christmas party. They could not hire a practical nurse. Family and friends who used to drop in stayed away. People whispered that the son had gay cancer . . . that it was lethal . . . that it could be caught from dishes, linens, a handshake, and breathing in the same air he breathed out.

In Athens, Alabama, the headline of the town's newspaper read, **"Athens doctor: 'I don't have AIDS.'"** This doctor, a prominent pediatrician in this town for 18 years, had to produce a public defense to dispel the gossip that he had AIDS. Because in a small town everybody knows everybody, the rumor spread with lightning speed to the town hospital, grocery store, hair salon, school, newspaper, and so on. The doctor offered a $2000 reward for any information about who began the rumor. To date no one has collected the money, but the townspeople have gathered to support him.

In Nebraska, a man sued a prominent woman for starting a **rumor** that he had AIDS. The Nebraska Supreme Court upheld a lower court ruling that the man was **slandered** and he received $25,350 in damage.

In Atlanta in March 1999, the CDC said it had received many inquiries about reports that drug users infected with HIV had left contaminated needles in public places. Some reports have falsely indicated that CDC confirmed the presence of HIV in the needles. But the CDC said in a statement, "CDC has not tested such needles. Nor has the CDC confirmed the presence or absence of

HIV in any samples related to these rumors. The majority of these reports and warnings appear to have no foundation in fact. CDC is not aware of any cases where HIV has been transmitted by a needle-stick injury outside a health-care setting."

Mathilde Krim of the American Foundation of AIDS Research said, "From the beginning, the people with AIDS have been a disposable group—gays, blacks and drug users. People don't care about them. They'd rather they wouldn't be here anyway." When the National Gay Rights Advocates asked the nation's 1000 biggest companies whether employee medical plans covered AIDS-related expenses, one anonymous answer read, "Just enough to defray the cost of the bullet." However, HIV has spread to infect most other groups of society and attitudes are slowly changing.

Good News, Bad News, and Late News

Good News— Good news is thinking and believing you're HIV-infected and you're not. There must be a reason to think you're infected, so not being infected is, as some would say, a new lease on life. All too often that feeling is soon forgotten and many people continue lifestyles that place them at risk for infection.

Bad News— Bad news is thinking you're HIV infected and you are. It is difficult to predict what a person sees, hears, or does after being told he or she is HIV positive. For example, some have contemplated suicide, some have committed suicide, others have become completely fatalistic and proceeded to live a reckless and careless lifestyle that endangered others. Some have said it's like death before you're dead.

You are never prepared to hear the bad news regardless of how sure you are that you're infected. For example, one man who had suffered from night sweats, fevers, weight loss, and other classic symptoms just knew he was infected. Yet when told of the positive test results he said "I got so angry, I ripped a shower out of the wall." Being told you are infected is totally devastating, said another infected person. "You feel that everyone is looking at you, everyone can tell you're dirty." Another person said, "The fact that I'm HIV-positive completely dominates my life. There is not a waking hour that I do not think about it. I feel like a leper. I live between hope and despair."

Still another said, "I did not leave the house for two days after being told I was HIV-positive. The initial shock was that I was contaminated— unhealthy, soiled, unclean. I carried this burden in isolation for over two years. After all, I had met people who had AIDS but never a person who said—I'm HIV-infected."

The bad news is not confined to those hearing they are HIV-infected; it touches everyone they know—lovers, family, friends, and employers. Nothing remains the same. The more symptomatic one becomes, the greater the social and human loss. One symptomatic mother said, "Whenever I tell my four-year-old I am going to the doctor, he screams because he knows I could be gone for weeks. I try to put him in another room playing with his sister when they come for me." This woman has died. Relatives care for her children.

Late News— Late news is remaining **asymptomatic** after infection. Asymptomatic can be defined as when no clinically recognizable symptoms appear that would indicate HIV infection. During this time period, the virus can be transmitted to sexual partners. By the time either antibodies and/or clinical symptoms appear, **the news is too late** for those who might have been spared infection had their sexual partner tested positive or demonstrated clinical symptoms early on.

Munchausen's Syndrome: When People Pretend to be HIV Positive or to Have AIDS

As Hector Gavin wrote in 1843 in his 400-page history *Of Feigned and Factitious Diseases*, "The monarch, the mendicant, the unhappy slave, the proud warrior, the lofty statesman, even the minister of religion . . . have sought to disguise their purposes, or to obtain their desires, by feigning mental or bodily infirmities."

Donald Craven (1994) reported that a growing number of people may pretend to have AIDS either because of emotional disorders or because they want to gain access to free housing, medical care, and disability income. In one case, seven patients with self-reported HIV infection were treated for an average of 9.2 months in a clinical AIDS program before their sero-negative status was discovered at the hospital (in general, hospitals in the United States do not require a written copy of the

BOX 13.6

TELLING STORIES ABOUT AIDS-RELATED EVENTS

At the International AIDS Society-USA course in New York in March 2001, Mary Fisher, a mother, author, AIDS activist, and diagnosed with AIDS in July 1991, reminded those in attendance of the importance of telling stories by and to the community of people affected by HIV and AIDS. She said that a community is defined by its stories; stories of victory and loss, of heroes and scapegoats, of tragedy and triumph. For the American AIDS community to become a community again, we must find ways to tell the stories again, to let others know that each story has a name, each with a purpose, each with a life. To that end she told her audience two of her favorite HIV/AIDS stories.

During Bill Clinton's last run for the presidency—1996—I was invited to speak at an AIDS-related event in Little Rock, Arkansas. It was an awards night for regional folk who'd made significant contributions to the fight against HIV. The room was packed with social workers, people with AIDS, family members, religious leaders, a few politicians, and journalists—in other words, the room was packed with Democrats. Out of deference to me, every speaker had been very discreet never to mention politics or Republicans, until the community awards were being handed out, and the last recipient wanted to talk. She was a wonderful, elderly public health nurse: bright, quick, tiny, 77 years old, and feisty. And you could hear every politically correct person in that room stop breathing when she reached up, grabbed the microphone and said, "I've had it with them dumb Republicans. For 15 years, I've talked to them dumb Republicans. Over and over, I've explained there ain't but three ways you can get AIDS.: swap needles or blood, have sex, or get born with it. And, for 15 years them dumb Republicans been askin', 'But can't you get it from mosquitoes?' " She paused for a moment, and then she said, "I'm telling y'all tonight that, from now on, I'm gonna tell 'em, 'Yep, you can get it from mosquitoes—but only in three states: Florida, Louisiana, and Arkansas. Cause them's the only places mosquitoes grow so big Republicans can have sex with 'em.' "

Her second story is taken from the book *I'll Go Quietly*. Billy Cox came out of his hospital bed in Birmingham, Alabama, to bring me a hug in Montgomery. I'd first met him a year earlier at the University of Alabama at Birmingham where I was visiting Michael Saag (Michael is known for

his work with antiretroviral drug therapies). Michael wanted me to meet Billy, to see his spunk and spirit. "Billy is the boxer in the ring," Michael once observed. "The doctors and nurses and medical staff, we're just the trainers in his corner. His friends and family are his fans, cheering him on." Now, a year later, I'd come to Montgomery to speak. But what I said there was not as eloquent as the events that soon played out in the life of Boxer Billy and Cousin Michael. Six weeks after he'd brought his hug to Montgomery— 7 years, 4 months, and 3 days after testing positive of the AIDS virus—Billy Cox died on November 23, 1994. On Billy's last day, Michael Saag was leaving town for a few days and stopped in just to say good-bye. When he heard Billy's labored breathing, he called the family together and told them the end was near. And then—as nurses and old friends and Billy's family crowded into the room forming a remarkable community bound only by love for the boxer—Michael rested his head on Billy's chest and, unashamed, before the crowd, sobbed, "I'm sorry, I'm sorry." Science has limits. Even community has bounds. But no one will ever know what love might do.

For those who want to become a part of the HIV/AIDS community through stories, here are a few more stories.

She was totally unprepared for the catastrophe that befell her and her family five years ago. She is a clever, articulate woman who has held a senior position in a multinational corporation, run her own business, and brought up two children. She was enjoying a happy and comfortable life with her husband of four years in South Africa, when suddenly and unexpectedly he became very ill. Within months he was dead, at the age of 58. He had died of AIDS. Never in her life had she imagined such an eventuality. Later on, she found out that she was HIV positive. "I don't think there is even a word to explain what it is like when you find out. It was devastating. I thought it happened to other people, I thought it happened to gay people, I thought it happened to black people, and I thought it happened to intravenous drug users. I certainly didn't think it could happen to me." She was living in a country where about 4.9 million adults and children are now estimated to be HIV positive but where the stigma attached to HIV is enormous and where the government was in denial—insisting that poverty rather than the virus was the cause

BOX 13.6 *(continued)*

of AIDS. She had no idea how to deal with this terrible new knowledge and there was no one to turn to. "My husband walked into the hospital in April and came out in a wheelchair and just gave up and died in August. He didn't want to live anymore when he found out. At that time the only drug available was AZT and it was as good as useless." She did not ask her husband, who had been married before how he became HIV positive. "At the end of the day it didn't matter how he got it." When he died, she did not tell people he had AIDS. "I told everybody my husband died of cancer because I hadn't told my children, and I'd lost my husband—from diagnoses to losing him was only a short time and I was having to come to terms with that and my own diagnosis. I couldn't deal with telling anybody at that time. But I confided in somebody who actually told other people so I realized that I would have to tell my children quickly before somebody else told them." That was tough. She had to explain the tragedy over the phone to her 22-year-old daughter who was overseas. More distressing still was the talk with her 14-year-old son and the impact the news had on him. "He stopped smiling. If your mother tells you your deeply loved stepfather had died of AIDS, you would probably stop smiling for a long time. It was terrible. It was terrible because of the social issues. He couldn't tell anybody. Teenagers have such problems just being teenagers." They left South Africa for the UK. "Like most people when they are diagnosed, I thought I was going to die soon. I'd heard about the new drugs on the market and thought if I could get access to those I could see my kids grow up." Four years later, she is well and not yet on medication, thanks to Body and Soul, the British support organization that dedicates itself to helping heterosexual people who are HIV positive and their families. She knows now that the toxic antiretroviral drugs should not be used until there is no alternative, and both she and her son have learned how to cope with her terminal diagnosis among people who understand and will not treat them as pariahs. She wanted to speak out about her HIV status long ago. She was deeply moved by the speech given to the Durban HIV/AIDS conference last year by Nkosi Johnson, the little boy who did more to break the silence around the disease in South Africa than almost anyone else—and is now dead. But fear of what it might do to her family made her wait until they were old enough and strong enough to deal with the repercussions. Eventually she spoke out to an audience at a recent theatre benefit to raise money for Body and Soul. "The love and support that surrounds other illness isn't there for people with HIV. For four years, we've discussed my talking about it because none of us feel any of us has done anything wrong, but just getting to the point where we all felt that I actually could speak out was really terrible. Why should that be, because if I was speaking up for instance about breast cancer awareness we'd be surrounded by all the love and support in the world. Why should it be any different for HIV? After all, it's just an illness."

In Sacramento, California, the wife of a minister taught Sunday school. She never gave HIV/AIDS a second thought. How could she be infected?—she was a loyal, faithful, monogamous wife. Her husband was her only sexual experience. Just before her second wedding anniversary, however, she learned that her husband had AIDS and that he had infected her. "I didn't know my husband was living a secret lifestyle." Homosexuality is not allowed in his church, so he hid it from everyone, including her. On his deathbed, he confessed to her. "Ava, I did what I did to you purposely because I didn't want to die by myself."

Uganda—When Lukio was 10 years old she watched as her big sister was forced to leave their home in disgrace. Their mother cried out that her unmarried daughter was pregnant. Shameful as the sight of a pregnant 18-year-old might be, it was a lie invented to hide what was considered an even greater horror—for the sister, Hasifa, was infected with HIV. She was banished, left to survive on her own. And Lukio had barely celebrated her 12th birthday when Hasifa's old boyfriend raped Lukio. Hasifa is now 27, battling not only AIDS but also tuberculosis that has infected her lungs. And Lukio, a shy 19, also has AIDS, which she says gives her sharp headaches and makes her tire easily. Lukio and Hasifa share an uneasy sisterhood. Though both girls were virgins when they met the man, it is not he who has paid the price for their HIV infections. To survive, Lukio sews people's clothing, repairing tears and replacing buttons to earn the 6000 shillings (about $4) a month that she needs for water and rent for a 6'×6' windowless cell that fills with water during the rains and smells of mold in the dry season. She has no toilet, bath, or electricity. Older Hasifa lives only slightly better thanks to her sales of macramé pot

BOX 13.6 *(continued)*

hangers. Neither have access to drug therapy and will die prematurely.

Lastly, in 1986, not long after his guerilla force seized power in Uganda, Yoweri Museveni sent 60 top officers from his bush army to Cuba for training. Several months later Fidel Castro approached Museveni at a conference in Zimbabwe with a staggering bit of news. Medical exams in Cuba revealed that 18 of the 60 officers, or 30%, were HIV positive. Castro said, "Brother Museveni, you have a problem." That was truly an understatement. Years of war, displacement, pillage, and rape had entrenched HIV in Uganda as early as the late 1970s. Museveni took Castro's warning to heart. Within one year he lead a nationwide mobilization against AIDS that drew in bishops, imams, and public health experts, as well as thousands of small community groups nationwide. The program would become known as ABC, for "Abstain, Be Faithful, or wear a Condom"— very much in order of emphasis. Vinand Nantulya, an infectious disease specialist who helped

advise Museveni said, "Ugandans really never took to condoms." Instead, the message, promoted everywhere from Museveni's speeches to elementary school curricula, was that children should abstain from sex until marriage and then practice "zero grazing"—i.e., fidelity. Billboards with this message are everywhere in Uganda. By 2001, the number of pregnant Ugandan women testing positive for HIV antibodies had fallen from 22% at the height of the epidemic in 1991 to 6.2%. By contrast, in neighboring Kenya the rate for HIV-infected women is about 15%; in Zimbabwe it stands at 32%; and in Botswana 38%. Because Uganda's success is nearly unique in sub-Saharan Africa, more and more people are asking how it can be duplicated. Clearly, Museveni's strong leadership was key. But researchers have begun to unravel the reasons for Uganda's success; controversy has dogged their work, perhaps because most of them agree on one troublesome fact: condoms had relatively little to do with lowering the HIV infection rate.

HIV test results proving that someone is HIV positive). Craven noted that "because patients with AIDS often have preferred access to drug treatment, prescription drugs, social security disability insurance, housing and comprehensive medical care, the rate of malingering may increase and reach extremes."

Another doctor who treats many AIDS patients said that he and his colleagues have seen many patients who repeatedly come to their offices fearing that they have AIDS, even though multiple tests have shown that they do not (Zuger, 1995).

An Oklahoma physician has written about the AIDS **Munchausen's syndrome**—an emotional disorder in which people pretend to have the disease simply to get attention from doctors. Confidentiality requirements make AIDS a perfect illness for people suffering from Munchausen syndrome because the laws shield them from being discovered.

Physicians' Public Duty: An Historical Perspective of Professional Obligation

Physicians enjoy a virtual monopoly on medical care, social status, and generous financial remuneration. Thus the medical profession is uniquely

entrusted with the knowledge to care for those with HIV disease/AIDS or any other contagious disease and has a clear responsibility to do so, absent compelling considerations to the contrary. A fair and reasonable share of medical risk just naturally goes with the professional territory.

Robert Fulton and Greg Owen (1988) stated that throughout history, plagues and pestilences have challenged humankind. In his book, *Plagues and People*, William McNeill (1976) cited the many death-dealing epidemics in Europe. He wrote that one advantage the West had over the East in the face of deadly epidemics was that caring for the sick was a recognized duty among Christians. The effect of a prolonged epidemic more often than not strengthened the Church when other social institutions were discredited for not providing needed services. McNeill further observed that the teachings of Christianity made life meaningful, even in the immediate face of death: Not only would survivors find spiritual consolation in the vision of heavenly reunion with their dead relatives or friends, but God's hand was also seen in the work of the life-risking caregivers.

The United States has also had its share of plagues and epidemics; one of the most notable was the outbreak of yellow fever in Philadelphia in 1793. Thousands of citizens of the capital city perished. William Powell (1965), in his book *Bring Out Your Dead*, describes Philadelphia at the time of the yellow fever plague: the dying were abandoned, the dead left unburied, orphaned children and the elderly wandered the streets in search of food and shelter. Nearly all who could fled the city, including the President, leaving the victims of the fever to their fate. Among those who remained, however, were Benjamin Rush, M.D., the mayor, a handful of medical colleagues and their assistants, and a number of clergy. With the help of a small group of laborers and crafts-men, they undertook the enormous tasks of maintaining law and order, providing medical care, food and shelter to the sick and helpless, as well as gathering up and burying the dead.

Dr. Rush and the others remained at their posts because of their overriding sense of profes-sional obligation along with a conviction inspired by the precept of the New Testament **"Blessed are the merciful, for they shall obtain mercy"** (Matthew 5:9).

But this vision, shared by Christians for cen-turies, along with a sense of professional com-mitment, may not be sufficient to persuade contemporary health care workers to stay at their posts.

The baby boom generation, well-educated and self-oriented, has learned to blame AIDS on groups whom society defines as deviant: homo-sexuals, prostitutes, and drug abusers. There is a significant probability, therefore, that today's young health care practitioner may turn away from HIV/AIDS patients despite the fact that a 1981 Gallup Poll of the religious beliefs and prac-tices of 14 countries showed that the United States leads the world not only in church membership but also in charitable services.

According to an article in the November 13, 1987, issue of *The Wall Street Journal*, Arthur Ca-plan, a director for the Center of Biomedical Ethics at the University of Minnesota in Min-neapolis, believes that doctors and nurses who refuse to treat AIDS patients do so out of disap-proval. "They know how to deal with violent pa-tients and infectious diseases like hepatitis." So why not treat someone with AIDS? "It's more than fear. They're making a value . . . judgment about AIDS victims. They're saying they won't treat peo-ple (they find) disgusting." Others refuse to place

their lives at risk for someone who became HIV-infected through immoral behavior. **C. Everett Koop said the refusal by some medical person-nel to treat AIDS patients "threatens the very fabric of health care in this country." DO YOU AGREE?**

Medical Moral Issues

HIV/AIDS represents a new era in medicine, one in which physicians are faced with complex moral issues. When the American Medical Association (AMA) issued a statement to the effect that it is unethical to refuse to treat HIV/AIDS patients, that statement reflected a deep concern in the medical community about the possibility of their becoming infected by treating patients with HIV/AIDS.

The AMA statement for an ethical call to arms is unprecedented in this century. It is the result of a spreading fear that HIV/AIDS is too contagious to tolerate in spite of the knowledge that the virus is not transmitted via casual con-tact. **Emotions, not education, are in control of those whose fears exceed reality.** But these emo-tions are real and they are having an impact on the medical community.

There is an ongoing dilemma concerning the rights of the physician and other health care workers to practice medicine in a safe environ-ment as opposed to the rights of HIV-infected and AIDS patients to receive care and medical support. Although the risk of HIV transmission through medical occupational exposure appears to be quite low, the fact that it is possible at all, coupled with the uniformly fatal prognosis asso-ciated with AIDS, suggests that physicians, nurses, and other health care workers have legitimate concerns about risk to their health.

In a report by C.E. Lewis and colleagues (1992), almost half the primary care physicians in the Los Angeles area had refused to treat HIV-infected pa-tients or had planned not to accept them as regu-lar patients.

In a more recent survey of American doctors in residency training, 39% said that a surgeon or other specialist had refused to treat a patient with AIDS in the resident's care. In Canada, only 13% reported a specialist had refused to treat a patient with AIDS; in France, only 8% said a specialist had rejected care.

DEALING WITH DISCRIMINATION: THE AMERICANS WITH DISABLILITIES ACT

Although incidents of discrimination are disheartening, they are only a part of the story. Another part of the story is how discrimination has been fought and how courts, legislatures, and other social institutions have responded with attempts to reduce HIV/AIDS discrimination and to minimize its impact. To this end a brief synopsis of the Americans with Disabilities Act is presented along with the first U.S. Supreme Court ruling based on this act.

AMERICANS WITH DISABILITIES ACT

The primary federal nondiscrimination statute that prohibits discrimination on the basis of a person's disability or health status is the **Americans with Disabilities Act (ADA) of 1990.** The ADA provides that no individual **"shall be discriminated against on the basis of disability in the full and equal enjoyment of the goods, services, facilities, privileges, advantages or accommodations of any place of public accommodation."** The ADA's definition of "public accommodation" specifically includes hospitals and professional offices of health care providers. A critically important issue under the ADA is whether persons with **asymptomatic** HIV infection have a disability and thus are protected under the ADA. **Disability is defined as a physical or mental impairment that substantially limits one or more of the major life activities of the individual, a record of such impairment, or being regarded as having an impairment.** In the past, many courts have ruled or assumed as undisputed that HIV infection, as the underlying cause of a life-threatening illness, is a disability. However, several recent court decisions have held that HIV does not automatically qualify as a disability, and in each case there must be an individualized determination as to whether the infection actually limits, in a substantial way, a major life activity. The ADA's legislative history, however, indicates that Congress intended to include HIV infection within the definition of disability, and the Equal Employment Opportunity Commission's regulations embody that view. **In its first AIDS case ever, the Supreme Court had to decide whether and to what extent persons with HIV infection are protected under the ADA.**

THE CASE OF *BRAGDON V. ABBOTT*: UNITED STATES SUPREME COURT

1998

In the 17-year history of the HIV/AIDS pandemic, the U.S. Supreme Court has never considered a case directly involving HIV or AIDS. That changed on Monday, March 30, 1998, when oral arguments began in the case of *Bragdon v. Abbott*. The *Bragdon* case is also the first time the court has ever heard a case involving the ADA. On September 16, 1994, Sidney Abbott, age 37, went to her dentist in Bangor, Maine, to get a cavity filled. Dr. Randon Bragdon refused to fill a gum line cavity in his office when he read on her medical form that she was HIV positive. He told her he could do the procedure in a hospital, a change of venue that would have added approximately $150 to the bill. According to a **cover story** about the case in the *American Bar Association Journal*, Dr. Bragdon did not have privileges to practice in any area hospitals, nor had he applied for them. Dr. Bragdon maintains that he could have sought and received permission to perform occasional procedures without having been granted full privileges.

Abbott's Lawsuit

Her lawsuit argues that in refusing to treat her in his office, Bragdon violated the ADA and the Maine Human Rights Act. Federal district and appeals courts both agreed with her.

United States Supreme Court: Decision June 25, 1998

The Supreme Court ruled 5 to 4, upholding the District Court and the First Circuit Court of Appeals, finding that **Bragdon** violated Abbott's rights to treatment under the provisions of the ADA of 1990. Abbott's HIV infection constituted **a disability** under the ADA in that her HIV infection **"substantially limits"** a major life activity—her ability to reproduce and bear children (to have a child she places her husband at risk for HIV infection and risks infecting her child). **Justice Kennedy** in delivering the opinion of the court held that from the moment of infection and throughout every stage of the disease, HIV infection satisfies the statutory and regulatory definition of a "physical impairment." Applicable Rehabilitation Act regulations define "physical or mental impairment" to mean "any physiological disorder or condition affecting the body['s] hemic and lymphatic [systems]." HIV infection falls well within that definition. The medical literature reveals that the disease follows a predictable and unalterable course from infection to inevitable death. It causes immediate abnormalities in a person's blood, and the infected person's white cell count continues to drop throughout the course of the disease, even during the intermediate stage when its attack is concentrated in the lymph nodes. Thus, HIV infection must be regarded as a physiological disorder with an immediate, constant, and detrimental effect on the hemic and lymphatic systems.

DISSENT IN PART

Justice O'Conner stated that Abbott's claim of a disability should be evaluated on an individual basis and that she has not proven that her symptomatic HIV status substantially limited one or more of her major life activities. "In my view, the act of giving birth to a child, while a very important part of the lives of many women, is not generally the same as the representative major life activities of all persons—caring for one's self, performing manual tasks, walking, seeing, hearing, speaking, breathing, learning, and working"— listed in regulations relevant to the Americans with Disabilities Act of 1990. Based on that conclusion, there is no need to address whether other aspects of intimate or family relationships not raised in this case could constitute major life activities; nor is there reason to consider whether HIV status would impose a substantial limitation on one's ability to reproduce if reproduction were a major life activity.

U.S. SUPREME COURT RULES ON INSURANCE COVERAGE CAP FOR HIV/AIDS TREATMENT

January 2000. The U.S. Supreme Court let stand a ruling that allowed an insurance company to provide less coverage for AIDS-related illnesses than for other conditions under the same policy. The high court, without comment, refused to hear the appeal brought by two HIV-positive

Chicago men who claimed that their insurance company's policies violate the Americans with Disabilities Act. The two policies in question were issued by Mutual of Omaha. One policy set a $25,000 lifetime coverage limit for AIDS-related illnesses and the other contained a $100,000 cap, while both allowed a $1 million cap for other illnesses. Attorneys for Mutual of Omaha argued that the insurance company had not discriminated because it offered the men the same coverage offered to other customers. In 1998, the federal judge in Chicago ruled in favor of the two men, but the 7th U.S. Circuit Court of Appeals reversed that ruling. **The appeals court said the ADA guarantees access to insurance but does not regulate the content of coverage.**

NATIONAL SURVEY OF DENTISTS IN CANADA: REFUSAL TO TREAT HIV-INFECTED PATIENTS

According to the report by Gillian McCarthy and colleagues (1999) there are about 15,232 dentists in Canada. A random sample of 6444 answered a survey on whether they would refuse to treat HIV-infected patients. Some 4281 dentists responded. The conclusion presented by the investigators was that 1 in 6 (or 17%) would **refuse to treat** an HIV-infected patient. The refusal was associated with the respondent's lack of belief in an ethical responsibility to treat patients with HIV and his or her fears of becoming infected from their patients.

Class Discussion: Clearly a 5 to 4 ruling is not an overwhelming mandate to support Abbott's lawsuit. Do you feel that a simple majority, 55% in this case, is sufficient or because this case has vast implications, should it require a two-thirds majority, 6 in favor–3 against (67%)? What are the legal and moral issues in accepting a simple majority versus a two-thirds ruling?

Bragdon raised a question for you to consider as you research the question above. Looking at **MAGIC JOHNSON**—he asks if it really makes sense to consider someone "disabled" who can earn millions of dollars playing professional basketball, or go to work, or otherwise perform the tasks of daily living. YOUR RESPONSE IS . . .

Further, 23% of American doctors would not care for AIDS patients if they had a choice as compared with 14% of Canadian physicians and 4% of French doctors.

The survey results may be a disturbing indicator of how American physicians view their work and a reflection of cultural and political attitudes here that view with veiled hostility those with AIDS.

HIV TRANSMITTED BY AUSTRALIAN AND FRENCH SURGEONS

A breakdown in infection control procedures is being blamed for the transmission of HIV to five patients of an Australian surgeon. It's believed the virus was transmitted from one patient to four others during minor skin surgery on a single day in November, 1989. Health officials say one patient, a gay man, is believed to have been the infection source. **The CDC calls the case the first known patient-to-patient transmissions of HIV in a health care setting** (*American Medical News.* 1994 37:2.) In October 1995, after the HIV seropositive status of an orthopedic surgeon in Saint Germain en Laye (west suburb of Paris) was announced in the medical press, the French director of general health decided to inform and offer testing to the patients operated on by this surgeon. Review of the medical history of the surgeon suggests that he most probably became infected with HIV in May 1983. The diagnosis of HIV infection and AIDS were made simultaneously in May 1994. This investigation identified 3004 patients who had undergone at least one invasive procedure by the surgeon; 2458 patients were able to be contacted by mail. The serologic status of 968 patients was ascertained; 967 are negative. Only one patient, who was negative before prolonged operation performed by the surgeon in 1992 (10 hours) is HIV positive. Typing of the viral strains of the patient and the surgeon comparing nucleotide sequences of two viruses showed they are closely related. In February 2000, the surgeon was ordered to pay $107,000 to the infected patient. Similar to the more recent dentist-Bergalis case, the source of HIV in these cases will most likely never be documented to everyone's satisfaction.

In only the **third** known case of HIV being transmitted to a patient by a health care worker, a 61-year-old female patient became infected. At the **Free University of Brussels,** in July of 1996 the woman developed severe symptoms of HIV infection. Viral RNA sequence studies showed the virus came from her nurse who at the time had advanced HIV disease but did not know she was infected (Goujan, 2000).

To combat that fear, medical schools are now providing their students with disability insurance that covers AIDS. Hospitals have adopted policies that require physicians to treat AIDS patients or face dismissal.

Risk Protection of the Patient: Political Dimensions— The American Medical Association's position is that HIV/AIDS doctors "should consult colleagues as to which activities the physician can pursue without creating a risk to patients."

There must be a rational relationship between the degree of risk, the morbidity and mortality of the disease, and the consequences of policies and procedures implemented to reduce the risk. Invasive surgery involves many risks. There is an overriding ethical obligation to reduce these risks in ways that do not create more harm than good. The justification of policies to prevent life-threatening illnesses with a risk factor of 1 in 10,000 is significantly greater than those with a risk factor of 1 in 100,000. More lives can be saved by innovative approaches to preventing the kind of injuries that have accounted for 75% of all cases of occupationally related HIV infection than by preventing HIV-infected health care workers from performing invasive surgery.

The risk of HIV infection by an HIV-infected surgeon is only one-tenth the chance of being killed by lightning, one-fourth the chance of being killed by a bee, and half the chance of being hit by a falling aircraft. The 1 in 100,000 risk of transmission from an infected surgeon equals the probability of death we face bicycling 2 miles each way to school for one month, or commuting 15 miles round-trip by car for a year.

Similarly, our chance of dying from anesthesia during an operation is roughly 10 times our chance of being infected by a surgeon known to be infected with HIV. A mother who approves a penicillin injection for her toddler with pharyngitis accepts a 1 in 100,000 risk of death from anaphylactic shock. In one study, the most successful coronary artery bypass graft surgeon surveyed had a 1.9% mortality rate, while the least successful had a 9.2% mortality rate. Patients selecting the least successful surgeon thus face 7300 times the extra risk of death posed by an HIV-infected surgeon. The risk to a person undergoing invasive surgery by a surgeon of **unknown** HIV status is about 1 in 20 million of becoming HIV-infected (Daniels, 1992). The CDC estimates the risk to a patient by an **HIV-infected surgeon** to be between 1 in 42,000 and 1 in 420,000 (Lo et al., 1992).

Finally, to place the risk of the patient's HIV infection/death in perspective, the National Academy of Science reported that each year in America, as many as 98,000 Americans die from medical mistakes made by physicians, pharmacists, and other health care professionals. More Americans die from medical mistakes than from breast cancer, highway accidents, or AIDS (Weiss, 1999). According to a study released in January 2000 by the Canadian Public Health Journal, *Tobacco Control,* 10,000 people die worldwide every day due to smoking.

Patients' Right to Know if Their Physician has HIV/AIDS—

In a 1987 Gallup Poll, 86% of those polled felt that they had the right to know if a health care worker treating them was HIV-infected. Many lawyers also take this position. The courts appear to be moving toward an interpretation of the doctrine of informed patient consent as **"what a reasonable patient would want to know,"** rather than "what a reasonable physician would disclose." Because it is so difficult for surgeons to avoid occasionally cutting themselves during surgery, it has been suggested that the best solution is not to have HIV-infected surgeons perform surgery at all.

Public anxiety on HIV/AIDS and medical care is becoming increasingly tinged with hysteria. A national Gallup Poll undertaken for *Newsweek* (June 20, 1991) asked a representative sample of 618 adults, "Which of the following kinds of health care workers should be required to tell patients if they are infected with the AIDS virus?"

The answers were: surgeons 95%; all physicians 94%; dentists 94%; all health care workers 90%.

Clearly, people do not differentiate between doctors who perform invasive procedures and those who do not. However, the patient could ask what the probability is of a single dentist (Acer) infecting six of his patients (Bergalis, Web, and four others). Extremely low, **yet it did happen!** The lowest of probabilities and best of guidelines and precautions do not stop the fire of fear. It must also be mentioned that the same *Newsweek* poll found that 97% of those interviewed felt that

HIV-infected patients should tell their health care workers that they are infected.

There is one important aspect related to this poll that needs to be addressed. That is, many of the people interviewed stated that if they **knew** their surgeon was HIV-infected, they would "get another surgeon." This *switching dilemma* may, at some point, have the majority of the population needing surgery standing in line for the uninfected surgeons. Services provided by the reduced number of surgeons, it could be claimed, at some point, result in increased costs and diminished quality.

HIV-Infected Health Care Professional's Duty to Disclose—

Several courts have held that health care professionals have a duty to disclose their HIV status to patients or health authorities, assuming that their professional activities pose a risk of transmission to patients. The Maryland Court of Appeals ruled that a surgeon has a duty to inform his patients of his infection; even if the patient has not actually been exposed and tests HIV negative, the contact with the surgeon may subsequently give rise to a claim for their infliction of mental distress due to fear of transmission. Courts justify orders to disclose based on a duty to protect patients and on the doctrine of informed consent. Requiring disclosure to patients, of course, can severely jeopardize a health care professional's career. To avoid this result, some states allow the professional to continue practicing, with appropriate restrictions and supervision, but without disclosing his or her HIV status (Gostin, et al., 1998).

Physician–Patient Relationships

In most states, physicians may **not test** a patient for HIV antibodies without written permission from the patient. Physicians can run tests for any other infectious diseases without written permission.

CLASS QUESTION: Do you think this is fair and equal medical practice?

Because the majority of HIV-infected patients are asymptomatic, there is no way of telling **who** is or is **not** infected. Therefore, for the protection of health care workers, everyone must be treated as though they were HIV-infected.

HIV has been a silent medical threat for 22 years and continues into the new millennium. Wherever blood is drawn, a wound is examined, a dressing is changed, or anything that involves blood, needles, or surgery is done, there is an unspoken fear that HIV might be present. The patient sees this preventive attitude of physicians and other health care workers by the new look: wraparound smocks, gloved hands, and masks. The patient wonders whether his or her physician is an HIV carrier and the physician assumes that the patient may be a carrier. A recent Associated Press article presented some examples of how the AIDS pandemic has changed doctor–patient relationships:

1. In many operating rooms, doctors and nurses wear wraparound glasses in case of blood splashes.

2. In many emergency rooms, health care workers cover themselves with caps, goggles, masks, gowns, gloves, shoe covers, and blood-proof aprons.

3. Infection control specialists must spend time convincing hospital workers it is safe to enter an HIV/AIDS patient's room to perform normal duties ranging from picking up dinner trays to fixing the plumbing.

4. At some hospitals, all emergency room trash, no matter how innocuous, is treated as hazardous waste.

5. Many doctors and nurses routinely pull on gloves whenever they give an injection or draw blood.

6. Mouth-to-mouth resuscitation is simply not done at many hospitals. Instead a mask and valve device is used to avoid direct contact with the patient's mouth.

7. A surgeon at San Francisco General Hospital takes the AIDS drug zidovudine whenever he operates on people he thinks are infected.

8. Physicians are increasing life insurance policies to provide for their families in case they become HIV-infected.

The health care professionals' fear of getting AIDS will persist as long as there is a risk that HIV can be transmitted in the workplace. **The goal is not to eradicate that fear, but to prevent it from compromising the quality of patient care and from threatening the health professional's own well-being** (Gerbert et al., 1988).

In early 1990, Lorraine Day quit her post as chairperson of the orthopedics department at San Francisco General Hospital and abandoned her surgical practice because of her fear of exposure to HIV. "I have two children to think about and operating was too dangerous. If I was a skydiver, people would say I was an irresponsible mother, but to me, surgery now, it was just as risky."

BOX 13.7

MY FIRST AIDS EXPERIENCE

"A man was waiting for his mother in my office while she consulted me about a back problem," reports a family practitioner in a Gulf state city. "He had a grand mal seizure, bit his tongue and bled quite a bit. I put a tape-wrapped tongue depressor into his mouth to keep him from further injuring his tongue and then just supported him until the seizure was over. Later the physician who had been caring for him at a hospital clinic called to ask that I confirm the seizure, adding, **"By the way, this man has AIDS."** I never gave a thought to AIDS in this situation," continues the family practitioner. "It was my first experience in dealing with an AIDS patient" (Polder et al., 1989).

Dr. Day said during a TV interview, "Our risk is one in 200 per single (needle) stick with AIDS blood and it can be the first one—it doesn't take 200. And I ask you, if you came to work every day and flipped the light switch on in your office and only one out of 200 times you were electrocuted would you consider that low-risk?"

While Dr. Day has been called a scaremonger, many surgeons in private conversations call her a "hero" for raising the risk issue.

Physicians with AIDS

According to Mandelbaum-Schmid (1990), one overriding issue facing physicians who become HIV-infected is that there is no support system to compensate them once they become too sick to work. For example, a 32-year-old gastroenterologist claimed she was infected with HIV in 1983 when she accidently pricked herself with a needle that an intern had used to draw blood from an AIDS patient. She was working at the time at Brooklyn's Kings County Hospital.

She tested HIV positive in 1985. On subsequent consultations with physicians at the National Institutes of Health (NIH), she was told that she was a healthy carrier of the virus who could become ill. She continued training at Kings County, completing a residency in internal medicine and a fellowship in gastroenterology.

She became symptomatic in 1987. A year later, she filed a $175 million lawsuit charging that the hospital's negligence had caused her illness. At the

CURRENT VIEW OF HEALTH CARE WORKERS WHO ARE HIV INFECTED

The legal system traditionally has been reluctant to challenge the professional autonomy of physicians by removing or altering their choice of medical decisions. In this light, neither the courts, legislatures, nor public health agencies have produced clear, binding rules for the treatment of HIV-positive health care workers (HCWs). The legal developments of the last several years return the question of HIV-infected HCWs to the HCWs themselves, to the institutions that employ them, and therefore to the colleagues and professional organizations with whom HIV-infected HCWs are associated.

What Is the Medical Profession Doing with This Authority Relative to HIV Infection/AIDS?

Individual HCWs have evidently concluded that they should keep their infections secret for as long as possible, while **many institutions seem to have adopted a "don't ask, don't tell" policy.** When a HCW's HIV infection is discovered, most institutions evaluate the worker under applicable guidelines and negotiate a mutually acceptable course of action, all in strict confidence. Few institutions go public; in some cases the HCW has no option but to sue (Burris, 1996).

time of the trial, her life expectancy was estimated at less than a year. Following a stormy two-month trial that challenged the integrity of all the physicians and expert witnesses who testified, she reportedly settled for just under $2 million.

Another pressing issue pointed out by Mandelbaum-Schmid is that HIV-infected doctors are not protected against discrimination. The experience of an otolaryngologist who died of AIDS in June, 1989, at the age of 46, set an unwelcome precedent. Before his illness, he had a thriving practice in Princeton, New Jersey. He believed he was infected in 1984 after being splashed in the face with blood while performing an emergency tracheotomy. He became ill with an undifferentiated pneumonia in 1987. Physicians performed a bronchoscopy and gave him an HIV test without telling him.

Word of his positive HIV test soon spread through the hospital and soon after into his community. By the time he was released from the hospital, his telephone lines were jammed with calls

from hysterical patients. He eventually lost about half his practice. When he tried to schedule operating room time, the hospital's president convened an emergency meeting of trustees. They made the unprecedented decision that he may operate but only with the informed consent of his patients.

He filed a lawsuit based on breach of ethics and doctor–patient confidentiality—his diagnosis had been leaked by the hospital laboratory—and violation of antidiscrimination laws. In April 1991, New Jersey Superior Court Judge Philip S. Carchman ruled that the Medical Center of Princeton, after learning the doctor had AIDS, made a "reasoned and informed response" in barring him from performing surgery without informed consent of his patients.

The last example of the plight of a physician with AIDS involves a physician at Johns Hopkins Medical Center. He contracted an HIV infection from a patient in 1983 while working as a resident in the bone marrow transplantation unit. He had an accident with the blood of a young leukemia patient who had been transfused many times. The accident was followed three weeks later by an acute febrile illness with cough, sore throat, rash, and lymphadenopathy. After this, he was in good health for the next three years. He completed his residency and became a chief resident and a fellow in cardiology. He married and had a daughter. In November of 1986, unexplained weight loss led him to be HIV tested. He tested positive for HIV.

The hospital's reaction was unexpected. He had to sue the institution and some members of the faculty in an effort to defend his reputation and obtain appropriate benefits. After endless months of legal battle, Johns Hopkins proposed a settlement three weeks before the trial date.

He said, "By actions like this, medical institutions send an awful message to the health care worker: we ask you to be in the front lines, but if something happens to you, we will not stand behind you, you will be abandoned, and you will be deprived of the privilege of practicing medicine" (Aoun, 1990). He died of AIDS in February of 1992, nine years after becoming infected with HIV.

FEDERAL AND PRIVATE SECTOR FINANCING: CREATION OF AN AIDS INDUSTRY

Twenty years ago, when the public was just learning about a new disease that would be called AIDS, the scientists tracking down the cause were already thinking about how their research could be marketed. French and American groups eventually claimed to have codiscovered HIV independently and in different ways. In one respect their approach was the same: Shortly before announcing their discoveries, both rushed to file patents that described how to determine whether a person's blood harbored the virus. By doing this, they gave birth to the HIV/AIDS industry. (Figure 13-4)

Federal Government

The federal government has responded to the challenges presented by the HIV/AIDS epidemic with the expenditure of federal funds and the enactment of a series of laws authorizing activities to foster research, prevention, treatment, and care related to HIV/AIDS. Much of the federal response has been accomplished through the annual appropriations process and through the general authorities of the federal agencies involved—primarily in the Department of Health and Human Services (for example, the National Institutes of Health, the Centers of Disease Control and Prevention, the Health Resources and Services Administration, and the Substance Abuse and Mental Health Services Administration) and also at the Departments

of Defense, Veterans Affairs, Housing and Urban Development, and the Agency for International Development. In addition to these discretionary spending accounts, the federal government has expended a significant amount through entitlement programs, including Medicaid, Medicare, Social Security Disability Insurance (SSDI), and Supplemental Security Income (SSI).

Financing the AIDS Industry

Federal— In 1990, the U.S. Congress did something quite rare: **It allocated money specifically for the treatment of one disease—HIV/AIDS.** In some ways the increased commitment of federal and state government to cancer research and treatment in the early 1970s is similar to what has happened in the war on AIDS in the 1980s. In both decades, there was a major funding surge to stimulate research, therapy, and prevention. A major difference, however, is that dollars for cancer came more slowly over a longer time period that began well before the 1970s. With AIDS, federal funding began in 1981 (Figure 13-5) and has increased at an unprecedented rate. During the 22 years from 1982 through 2003, federal spending on AIDS-related projects increased from $8 million in 1982 to $15.8 billion for 2003. The Presidential Advisory Council on HIV/AIDS provided the president with six AIDS goals that will be funded with the federal budget for AIDS. The goals are to: (1) develop a cure, (2) reduce/eliminate new infections, (3) guarantee care/service for the HIV-infected, (4) fight against HIV/ AIDS discrimination, (5) quickly translate scientific advances into improved care/ prevention, and (6) provide support for international AIDS efforts. (See Figure 13-6).

Private sector funding— In addition to the money spent by the federal government, collectively the states also spend between $6 billion and $8 billion each year. The private sector spends about $5 billion a year. By the end of 2003, the federal government spent about $128 billion for HIV/AIDS-related work, and the states and private sector spent about the same. In reality, adding in unspecified federal dollars that went to AIDS-related projects and the dollars spent in the private sector would most likely bring the total AIDS-related expenditures to between $250 billion and $300 billion. Yet, in spite of this massive expenditure on HIV/AIDS, the United States still does not have the underpinning of a uniform health care system

FIGURE 13-4 Representation of the Enormous Sum of Federal, State, and Private Sector Monies Spent on HIV/AIDS Has Made This Disease an Industry unto Itself.

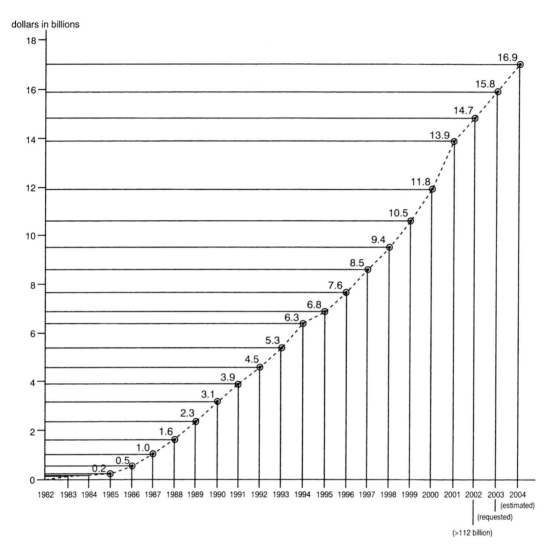

dollars in billions

FIGURE 13-5 Federal Government AIDS Expenditures to the Year 2003. Note the sharp rise in monies spent on AIDS-related projects by the Public Health Services. Federal expenditures were $1 billion in 1987, and $15.8 billion for 2003. Bernhard Schwartlander of UNAIDS said that the United States actually spends over $20 billion a year on prevention, care, and research. Ending 2004 the United States will have spent about $150 billion over 23 years on this disease.

to provide an organized, controlled use of AIDS funds. The current funding is **heterogeneous** and provides **unequal access** to HIV/AIDS care.

AIDS Costs as a Percentage of the National Health Care Budget Placed in Perspective

The $15.8 billion for 2003 represents about 0.6% of the $2 trillion, 16 billion federal budget. For 2003, the total expenditures for HIV/AIDS will be about 7% of the U.S. health care budget of $215 billion. To place health care and AIDS expenditures in perspective, in 1989 the federal government allocated $166 billion to "bail out" the savings and loan industry through year 2000. It is estimated that $500 billion will be needed over the next 40 years. In 1989, the Department of Energy estimated it would take 30 years and over $1 trillion to clean up nuclear waste dumps across

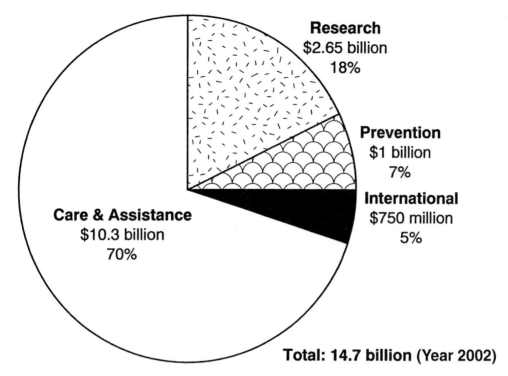

Research
$2.65 billion
18%

Prevention
$1 billion
7%

International
$750 million
5%

Care & Assistance
$10.3 billion
70%

Total: 14.7 billion (Year 2002)

FIGURE 13-6   Total Federal HIV/AIDS Spending by Category FY 2003. Federal HIV/AIDS spending are divided generally into four categories: Care and Assistance, Research, Prevention, and International.

Programs under **Care and Assistance** are those that deliver health care services, support services, and disability assistance to individuals with HIV/AIDS. Major health care programs in this category include Medicaid, Medicare, Supplemental Security Income (SSI), Social Security Disability Income (SSDI), Ryan White CARE Act, Ricky Ray Hemophilia Relief Fund, Housing Opportunities for People with AIDS (HOPWA).

Research programs are those that address the range of biomedical, epidemiological, behavioral, health services, and social science research activities. These programs include those operated within the Department of Health and Human Services (HHS) (including the National Institutes of Health (NIH), the Food and Drug Administration (FDA), and the Agency for Healthcare Research and Quality (AHRQ), and the Department of Defense (DOD).

The **Prevention** category includes programs designed to provide information, education, counseling, and risk reduction regarding HIV; to reduce the number of HIV infections through perinatal transmission, from workplace accidents, among immigrants, in public housing, and throughout the prison system; and to ensure the safety of the blood supply. Most of these programs are run through the HHS/Centers for Disease Control and Prevention (CDC).

International programs include efforts to cooperate with other nations on research, to coordinate international activities, to provide training and education in skills to prevent the spread of HIV, to encourage the use of non-governmental organization networks and community-based organizations to implement prevention and care programs, and to disseminate information via multi-language television, radio, and texts distributed overseas. International programs are primarily conducted by the U.S. Agency for International Development. *(Source: Kaiser Family Foundation, Federal HIV/AIDS Spending: A Budget Chartbook, Fiscal Year 2001 Updated)*

A VIEW OF HIV/AIDS FUNDING

It should be noted that only about half of all federal HIV/AIDS funding is specifically designated for HIV/AIDS programs. Most of the federal help comes from programs such as Medicaid or Medicare that are intended to provide care and services to any qualifying person, based on his or her medical, functional, and income status. People with HIV/AIDS qualify for these programs in much the same manner as people with cancer or heart disease do. The level of support that is identified as "for HIV/AIDS" is an estimate of what portion of the overall national spending goes for HIV/AIDS care. In addition, there are other federal programs that are not specifically designed for HIV/AIDS services and that serve people with HIV/AIDS, but for which HIV/AIDS-related spending estimates cannot be provided. For example, federally supported tuberculosis control programs are undoubtedly used by people with HIV/AIDS, but estimates of the proportionate spending are not available. Likewise, people with HIV/AIDS buy Treasury bills, take out federal flood insurance policies, go to government-subsidized museums, and pay taxes, but, since such activities are not HIV-related, no data is gathered on the basis of HIV infection status. Estimates of funding for these programs that may be used by many people with HIV/AIDS are not included. Spending by the federal government as an employer providing health insurance to its workers with HIV/AIDS through the Federal Employee Health Benefits Program (FEHBP) is also not included in total federal spending data. In addition, federal funding is not the only funding for HIV/AIDS programs. States supply a substantial portion of overall Medicaid spending, ranging from a maximum of 50% of the total Medicaid funding in comparatively affluent states to a minimum of 17% in the poorest states. States are also required to make matching payments for some federal programs including the Ryan White CARE Act. In the Supplemental Security Income (SSI) program, many states make the supplemental payments to raise disability cash assistance above the federal minimum. Many states also operate HIV/AIDS programs of their own. Beyond federal and state funding, many local governments, foundations, and charities also provide HIV/AIDS services. Public hospitals, for example, are usually supported by counties or cities and are often the sites of much clinical HIV/AIDS care. Likewise, free clinics and specialized HIV/AIDS service organizations provide both care and prevention services. Several foundations have made substantial contributions to HIV/AIDS programs. Federal funds have, nonetheless, remained predominant during the HIV/AIDS pandemic.

It is difficult to estimate overall HIV/AIDS spending. Just trying to work with federal dollars for any individual fiscal year is difficult. For example, the federal budget for any individual fiscal year takes several years to prepare, carry out, and audit. For instance, on preparing this textbook (mid-2002), final accounts of what was spent in FY 2001 have closed; the Congress has finished appropriations for FY 2002; the President had delivered his budget for FY 2003 to the Congress; and the Executive Branch agencies are preparing their recommended budget proposals for FY 2004!

the United States. The government spends about $300 billion annually on its military machines.

AIDS Expenditures Compared to Other Major Diseases

Federal spending for AIDS research, educational programs, counselor training, testing, and prevention programs has been compared with federal spending for other diseases. There is a discrepancy between the total federal dollars spent on certain diseases and the number of deaths they cause. In 2000, with about 15,000 deaths, HIV/AIDS received $11.8 billion. That's equivalent to about **$790,000** per AIDS-related death! In 2000, cancer caused about 560,000 deaths (about 1500 people/day) and received $3.3 billion or about $5900/death. During the same time, there were 1,220,000 new cases of cancer in the United States; 183,000 were new cases of breast cancer and there were over 42,000 breast cancer-associated deaths. One in seven to nine women will get breast cancer. Heart disease, which caused some 950,000 deaths in 2000 (43% of all deaths for the year), received about $1.5 billion or about $1580/death. Some 2 million Americans require insulin injections for type I diabetes and perhaps as many as 14 million have type II diabetes (diet controlled). Diabetes, a severe progressive disorder, received $541 million, or about 5% of the AIDS budget in 2000 or about $2847/death. It is estimated that 190,000 people will die annually because of diabetes complications. Stroke, which affects millions of Americans and is involved in about 160,000 deaths per year, received $212 million or $1325/death. Overall, between 1981 and the beginning of 2003, while 480,000 people died of AIDS, 17 million died of heart disease and 9.3 million died of cancer. For the year 2003 15.8 billion federal dollars were allocated for HIV/AIDS programs. There will be about 15,000 AIDS-related deaths or over $1 million/death! **This is the most expensive disease in history relative to time, 1981 through 2003.**

BOX 13.8

AIDS PROGRAMS: AN EPIDEMIC OF WASTE?

Through the year 2002 there has been constant pressure on politicians and leaders of private industry to contribute higher levels of money in the fight against HIV/AIDS. In 2002, AIDS activists marched in Washington in an attempt to get Congress to allocate $2.5 billion to the Global AIDS, Tuberculosis, and Malaria Fund. Their belief is that America is not spending enough money at home or globally on HIV/AIDS. Others, however, protest this notion and feel that if graft and corruption were eliminated there would be sufficient money such that yearly increases in the federal HIV/AIDS program would not be called for. To support this belief, a group called "Citizens Against Government Waste" (CAGW) released a report in February 2002 on **"AIDS Programs: An Epidemic of Waste"** (www.cagw.org). Citizens Against Government Waste is the nation's largest nonpartisan, nonprofit organization dedicated to eliminating waste, fraud, abuse, and mismanagement in government. Some of the fraud found by this group is listed exactly as it is presented in their report:

♦ CAGW has obtained a copy of a $20,000 grant to the Vermont Department of Public Health from the Twin State Women's Network (TSWN) to be used for a weekend retreat. Topics for the weekend included "Toys 4 Us" and "Self Loving/Self Healing: Discussing the Role of Masturbation as a Tool for Healing." TSWN also received: $1,500 for long distance phone calls; $1,000 for books, including "The New Good Vibrations for Sex" manual; and $250 for videos, choices of which included "Fire in the Valley: A Guide to Masturbation for Women" and "Fire in the Valley: A Guide to Masturbation for Men." Each participant received a welcome bag filled with mints and chocolate and each room was equipped with welcome packets containing condoms, lubricant, candles, massage lotion, and lip balm. TSWN received 86% of its funds from government sources, including the Centers for Disease Control (CDC).

♦ Positive Force in San Francisco receives $1 million a year from the CDC. The group offers flirting classes and, last July, hosted a workshop on how to have anal intercourse if you suffer from diarrhea. (Diarrhea is a common side effect of AIDS.)

♦ On February 28, 2002, the Stop AIDS Project of San Francisco, which received nearly $700,000 from the CDC in fiscal 2001, will sponsor "GUYWATCH: Blow by Blow." The advertisement for the seminar reads, in part: "What tricks do you want to share to make your man tremble with delight?"

♦ A Central Florida AIDS Unified Resources (CENTAUR) staffer spent $600,000 in Ryan White CARE Act money on tickets to Disney World, hotels, and restaurants.

♦ In April 2001, *The New York Post* revealed New York City was spending nearly $180,000 a week ($9 million a year) on hotel rooms for HIV and AIDS patients. That month, the city had reserved 20 rooms at the Sofitel Hotel in Midtown Manhattan at $329 apiece. Advocates say DASIS must use the expensive hotels because it has ruined its relationship with lower-cost hotels by not paying bills on time. New York city received $52.6 million in Housing Opportunities for People With AIDS (HOPWA) program funding in fiscal 2001.

♦ The University of California-San Francisco AIDS Health Project (AHP), which received a $633,765 grant from the CDC prevention in fiscal 2001 and continually receives nearly

BOX 13.8 *(continued)*

85% of its funding from government sources, sponsored a workshop in November in physical intimacy, focusing on "holding, kissing, licking, sucking, and . . ."

♦ A doctor in Puerto Rico used $2.2 million in federal funds to buy luxury items like cars and jet skis, while severely neglecting the AIDS patients in his care.

♦ More than $20 million in grant money intended to help house AIDS patients was collected—but never spent—in Los Angeles.

♦ AID Atlanta, Inc., which received more than $3.5 million from the government in fiscal 2000 and only $1.2 million in private contributions, sponsors "Deeper Love: A Workshop for Gay and Bisexual Men of African Descent" that addresses such subjects as dating, relationships, and erotica. The program lists the following topics of discussion: "Dirty talk: what makes it good; Tossing salad; Strollin' in the park, through the trails; The art of latex; Safety versus trust." AID Atlanta, Inc. also sponsors "Slipping and Sliding" where men can explore their needs and desires and learn how to fulfill them.

♦ FBI investigation into the South Dallas Health Clinic revealed that more than $60,000 in the Title I funds had been spent on calls to psychic hotlines and on shopping trips to Neiman Marcus.

♦ The non-profit Tampa Hillsborough Action Plan (THAP) gives its top executives plenty of perks despite its financial woes. THAP boss and THAP Chief Executive Officer rang up nearly $1,000 in meal charges in a three-week period and were also afforded the use of sport utility vehicles. THAP boss received up to $45,000 a year annually for the maintenance of his vehicles. THAP's top executives also received four season tickets for Tampa Bay Buccaneers games and two season tickets for both the Tampa Bay Devil Rays and the Tampa Bay Lightning. Meanwhile, THAP owed nearly $25,000 in delinquent payroll taxes. THAP receives $450,000 a year from the federal government to provide housing to people with AIDS.

♦ Not in the CAGW investigation is the Los Angeles County Auditor Controller's Office report that states "officials in the county's Office of AIDS Programs and Policy cannot account for $83 million it spent in 2001. That is more money than the budget for many American cities.

CONCLUSION OF CAGW

Before new resources are added to the $13 billion in federal money currently allotted for AIDS-related programs, the Departments of Health and Human Services and Housing and Urban Development should conduct extensive audits of the Ryan White CARE Act Title I and the HOPWA program. Such audits will give Congress more incentive to reform or eliminate these antiquated and duplicated social programs. Congress should redirect many CDC prevention grants to international AIDS relief efforts or increased funds for researching an AIDS cure. Many CARE Act programs, including all of Title I, should be phased out and incorporated into existing federal safety net programs such as Medicaid and Medicare. This would ensure necessary, life-saving medical care to those with HIV and AIDS who are low-income or uninsured, while also eliminating nonessential AIDS services. It would also save money to bolster the AIDS Drug Assistance Program.

UPDATE 2002 In May 2002, U.S. Treasury Secretary Paul O'Neill took a 10-day tour of Africa. On his return, he called for increased access to HIV/AIDS treatment and greater accountability for assistance programs. O'Neill went to Chris Hani Baragwanath Hospital in Soweto where he met with HIV-positive women whose children had been treated at birth with the antiretroviral drug nevirapine to reduce the risk of vertical HIV transmission. O'Neill, who has been critical of foreign aid in the past, asked why the South African government was not providing treatment to all HIV-positive pregnant women. O'Neill said, "This whole business about having so much money . . . and it not going primarily to treatment is just a stunning revelation." In an interview with ABC's "This Week," on May 26th, O'Neill echoed his call for greater accountability. "My problem is that it isn't clear why we aren't getting better choices about the priority use of the money that is already there. For me, this is about getting real results on the ground."

Question: Do you think in Africa, there is at least an equal amount of fraud and corruption as found in America with regard to the allocation and spending of HIV/AIDS dollars donated for the prevention and treatment of HIV/AIDS? Support your opinions with examples.

U.S. GOVERNMENT BELIEVES HIV/AIDS IS A THREAT TO NATIONAL SECURITY

In addition to spending enormous sums of money on HIV/AIDS, the federal government declared in May 2000 that "AIDS is a threat to our national security." U.S. Secretary of Health Donna Shalala said, "We know that infectious diseases know no borders, that they can affect this country, and in this case it is both in our economic interest and in our national security interest to work on these infectious diseases abroad. The high rates of AIDS in Africa are putting security and stability at risk by disabling national armies, disrupting economies and killing off people who might become the next generation of leaders. Basically AIDS is uncoupling the economic gains in Africa as African countries are forced to shift more resources to their health care systems from their economic investments." Shalala also said that countries in other parts of the world face a growing HIV/AIDS crisis. "Eastern Europe has an AIDS problem, Russia has it, India has it, every country in the world that we do business with, but more importantly our need to be politically stable, is suffering from this huge onslaught of AIDS. And that makes the relationship economically and from the security point of view relevant to America's national security."

Class Discussion: Present reasons that agree or disagree with the federal government's declaration that HIV/AIDS is a threat to America's national security.

GLOBAL HIV/AIDS FUNDING FOR UNDERDEVELOPED NATIONS

In many ways, we are of one world. Africa's destiny is our destiny. There is hope on the horizon, but that hope will only be realized if the developed nations take constructive action together. As South Africa's Archbishop Desmond Tutu said: "If we wage this holy war together—we will win."

The bottom line is this: There is no vaccine or cure for AIDS in sight, and the world is at the beginning of a global pandemic, not the end. What is happening in Africa now is just the tip of the iceberg. As goes Africa, so will go India and the Newly Independent States of the former Soviet Union. There must be a sense of urgency for the developed world to work together; to learn from their failures and successes, and to share their experience with those countries that now stand on the brink of disaster. Millions of lives—perhaps hundreds of millions of lives—hang in the balance. AIDS is a devastating human tragedy that requires global help.

HINDSIGHT Thirteen years ago, when the AIDS death toll in the United States crossed 100,000, few paid heed to a grim prediction by the World Health Organization (WHO) that "by the year 2000, 40 million persons may be infected with HIV." In the developed world, AIDS was seen as a serious but small disease, restricted to gay men, drug users, hemophiliacs, and the infants of all three. In the developing world, just a few courageous voices were warning about the silent spread of a deadly new plague. In retrospect, WHO's grim prediction was 15 million too low! Africa is in crisis. In some countries, over 35% of the adult population is infected. Many millions have died, and millions more will follow, leaving their societies trapped in poverty, burdened with a generation of orphans, and facing demographic catastrophe. The grim statistics are not confined to Africa. Asia and the Caribbean face explosive HIV epidemics, while the nations of the former Soviet empire are looking at an overwhelming increase of drug addiction, untreated sexual diseases, and the unchecked spread of HIV. Finally the world has begun to take notice. In January 2000, the United Nations Security Council held a precedent-setting special session, in which for the first time it identified a disease—AIDS—as a global security threat. A second UN-HIV/AIDS special session of the General Assembly was held on June 25–27, 2001 (Figure 13-7).

The Productive Years

HIV kills young people in their most productive years. In a growing number of countries, many thousands of workers, teachers, nurses, civil servants, and others have died and are dying. The backbone of civil society is threatened in many nations, and that threat remains uncontrolled. The security threat is real, but only half the story. HIV began as an obscure simian virus in equatorial Africa in the first half of the 20th century and within 50 years had spread throughout the world. The

EARLY GLOBAL RESPONSE TO AIDS AND NATIONAL SECURITY

As national intelligence office at large, Katherine Hall supervised the CIA's taxonomy of upheaval overseas. What signs forecast a government's collapse, an economy's ruin, a civil war? Hall and her staff had a hunch that conventional indicators, heavy on politics and money, were missing something. In 1990, after three years of frustrated lobbying, she received permission to study the rapidly expanding growth of HIV/AIDS, particularly in Africa. When Hall first proposed to study the AIDS phenomenon in 1987, she could not obtain CIA approval for use of personnel and computer-modeling resources. Internal critics declared global AIDS an unfit subject of intelligence, or said the impact on U.S. interests would be benign. However, an Interagency Intelligence Memorandum, distributed in classified channels in July 1991 foretold one of the deadliest calamities in human experience. Titled simply, **"The Global AIDS Disaster,"** the report projected 45 million infections by 2000—inexorably fatal—the great majority in Africa. The number lacked comparison. Not that many combatants were killed in World War I, World War II, Korea, and Vietnam combined. Unlike the Black Death in 14th-century Europe, which took half as many lives, the means of controlling AIDS were known. Yet African and foreign governments, the report said, were making no more than a "modest level of effort." The same might have been said for the intelligence memorandum that landed near the top of the pile of incoming intelligence at the White House and Cabinet agencies.

The reaction was "indifference—that's the right word." Hall and others prepared for the flurry of briefings that accompanies the release of a major intelligence product. Surprise, surprise, except for then-Surgeon General C. Everett Koop, no one asked about the memorandum.

Nine years later, a highly public awakening played out in the Clinton administration, Congress, foreign capitals, the United Nations system, and the offices of drug manufacturers. The premise of their new commitments on AIDS was that they were confronted for the **first time** with the magnitude of the disaster. Yet for a decade, the world knew the dimensions of the coming catastrophe and the means available to slow it. Estimates ranged widely, but the World Health Organization in 1990 and 1991 projected a caseload, and eventual death toll, in the tens of millions by 2000. Individually and collectively, most of those with power decided not to act. As for Hall's predictions of 45 million HIV infection by 2000, she was about 10 million short.

UPDATE 2002—A senior U.S. intelligence officer being interviewed at the CIA in Langley, Virginia said, "The HIV/AIDS crisis is entering a larger breakout phase." Analysis from the National Intelligence Council said, "In Africa, roughly 23 million people were infected with the disease in 1997, according to UNAIDS, the joint United Nations program for HIV/AIDS. The figure is 30 million now, a 30% increase over the previous five-year period. A doubling of cases in Africa in the next five years would push the number of people infected there to 60 million by 2007!" Senior policymakers at the World Health Organization, World Bank, and UNAIDS said that while they had not heard about U.S. intelligence's new projections, they believed the forecast could be on target. The U.S. Defense Intelligence Agency issued a report in July 2002 concluding that global security is imperiled by AIDS; that more than half of Congo and Angola's armies are infected, along with upwards of 75% of the Zimbabwe and Malawi forces. UNAIDS also reported in July 2002 that Africa's economy is declining by 4% annually due to AIDS; that labor productivity in hard-hit countries is down by 50%, and half the continent's population lives on less than $1 day. And it found that economic development and life expectancy on most of the continent has returned to World War II levels. Last year, according to the International Monetary Fund, the continent contributed less than 4% of the world domestic product.

forces that brought HIV to America in the 1970s— world travel, globalization, and urbanization—are accelerating. One need only look at the number of variant strains of HIV-1 spreading worldwide or at the number of HIV-2 cases now emerging in New York and other gateway American cities to see how the forces of globalization are adding new ingredients to America's HIV/AIDS problems. When HIV remains unchecked in large regions of the globe, as it does, no country is safe, including America. Fighting AIDS abroad is in America's own interest.

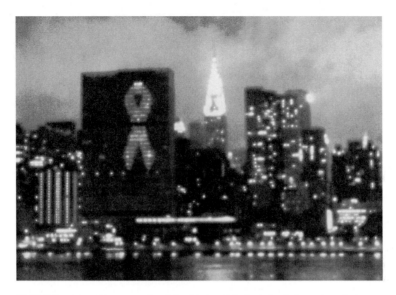

FIGURE 13-7 Photograph of the United Nations building after dark. On the evenings of June 25, 26, 27, 2001, all lights were turned off. Only in the rooms where windows were fitted with red plastic panels, were the lights left on. This gave the image of the AIDS ribbon. On Sept. 11, 2001, this skyline was shattered by terrorists who destroyed the World Trade Center Twin Towers. Less than a month later, that attack drastically affected HIV/AIDS fundraising, already dropping due to a slow economy. *(Photograph courtesy of Archive Photos)*

United Nations Secretary-General Kofi Annan Calls for Large-Scale Mobilization in Fight against AIDS, Tuberculosis, and Malaria

In mid-2001, calling the battle his personal priority, the secretary-general outlined five priority areas for the global campaign.

1. Preventing further spread of the epidemic, especially by giving young people the knowledge and power to protect themselves.
2. Reducing HIV transmission from mother to child, which he called "the cruelest, most unjust" infections of all.
3. Ensuring that care and treatment is within reach of all.
4. Delivering scientific breakthroughs. Finding a cure and vaccine for HIV/AIDS must be given increased priority in scientific budgets.
5. Protecting those made most vulnerable by the epidemic, especially orphans.

To achieve these five goals, Annan called world leaders to help finance the campaign against AIDS, tuberculosis, and malaria in Africa. In April of 2001, he said, "a war chest of 7 billion to 10 billion U.S. dollars is needed annually, over an extended period of time, to wage an effective global campaign against AIDS. In July 2001 the Group of Eight (G8) industralized countries (Britian, Canada, France, Germany, Italy, Japan, Russia and USA) proposed the creation of a new Global Fund to obtain $10 billion a year dedicated to the battle against HIV/AIDS and other infectious diseases. Current spending on AIDS in developing countries totals around $1 billion annually." This is many billions of dollars less than they spend on their military. Although Annan's figure of $10 billion for combating AIDS seems like a large sum, it is equivalent to:

◆ Four days of global military spending.
◆ Ten days of running the Organization for Economic Cooperation and Development (OECD).
◆ The cost of 100 Eurofighters (jet fighting planes).

A contribution of $10 billion a year would be equivalent to the amount of money spent in 60 days

---
BOX 13.9

FORMS OF U.S. FOREIGN MONETARY AND OTHER ASSISTANCE FOR HIV/AIDS

U.S. Agency Activity—Several U.S. agencies oversee and engage in global AIDS activities and programs, including the State Department, USAID, CDC, NIH, and the Peace Corps. The State Department provides overall direction for U.S. global HIV/AIDS policies, including policy guidance to USAID, an independent agency. USAID implements U.S. foreign economic and humanitarian assistance programs, and provides the bulk of bilateral assistance for addressing the epidemic in developing countries. The CDC supports HIV/AIDS prevention and prevention research activities around the world as part of the U.S. response to the global pandemic. Much of CDC's activities involve technical assistance conducted in partnership with USAID. NIH conducts and funds international HIV/AIDS research efforts. The Peace Corps, which places volunteers around the world, recently launched a new education effort to train volunteers to provide HIV prevention and care services.

Direct Assistance Through Government-to-Government Agreements and Bilateral Aid—A key strategy of USAID is to form bilateral working relationships with governments around the world to cooperatively conduct prevention, care, and research programs. This approach to development assistance is based on promoting broad-based economic growth through policy analyses, technical assistance, and training. In addition, emergency relief is structured to help nations make the transition to sustainable development. In addition to developing working relationships, the United States also provides bilateral support directly to governments to address HIV/AIDS.

Contributions to Multilateral Programs—The United States also contributes to multilateral programs, such as UNAIDS, the World Bank, and the Pan American Health Organization. The newly proposed Global Fund represents the creation of a new multilateral program. The Global Fund has received pledged contributions from the United States and other country donors as well as the private sector.

Loans to Developing Countries—Loans are another mechanism used by the United States and others to provide international assistance. Last year, the United States Export-Import (Ex-Im) Bank announced plans to provide $1 billion in loans per year for five years to support the purchase of HIV/AIDS medications made in the United States. The Ex-Im Bank also announced that it would increase the standard repayment terms for HIV/AIDS pharmaceutical sales in these countries from six months to five years.

Debt Relief—According to the World Bank, 33 of the world's 41 most heavily-indebted countries are in Africa with a total debt of $230 billion. There is a growing movement on the part of developed nations to forgive all or part of that debt. Debt relief can enable developing nations to spend more of the resources on health programs addressing HIV/AIDS. Such efforts are also focusing on ways to ensure that debt relief results in commitments by host countries to use resources for health-related initiatives. Last year, Congress approved nearly $450 million in debt relief for developing nations, primarily in sub-Saharan Africa. Pending legislation—the Debt Cancellation for HIV/AIDS Response Act (H.R. 1567)—would allow the United States to instruct its directors at the World Bank and the International Monetary Fund to advocate for debt relief efforts.

Direct Assistance to Non-Governmental Organizations (NGOs)—Non-governmental Organizations (NGOs) play a critical role in many nations' response to the epidemic. Providing financial and non-financial assistance to such organizations enhances their ability to respond to local needs and ensures more accountability for U.S. resources. Many of USAID's activities, for example, target non-government organizations (NGOs) either directly or through other organizations in an effort to build their capacity and provide technical assistance. Some U.S. NGOs have also begun to form partnerships with NGOs in other nations.

Source: Kaiser Daily HIV/AIDS-AIDS at 20 at Kaisernetwork.org.

---

in the United States on soft drinks or in 35 days on fast foods.

Annan also wants all antiretroviral drugs to be sold to underdeveloped nations at 5% of the cost to people in the developed world. Should

Africa receive $10 billion annually from the developed world, it would average out that each living HIV-infected African would receive $333 per year ($10 billion divided by 30 million HIV-infected) for as long as the money was provided.

THE GLOBAL FUND TO FIGHT HIV/AIDS, TB, AND MALARIA

This fund was set up in response to widespread public criticism of governments' apathy to the health crisis in developing countries, especially concerning HIV/AIDS. The health status of the poor, women, men, and children is deteriorating in many parts of the world, and the fund is a unique opportunity to mobilize international political will and resources to address this crisis in a new way, rather than continuing with "business as usual."

The Global Fund was initiated through the United Nations General Assembly Special Session on AIDS (UNGASS) in June of 2001. The year 2001 will be recorded in AIDS history as the year when political commitment to the disease moved to center stage. UNGASS demanded real political commitment, and activists had to think on their feet as they adjusted to the opaque UN negotiations.

Countries/Others	$ Million
United States	1,750
Germany	131
France	127
Norway	110
United Kingdom	200
Japan	200
Canada	100
Nigeria	10
Uganda	2
Austria	1
Zimbabwe	1
Bill and Melinda Gates Foundation	100
Winterthur Insurance Agency	1

Total as of December 2002 was about $3.73 billion (U.S. dollars)

Legislators in the U.S. Congress are committed to adding $1 billion in 2003. According to the July 2002 Henry J. Kaiser Foundation Report, the United States spent about $2.9 billion on Global HIV/AIDS programs from 1996 through 2002. An additional $1.1 billion will be added in 2003. From 1996 through 2002, the World Bank, the second largest donor, gave $2.7 billion.

Comments Relative to the War Chest

In August 2001, Kofi Annan appointed Crispus Kiyonga, a former Ugandan health and finance minister, to chair the Global AIDS and Health Fund. Kofi Annan's war chest is unprecedented in the world of global public health. Many nations refuse to pledge money because there is no mechanism in place to decide who will handle the funds, how corruption will be avoided, how funds will be dispersed, who besides Africa will receive any of the funds, and what the money will be spent for. For example, there remains a large division among the 184 countries of the United Nations General Assembly on whether most of the money should be spent on prevention rather than antiretroviral drugs. Many members of the General Assembly felt that about half the $10 billion should be spent on drugs for Africa and the other half be spent on prevention programs in Asia and the former Soviet nations where the epidemic is expanding out of control. Clearly there are no easy choices, but choices must be made. The United States was the first and only country by mid-2001 to offer Annan $200 million toward his global AIDS fund. Ten other nations quickly followed. The U.S. pledge

This would occur only if the money was actually given to the people. This money, along with free or very low drug costs could be of considerable help, especially since many of the African countries spend less than $5 to $10 per person a year on public health. But, used in this way, this large sum of money would not be available to build needed medical facilities or import the thousands of doctors necessary to treat the HIV-infected. That will take a few hundred billion more dollars.

As this book goes to press, Kofi Annan received great applause for his work at the special General Assembly for his work on HIV/AIDS, but the growth of the war chest of money is in danger of stalling long before it reaches its $10 billion in 2005. A recent study shows that the developing nations need $10 billion a year now! An article on "Estimating the Cost of Expanded AIDS Treatment in Africa," that appeared in the June 2001 issue of *Topics in HIV Medicine,* states that it would cost $1.12 billion/year to treat 1 million HIV-infected Africans. Beginning 2003 there will be an estimated 30 million Africans living with HIV. The cost, based on information presented in the article, would be about $33 billion/year if all were to be treated equally. To date, those who have pledged money to the global fund through 2002 are:

is in addition to the $760 million already pledged for the year 2001 and 1 billion in 2002. No single nation has spent more on the African HIV/AIDS problem than the United States.

The Problem in Perspective

According to the UNAIDS chief epidemiologist, ending 2003 there will be 44 million living HIV-infected people globally. About 39 million of these people are poor. They live on less than $2 a day. There is an overwhelming problem of poverty. An HIV-positive American can focus on his T cell counts; an HIV-positive African in a rural village still has to focus on finding clean water and food.

Politicians, economists, and AIDS specialists rarely say this bluntly, but the truth is that most of those 44 million people have simply been written off because the first priority for the first few billion dollars is prevention, not treatment. An economist who studies AIDS in South Africa, which has the world's fastest growing epidemic, said, "You can't give up on the infected because of the message it sends. But if he had $1 billion to spend most wisely, I would spend it on giving women more power, caring for orphans, and getting them education."

FINALLY, THE QUESTION: How much would it cost to contain the global AIDS pandemic? The answer is: How much have you got? How much would it cost to banish ignorance, to deaden lust, to shame rape, to stop war, to enrich the poor, to empower women, to defend children, to make decent medical care as globally ubiquitous as Coca-Cola—in short, to get rid of all the underlying causes of the epidemic in the developing nations. Much of the world at risk for HIV/AIDS can't read. Most of the world at risk has never used a condom. Most of the world at risk has never heard of Act Up and wouldn't dare heckle a president. And most of the world with AIDS thinks it doesn't have the disease and doesn't know anyone who does, because 95% of those infected in the developing nations have never been tested. (Most estimates come from anonymous testing at prenatal clinics.) Most of the world cannot afford the antiretroviral drugs.

For Class Reflection and Discussion:

ONE—It has been estimated that the United States spent $225 billion on the Y2K problem. All nations, globally, spent about $600 billion on Y2K. Why isn't there as much fear of AIDS, a transmissible death-causing disease, around the world as there was for the potential Y2K problem?

TWO—The CDC in 2002 estimated the nation's total cost of smoking at $3391 a year for every smoker or a total $157.7 billion. The agency estimated the nation's smoking-related medical costs at $3.45 a pack, and said job productivity lost because of premature death from smoking amounted to $3.73 a pack, for a total of $7.18. The average cost of a pack of cigarettes in 2002 was $2.92. Americans buy about 22 billion packs of cigarettes annually which results in about 440,000 smoking-related deaths a year.

Comment: Smoking, like HIV infection, is preventable. Why is there no public outcry about the large cost of a bad habit to the taxpayer, as there is about the costs for HIV/AID expenditures?

THREE—Scientists and economists have estimated a need of $10 billion a year to halt rising death tolls and HIV infection rates. The global AIDS fund will be fortunate if it reaches $10 billion in commitments by 2005. And this was before September 11, 2001, when terrorists destroyed the World Trade Center towers and a section of the Pentagon. Following September 11th, the donations to HIV/AIDS funds dropped by many millions of dollars across the United States. The federal government decided to flat line AIDS expenditures, yet within two weeks after September 11th, President Bush committed about $40 billion to deal with the September 11 disaster and punish those responsible for the terror attacks against the United States.

Question: Because HIV/AIDS kills about 8000 people every day, worldwide, should the United States, regardless of what other countries do, commit a larger sum of money to the global AIDS fund?

Global Funds for AIDS, Tuberculosis, and Malaria Announces the First Grant Recipients (It should be noted that when resources are limited, choices must be made)

About $700 million was available for grants in 2002. During the first round of grants (April 2002), $378 million was awarded to 40 programs in 31 countries for use over a two-year period. Over 300 proposals requesting over $5 billion were reviewed for funding.

The Breakdown— Programs in African nations received 52% of the total grants awarded; 13% went to programs in the Americas; 8% to programs in Eastern Europe and Central Asia; 12% to programs in Southeast Asia, and 14% to programs in the Western Pacific. Nations receiving the most money were South Africa with $25 million, Zambia with almost $20 million, China with $15 million, and Zimbabwe and Haiti with $10 million each. Most of the grants will fund programs that incorporate a combination of prevention and treatment, and 21 of the 28 HIV/AIDS-specific grants specifically include money to buy antiretroviral drugs. A second round of grant funding is set for September 2002.

Criticism: The Global Fund has given $66 million over five years to two of the region's wealthiest nations—Chile and Argentina, but nothing to countries such as Nicaragua, Ecuador, Peru, Belize, or the Dominican Republic.

As of October 2002, none of the first round grants awarded had been funded!

UPDATE 2002 In June 2002, the Organization of Petroleum Exporting Countries (OPEC) joined forces with the World Health Organizations to fight HIV/AIDS in Africa. The OPEC Fund for International Development has prepared a first grant of $8.1 million to help fund WHO projects in 12 hard-hit nations in sub-Saharan Africa.

The Antiretroviral Drug War of 2001

The public opinion storm that erupted against the 39 international pharmaceutical companies brought the spotlight on the AIDS catastrophe in Africa front and center. After the dust has settled,

the major pharmaceutical firms backed down. The international court trial in Peoria, South Africa, was cancelled. In short, the drug firms agreed to supply the antiretrovirals at cost or below in some cases to Africa and a select few other underdeveloped countries hit hard by the HIV/AIDS. In addition, the drug companies have consented for these same countries to import cheaper antiretroviral drugs if available from competing nations who say they can produce generic versions of the antiretrovirals.

The Surprise! After all the legal threats, charges of discrimination, and maligning of the international drug companies to drop their prices, and after winning the drug supply and price war, South Africa, the leading drug pharmaceutical foe, announced that it has no intention of buying the antiretroviral drugs from anyone. Manto Tshabalala-Msimang, health minister of South Africa, said instead of investing in the antiretrovirals to keep those with HIV/AIDS alive, her government will seek to obtain cheap antibiotics for tuberculosis and other infections that kill people whose immune systems are damaged by HIV.

Surprised Again! In May of 2002, the President of South Africa, Thabo Mbeki (see Chapter 2), in a major departure from his controversial stance on AIDS made a dramatic announcement that his government will put in place a plan for a universal roll-out of antiretroviral drugs for HIV-positive pregnant women, rape survivors, and people infected through needle stick injuries. This program is to begin in January 2003.

SUMMARY

In 1981, the CDC announced a new disease affecting the homosexual population. This disease was later called AIDS. Many religious people believed this was a sign that homosexuality should be punished. The few facts available at that time gave rise to a great deal of fantasy and fear. Affected people were either innocent victims or they deserved the disease. Contracting AIDS labeled a person as less than desirable, a homosexual, or one who practiced deviant forms of sexual behavior. But even the so-called innocent victims, the children, the hemophiliacs, and the recipients of blood transfusions were not spared social ostracism. If you had AIDS, you were twice the victim—first of the virus and second of the social behavior.

Children were barred from attending school, adults from their jobs, and both from adequate medical care. For example, there are still relatively few dentists who will treat AIDS patients and a significant number of surgeons refuse to operate on AIDS patients. Years have passed, but many misconceptions about HIV/ AIDS linger on.

Fear is being casually transmitted rather than the virus. A significant number of people, after years of broad-scale education, still believe that the AIDS virus can be casually transmitted from toilet seats, drinking glasses, and even by donating blood.

The fallout from the fear of the AIDS pandemic has been a major change in sexual language in

TV advertisements, magazines, and radio. Condoms once spoken about only in hushed tones in conversations and kept under the counter in most drug stores, are now spoken of everywhere as a means of safer sex. AIDS, perhaps more than any other disease, has demonstrated that ignorance leads to fear and knowledge can lead to compassion.

To achieve understanding and compassion, people must be educated as to their HIV risk status and how they can keep it low. Many hundreds of millions of dollars have been spent to inform the public of the kinds of behavior that either place them at risk or reduce their risk for HIV infection. The problem is that although people are getting the information, too many refuse to act on it. Former Surgeon General C. Everett Koop's office mailed 107 million copies of the brochure "Understanding AIDS" to households in the United States. Fifty-one percent of those who received it said they never read it. Even among those who read the brochure are those who refuse to change their sexual behavior. Old habits are difficult to break.

To date, the hard evidence shows that only the homosexual population has significantly modified their sexual behavior as evidenced by the drop in the number of new cases of AIDS among them from 1988 through 2002.

A major problem looming on the horizon is the prospect of HIV being spread in the teenage population. Large numbers of teens use drugs and alcohol, have multiple sex partners, and believe they are invulnerable to infection.

The AMA stated in 1988 that physicians may not refuse to care for patients with AIDS because of actual risk or fear of contracting the disease. Some physicians get around this through referral to other physicians who will treat AIDS patients. There is one area of medicine that takes issue at having to treat AIDS patients. That area is surgery. Because it is difficult not to accidently get cut during surgery, surgeons have been the leading advocates for HIV testing of all surgical patients so they will know their risks before performing surgery.

On the other hand, patients feel they have a right to know if their physician, especially a surgeon, is HIV-infected. Surveys indicate that most people would not want to be treated by an HIV-infected physician.

On June 25, 1998, the U.S. Supreme Court ruled that the Americans with Disabilities Act protected HIV-infected people. Even though they experienced **no symptoms,** they are to be treated as handicapped.

Global AIDS, Tuberculosis, and Malaria Fund

Kofi Annan's request for $7 billion to $10 billion by 2005 has reached about $3.7 billion beginning 2003. The September 11th terrorist attack on the World Trade Center towers has impeded donations.

REVIEW QUESTIONS

(Answers to the Review Questions are on page 489.)

1. Name three major sources of information that contributed to the early panic and hysteria about the spread of AIDS.

2. Give three examples of unfounded public fears to AIDS infection.

3. Fear of the casual transmission of AIDS parallels what other earlier STD epidemic?

4. What evidence is there that it is difficult to get people to change their behavior even though they know it is harmful to their well-being?

5. What is the major thrust of AIDS education in the United States?

6. If education is the key to preventing HIV infection and new cases of AIDS, and most people interviewed say they have been 'educated,' why is it not working?

7. Why are today's teenagers in danger of contracting and spreading HIV?

8. Yes or No: Do physicians have a right to refuse to treat AIDS patients? Support your answer.

9. Do patients have a right to know if their physician is HIV-infected or has AIDS?

10. What is the primary means of offsetting the bias toward people with AIDS in the workplace?

11. Who is the current Secretary of the United Nations and how much money does he believe is needed to fight AIDS globally/year.

12. About how much money has been pledged to the global AIDS fund through 2002?

Epilogue

Albert Camus' closing reflection in his novel *The Plague*: "What we learn in a time of pestilence is that there are more things to admire in men than to despise."

Year 2003 is the 22nd year of the struggle with and against HIV. The assault on HIV has been, at times, courageous, insulting, and failing. This virus has caused irreversible emotional, spiritual, and economical devastation worldwide. Even though millions of people have died from it, millions live with it and many millions more are involved in preventing its spread. Is AIDS on planet earth serving some higher purpose? If so, how many people more must die before we realize what that purpose is?

Having reviewed to some degree what is known about AIDS and having presented you with some staggering statistics about the spread of HIV worldwide and in the United States, we now recognize that what began as a few cases of a new disease among gay men in the United States in 1980 has become a global pandemic of such proportions that is clearly ranks as one of the most destructive infectious diseases in history. We are at a pivotal point in the evolution of this historic disease as we move forward in the new millennium. Unless methods of prevention, with or without a vaccine, are successful, the worst of the global pandemic will occur in the 21st century having by far the greatest global impact in our lifetimes. HIV has fueled a global resurgence of TB and has given new and emerging microbes a great opportunity to adapt to humans—and AIDS has yet to run its course!

Responsibility

No one person is responsible for the existence of the AIDS pandemic. Yet, ultimately, all people must accept the task of dealing with its consequences. AIDS is intimately bound with health care in general, racism, homophobia, sexism, religion, and class issues. But the virus doesn't care. It's only interested in replicating. While the achievements of the global response to date should not be underestimated, neither should

the challenge ahead. HIV/AIDS is a catastrophe in slow motion, and it is essential that the world community pace itself for the long haul. The task ahead calls for clear vision, renewed will, and greatly increased resources. It also calls for greater determination to use the resources in the interest of everyone: HIV disease or AIDS must not be allowed to join the list of problems, like poverty and hunger, that this world has learned to live with because the powerful have lost interest, and the powerless have no choice. Whatever we do now, the die is already cast for many millions of people. The HIV/ AIDS epidemic will exact an enormous toll. What is at stake is the possibility of shaping the future course of the pandemic, of moderating or lessening the suffering that inevitably will occur as a result of the infections that already exist. **An epidemiological catastrophe is unavoidable. What can be limited are the dimensions of the catastrophe.**

In the United States, beginning 2003, through 22 years of the HIV/AIDS epidemic, we can reflect on the fact that we have learned a lot about this new disease but there is a long way to go. While it is easy to criticize, condemn, ridicule, and find mistakes in the way the HIV/AIDS pandemic has been handled, society should not lose sight of the outstanding scientific and social achievements made since HIV/AIDS was discovered. Excellent progress has been made in understanding the biology of HIV, its transmission, therapy, and its relationship to the progression of AIDS. If the 1980s are to be remembered as the period of AIDS violence, hatred, and irrational fears, the 1990s will hopefully be remembered as the time of optimism.

Will the years from 2000 to 2010 be known as the years of global cooperation against HIV/AIDS? HIV disease has become a more treatable illness wherein the quality and duration of life are being extended. Promising antiviral treatments are now in use and vaccines for the prevention of HIV infection are in field trials. HIV/AIDS education will soon reach every grade school, high school, and workplace in the United States. Courts have affirmed the rights of HIV-infected/AIDS patients to a public education and to remain at their jobs.

Recently, the world's leaders resolved that by 2015, we will have halted and begun to reverse the spread of HIV/AIDS. In June, 2001 we had an unprecedented opportunity to follow up on that resolve. The General Assembly of the United Nations convened a special session to review all aspects of the AIDS problem and to secure a coordinated global commitment in the struggle against it. This special session provided us with an occasion as never before to face up to our responsibility to future generations, and take decisive action how to turn back the progress of this terrible disease.

To the Future

Despite the gains against HIV, we are somewhere between the end of the beginning and the beginning of the end of AIDS. Exactly where depends on our willingness to make the most of our opportunities. The things we still need to do about HIV also illustrate a fundamental truth: Fighting HIV isn't only about HIV. It's about our vision of a better society where we are clearer about our responsibilities to ourselves and one another, and act accordingly. There is great hope that in the early years of the new millennium, the diagnosis of HIV infection will not indicate the almost certain destruction of the immune system, the onset of AIDS, and death. It is hoped that HIV will be just another controllable viral infection. **The divisiveness that has marked the 1980s and the 1990s has been too costly, the human toll too great. We can spend the present debating the past but we must look to the future—we must go forward from where we are.** Let history be history—learn from it and move on! The way for us to get through this crisis is hand in hand. **Humans shall overcome HIV!**

Answers to Review Questions

CHAPTER 1

1. Acquired Immune Deficiency Syndrome
2. No. AIDS is a syndrome. A syndrome is made up of a collection of signs and symptoms of one or more diseases. AIDS patients have a collection of opportunistic infections and cancers. Collectively they are mistakenly referred to as the AIDS disease.
3. In 1983 by Luc Montagnier
4. 1981
5. LAV
6. Five; 1982, 1983, 1985, 1987, and 1993
7. The ARC or AIDS Related Complex definition was a middle ground used before AIDS was better understood. It became meaningless after the 1985 expanded definition listed organisms and symptoms which indicated that two states existed: HIV infection and progression to AIDS.
8. It allows HIV-infected persons earlier access into federal and state medical and social programs.

CHAPTER 2

1. The unbroken transmission of infection from an infected person to an uninfected person.
2. The answer to both questions is unknown at this time.

CHAPTER 3

1. Because it contains RNA as its genetic message and a reverse transcriptase enzyme to make DNA from RNA
2. GAG-POL-ENV; at least six
3. Because HIV has demonstrated an unusually high rate of genetic mutations; (1) the reverse transcriptase enzyme in HIV is highly error prone (makes transcription errors), and (2) a variety of HIV mutants have been found within a single HIV-infected individual.
4. The reverse transcriptase enzyme is highly error prone, making at least one, and in many cases

more than one, deletion, addition, or substitution per round of proviral replication.

CHAPTER 4

1. Not really, because there is no way as yet to remove the provirus from the cell's DNA.
2. A physiological measurement that serves as a substitute for a major clinical event.
3. March; February, 17
4. 7
5. Zidovudine, didanosine, zalcitabine, stavudine, lamivudine.
6. Becoming incorporated into DNA as it is being synthesized, thereby stopping reverse transcriptase from attaching the next nucleotide.
7. (a) Clinical biological side effects; (b) the selection of drug-resistant HIV mutants.
8. (a) The number of copies of HIV RNA present in the plasma; (b) this number indicates the reproductive activity of HIV at the time and, if therapy is being used, the effect of the therapy on the reproductive ability of the virus.
9. Saquinavir mesylate, saquinavir (Fortovase) ritonavir, indinavir, nelfinavir, amprenavir, kaletra.
10. Indinavir, because either as a monotherapy or in combination, it is the most successful at dropping the viral load.
11. They physically interact with the reverse transcriptase enzyme and interfere with its function.
12. To suppress HIV replication, thereby reducing the number of mutant RNA strands produced.
13. A
14. B
15. To be determined by the instructor.
16. Answer depends on the credible facts the student presents.

CHAPTER 5

1. T4 helper cells; because T4 cells are crucial for the production of antibodies, a depletion of T4 cells

489

results in immunosuppression, which results in OIs.

2. CD4 is a receptor protein (antigen) secreted by certain cells of the immune system, for example, monocytes, macrophages, and T4 helper cells. It becomes located on the exterior of the cellular membrane and happens to be a compatible receptor for the HIV to attach and infect the CD4-carrying cell.

3. The question of true latency after HIV infection has not been settled. Most HIV/AIDS investigators currently believe there is a latent period, a time of few if any clinical symptoms and low levels of HIV in the blood. Other scientists, currently the minority, believe there is no true latency. The virus hides out in the lymph nodes slowly reproducing, and slowly killing off the T4 cells. The virus is always present, increasing slowly in numbers over time.

4. True
5. False
6. True
7. False
8. False
9. True
10. False
11. True
12. True
13. True
14. B, assessing risk of disease progression.

CHAPTER 6

1. OI is caused by organisms that are normally within the body and held in check by an active immune system. When the immune system becomes suppressed, for whatever reason, these agents can multiply and produce disease.

2. *Pneumocystis carinii;* lungs, pneumonia

3. *Isospora belli*

4. *Mycobacterium avium intracellulare*

5. False. HIV has not been found in KS tissue. KS is believed to develop as a result of a suppressed immune system and not the virus *per se.*

6. Classic KS, as described by Moritz Kaposi; and KS associated with AIDS

7. False. KS normally affects gay males. It is highly unusual to find KS in hemophiliacs, injection drug users and female AIDS patients.

8. True
9. True
10. True (Answer provided in POI 6.1)

CHAPTER 7

1. The 6-stage Walter Reed System and the 4-group CDC system

2. About 30%; about 90%

3. AIDS dementia complex

4. Skin—Kaposi's sarcoma
   Eyes—CMV retinitis
   Mouth—thrush or hairy leukoplakia
   Lungs—pneumocystis pneumonia
   Intestines—diarrhea

5. True

6. False. The average time is 6 to 18 weeks.

7. False. HIV infection leads to HIV disease. AIDS is the result of a weakened immune system that allows opportunistic infections to occur.

8. False. The average length of time is about 10 to 11 years.

9. Instructor's evaluation

10. Answer is E (all of the above).

CHAPTER 8

1. False. The United States currently **reports** most of the world's AIDS cases.

2. Cases of AIDS-related death, according to the CDC definition, can be traced back to 1952 in the United States and to the mid-1950s in Africa.

3. HIV-1 and HIV-2 show a 40% to 50% genetic relationship to each other.

4. False. HIV-1 and HIV-2 are both transmitted via the same routes. HIV-2 is spreading globally in similar fashion to HIV-1.

5. True. All scientific and empirical evidence to date indicates that HIV is **not** casually transmitted.

6. Through sexual activities: exchange of certain body fluids—blood and blood products, semen and vaginal secretions; and from mother to fetus or newborn by breast milk.

7. False. There is only one documented case of HIV infection caused by deep kissing. HIV has been found in the saliva of infected people in very low concentration, and saliva has been shown to have anti-HIV properties.

8. True; but this assertion has been proven to be untrue. Insects, in particular mosquitoes, have not been shown to transmit HIV successfully.

9. False. According to studies involving the sexual partners of injection drug users and hemophiliacs, HIV transmission from male to female is the more efficient route. This is believed to be due to a greater concentration of HIV found in semen than in vaginal fluid.

10. The answer may be True or False. There have been cases in which a single act of intercourse has resulted in HIV infection. However, the majority of surveys on the sexual partners of injection drug users and hemophiliacs indicate that the number of sexual encounters may increase the risk of HIV infection but does not guarantee infection. Sexual partners of infected people have remained HIV-free after years of unprotected penis-vagina or penis-anus intercourse.

11. The percentage of fetal risk varies widely in a number of hospital studies. At the moment, the risk as reported without zidovudine therapy, varies from less than 30%. For Africa the figures most commonly used are 30% to 50%. With the use of zidovudine therapy, the risk has been cut to about 8%. Using zidovudine and a cesarean section reduces HIV transmission to about 2%.

12. E, all of the above

13. True

14. True

15. True

16. True

17. True

18. False

19. True

20. True

21. False

22. True

23. True

24. True

25. B, mosquito bites

26. HIV/AIDS word unscrambled

ABMETARUTS	MASTURBATE
ACIPMDEN	PANDEMIC
AERIBRR	BARRIER
AGSEASM	MASSAGE
ANLA	ANAL
ATOUNITM	MUTATION
BENSTCENIA	ABSTINENCE
BLAUEXSI	BISEXUAL
BLMSKRITAE	BREASTMILK
BYUDILSFOD	BODYFLUIDS
CDRLSAIIMEP	SPERMICIDAL
DBOOL	BLOOD
DEIPCIME	EPIDEMIC
EGEIVTAN	NEGATIVE
FOCTNEINI	INFECTION
HEHALIIMPO	HEMOPHILIA
HREUSALXEOET	HETEROSEXUAL
IAVLNAG	VAGINAL
IDSA	AIDS
IVH	HIV
LSNCMIAOOO	NOSOCOMIAL
MEENS	SEMEN
MNTSNAOISISR	TRANSMISSION
MREPS	SPERM
NCEIALBCUMMO	COMMUNICABLE
NITSARS	STRAINS
NOEUTESRIRC	INTERCOURSE
OEULXMASOH	HOMOSEXUAL
OMODNC	CONDOM
PESREH	HERPES
PRLIATANE	PERINATAL
RSNIAUVONET	INTRAVENOUS
SAXELU	SEXUAL
SDT	STD
SILAAV	SALIVA
SIPEN	PENIS
SNRISEGY	SYRINGES
TFYELSEIL	LIFESTYLE
TLACER	RECTAL
UNOASNISFTR	TRANSFUSION
VPIETISO	POSITIVE
VSURI	VIRUS

CHAPTER 9

1. Latex condoms. They are known to stop the transmission of viruses. This may not be true for animal intestine condoms.

2. Water-based lubricants. Oil-based lubricants weaken the latex rubber causing them to leak or break under stress.

3. Safer sex is having sexual intercourse with an *uninfected* partner while using a condom.

4. The answer may be True or False. There have been cases where a single act of intercourse resulted in HIV infection. However, the majority of surveys completed by sexual partners of injection drug users and hemophiliacs indicate that the number of sexual encounters may increase the risk of HIV infection but does not guarantee infection. Sexual partners of infected persons have remained HIV-free after years of unprotected penis-vagina intercourse.

5. No. IDUs exist between "fixes." They lose things, they may not care to pick up new equipment— they need the "fix" now, it may be easier to share. Circumstances vary considerably among the IDU. Just giving them free equipment is no assurance that they will use it.

6. Between 1 in 39,000 and 1 in 200,000.

7. Have several students read their answers for promoting class discussion. Compare their response to that given in the text (that they should be punished).

8. Because attenuated HIV may mutate to a virulent form causing an HIV infection; there is no absolute guarantee that 100% of HIV are inactivated.

9. Because at no time will a whole HIV be present in the vaccine. Only a specific subunit of the HIV will be present in pure form so the vaccine should be free of any contaminating proteins that might prove toxic to one or more persons receiving the vaccine.

10. It is a situation wherein HIV antibodies might predispose the host to become more easily HIV-infected. For whatever reason, it appears that the HIV antibody complex enters the cell more easily than HIV alone.

11. Because of the severe forms of social ostracism that occur when it is learned that someone is HIV positive or belongs to a high-risk group (gay, injection drug user, bisexual).

12. Universal precautions are a list of rules and regulations provided by the CDC to help prevent HIV infection in health care workers.

13. False

14. False

15. True

16. True

17. True

18. False

19. False

20. False, 1998

21. Instructor evaluation

22. HIV/AIDS SEARCH-A-WORD

CHAPTER 10

1. The CDC said for each AIDS case there are from 50 to 100 HIV-infected people in the population. They got the 1 to 1.5 million figure using the 50 HIV-infected/AIDS cases; 1986; they are believed to be within plus or minus 10%.

2. Because their social and sexual behaviors and medical needs place these people at a greater risk for HIV exposure than those not practicing these social and sexual behaviors or who do not need blood or blood products.

3. False. Studies show that the time for progression from HIV infection to AIDS is the same regardless of parameters.

4. 52%

5. 30% to 50%

6. 99%

7. Two per 1000 students; more: the rate for military personnel is 1.4 per 1000.

8. College students 2/1000, general population 0.2/1000; this means the rate of HIV infection on college campuses is about 10 times higher than in the general population.

9. One in 20 to 300

10. Needle stick injuries

11. 3.5%

12. Hepatitis B virus

13. GAO—300,000 to 485,000
    CDC—270,000

14. Student's answer; text says no. People most often do not tell the truth—much depends on where, when, why, and who is doing the survey. There are just too many variables involved to believe sexual surveys.

15. Worldwide about 26 million, United States about 495,000.

16. 56% $\dfrac{480,000}{850,000}$

CHAPTER 11

1. Approximately 29 million women and 41 million men

2. About 50%

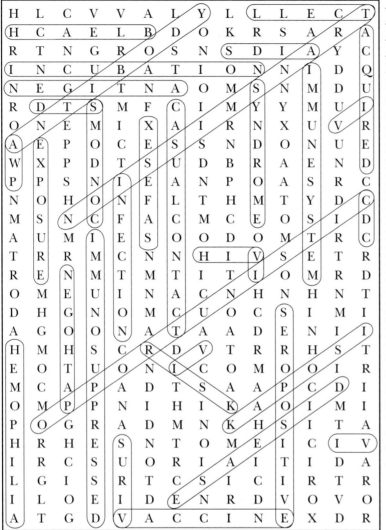

ACQUIRED
AIDS
ANTIBODY
ANTIGEN
BLEACH
CASUAL CONTACT
CDC
CONDOMS
DISEASE
EXPOSURE
HEMOPHILIA
HIV
IMMUNE SYSTEM
INCUBATION
IMMUNOSUPPRESSED
INFECTION
IV
KAPOSI
OPPORTUNISTIC
PATHOGEN
PWA
RISK
SAFE SEX
SEROPOSITIVE
STD
SYNDROME
T-CELL
TRANSMISSION
VACCINE
VIRUS

3. Injection drug use, being a sexual partner of an IDU, and through heterosexual contact.

4. IDU

5. Over 2 million; 1.3 million

6. Leading; 25 and 34; fifth; white; 25 and 44; leading; 25 and 44

7. An estimated 100,000

8. None, all states now have reported pediatric cases.

9. Virtually all—100%

10. (1) maternal viral load; (2) route of delivery, and (3) duration of early membrane rupture.

11. Most orphaned AIDS children have mothers who are IDUs and are themselves HIV-infected. They are AIDS orphans because (1) their parents abandon them due to illness or death; and (2) these children are HIV-infected or demonstrate AIDS and therefore no one wants them.

12. Over 50%

13. Two; 300

14. 28 million

15. Teenage gay men and teenage women; 75%

16. 25%

17. About 500,000

18. Yes; black and Latinos

19. One-third or about 14.5 million

20. 1-800-234-8336

CHAPTER 12

1. ELISA; enzyme-linked immunosorbent assay

2. That the body will produce antibody against antigenic components of the HIV virus after infection occurs.

3. No; a positive antibody result must be repeated in duplicate and if still positive, a confirmatory test is performed prior to telling people they are HIV-infected.

4. No; AIDS is medically diagnosed after certain signs and symptoms of specific diseases occur.

5. Western blot

6. Indirect immunofluorescent assay

7. By a color change in the reaction tube; the peroxidase enzyme oxidizes a clear chromogen into color formation. This occurs if the HIV antibody–antigen enzyme complex is present in the reaction tube.

8. False. Some newborns receive the HIV antibody passively during pregnancy. About 30% to 50% of HIV-positive newborns are truly HIV positive; it is unknown whether all HIV-positive newborns go on to develop AIDS. Not all have been discovered and it has not been determined whether 100% of HIV-infected adults or babies will develop AIDS.

9. They are not 100% accurate.

10. Determining that positive and negative tests are truly positive and negative and not falsely positive or negative.

11. Using either too high or too low cut-off points in the spectrophotometer and the presence of cross-reacting antibodies.

12. The percentage of false positives will increase as the prevalence of HIV-infected people in a population decreases.

13. It is a screening test value that represents the probability that a positive HIV test is truly positive; because screening tests are not 100% accurate.

14. Western blot

15. There is no standardized WB test interpretation. Different agencies use different WB results (reactive bands) to determine that the test sample is positive.

16. Because the PCR allows for the detection of proviral DNA in cells before the body produces detectable HIV antibody; PCR reactions can be used to determine if high-risk (or anybody) antibody-negative people are HIV-infected but not producing antibodies and whether newborns are truly HIV positive or passively HIV positive.

17. False. The FDA approved two home-use HIV antibody test kits in 1996 but one was withdrawn from the market.

18. Between 6 and 18 weeks after HIV infection.

19. As early as two weeks after infection.

20. (1) Changes in their lifestyles that reduce stress on their immune systems may delay the onset of illness.

(2) They can practice safer sex and hopefully not transmit the virus to others.

(3) The earlier the detection, the earlier they can enter into preventive therapy.

21. Mandatory with confidentiality; voluntary with confidentiality, anonymous, and blinded.

22. For anonymous testing no personal information is given; in blind tests, the name is deleted but the demographic data remain.

23. Because there are many example of breaches of confidence, which destroys trust and subjects people to social stigma.

24. False

25. True

CHAPTER 13

1. Newspapers, TV, radio, magazines, etc.

2. Barring children from public schools, police wearing rubber gloves during arrests, not going to a restaurant because someone who works there has AIDS, firing AIDS employees, etc.

3. Syphilis

4. Use of tobacco products, alcohol, drugs; nonuse of seat belts and motorcycle helmets, etc.

5. The ways by which one can become HIV-infected and how not to become HIV-infected.

6. Because most of the new cases of HIV infection and AIDS occur in high-risk groups that will not or cannot change sexual and drug practices.

7. Because a larger percentage of teenagers are sexually active with more than one partner, use drugs, use alcohol, and think that they are invulnerable to infection and death.

8. According to the AMA, no. Physicians may not refuse to care for patients with AIDS because of actual risk or fear of contracting the disease.

9. The CDC and AMA state that a patient's right to that information should be determined on a case-by-case basis where surgery will be performed. There is no legal requirement for physicians to tell their patients of their HIV status.

10. Worker information sessions that explain how the virus can and cannot be transmitted.

11. Kofi Annan; $7 billion to 10 billion

12. About $3.7 billion

Glossary

ACRONYMS

ACTG AIDS clinical trial group

ADA Americans With Disabilities Act

AIDS acquired immunodeficiency syndrome

AZT azathioprine (a misnomer for zidovudine or azidothymidine)

CD Cluster Differentiating Antigen

CD4 a protein imbedded on the surface of a T lymphocyte to which HIV most often binds—a CD4+ or T4 cell.

CD8 a protein imbedded on the surface of a T lymphocyte suppressor cell—a T8 cell.

CDC Centers for Disease Control and Prevention (part of PHS)

3TC Lamivudine; nucleoside analog

DHHS Department of Health and Human Services

DNA deoxyribonucleic acid

d4T stavudine; nucleoside analog

ddC dideoxycytosine; nucleoside analog

ddI dideoxyinosine; nucleoside analog

FDA Food and Drug Administration (part of PHS)

HAART Highly Active Antiretroviral Therapy

HIV Human Immunodeficiency Virus

IDU Injection Drug User

LAV lymphadenopathy-associated virus

NCI National Cancer Institute (part of NIH)

NIAID National Institute of Allergy and Infectious Diseases (part of NIH)

NIH National Institutes of Health (part of PHS)

NNRTI Non-nucleoside reverse transcriptase inhibitor

PCR (polymerase chain reaction) a very sensitive test used to detect the presence of HIV

PHS Public Health Service (part of DHHS)

PLWA Person Living With AIDS

RNA ribonucleic acid

ZDV Zidovudine; major drug in treating HIV/AIDS; nucleoside analog

For the newest anti-HIV drugs, names, and use, see Chapter 4.

TERMS

Acquired immunodeficiency syndrome (AIDS): A life-threatening disease caused by a virus and characterized by the breakdown of the body's immune defenses. (See AIDS.)

Acute: Sudden onset, Short-term with severe symptoms.

Acyclovir (Zovirax): Antiviral drug for herpes 1 and 2 and herpes zoster.

Adjuvant: The active ingredient in vaccines that improves the human immune system response by attracting immune cells into the region where the vaccine is injected.

AIDS (acquired immunodeficiency syndrome): A disease caused by a retrovirus called HIV and characterized by a deficiency of the immune system. The primary defect in AIDS is an acquired, persistent, quantitative functional depression within the T4 subset of lymphocytes. This depression often leads to infections caused by opportunistic microorganisms in HIV-infected individuals. A rare type of cancer (Kaposi's sarcoma) usually seen in elderly men or in individuals who are severely immunocompromised may also occur.

AIDS dementia: Neurological complications affecting thinking and behavior; intellectual impairment.

AIDSVAX: Trade name for all formulations of VAXGEN's vaccine.

Analog (analogue): A chemical molecule that closely resembles another one but which may function differently, thus altering a natural process.

Anemia: Low number of red blood cells.

Antibiotic: A chemical substance capable of destroying bacteria and other microorganisms.

Antibody: A blood protein produced by mammals in response to a specific antigen.

Antigen: A large molecule, usually a protein or carbohydrate, which when introduced into the body stimulates the production of an antibody that will react specifically with that antigen.

Antigen-presenting cells: B cells, cells of the monocyte lineage (including macrophages and dentritic cells) and various other body cells that 'present' antigen in a form that T cells can recognize.

Antigenemia: Presence of viral proteins (antigens).

Antiserum: Serum portion of the blood that carries the antibodies.

Antiviral: Means against virus; drugs that destroy or weaken virus.

Asymptomatic carrier: A host that is infected by an organism but does not demonstrate clinical signs or symptoms of the disease.

Asymptomatic seropositive: HIV positive without signs or symptoms of HIV disease.

Attenuated: Weakened.

Atypical: Irregular; not of typical character.

Autoimmunity: Antibodies made against self tissues.

B lymphocytes or B cells: Lymphocytes that produce antibodies. B lymphocytes proliferate under stimulation from factors released by T lymphocytes.

B- and T-cell lymphomas: Cancers caused by proliferation of the two principal types of white blood cells—B and T lymphocytes.

Bacterium: A microscopic organism composed of a single cell. Many but not all bacteria cause disease.

Blood count: A count of the number of red and white blood cells and platelets.

Bone marrow: Soft tissue located in the cavities of the bones. The bone marrow is the source of all blood cells.

Cancer: A large group of diseases characterized by uncontrolled growth and spread of abnormal cells.

Candida albicans: A fungus; the causative agent of vulvovaginal candidiasis or yeast infection.

Candidiasis: A fungal infection of the mucous membranes (commonly occurring in the mouth, where it is known as Thrush) characterized by whitish spots and/or a burning or painful sensation. It may also occur in the esophagus. It can also cause a red and itchy rash in moist areas, for example, the vagina.

Capsid: The protein coat of a virus particle.

CC-CKR-5 (CKR-5): Receptor for human chemokines and a necessary receptor for HIV entrance into macrophage.

CD: Cluster differentiating type antigens found on T lymphocytes. Each CD is assigned a number: CD1, CD2, etc.

CD4(T4 cell): White blood cell with type 4 protein embedded in the cell surface—target cell for HIV infection.

CD8 cell: Suppressor white blood cell with type 8 protein embedded in the cell surface.

Cell-mediated immunity: The reaction to antigenic material by specific defensive cells (macrophages) rather than antibodies.

Cellular immunity: A collection of cell types that provide protection against various antigens.

Chain of infection: A series of infections that are directly or immediately connected to a particular source.

Chemokines: Chemicals released by T cell lymphocytes and other cells of the immune system to attract a variety of cell types to sites of inflammation.

Chemotherapy: The use of chemicals that have a specific and toxic effect upon a disease-causing pathogen.

Chlamydia: A species of bacterium, the causative organism of *Lymphogranuloma venereum*, chlamydial urethritis, and most cases of newborn conjunctivitis.

Chromosomes: Physical structures in the cell's nucleus that house the genes. Each human cell has 22 pairs of autosomes and two sex chromosomes.

Chronic: Having a long and relatively mild course.

Clade: Related HIV variants classified by degree of genetic similarity; nine are known for HIV.

Cleavage Site: One of nine sites (peptide bond) within the gag-pol polyprotein (peptide precursor) that is cleaved by HIV-1 protease to form functional subunits of gag (p17, p7, p24) and pol (protease, reverse transcriptase, integrase).

Clinical latency: Infectious agent developing in a host without producing clinical symptoms.

Clinical manifestations: The signs of a disease as they pertain to or are observed in patients.

CMV: See cytomegalovirus

Cofactor: Factors or agents that are necessary or that increase the probability of the development of disease in the presence of the basic etiologic agent of that disease.

Cohort: A group of individuals with some characteristics in common.

Communicable: Able to spread from one diseased person or animal to another, either directly or indirectly.

Condylomata acuminatum (venereal warts): Viral warts of the genital and anogenital area.

Congenital: Acquired by the newborn before or at the time of birth.

Core proteins: Proteins that make up the internal structure or core of a virus.

Cross-resistance: Development of resistance to one agent as an antibiotic, that results in resistance to other, usually similar agents.

Cryptococcal meningitis: A fungal infection that affects the three membranes (meninges) surrounding the brain and spinal cord. Symptoms include severe headache, vertigo, nausea, anorexia, sight disorders, and mental deterioration.

Cryptococcosis: A fungal infectious disease often found in the lungs of AIDS patients. It characteristically spreads to the meninges and may also spread to the kidneys and skin. It is due to the fungus *Cryptococcus neoformans*.

Cryptosporidiosis: An infection caused by a protozoan parasite found in the intestines of animals. Acquired in some people by direct contact with the infected animal, it lodges in the intestines and causes severe diarrhea. It may be transmitted from person to person. This infection seems to be occurring more frequently in immunosuppressed people and can lead to prolonged symptoms that do not respond to medication.

Cutaneous: Having to do with the skin.

CXCR4 (FUSIN): Receptor for human chemokines and a necessary receptor for HIV entrance into T4 cells.

Cytokines: Powerful chemical substances secreted by cells. Cytokines include lymphokines produced by lymphocytes and monokines produced by monocytes and macrophages.

Cytomegalovirus (CMV): One of a group of highly host-specific herpes viruses that affect humans and other animals. Generally produces mild flu-like symptoms but can be more severe. In the immunosuppressed, it may cause pneumonia.

Cytopathic: Pertaining to or characterized by abnormal changes in cells.

Cytotoxic: Poisonous to cells.

Cytotoxic T cells: A subset of T lymphocytes that carry the T8 marker and can kill body cells infected by viruses or transformed by cancer.

Dementia: Chronic mental deterioration sufficient to significantly impair social and/or occupational function. Usually patients have memory and abstract thinking loss.

Dendritic cells: White blood cells found in the spleen and other lymphoid organs. Dendritic cells typically use threadlike tentacles to "hold" the antigen, which they present to T cells.

Didanosine: Also known as videx; see ddI-inhibits HIV Replication.

Dissemination: Spread of disease throughout the body.

DNA (deoxyribonucleic acid): A linear polymer, made up of deoxyribonucleotide repeating units. It is the carrier of genetic information in living organisms and some viruses.

DNA viruses: Contain DNA as their genetic material.

Dysentery: Inflammation of the intestines, especially the colon, producing pain in the abdomen and diarrhea containing blood and mucus.

Efficacy: Effectiveness.

ELISA test: A blood test that indicates the presence of antibodies to a given antigen. Various ELISA tests are used to detect a variety of infections. The HIV ELISA test does not detect AIDS but only indicates if viral infection has occurred.

Endemic: Prevalent in or peculiar to a community or group of people.

Enteric infections: Infections of the intestine.

ENV: HIV gene that codes for protein gp160.

Envelope proteins: Proteins that comprise the envelope or surface of a virus, gp120 and gp41.

Enzyme: A catalytic protein that is produced by living cells and promotes the chemical processes of life without itself being altered or destroyed.

Epidemiology: Science that deals with the incidence, distribution and control of disease in a population.

Epidemic: Affecting many persons at once, outbreak or rapid, sudden growth or development.

Epivir: See 3TC.

Epstein-Barr virus (EBV): A virus that causes infectious mononucleosis. It is spread by saliva. EBV lies dormant in the lymph glands and has been associated with Burkitt's lymphoma, a cancer of the lymph tissue.

Etiologic agent: The organism that causes a disease.

Etiology: The study of the cause of disease.

Extracellular: Found outside the cell wall.

Factor VIII: A naturally occurring protein in plasma that aids in the coagulation of blood. A congenital deficiency of Factor VIII results in the bleeding disorder known as hemophilia A.

Factor VIII concentrate: A concentrated preparation of Factor VIII that is used in the treatment of individuals with hemophilia A.

False negative: Failure of a test to demonstrate the disease or condition when present.

False positive: A positive test result caused by a disease or condition other than the disease for which the test is designed.

Fellatio: Oral sex involving the penis.

Fitness: The ability of an individual virus to replicate successfully under defined conditions.

Follicular dendritic cells: Found in germinal centers of lymphoid organs.

Fomite: An inanimate object that can hold infectious agents and transfers them from one individual to another.

Fortovase: A more easily assimilated form of saquinavir.

Fulminant: Rapid onset, severe.

Fungus: Member of a class of relatively primitive organisms. Fungi include mushrooms, yeasts, rusts, molds, and smuts.

Fusin: See CXCR4

Gammaglobulin: The antibody component of the serum.

Ganciclovir (DHPG): An experimental antiviral drug used in the treatment of CMV retinitis.

Gene: The basic unit of heredity; an ordered sequence of nucleotides. A gene contains the information for the synthesis of one polypeptide chain (protein).

Gene expression: The production of RNA and cellular proteins.

Genitourinary: Pertaining to the urinary and reproductive structures; sometimes called the GU tract or system.

Genome: The genetic endowment of an organism.

Genotype: The sequence of nucleotide bases that constitutes a gene.

GP41: Glycoprotein found in envelope of HIV.

GP120: Glycoprotein found in outer level of HIV envelope.

GP160: Precusor glycoprotein to forming gp41 and gp120.

Globulin: That portion of serum that contains the antibodies.

Glycoproteins: Proteins with carbohydrate groups attached at specific locations.

Gonococcus: The specific etiologic agent of gonorrhea discovered by Neisser and named *Neisseria gonorrhoeae*.

Granulocytes: Phagocytic white blood cells filled with granules containing potent chemicals that allow the cells to digest microorganisms. Neutrophils, eosinophils, basophils, and mast cells are examples of granulocytes.

Hemoglobin: The oxygen-carrying portion of red blood cells that gives them a red color.

Hemophilia: A hereditary bleeding disorder caused by a deficiency in the ability to synthesize one or more of the blood coagulation proteins, for example, Factor VIII (hemophilia A) or Factor IX (hemophilia B).

Hepatitis: Inflammation of the liver; due to many causes including viruses, several of which are transmissible through blood transfusions and sexual activities.

Hepatosplenomegaly: Enlargement of the liver and spleen.

Herpes simplex virus I (HSV-I): A virus that results in cold sores or fever blisters, most often on the mouth or around the eyes. Like all herpes viruses, it may lie dormant for months or years in nerve tissues and flare up in times of stress, trauma, infection, or immunosuppression. There is no cure for any of the herpes viruses.

Herpes simplex virus II (HSV-II): Causes painful sores on the genitals or anus. It is one of the most common sexually transmitted diseases in the United States.

Herpes varicella zoster virus (HVZ): The varicella virus causes chicken pox in children and may reappear in adulthood as herpes zoster. Herpes zoster, also called shingles, is characterized by small, painful blisters on the skin along nerve pathways.

Histoplasmosis: A disease caused by a fungal infection that can affect all the organs of the body. Symptoms usually include fever, shortness of breath, cough, weight loss and physical exhaustion.

HIV (human immunodeficiency virus): A newly discovered retrovirus that is said to cause AIDS. The target organ of HIV is the T4 or CD4 subset of T lymphocytes, which regulate the immune system.

HIV-positive: Presence of the human immunodeficiency virus in the body.

Homophobia: Negative bias toward or fear of individuals who are homosexual.

Human leukocyte antigens (HLA): Protein markers of self used in histocompatibility testing. Some HLA types also correlate with certain autoimmune diseases.

Humoral immunity: The production of antibodies for defense against infection or disease.

Immunity: Resistance to a disease because of a functioning immune system.

Immune complex: A cluster of interlocking antigens and antibodies.

Immune response: The reaction of the immune system to foreign substances.

Immune status: The state of the body's natural defense to diseases. It is influenced by heredity, age, past illness history, diet, and physical and mental health. It includes production of circulating and local antibodies and their mechanism of action.

Immunoassay: The use of antibodies to identify and quantify substances. Often the antibody is linked to a marker such as a fluorescent molecule, a radioactive molecule, or an enzyme.

Immunocompetent: Capable of developing an immune response.

Immunoglobulins: A family of large protein molecules, also known as antibodies.

Immunostimulant: Any agent that will trigger a body's defenses.

Immunosuppression: When the immune system is not working normally. This can be the result of illness or certain drugs (commonly those used to fight cancer).

Incidence: The total number of new cases of a disease in a given area within a specified time, usually one year.

Incubation period: The time between the actual entry of an infectious agent into the body and the onset of disease symptoms.

Indinavir: Crixivan, a protease inhibitor drug.

Infection: Invasion of the body by viruses or other organisms.

Infectious disease: A disease that is caused by microorganisms or viruses living in or on the body as parasites.

Inflammatory response: Redness, warmth, and swelling in response to infection; the result of increased blood flow and a gathering of immune cells and secretions.

Injection drug use: Use of drugs injected by needle into a vein or muscle tissue.

Innate immunity: Inborn or hereditary immunity.

Inoculation: The entry of an infectious organism or virus into the body.

Integrase: HIV enzyme used to insert HIV DNA into host cell DNA.

Interferon: A class of glycoproteins important in immune function and thought to inhibit viral infection.

Interleukins: Chemical messengers that travel from leukocytes to other white blood cells. Some promote cell development, others promote rapid cell division.

Intracellular: Found within the cell wall.

In utero: In the uterus.

In vitro: "In glass"—pertains to a biological reaction in an artificial medium.

In vivo: "In the living"—pertains to a biological reaction in a living organism.

IV: Intravenous.

Kaposi's sarcoma: A multifocal, spreading cancer of connective tissue, principally involving the skin; it usually begins on the toes or the feet as reddish blue or brownish soft nodules and tumors.

Lamivudine: Nucleoside analog inhibits HIV replication.

Langerhans cells: Dendritic cells in the skin that pick up antigen and transport it to lymph nodes.

Latency: A period when a virus or other organism is still in the body but in an inactive state.

Latent viral infection: The virion becomes part of the host cell's DNA.

Lentiviruses: Viruses that cause disease very slowly. HIV is believed to be this type of virus.

Lesion: Any abnormal change in tissue due to disease or injury.

Leukocyte: A white blood cell.

Leukopenia: A decrease in the white blood cell count.

Log: 10-fold difference.

Lymph: A transparent, slightly yellow fluid that carries lymphocytes, bathes the body tissues, and drains into the lymphatic vessels.

Lymph nodes: Gland-like structures in the lymphatic system that help to prevent spread of infection.

Lymphadenopathy: Enlargement of the lymph nodes.

Lymphadenopathy syndrome (LAS): A condition characterized by persistent, generalized, enlarged lymph nodes, sometimes with signs of minor illness such as fever and weight loss, which apparently represents a milder reaction to HIV infection.

Lymphatic system: A fluid system of vessels and glands that is important in controlling infections and limiting their spread.

Lymphocytes: Specialized white blood cells involved in the immune response.

Lymphoid organs: The organs of the immune system where lymphocytes develop and congregate. They include the bone marrow, thymus, lymph nodes, spleen, and other clusters of lymphoid tissue.

Lymphokines: Chemical messengers produced by T and B lymphocytes. They have a variety of protective functions.

Lymphoma: Tumor of lymphoid tissue, usually malignant.

Lymphosarcoma: A general term applied to malignant neoplastic disorders of lymphoid tissue, not including Hodgkin's disease.

Lytic infection: When a virus infects the cell, the cell produces new viruses and breaks open (lyse), releasing the viruses.

Macrophage: A large and versatile immune cell that acts as a microbe-devouring phagocyte, an antigen-presenting cell and an important source of immune secretions.

Major histocompatibility complex (MHC): A group of genes that controls several aspects of the immune response. MHC genes code for self markers on all body cells.

Malaise: A general feeling of discomfort or fatigue.

Malignant tumor: A tumor made up of cancerous cells. The tumors grow and invade surrounding tissue, then the cells break away and grow elsewhere.

Messenger RNA (mRNA): RNA that serves as the template for protein synthesis; it carries the information from the DNA to the protein synthesizing complex to direct protein synthesis.

Microbes: Minute living organisms including bacteria, viruses, fungi, and protozoa.

Microorganisms: Microscopic plants or animals.

Molecule: The smallest amount of a specific chemical substance that can exist alone. To break a molecule down into its constituent atoms is to change its character. A molecule of water, for instance, reverts to oxygen and hydrogen.

Monocyte: A large phagocytic white blood cell which, when it enters tissue, develops into a macrophage.

Monokines: Powerful chemical substances secreted by monocytes and macrophages. They help direct and regulate the immune response.

Morbidity: The proportion of people with a disease in a community.

Morphology: The study of the form and structure of organisms.

Mortality: The number of people who die as a result of a specific cause.

Mucosal immunity: Resistance to infection across mucous membranes.

Mucous membrane: The lining of the canals and cavities of the body that communicate with external air, such as the intestinal tract, respiratory tract, and the genitourinary tract.

Mucous patches: White, patchy growths, usually found in the mouth, that are symptoms of secondary syphilis and are highly infectious.

Mucus: A fluid secreted by membranes.

Mutant: A new strain of a virus or microorganism that arises as a result of change in the genes of an existing strain.

Natural killer cells (also called NK cells): Immune cells that kill infected cells directly within four hours of contact. NK cells differ from other killer cells, such as cytotoxic T lymphocytes, in that they do not require contact with antigen before they are activated.

Neisseria gonorrhoeae: The bacterium that causes gonorrhea.

Neonatal: Pertaining to the first four weeks of life.

Neoplasm: A new abnormal growth, such as a tumor.

Neuropathy: Group of nerve disorders—symptoms range from tingling sensation and numbness to paralysis.

Neutralizing Antibody: The kind of antibody that prevents a virus from entering a cell. It is hoped that a vaccine will produce neutralizing antibody because if HIV is prevented from entering cells, it cannot replicate and dies in the bloodstream within a few hours.

Nevirapine: Non-nucleostide analog inhibits HIV replication.

Notifiable disease: A notifiable disease is one that, when diagnosed, health providers are required, usually by law, to report to state or local public health officials. Notifiable diseases are those of public interest by reason of their contagiousness, severity, or frequency.

Nucleic acids: Large, naturally occurring molecules composed of chemical building blocks known as nucleotides. There are two kinds of nucleic acid, DNA and RNA.

Nucleoside analog: Synthetic compounds generally similar to one of the bases of DNA.

Nucleotide of DNA: Made up of one of four nitrogen-containing bases (adenine, cytosine, guanine, or thymine), a sugar, and a phosphate molecule.

Oncogenic: Anything that may give rise to tumors, especially malignant ones.

Opportunistic disease: Disease caused by normally benign microorganisms or viruses that become pathogenic when the immune system is impaired.

p24 antigen: A protein fragment of HIV. The p24 antigen test measures this fragment. A positive test result suggests active HIV replication and may mean the individual has a chance of developing AIDS in the near future.

Pandemic: Occurring over a wide geographic area and affecting a high proportion of the population.

Parenteral: Not taken in through the digestive system.

Parasite: A plant or animal that lives, grows, and feeds on another living organism.

Pathogen: Any disease-producing microorganism or substance.

Pathogenic: Giving rise to disease or causing symptoms of an illness.

Pathogenicity: Capable of causing a disease.

Pathology: The science of the essential nature of diseases, especially of the structural and functional changes in tissues and organs caused by disease.

Perianal glands: Glands located around the anus.

Perinatal: Occurring in the period during or just after birth.

Pestilence: A virulent, devastating contagious disease that is caused by a bacterium, e.g., *Yersina pestis*, which causes the plague.

Phagocytes: Large white blood cells that contribute to the immune defense by ingesting microbes or other cells and foreign particles.

Phenotype: A defined behavior; specifically drug susceptibility with regard to HIV drug resistance.

PID (pelvic inflammatory disease): Inflammation of the female pelvic organs; often the result of gonococcal or chlamydial infection.

Placebo: An inactive substance against which investigational treatments are compared to see how well the treatment worked.

Plague: A calamity; an epidemic of disease causing a high rate of mortality.

Plasma: The fluid portion of the blood that contains all the chemical constituents of whole blood except the cells.

Plasma cells: Derived from B cells, they produce antibodies.

Platelets: Small oval discs in blood that are necessary for blood to clot.

PLWA: Person Living With AIDS.

Polymerase chain reaction: Method to detect and amplify very small amounts of DNA in a sample.

Positive HIV test: A sample of blood that is reactive on an initial ELISA test, reactive on a second ELISA run of the same specimen, and reactive on Western blot, if available.

Pneumocystis carinii pneumonia **(PCP):** A rare type of pneumonia primarily found in infants and now common in patients with AIDS.

Prenatal: During pregnancy.

Prevalence: The total number of cases of a disease existing at any time in a given area.

Primary immune response: Production of antibodies about 7 to 10 days after an infection.

Prophylactic treatment: Medical treatment of patients exposed to a disease before the appearance of disease symptoms.

Protease: Enzyme that cuts proteins into peptides (breaks down proteins).

Protease inhibitors: Compounds that inhibit the action of protease.

Proteins: Organic compounds made up of amino acids. Proteins are one of the major constituents of plant and animal cells.

Protocol: Standardization of procedures so that results of treatment or experiments can be compared.

Protozoa: A group of one-celled animals, some of which cause human disease including malaria, sleeping sickness, and diarrhea.

Provirus: The genome of an animal virus integrated into the chromosome of the host cell, and thereby replicated in all of the host's daughter cells.

Quasispecies: A complex mixture of genetic variants of an RNA virus.

Race: Beginning in 1976 the federal government's data systems classified individuals into the following racial groups: American Indian or Alaskan Native, Asian or Pacific Islander, black, and white.

Rate: A rate is a measure of some event, disease, or condition in relation to a unit of population, along with some specification of time.

Receptors: Special molecules located on the surface membranes of cells that attract other molecules to attach to them. (For example CD4, CD8, and CC-CKR-5).

Recombinant DNA: DNA produced by joining pieces of DNA from different sources.

Recombinant DNA techniques: Techniques that allow specific segments of DNA to be isolated and inserted into a bacterium or other host (like, yeast or mammalian cells) in a form that will allow the DNA segment to be replicated and expressed as the cellular host multiplies.

Remission: The lessening of the severity of disease or the absence of symptoms over a period of time.

Retroviruses: Viruses that contain RNA and produce a DNA analog of their RNA using an enzyme known as reverse transcriptase.

Reverse transcriptase: An enzyme produced by retroviruses that allows them to produce a DNA analog of their RNA, which may then incorporate into the host cell.

Ritonavir: Novir, a protease inhibitor drug.

RNA (ribonucleic acid): Any of various nucleic acids that contain ribose and uracil as structural components and are associated with the control of cellular chemical activities.

RNA viruses: Contain RNA as their genetic material.

Sarcoma: A form of cancer that occurs in connective tissue, muscle, bone, and cartilage.

Saquinavir: Invirase, a protease inhibitor drug.

Secondary immune response: On repeat exposure to an antigen, there is an accelerated production of antibodies.

Sensitivity: The probability that a test will be positive when the infection is present.

Septicemia: A disease condition in which the infectious agent has spread throughout the lymphatic and blood systems, causing a general body infection.

Seroconversion: The point at which an individual exposed to the AIDS virus becomes serologically positive.

Serologic test: Laboratory test made on serum.

Serum: The clear portion of any animal liquid separated from its more solid elements, especially the clear liquid that separates in the clotting of blood (blood serum).

Shigella: A bacterium that can cause dysentery.

Specificity: The probability that a test will be negative when the infection is not present.

Spirochete: A corkscrew-shaped bacterium; for example, *Treponema pallidum.*

Spleen: A lymphoid organ in the abdominal cavity that is an important center for immune system activities.

Squamous: Scaly or plate-like; a type of cell.

Stavudine: Also known as Zerit; See d4T—inhibits HIV replication.

STD (sexually transmitted disease): Any disease that is transmitted primarily through sexual practices.

Subclinical infections: Infections with minimal or no apparent symptoms.

Subunit vaccine: A vaccine that uses only one component of an infectious agent rather than the whole to stimulate an immune response.

Suppressor T cells: A subset of T cells that carry the T8 marker and turn off antibody production and other immune responses.

Surrogate marker: A substitute; a person or agent that replaces another, an alternate.

Surveillance: The process of accumulating information about the incidence and prevalence of disease in an area.

Susceptible: Inability to resist an infection or disease.

Syndrome: A set of symptoms that occur together.

Systemic: Affecting the body as a whole.

T cell growth factor (TCGF, also known as interleukin-2): A glycoprotein that is released by T lymphocytes on stimulation by antigens and that functions as a T cell growth factor by inducing proliferation of activated T cells.

T Helper cells (also called T4 or CD4 cells): A subset of T cells that carry the CD4 marker and are essential for turning on antibody production, activating cytotoxic T cells, and initiating many other immune responses.

T lymphocytes or T cells: Lymphocytes that mature in the thymus and that mediate cellular immune reactions. T lymphocytes also release factors that induce proliferation of T lymphocytes and B lymphocytes.

T8 cells: A subset of T cells that may kill virus-infected cells and suppress immune function when the infection is over.

Thrush: A disease characterized by the formation of whitish spots in the mouth. It is caused by the fungus *Candida albicans* during times of immunosuppression.

Thymus: A primary lymphoid organ high in the chest where T lymphocytes proliferate and mature.

Titer: Level or amount.

Tolerance: A state of nonresponsiveness to a particular antigen or group of antigens.

Toxic reaction: A harmful side effect from a drug; it is dose dependent, that is, becomes more frequent and severe as the drug dose is increased. All drugs have toxic effects if given in a sufficiently large dose.

Toxoplasmosis: An infection with the protozoan *Taxoplasma gondii*, frequently causing focal encephalitis (inflammation of the brain). It may also involve the heart, lungs, adrenal glands, pancreas, and testes.

Transcription: The synthesis of messenger RNA on a DNA template; the resulting RNA sequence is complementary to the DNA sequence. This is the first step in gene expression.

Translation: The process by which the genetic code contained in a nucleotide sequence of messenger RNA directs the synthesis of a specific order of amino acids to produce a protein.

Treponema pallidum: The bacterial spirochete that causes syphilis.

Tropism: Involuntary turning, curving, or attraction to a source of stimulation.

Tumor: A swelling or enlargement; an abnormal mass that can be malignant or benign. It has no useful body function.

V3 loop: Section of the gp120 protein on the surface of HIV; appears to be important in stimulating neutralizing antibodies.

Vaccine: A preparation of dead organisms, attenuated live organisms, live virulent organisms, or parts of microorganisms that is administered to artificially increase immunity to a particular disease.

V.D.: Contagious disease usually acquired through sexual intercourse.

Vector: The means by which a disease is carried from one human to another.

Venereal: Venus = love, sexual desire; involves the sexual organs and related to sexual pleasure; comes through contact of sexual organs.

Venereal warts: Viral *Condylomata acuminata* on or near the anus or genitals.

Viral load: The total amount of virus in a person's blood.

Viremia: The presence of virus in the blood.

Virulence: The quality of expression or the expression of the disease.

Virus: Any of a large group of submicroscopic agents capable of infecting plants, animals, and bacteria; characterized by a total dependence on living cells for reproduction and by a lack of independent metabolism.

Western blot: A blood test used to detect antibodies to a given antigen. Compared to the ELISA test, the Western blot is more specific and more expensive. It can be used to confirm the results of the ELISA test.

Wild Type: A genotype or phenotype circulating prior to selection of drug resistance.

X-ray: Radiant energy of extremely short wavelength used to diagnose and treat cancer.

Zalcitabine: Also known as HIVID; see ddC—inhibits HIV replication.

Zidovudine: Also known as Retrovir; see ZDV—inhibits HIV replication. Mistakenly referred to as AZT.

References

CHAPTER 1

BARRE-SINOUSSI, FRANCOISE, et al. (1983). Isolation of a T-lymphocyte retrovirus from a patient at risk for acquired immune deficiency syndrome (AIDS). *Science*, 220:868–871.

GALLO, ROBERT C. (1987). The AIDS virus. *Sci. Am.*, 256:47–56.

HAHN, BEATRICE, et al. (2000). AIDS as a zoonosis: Scientific and public health implications. *Science*, 287:607–614.

HOBSON, SIMON WAIN, et al. (1991). LAV revisited: Origins of the early HIV-1 isolates from Institut Pasteur. *Science*, 252:961–965.

MARLINK, RICHARD, (1996), Lessons from the second AIDS virus HIV-2. *AIDS*, 10:689–699.

Morbidity and Mortality Weekly Report. (1981). Pneumocystis pneumonia Los Angeles, 30:250–252.

Morbidity and Mortality Weekly Report. (1982). Update on acquired immune deficiency syndrome (AIDS) United States, 31:507–508, 513–514.

Morbidity and Mortality Weekly Report. (1990). Surveillance for HIV-2 infection in blood donors United States, 1987–1989, 39:829–831.

Morbidity and Mortality Weekly Report. (1993). 1993 Revised classification system for HIV infection and expanded surveillance case definition for AIDS among adolescents and adults, 41:1–19.

Morbidity and Mortality Weekly Report. (1994). Update: Impact of the expanded AIDS surveillance case definition for adolescents and adults on case reporting—United States, 1993, 43:160–170.

SPRECHER, LORRIE. (1991). Women with AIDS: Dead but not disabled. *The Positive Woman*, 1:4.

STADTMAUER, GARY, et al. (1997). Primary Immune Deficiency Disorders that mimic AIDS. *Infections in Medicine*, 4:899–905.

CHAPTER 2

ANDREWS, CHARLA. (1995). "The Duesberg Phenomenon." What does it mean? *Science*, 267:157.

BALTER, MICHAEL. (1998). Virus from 1959 sample marks early years of HIV. *Science*, 279:801.

BAUM, RUDY. (1995). HIV link to AIDS strengthened by epidemiological study. *Chem. Eng. News*, 74:26.

BUIANOUCKAS, FRANCIS. (1995). HIV, an illusion. *Nature*, 375:197.

CDC Weekly. (1988). Extremists seek to blame AIDS on Jews. July 11.

CHERRY, MIKE. (1999). AZT critics swayed South African president. *Nature*, 402:225.

COHEN, JON. (1993). Keystone's blunt message: 'It's the virus, Stupid'. *Science*, 260:292–293.

CONNOR, EDWARD. (1994). Reduction of maternal infant transmission of HIV with zidovudine treatment (ACTG 076). *N. Engl. J. Med.*, 331: 1173–1180.

CULLITON, BARBARA J. (1992). The mysterious virus called "Isn't." *Nature*, 358:619.

DARBY, SARAH, et al. (1995). Mortality before and after HIV infection in the complete UK population of haemophiliacs. *Nature*, 377:79–82.

DICKSON, DAVID. (1994). Critic still lays blame for AIDS on lifestyle, not HIV. *Nature*, 369:434.

DUESBERG, PETER H. (1990). Duesberg replies [to the charges of Weiss and Jaffe]. *Nature*, 346:788.

DUESBERG, PETER H. (1993). HIV and AIDS. *Science*, 260:1705–1708.

DUESBERG, PETER H. (1995a). The Duesberg Phenomenon: Duesberg and other voices. *Science*, 267:313.

DUESBERG, PETER H. (1995b). Duesberg on AIDS causation: the culprit is noncontagious risk factors. *The Scientist*, 9:12.

DUESBERG, PETER H., et al. (1998). The AIDS Dilemma: drug diseases blamed on a passenger virus. *Genetica*, 104: 85–132.

EDITORIAL. (1995). More conviction on HIV and AIDS. *Nature*, 377:1.

GIBBS, WAYT. (2001). Dissident or Don Quixote? *Scientific American*, 285:30–32.

GILKS, CHARLES. (1991). AIDS, monkeys and malaria. *Nature*, 354:262.

GILKS, CHARLES. (1992). AIDS and malaria experiments. *Nature*, 355:305.

GRMEK, MIRKO. (1990). *History of AIDS: Emergence and Origin of a Modern Pandemic.* Princeton, NJ: Princeton University Press.

HAHN, BEATRICE, et al. (1999). Origin of HIV-1 in the chimpanzee Pan troglodytes troglodytes. *Nature*, 397: 436–441.

HAHN, BEATRICE, et al. (2000). AIDS as a zoonosis: scientific and public health implications. *Science*, 287: 607–614.

HARRIS, STEVEN. (1995). The AIDS heresies: A case study in skepticism taken too far. *Skeptic.* 3, no. 2: 42–58.

HIRSCH, VANESSA, et al. (1995). Phylogeny and natural history of the primate lentiviruses, SIV and HIV. *Current Opinion Genetic Development*, 5: 798–806.

HOLDER, CONSTANCE. (1988). Curbing Soviet disinformation. *Science*, 242:665.

KARPAS, ABRAHAM. (1994). AIDS plagued by journalists. *Nature*, 368:387.

KOPROWSKI, HILARY. (1992). AIDS and the polio vaccine. *Science*, 257:1024–1026.

KORBER, BETTE, et al. (1998). Limitations of a molecular clock applied to considerations of the origin of HIV-1. *Science*, 280:1868–1871.

KORBER, BETTE, et al. (2000). Timing the ancestor of the HIV-1 pandemic strains. *Science*, 288: 1789–1796.

KORBER, BETTE, et al. (2000). Timing the origin of the HIV-1 pandemic. Programs and abstracts of the 7th Conference on Retroviruses and Opportunistic Infections, January 30–February 2, San Francisco. Abstract L5.

LEVY, JAY. (1995). *HIV and the Pathogenesis of AIDS*. Washington, DC: ASM Press.

MOORE, JOHN. (1996). À Duesberg, adieu! *Nature*, 380:293–294.

NATIONAL INSTITUTE OF ALLERGY AND INFECTIOUS DISEASES. (1995). The relationship between the human immunodeficiency virus and the acquired immunodeficiency syndrome. *National Institutes of Health*, 1–61.

PEETERS, MARTINE, et al. (2002). Risk to human health from a plethora of simian immunodeficiency viruses in primate bushmeat. *Emerging Infectious Diseases*, 8:451–457.

ROOT-BERNSTEIN, ROBERT. (1993). *Rethinking AIDS*. New York: Free Press.

SALEMI, MARCO, et al. (2000). Dating the common ancestor of SIVcpz and HIV-1 group M and origin of HIV-1 subtypes by using a new method to uncover clock-like molecular evolution. *Federation American Societies Experimental Biology*, 15: 276–278.

SANTIGO, MARIO, et al. (2002). SIVcpz in wild chimpanzees. *Science*, 795:465.

STONE, RICHARD. (1995). Congressman uncovers the HIV conspiracy. *Science*, 268:191.

SULLIVAN, JOHN, et al. (1995). HIV and AIDS. *Nature*, 378:10.

VANGROENWEGHE, DANIEL. (2001). The earliest cases of human immunodeficiency virus type 1 group M in Congo-Kinshasa, Rwanda and Burundi and the origin of acquired immune deficiency syndrome. *Philos Trans R Soc Lond B Biol Sci;* 356 (1410):923–925.

VIDAL, NICOLE, et al. (2000) Unprecented degree of HIV-1 Group M genetic diversity in the Democratic Republic of Congo suggests HIV-1 pandemic originated in Central Africa. *J. Virology* 74: 10,498–10,507.

WEISS, ROBIN A., et al. (1990). Duesberg, HIV and AIDS. *Nature*, 345:659–660.

CHAPTER 3

BONHOEFFER, SEBASTIAN, et al. (1995). Causes of HIV diversity. *Nature*, 376:125.

BRIX, DEBORAH, et al. (1996). Summary of track A: Basic science. *AIDS*, 10 (suppl. 3): S85–S106.

BRODINE, STEPHANIE, et al. (1997). Genotypic variation and molecular epidemiology of HIV. *Infect. Med.*, 14:739–748.

COHEN, JON. (1997). Looking for leads in HIV's battle with immune system. *Science*, 276:1196–1197.

COHEN, MITCHELL, et al. (1994). When bugs outsmart drugs. *Patient Care*, 28:135–146.

COLLINS, KATHLEEN, et al. (1998). HIV-1 Nef protein protects infected primary cells against killing by cytotoxic T Lymphocytes. *Nature*, 391:397–401.

DELWART, ERIC, et al. (1993). Genetic relationships determined by a DNA heteroduplex mobility assay: Analysis of HIV envGenes. *Science*, 262:1257–1262.

DEVEREUX, HELEN, et al. (2002). In vitro HIV-1 compartmentalisation: drug resistance associated mutation distribution. *J Med. Virology*, 66:8–12.

DIAZ, RICARDO, et al. (1997). Divergence of HIV quasispecies in an epidemiology cluster. *AIDS*, 11:415–422.

DIMMROCK, N.J., and PRIMROSE, S.B. (1987). *Introduction to Modern Virology*, 3rd ed. Oxford: Blackwell Scientific Publications.

ESSEX, MAX. (1996). Deciphering the mysteries of subtypes: communities of color, Spring/Summer: *Harvard AIDS Rev.*, 18–19.

FIELDS, BERNARD. (1994). AIDS: Time to turn to basic science. *Nature*, 369:95–96.

FISCHL, MARGARET. (1984). Combination retroviral therapy for HIV infection. *Hosp. Pract.*, 29:43–48.

FRITZ, CHRISTIAN, et al. (1995). A human nucleoprotein-like protein that specifically interacts with HIV-Rev. *Nature*, 376:530–533.

GAO FENG, et al., (1999). Origin of HIV-1 in the chimpanzee Pan troglodytes troglodytes. *Nature*, 397:436–441.

GAO FENG, et al., (1992). Human infection by genetically diverse SIVSM-related HIV-2 in west Africa. *Nature;* 358:495–499.

GARRUS, JENNIFER, et al. (2001). Tsg 101 and the vacuolar protein sorting pathway are essential for HIV-1 budding. *Cell*, 107:55–65.

GREENE, WARNER. (1993). AIDS and the immune system. *Sci. Am.*, 269:99–105.

HILDRETH, JAMES. (2001). Adhesion molecules, lipid rafts and HIV pathogenesis. HIV Pathogenesis Keystone Symposium, March 28–April 3, Presentation 038.

HU, DALE, et al. (1996). The emerging genetic diversity of HIV. *JAMA*, 275:210–216.

JETZT, AMANDA, et al. (2000). High rate of recombination throughout the HIV genome. *Journal of Virology*, 74:1234–1240.

JUNG, ANDREAS, et al. (2002). Recombination: Multiply infected spleen cells in HIV patients. *Nature*, 418:144–147.

KOHLEISEN, MARKUS, et al. (1992). Cellular localization of Nef expressed in persistently HIV-1 infected low-producer astrocytes. *AIDS*, 6:1427–1436.

LAURENCE, JEFFREY. (1997). HIV vaccine conundrum. *Aids Reader*, 7:1–2, 27.

LENNOX, JEFFREY, (1995). Approaches to gene therapy. *International AIDS Society—USA*, 3:13–16.

LEVIN, BRUCE, et al. (2001). Epidemology, evalution and future of the HIV/AIDS pandemic. *Emerging Infectious Diseases*, 7:505–511.

LI, CHIANG. (1997). Tat protein perpetuates HIV-1 infection. *Proc. Natl. Acad. Sci. USA*, 94:8116–8120.

MARX, PRESTON, et al. (2001). Serial human passage of simian immunodeficiency virus by unsterile injections and the emergence of epidemic HIV in Africa. *Philos Trans R Soc Lond B Biol Sci*, 356:911–920.

MATSUYA, HIROAKI, et al. (1990). Molecular targets for AIDS therapy. *Science*, 249:1533–1543.

MATTHEWS, STEPHEN, et al. (1994). Structural similarity between p17 matrix protein of HIV and interferon-2. *Nature*, 370:666–668.

MOORE, JOHN, et al. (1994). The who and why of HIV vaccine trials. *Nature*, 372:313–314.

Morbidity and Mortality Weekly Report. (1993). Nosocomial enterococci resistant to vancomycin—United States, 1989–1993, 42:597–599.

NOWAK, MARTIN A. (1990). HIV mutation rate. *Nature*, 347:522.

NOWAK, MARTIN A., et al. (1991). Antigenic diversity thresholds and the development of AIDS. *Science*, 254:963–969.

NOWAK, RACHEL. (1995). How the parasite disguises itself. *Science*, 269:755.

PATRUSKY, BEN. (1992). The Intron story. *Mosaic*, 23:20–33.

POTASH, MARY JANE, et al. (1998). Peptid inhibitors of HIV-1 protease and viral infection of peripheral blood lymphocytes based on HIV-1 ViF. *Proc. National Academy of Science*, 95:13,865–13,868.

PRESTON, BRADLEY D., et al. (1988). Fidelity of HIV-1 reverse transcriptase. *Science*, 242:1168–1171.

ROBERTSON, DAVID, et al. (1995). Recombination in HIV 1. *Nature*, 374:124–126.

ROSEN, CRAIG A. (1991). Regulation of HIV gene expression by RNA-protein interactions. *Trends Genet.*, 7:9–14.

SAGG, MICHAEL S., et al. (1988). Extensive variation of human immunodeficiency virus Type-1 *in vivo*. *Nature*, 334:440–444.

SAGG, MICHAEL S., et al. (1995). Improving the management of HIV disease. *Advanced Causes in HIV Pathogenesis*, pp. 1–30. February 25, Swissotel, Atlanta (Michael Sagg, Program Chair).

SIMON, FRANCOIS, et al. (1998). Identification of a New Human Immunodeficiency Virus Type I Distinct from Group M and Group O. *Nature Medicine*, 4:1032.

SOMASUNDARAN, M., et al. (1988). Unexpectedly high levels of HIV-1 RNA and protein synthesis in a cytocidal infection. *Science*, 242:1554–1557.

SOTO-RAMIREZ, LUIS, et al. (1996). HIV-Langerhans' cell tropism associated with heterosexual transmission of HIV. *Science*, 271:1291–1293.

STEVENSON, MARIO. (1998). Basic Science: Highlights of the 5th Retrovirus Conference. *Improving the Management of HIV Disease*, 6:4–10.

TORRES, YOLANDA, et al. (1996). Cytokine network and HIV syncytium-inducing phenotype shift. *AIDS*, 10:1053–1055.

UNAIDS. (1997). Implications of HIV variability for transmission: Scientific and policy issues. *AIDS*, 11:1–15.

VARTANIAN, JEAN-PIERRE, et al. (1992). High-resolution structure of an HIV-1 quasispecies: Identification of novel coding sequences. *AIDS*, 6:1095–1098.

WILLS, JOHN W., et al. (1991). Form, function and use of retroviral Gag protein. *AIDS*, 5:639–654.

Workshop Report from the European Commission/Joint United Nations Program on HIV/AIDS. (1997). HIV-1 subtypes: Implications for epidemiology, pathogenicity, vaccines, and diagnostics. *AIDS*, 11:17–36.

WU, YUNTAO, et al. (2001). Selective transcription and modulation of resting T cell activity by preintegrated HIV DNA. *Science*, 293:1503–1506.

CHAPTER 4

AIDS CLINICAL CARE. (1998). Report on the Fifth Conference on Retroviruses and Opportunistic Infections. 10:27–29.

AUTRAN, BRIGITTE, et al. (1997). Positive effects of combined antiretroviral therapy on CD4+ T cell homeostasis and function in advanced HIV disease. *Science*, 277:112–116.

BACK, DAVID. (2001). Pharmacology to the fore. *PRN NOTE-BOOK*, 6:11–14.

BALTER, MICHAEL. (1997). HIV Survives Drug On-slaught by Hiding Out in T Cells. *Science*, 278: 1227.

BARTHWELL, ANDREA. (1997). Substance use and the puzzle of adherence. *FOCUS*, 12:1–4.

BEEKER, AMANDA STEPHEN, et al. (2002). Young HIV-infected adults are at greater risk for medication nonadherence. *Medscape HIV/AIDS eJournal* B(4).

BLANKSTON, JOEL, et al. (2001). Structured therapeutic interruptions: A Review. *Hopkins HIV Report*, 13. 1, 8–9, 13.

BOZZETTE, SAMUEL, et al. (2001). Expenditures for the care of HIV infected patients in the era of HAART. *N. Eng. J. Med.*, 344: 817–823.

British Guidelines Coordinating Committee. (1997). British HIV Association guidelines for antiretroviral treatment of HIV seropositive individuals. *Lancet*, 349:1086–1091.

BURMAN, WILLIAM, et al. (1998). The Case for Conservative Management of Early HIV Disease. *JAMA*, 280:93–95.

CARPENTER, CHARLES, et al. (1997). Antiviral therapy for HIV infection in 1997. *JAMA*, 277:1962–1969.

CARPENTER, CHARLES, et al. (2000). Antiretroviral therapy for Adults: Updated recommendations of the International AIDS Society—USA Panel. *JAMA*, 283:381–390.

CARR, ANDREW, et al. (1998). Pathogenesis of HIV protease inhibitor-associated peripheral lipodystrophy, hyperlipidemia and insulin resistance. *Lancet*, 351:1881–1883.

CARR, ANDREW, et al. (1998a). A syndrome of peripheral lipodystrophy, hyperlipidemia and insulin resistance in patients receiving HIV protease inhibitors. *AIDS*, 12: F51–58.

CARR, ANDREW, et al. (1998b). Lipodystrophy associated with an HIV protease inhibitor. (Images in Clinical Medicine) *N. Engl. J. Med.*, 339:1296.

CARR, ANDREW, et al. (1998c). Abnormal fat distribution and use of protease inhibitors. *Lancet*, 351:1736 (letter).

CARR, ANDREW, et al. (1998d). Pathogenesis of HIV-1 protease inhibitor-associated peripheral lipodystrophy, hyperlipidaemia and insulin resistance. *Lancet*, 351:1881–1883.

CASCADE COLLABORATION (2000). Survival after the introduction of HAART in people with known duration of HIV-1 infection. 355:1158–1159.

CASPER, TONY. (2000). How to make billions out of the misery of millions. Online. Available: http://www.dispatch.co.2a [2000, May 18].

CHUN, TAE-WOOK, et al., (2000). Relationship between pre-existing viral reservoirs and the re-emergence of plasma viremia after discontinuation of highly active anti-retroviral therapy. *Nature Medicine*, 6: 757–762.

CLARK, DAWN, et al. (1999). T cell renewal impaired in HIV-1 infected individuals. Presented at: 6th Conference on Retroviruses and Opportunistic Infections; January 31–February 4, Chicago. Abstract 22.

CLOUGH, LISA, et al. (1999). Factors that predict incomplete virological response to protease inhibitors-based antiretroviral therapy. *Clinical Infections Diseases.* 29:75–81.

CLUMECK, NATHAN. (1995). Summary to the use of saquinavir for HIV therapy. *AIDS*, 9(Suppl. 2): 533–534.

COFFIN, JOHN. (1995). HIV population dynamics *in vivo*: Implications for genetic variation, pathogenesis and therapy. *Science*, 267:483–489.

DANNER, SVEN, et al. (1995). Short term study of the safety, pharmacokinetics and efficacy of ritonavir. *N. Engl. J. Med.*, 333:1528–1533.

DEEKS, STEVEN, et al. (1997). Genotypic-resistance assays and anti-retroviral therapy. *Lancet*, 349: 1489–1490.

DEEKS, STEVEN, et al. (1999). HIV RNA and CD4 cell count response to protease inhibitor therapy in an urban AIDS clinic: Response to both initial and salvage therapy. *AIDS*, 13:F35–F43.

DE MARTINO, MAURIZIO. (1995). Redox potential status in children with perinatal HIV-1 infection treated with zidovudine. *AIDS*, 9:1381–1383.

DICKOVER, RUTH, et al. (1996). Identification of levels of maternal HIV-RNA associated with risk of perinatal transmission. *JAMA*, 275:599–605.

DOBKIN, JAY. (1997). Fortovase: Son of Invirase. *Infections in Medicine.* 14:926, 934.

D'SOUZA, M. PATRICIA, et al. (2000). Current evidence and future directions for targeting HIV entry. *JAMA*, 284: 215–222.

DUBÉ, MICHAEL, et al. (1997). Protease associated hyperglycaemia. *Lancet*, 350:713–714.

ERICKSON, JOHN, et al. (1990). Design, activity, and 2.8 angstrom crystal structure of a C_2 symmetric inhibitor complexed to HIV protease. *Science*, 249:527–533.

FINZI, DIANA, et al. (1999). Latent infection of CD4(+) T cells provides a mechanism for life-long persistence of HIV-1, even in patients on effective combination therapy. *Nature Medicine*, 5:512–517.

FLEXNER, CHARLES. (1996). Pharmacokinetics and pharmacodynamics of HIV protease inhibitors. *Infect. Med.*, 13:16–23.

FREEDBERG, KENNETH, et al. (2001). The cost effectiveness of combination antiretroviral therapy for HIV disease. *N. Eng. J. Med.* 344: 824–831.

GERBER, JOHN. (1996). Drug interactions with HIV protease inhibitors. *Improv. Manage. HIV Dis.*, 4:20–23.

GERVASONI, CRISTINA, et al. (1999). Redistribution of body fat in HIV-infected women undergoing combined antiretroviral therapy. *AIDS* 13:465–472.

GOLDSCHMIDT, RONALD, et al. (1995). Antiretroviral strategies revisited. *J. Am. Board Fam. Pract.*, 8:62–69.

GOLDSCHMIDT, RONALD, et al. (1998). Individualized strategies in the era of combination antiretroviral therapy. *J.A.M. Board Family Practice*, 11:158–164.

Guidelines for the Use of Antiretroviral Agents in HIV-Infected Adults and Adolescents. (1999). *MMWR* 47:1–63 No. RR–5.

Guidelines for the Use of Antiretroviral Agents in Pediatric HIV Infection (1998). *MMWR* 47:1–38 No. RR4.

HELLERSTEIN, MARC, et al. (1999). Directly measured kinetics of circulating T lymphocytes in normal and HIV-infected humans. *Nat Med.*, 5:83–89.

HENDERSON, DAVID, et al. (2001). HIV postexposure prophylaxis in the 21st Century. *Emerging Infectious Diseases*, 7:254–258.

HENRARD, DENIS, et al. (1995). Natural history of HIV cell-free viremia. *JAMA*, 274:554–558.

HIRSCHEL, BERNARD et al. (1998). Progress and Problems in the Fight Against AIDS. *N. Engl. J. Med.*, 338:906–908.

HO, DAVID, et al. (1995). Rapid turnover of plasma virions and CD4 lymphocytes in HIV-1 infection. *Nature*, 373:123–126.

HU, DALE, et al. (1996). The emerging genetic diversity of HIV. *JAMA*, 275:210–216.

JACOBSEN, HELMUT, et al. (1995). Reduced sensitivity to saquinavir: An update from genotyping from phase I/II trials. 4th International Workshop on HIV Drug Resistance, Sardinia.

JOHN, PATRICIA, et al. (1996). Predictive value of viral load measurements in asymptomatic untreated HIV infection: A mathematical model. *AIDS*, 10:255–262.

JURRIAANS, SUZANNE, et al. (1994). The natural history of HIV infection: Virus load and virus phenotype independent determinants of viral course? *Virology*, 204:223–233.

KAISER FAMILY FOUNDATION. (1999). National monitoring project: *Annual Report* 1–45 and Appendix 1–14.

KATZ, MARK. (2000). Top 10 HIV/AID stories of 2000. *Being Alive Newsletter*, Feb 01. http://www.beingalivela.org.

KAUFMANN, DANIEL, et al. (1998). CD4-cell count in HIV-1 infected individuals remaining viraemic with HAART. (Swiss HW Cohort Study) *Lancet*, 351:723–724.

KENYON, GEORGE. (2001). Resistance study to re-evaluate HAART, *Nature*, 7:515.

LAURENCE, JEFFREY. (1996). The clinical promise of HIV protease inhibitors. *AIDS Reader*, 6:39–41, 71.

LEE HUANG, SYLVIA, et al. (1999). Lysozyme and RNases as anti-HIV components in beta-core preparations of human chorionic gonadotropin. Proceedings of the National Academy of Sciences. 96:2678–2681.

LIPSKY, JAMES. (1998). Abnormal Fat Accumulation in Patients with HIV-I Infection. *Lancet*, 351:847–848.

LITTLE, SUSAN, et al. (1999). Reduced antiretroviral drug susceptibility among patients with primary HIV infection. *JAMA*, 282:1142–1149.

LO, JOAN, et al. (1998). "Buffalo Hump" in Men with HIV-1 Infection. *Lancet*, 351:867–870.

MARKOWITZ, MARTIN, et al. (1995). A preliminary study of ritonavir, an inhibitor of HIV protease. *N. Engl. J. Med.*, 333:1534–1539.

MAYERS, DOUGLAS. (1996). Rational approaches to resistance: Nucleoside analogues. *AIDS*, 10 (Suppl. 1):S9–S13.

MELLORS, JOHN, et al. (1995). Quantitation of HIV-1 RNA in plasma predict outcome after seroconversion. *Ann. Intern. Med.*, 122:573–579.

MELLORS, JOHN. (1996). Clinical implications of resistance and cross-resistance to HIV protease inhibitors. *Infect. Med.*, 13:32–38.

MERRICK, SAMUEL. (1997). Managing antiretrovirals in HIV-infected patients. *AIDS Reader*, 7:16–27.

MILLER, KIRK, et al. (1998). Visceral abdominal-fat accumulation associated with use of indinavir. *Lancet*, 351:871–875.

Morbidity and Mortality Weekly Report. (1994). Zidovudine for the prevention of HIV transmission from mother to infant. 43:285–287.

MOYLE, GRACME. (1995). Resistance to antiretroviral compounds: Implications for the clinical management of HIV infection. *Immunol. Infect. Dis.*, 5:170–182.

NIGHTINGALE, STUART. (1996). From the Food and Drug Administration: First protease inhibitor approved. *JAMA*, 275:273.

NOWAK, MARTIN. (1995). How HIV defeats the immune system. *Sci. Am.*, 273:58–64.

PALELLA, FRANK, et al. (1998). Declining morbidity and mortality among patients with advanced HIV infection. *N. Engl. J. Med.*, 338:853–860.

PERRIN, LUC, et al. (1998). HIV treatment failure: Testing for HIV resistance in clinical practice. *Science*, 280:1871–1873.

PIATAK, MICHAEL, et al. (1993). High levels of HIV-1 in plasma during all stages of infection determined by competitive PCR. *Science*, 259:1749–1754.

RICH, JOSIAH, et al. (1999). Misdiagnosis of HIV infection by HIV plasma viral load testing: A case series. *Annals of Internal Medicine Online* (1/5/99) 130:37.

ROBERTS, JOHN, et al. (1988). The accuracy of reverse transcriptase from HIV-1. *Science*, 242: 1171–1173.

SAKSELA, KALLE, et al. (1994). Human immunodeficiency virus type 1 mRNA expression in peripheral blood cells predicts disease progression independently of the number of CF4+ lymphocytes. *Proc. Natl. Acad. Sci. USA*, 91:1104–1108.

SCHMIT, JEAN-CLAUDE, et al. (1996). Resistance-related mutations in the HIV protease gene of patients treated for 1-year with protease inhibitor ritonavir. *AIDS*, 10:995–999.

SCHRAGER, LEWIS, et al. (1998). Cellular and anatomical reservoirs of HIV in patients receiving potent antiretroviral combination therapy. *JAMA*, 280:67–71.

SIMBERKOFF, MICHAEL. (1996). Long-term follow-up of symptomatic HIV-infected patients originally randomized to early vs. later zidovudine treatment: Report of a Veterans Affairs cooperative study. *AIDS*, 11:142–150.

STEPHENSON, JOAN. (1996). New anti-HIV drugs and treatment strategies buoy AIDS researchers. *JAMA*, 275:579–580.

TELENTI, AMALIO, et al. for the Swiss HIV Cohort Study. (1998). CD4 T cell counts in HIV-infected individuals remaining viraemic with highly active antiretroviral therapy followed in the Swiss HIV Cohort Study (SHCS). *Antiviral Ther.*, 3 (suppl 1):53.

VALDEZ, HERNAN, et al. (1999). Human immunodeficiency virus 1 protease inhibitors in clinical practice. Archives of *Internal Medicine*. 159:1771–1776.

VELLA, STEFANO. (1995). Clinical experience with saquinavir. *AIDS*, 9(Suppl 2):S21–S25.

VELLA, STEFANO. (1997). Clinical implications of resistance to antiretroviral drugs. *AIDS Clin. Care*, 9:45–47, 49.

VELLA, STEFANO, et al. (1996). HIV resistance to antiretroviral drugs. *Improv. Manage. HIV Dis.*, 4:15–18.

WAIN-HOBSON, SIMON. (1995). Virologies mayhem [editorial]. *Nature*, 373:102.

WALKER, BRUCE, et al. (1998). Treat HIV infection like other infections—Treat it. *JAMA*, 208:91–93.

WEI, XIPING, et al. (1995). Viral dynamics in human immunodeficiency virus type 1 infection. *Nature*, 373:117–122.

WEI, XIPING, et al. (2002). Emergence of resistant human immunodeficiency virus type 1 in patients receiving fusion inhibitor (T-20) monotherapy. *Antimicrob Agents Chemother*, 46(6):1896–1905.

WONG, JOSEPH, et al. (1997). Recovery of replication-competent HIV despite prolonged suppression of plasma viremia. *Science*, 278:1291–1294.

WONG, JOSEPH, et al. (2000). Primary infection with HIV-1 with reduced drug susceptibility does not appear to result from point source transmission. Program abstracts of the 7th Conference on Retroviruses and Opportunistic Infections; January 30–February 2, San Francisco. Abstract 212.

CHAPTER 5

AMEISEN, JEAN CLAUDE. (1994). Programmed cell death apoptosis and cell survival regulation: relavance to cancer. *AIDS*, 8:1197–1213.

AMIGORENA, SEBASTIAN et al., (1994). Transient accumulation of new class II MHC molecules in a novel endocytic compartment in B lymphocytes. *Nature*, 369:113–120.

BAKKER, LEENDERT J., et al. (1992). Antibodies and complement enhance binding and uptake of HIV-1 by human monocytes. *AIDS*, 6:35–41.

BARR, PHILIP, et al. (1994). Apoptosis and its role in human disease. *BioTechnology*, 12:487–494.

BAXENA, S., et al. (1985). Immunosuppression by human seminal plasma. *Immunol. Invest.*, 14: 255–269.

BERKMAN, S. (1984). Infectious complications of blood transfusions. *Sem. Oncol.*, 11:68–75.

BLEUL, CONRAD, et al. (1996). The lymphocyte chemoattractant SDF-1 is a ligand for LESTR/fusin and blocks HIV entry. *Nature*, 382:829–833.

BLUMBERG, N., et al. (1985). A retrospective study of transfusions. *Br. Med. J.*, 290:1037–1039.

BOLOGNESI, DANI P. (1989). Prospects for prevention of and early intervention against HIV. *JAMA*, 261:3007–3013.

CALLEBAUT, CHRISTIAN, et al. (1993). T cell activation antigen, CD26 as a cofactor for entry of HIV in CD4+ cells. *Science*, 262:2045–2050.

CHEN, SI-YI, et al. (1997). Second major HIV coreceptor inactivated by intrakine gene therapy. *Proc. Natl. Acad. Sci. USA*, 94:11,567–11,572.

COHEN, JON. (1993). Keystone's blunt message: "It's the virus stupid." *Science*, 260:292–293.

COHEN, JON. (1993). HIV cofactor comes in for more heavy fire. *Science*, 262:1971–1972.

COHEN, JON. (1997). Exploiting the HIV-chemokine nexus. *Science*, 275:1261–1264.

CONNER, RUTH, et al. (1994). Human immunodeficiency virus type 1 variants with increased replicative capacity develop during the asymptomatic stage before disease progression. *J. Virol.*, 68: 4400–4408.

CORBEIL, JACQUES, et al. (2001). Temperal gene regulation during HIV-1 infection of human CD4+ T cells. *Genome Research*, 11:1198–1204.

DEAN, MICHAEL, et al. (1996). Genetic restriction of HIV infection and progression to AIDS by a deletion allele of the CKR5 structural gene. *Science*, 273:1856–1861.

DENG, HONGKUI, et al. (1996). Identification of a major coreceptor for primary isolates of HIV-1. *Nature*, 381:661–666.

DOHERTY, PETER. (1995). The keys to cell-mediated immunity. *JAMA*, 274:1067–1068.

DRAGIC, TATJANA, et al. (1996). HIV-1 entry into CD4+ cells is mediated by the chemokine receptor CC-CKR-5. *Nature*, 381:667–673.

EDGINGTON, STEPHEN M. (1993). HIV no longer latent, says NIAID's Fauci. *BioTechnology*, 11:16–17.

EMBRETSON, JANET, et al. (1993). Massive covert infection of helper T lymphocytes and macrophages by HIV during the incubation period of AIDS. *Nature*, 362:359–362.

Eugen-Olsen, Jesper, et al. (1997). Heterozygosity for a deletion in the CKR5 gene leads to prolonged AIDS-free survival and slower CD4 T-cell decline. *AIDS*, 11:305–310.

Fauci, Anthony, et al. (1995). Trapped but still dangerous. *Nature*, 337:680–681.

Fitzgerald, Lynn. (1988). Exercise and the immune system. *Trends Genet.*, 2:1–12.

Foster, R., et al. (1985). Adverse effects of blood transfusions in lung cancer. *Cancer*, 55:11,951–12,202.

Fox, Cecil H., et al. (1991). Lymphoid germinal centers for reservoirs of HIV type I RNA. *J. Infect. Dis.*, 164:1051–1057.

Fox, Cecil. (1996). How HIV causes disease. *Carolina Tips*, 59:9–11.

Geijtenbeek, Teunis, et al. (2000). Identification of DC-SIGN, a novel dendritic cell specific ICAM-3 receptor that supports primary immune response. *Cell*, 100:575–585.

Gelderblom, H.R., et al. (1985). Loss of envelope antigens of HTLV III/LAV, a factor in AIDS pathogenesis. *Lancet*, 2:1016–1017.

Groenink, Martijin, et al. (1993). Relation of phenotype evolution of HIV to envelope V2 configuration. *Science*, 260:1513–1516.

Haase, Ashley, et al. (1996). Quantitative image analysis of HIV infection in lymphoid tissue. *Science*, 274:985–990.

Heath, Sonya, et al. (1995). Follicular dendritic cells and HIV infectivity. *Nature*, 377:740–744.

Hengartner, Michael. (1995). Life and death decisions: Ced-9 programmed cell death in *C. elegans*. *Science*, 270:931.

Hill, Mark, et al. (1996). Natural resistance to HIV. *Nature*, 382:668–669.

Ho, David. (1995). Pathogenesis of HIV infection. *International AIDS Society–USA*, 3:9–12.

Ho, David, et al. (1995). Rapid turnover of plasma virons and CD4 lymphocytes in HIV infection. *Nature*, 373:123–126.

Kingsley, L., et al. (1987). Risk factors for seroconversion to HIV among male homosexuals. *Lancet*, 8529:345–348.

Kion, Tracy, et al. (1991). Anti-HIV and Anti-Anti-MHC antibodies in alloimmune and auto-immune mice. *Science*, 253:1138–1140.

Klein, Jan, et al. (2000). (a) The HLA System: Part I. *NEJM*, 343: 702–709.

Klein, Jan, et al. (2000). (b) The HLA System: Part II. *NEJM*, 343: 782–786.

Knight, Stella. (1996). Bone-marrow-derived dendritic cells and the pathogenesis of AIDS. *AIDS*, 10:807–817.

Kunal, Saha, et al. (2001). Isolation of primary HIV-1 that target CD8+ lymphocytes using CD8 as a receptor. *Nature Medicine*, 7: 65–72.

Kwong, Peter, et al. (1998). Structure of an HIV gp120 envelope glycoprotein in complex with the CD4 receptor and a neutralizing human antibody. *Nature:* 648–659.

LaPierre, A., et al. (1992). Exercise and health maintenance in AIDS. In Galantino, M.L. (ed.), *Clinical Assessment and Treatment in HIV: Rehabilitation of a Chronic Illness*, Chap. 7. Thorofare NJ: Slack, Inc.

Laurence, Jeffrey. (1996). Where do we go from here? *AIDS Reader*, 6:3–4, 36.

Liu, Rong, et al. (1996). Homozygous defect in HIV-1 coreceptor accounts for resistance of some multiple-exposed individuals to HIV-1 infection. *Cell*, 86:367–377.

Marmor, Michael, et al. (2001). Homozygous and heterozygous CCR5-32 genotypes are associated with resistance to HIV infection. *J Acq. Immune Def Syndromes*, 27:472–481.

McDermott, David, et al. (2000). Chemokine promoter polymorphism affects risk of both HIV infection and disease progression in Multicenter AIDS Cohort Study. *AIDS*, 14: 2671–2678.

McNicholl, Janet, et al. (1997). Host genes and HIV: The role of the chemokine receptor gene CCR5 and its allele (Δ32CCR5). *Emerg. Infect. Dis.*, 3:261–271.

Moir, Susan, et al. (2000). B cells of HIV-1 infected patients bind virons through CD21-complement interactions and transmit infectious virus to activated T cells. *J Exp Med*, 192: 637–646. Published online August 28, at http://www.jem.org.

Moir, Susan, et al. (2001). HIV induces phenotypic and functional perturbations of B cells in chronically infected individuals. *PNAS*, 98: 10362–10367.

Moore, John. (1997). Coreceptors: Implications for HIV pathogenesis and therapy. *Science*, 276: 51–52.

Mountain-Plains Regional HIV/AIDS Curriculum, 4th ed. (1992). Mountain-Plains Regional AIDS Office, University of Colorado Health Sciences Center, Denver, CO 80262.

Nowak, Martin, et al. (1995). HIV results in the frame: Results confirmed. *Nature*, 375:193.

O'Brien, Stephen. (1998). AIDS: A role for host genes. *Hospital Practice*, 33:53–79.

Olinger, Gene, et al. (2000). CD4-negative cells bind HIV-1 and efficiently transfer virus to T cells. *J Virol*, 74: 8550–8557.

Pantaleo, G., et al. (1993). HIV infection is active and progressive in lymphoid tissue during the clinically latent stage of disease. *Nature*, 362: 355–358.

Pennisi, Elizabeth. (1994). A room of their own. *Science News*, 145:335.

Pianz, Oliver, et al. (1996). Specific cytotoxic T Cells eliminate cells producing neutralizing antibodies. *Nature*, 382:726–729.

Rizzuto, Carlo, et al. (1998). A conserved HIV gp120 glycoprotein structure involved in chemokine receptor binding. *Science*, 280:1949–1953.

Samson, Michel, et al. (1996). Resistance to HIV-1 infection in Caucasian individuals bearing mutant alleles of the CCR-5 chemokine gene. *Nature*, 382:722–725.

SCHMID, SANDRA, et al. (1994). Making class II presentable. *Nature*, 369:103–104.

SCHNITTMAN, STEVEN M., et al. (1989). The reservoir for HIV-1 in human peripheral blood is a T cell that maintains expression of CD4. *Science*, 245:305–308.

SINHA, ANIMESH, et al. (1990). Autoimmune diseases: The failure of self-tolerance. *Science*, 248: 1380–1387.

SPRENT, JONATHAN, et al. (1994). Lymphocyte life-span and memory. *Science*, 265:1395–1400.

STEINMAN, RALPH. (2000). DC-SIGN: A guide to some mysteries of dendritic cells. *Cell*, 100:491–494.

STROMINGER, JACK, et al. (1995). The Class I and Class II proteins of the Human major histocompatibility complex. *JAMA*, 274:1074–1076.

TULP, ABRAHAM, et al. (1994). Isolation and characterization of the intracellular MHC class II compartment. *Nature*, 369:120–126.

UNANUE, EMIL. (1995). The concept of antigen processing and presentation. *JAMA*, 274:1071–1073.

WEI, XIPING, et al. (1995). Viral dynamics in HIV type I infection. *Nature*, 373:117–122.

WEISS, ROBIN, et al. (1996). Hot fusion of HIV. *Nature*, 381:647–648.

WITKIN, S., and SONNABEND, J. (1983). Immune responses to spermatozoa in homosexual men. *Fertil. Steril.*, 39:337–341.

WYATT, RICHARD, et al. (1998). The antigenic structure of the HIV gp120 envelope glycoprotein. *Nature*, 705–711.

YEH, EDWARD. (1998). Life and Death of a Cell. *Hospital Practice*, 33:85–92.

ZHU, TOUFU. (1993). Genotypic and phenotypic characterization of HIV-1 patients with primary infection. *Science*, 261:1179–1181.

ZINKERNAGEL, ROLF. (1995). MHC-restricted T-cell recognition: The basis of immune surveillance. *JAMA*, 274:1069–1071.

CHAPTER 6

AMIN, NAVIN M. (1987). Acquired immunodeficiency syndrome, Part 2: The spectrum of disease. *Fam. Pract. Recert.*, 9:84–118.

ANTMAN, KAREN, et al. (2000). Karposi's Sarcoma. *NEJM*, 342:1027–1038.

AWE, ROBERT J. (1988). Benefits, promises and limitations of zidovudine (AZT). *Consultant*, 28: 57–72.

BALFOUR, HENRY. (1995). Cytomegolovirus retinitis in persons with AIDS. *Postgrad. Med.*, 97:109–118.

BARTLETT, JOHN. (2002). Report from IAAC: Update on opportunistic infections. *Hopkins HIV Report*, 14:1–13.

BERMEJO, ALVERO, et al. (1992). Tuberculosis incidence in developing countries with high prevalence of HIV infection. *AIDS*, 6:1203–1206.

BROOKE, GRACE LEE, et al. (1990). HIV disease: A review for the family physician Part II. Secondary infections, malignancy and experimental therapy. *Am. Fam. Pract.*, 42:1299–1308.

BUCHANAN, KENT, et al. (1998) What makes *Cryptococcus neoformans* a pathogen? *Emerging Infectious Diseases*, 4:71–83.

CHANG, YUAN, et al. (1994). Identification of Herpes virus-like DNA sequences in AIDS-Associated Kaposi's Sarcoma. *Science*, 266:1865–1869.

CHIN, DANIEL. (1992). Mycobacterium avium complex infection. *AIDS File: Clin. Notes*, 6:7–8.

Coalition News. (1993). Pet guidelines for people with HIV. 2:4–5.

CURRIER, JUDITH, et al. (1997). Pathogenesis, prevention and treatment of opportunistic complications. *Improv. Manage. HIV Dis.*, 4: S17–S18.

DALEY, CHARLES L. (1992). Epidemiology of tuberculosis in the AIDS era. *AIDS File: Clin. Notes*, 6:1–2.

DANNENBERG, ARTHUR M. (1993). Immunopathogenesis of pulmonary tuberculosis. *Hosp. Pract.*, 28:51–58.

DEHOVITZ, JACK A. (1988). Management of *Isospora belli* infections in AIDS patients. *Infect. Med.*, 5:437–440.

DEWIT, STEPHANE, et al. (1991). Fungal infections in AIDS patients. *Clin. Adv. Treatment Fungal Infect.*, 2:1–11.

ENNIS, DAVID M., et al. (1993). Cryptococcal meningitis in AIDS. *Hosp. Pract.*, 28:99–112.

Emergency Medicine. (1989). Fighting opportunistic infections in AIDS. 21:24–38.

ERNST, JEROME. (1990). Recognize the early symptoms of PCP. *Med. Asp. Hum. Sexuality*, 24:45–47.

EZZELL, CAROL. (1993). Captain of the men of death. *Science News*, 143:90–92.

GANEM, DONALD. (1996) Kaposi's sarcoma-associated herpesvirus. *Improv. Manage. HIV Dis.*, 4(3):8–10.

GOTTLIEB, MICHAEL S., et al. (1987). Opportunistic viruses in AIDS. *Patient Care*, 23:139–154.

GROSS, DAVID J., et al. (1989). Update on AIDS. *Hosp. Pract.*, 25:19–47.

GROSSMAN, RONALD J., et al. (1989). PCP and other protozoal infections. *Patient Care*, 23:89–116.

GRULICH, ANDREW. (2000). Cancer risk in persons with HIV/AIDS in the era of combination antiretroviral therapy. *AIDS Reader*, 10:341–346.

GUARINO, M., et al. (1995). Progressive multifocal leucoencephalopathy in AIDS: Treatment with cytosine arabinoside. *AIDS*, 9:819–820.

Guidelines, U.S. Public Health Service, (1995). Preventing OIs in persons with HIV disease. *AIDS Reader*, 5:172–179.

HARDEN, C.L., et al. (1994). Diagnosis of central nervous system toxoplasmosis in AIDS patients confirmed by autopsy. *AIDS*, 8:1188–1189.

HARDY, DAVID. (1996). Lessons learned from HIV pathogenesis and therapy: Implications for better management of cytomegalovirus disease. *AIDS*, 10 (Suppl, 1): S31–S35.

HARRIS, CHARLES. (1993). TB and HIV: The boundaries collide. *Medical World News*, 34:63.

Harvard AIDS, Institute, (1994). *Special Report—Opportunistic Infections.* Fall issue:1–14.

HAY, R.J. (1991). Oropharyngeal candidiasis in the AIDS patient. *Clin. Adv. Treatment Fungal Infect.*, 2:10–12.

HERNDIER, BRIAN, et al. (1994). Pathogenesis of AIDS lymphomas. *AIDS*, 8:1025–1049.

HESSOL, NANCY. (1998). The changing epidemology of HIV related cancers. *The AIDS Reader*, 8:45–49.

HUGHES, WALTER. (1994). Opportunistic infections in AIDS patients. *Postgrad. Med.*, 95:81–86.

HIV/AIDS Surveillance Report, Year End. (1997). 9:1–44.

JACOBSON, MARK A., et al. (1988). Serious cytomegalovirus disease in the acquired immunodeficiency syndrome (AIDS): Clinical findings, diagnosis, and treatment. *Ann. Intern. Med.*, 108:585–594.

JACOBSON, MARK A., et al. (1992). CMV disease in patients with AIDS: Introduction. *Clin. Notes*, 6(2):1–11.

JOINER, K.A., et al. (1990). Toxoplasma gondii: Fusion competence of parasitophorous vacuoles in Fe receptor-transfected fibroblasts. *J. Cell Biol.*, 109:2771.

KLEDAL, THOMAS, et al. (1997). A broad spectrum chemokine antagonist encoded by KS-associated herpesvirus. *Science*, 277:1656–1659.

LAURENCE, JEFFREY. (1995). Evolving management of OIs. *AIDS Reader*, 5:187–188, 208.

LAURENCE, JEFFREY. (1996). Where do we go from here? *AIDS Reader*, 6:3–4, 36.

LEDERGERBER, BRUNO, et al. (1999). AIDS-related OI occurring after initiation of potent antiretroviral therapy: A Swiss cohort study. *JAMA*, 282:2220–2226.

LOONEY, DAVID, (1996). Kaposi's sarcoma. *Improv. Manage. HIV Dis.*, 4:21–24.

LYNCH, JOSEPH P. (1989). When opportunistic viruses infiltrate the lung. *J. Resp. Dis.*, 10:25–30.

MARTIN, JEFFREY, et al. (1998). Sexual transmission and the natural history of human herpesvirus 8 infection. *N. Engl. J. Med.*, 338:948–954.

MCGRATH, MICHAEL, et al. (1994). Identification of a common clonal human immunodeficiency virus integration site in human immunodeficiency virus-associated lymphomas. *Cancer Res.*, 54:2069.

MEDOFF, GERALD, et al. (1991). Systemic fungal infections: An overview. *Hosp. Pract.*, 26:41–52.

MONETTE, PAUL. (1988). *Borrowed Time: An AIDS Memoir.* New York: Avon Books.

MONFORTE, ANTONELLA D'ARMINIO, et al. (1992). AIDS-defining diseases in 250 HIV-infected patients: A comparative study of clinical and autopsy diagnoses. *AIDS*, 6:1159–1164.

MONTGOMERY, BRUCE A. (1992). *Pneumocystis carinii* pneumonia prophylaxis: Past, present and future. *AIDS*, 6:227–228.

Morbidity and Mortality Weekly Report. (1993). Estimates of future global TB morbidity and mortality. 4:961–964.

Morbidity and Mortality Weekly Report. (1995). USPHS/IDSA guidelines for the prevention of opportunistic infections in persons infected with HIV: A summary. 44:1–34.

Morbidity and Mortality Weekly Report. (1995). 1995 Revised guidelines for prophylaxis against PCP for children infected with or perinatally exposed to HIV. 44:1–10.

Morbidity and Mortality Weekly Report. (1997). 1997 USPHS/IDSA guidelines for the prevention of OIs in persons infected with HIV. 46:1–46.

Morbidity and Mortality Weekly Report. (1999). USPHS/IDSA Guidelines for the prevention of opportunistic infections in persons infected with HIV. 48:1–59.

MURPHY, ROBERT. (1994). Opportunistic infection prophylaxis. *Int. AIDS Soc.–USA*, 2:7–8.

NEWTON, HERBERT. (1995). Common neurologic complications of HIV infection and AIDS. *Am. Fam. Phys.*, 51:387–398.

O'BRIEN, THOMAS, et al. (1999). Evidence for concurrent epidemics of HHB and HIV type 1 in US homosexual men: Rates, risk factors, and relationship to KS. *J. Infectious Disease*, 180:1010–1017.

OSMOND, DENNIS, et al. (2002). Prevalance of Kaposi Sarcoma-associated herpes virus infection in homosexual men at the beginning of and during the HIV epidemic. *JAMA*, 287:221–225.

PHAIR, JOHN, et al. (1990). The risk of *Pneumocystis carinii* among men infected with HIV-1. *N Engl. J Med.*, 322:161–165.

POWDERLY, WILLIAM G., et al. (1992). Molecular typing of Candida albicans isolated from oral lesions of HIV-infected individuals. *AIDS*, 6:81–84.

POWDERLY, WILLIAM, et al. (1998). Recovery of the immune system with antiretroviral therapy: the end of opportunism? *JAMA*, 280:72–77.

RINALD, CHARLES, et al. (2001). Primary human herpesvirus 8 infection generates a broadly specific CD8+ T cell response to viral lytic cycle proteins. *Blood*, 97:2366–2373.

ROSSITCH, EUGENE, et al. (1990). Cerebral toxoplasmosis in patients with AIDS. *Am. Fam. Pract.*, 41:867–873.

RUSSELL, JAMES. (1990). Study focuses on eyes and AIDS. *Baylor Med.*, 21:3.

SAID, JONATHAN, et al. (1997). KS-associated herpesvirus/ human herpesvirus type 8 encephalitis in HIV-positive and -negative individuals. *AIDS*, 11:1119–1122.

SEPKOWITZ, KENT. (1998). Effect of HAART on natural history of AIDS-related opportunistic disorders. *Lancet*, 351:228–230.

SIBLEY, L. DAVID. (1992). Virulent strains of *Toxoplasma gondii* comprise single clonal linage. *Nature*, 359:82–85.

SMALL, PETER. (1996). Tuberculosis research: Balancing the portfolio. *JAMA*, 276:1512–1513.

SOLOWAY, BRUCE. (1998). Report on the Fifth Conference on Retroviruses and Opportunistic Infections. *AIDS Clinical Care*, 10:27–29.

STANFORD, J.L., et al. (1993). Old plague, new plague, and a treatment for both? *AIDS*, 7:1275–1276.

STRINGER, JAMES, et al. (1996). Molecular biology and epidemiology of pneumocystis carinii infections in AIDS. *AIDS*, 10:561–571.

TUAZON, CARMELITA, et al. (1991). Diagnosing and treating opportunistic CNS infections in patients with AIDS. *Drug Therapy*, 21:43–53.

United States Public Health Service and Infectious Diseases Society of America. (2001). Guidelines for the prevention of opportunistic infections in persons infected with human immunodeficiency virus. *MMWR*, November 28, 1–65.

WALLACE, MARK R., et al. (1993). Cats and toxoplasmosis risk in HIV-infected adults. *JAMA*, 269:76–77.

WALZER, PETER D. (1993). *Pneumocystis carinii*: Recent advances in basic biology and their clinical application. *AIDS*, 7:1293–1305.

WHEAT, L. JOSEPH. (1992). Histoplasmosis in AIDS. *AIDS Clin. Care*, 4:1–4.

ZOLER, MITCHELL L. (1991). OI's widening realm. *Medical World News*, 32:38–44.

CHAPTER 7

ABOULKER, JEAN-PIERRE, et al. (1993). Preliminary analysis of the concorde trial. *Lancet*, 341:889–890.

ANDERSON, ROBERT E., et al. (1991). CD8 T lymphocytes and progression to AIDS in HIV-infected men: Some observations. *AIDS*, 5:213–215.

BALTER, MICHAEL. (1998). Chemokine mutation slows progression. *Science*, 279:327.

BALTIMORE, DAVID. (1995). Lessons from people with nonprogressive HIV infection. *N. Engl. J. Med.*, 332: 259–260.

BARNHART, HUIMAN, et al. (1995). *Abstracts of the 2nd National Conference on Human Retroviruses*, Washington, D.C., p. 161, abstr. 575.

BARTLETT, JOHN, et al. (1998). Primary care of HIV infection. *Hospital Practice*, 33:53–55.

BOLOGNESI, DANI P. (1989). Prospects for prevention of and early intervention against HIV. *JAMA*, 261: 3007–3013.

BRYSON, YVONNE J., et al. (1995). Clearance of HIV infection in a prenatally infected infant. *N. Engl. J. Med.*, 332:833–838.

BUCHBINDER, SUSAN P., et al. (1992). Healthy long-term positives: Men infected with HIV for more than 10 years with CD4 counts of 500 cells. *Eighth International Conference on AIDS*, Amsterdam, July 1992, abstr. TUCO572.

BUCHBINDER, SUSAN P., et al. (1994). Long-term HIV infection without immunologic progression. *AIDS*, 8: 1123–1128.

BUCY, R. PAT. (1999). Viral and cellular dynamics in HIV-1 disease. *Improving Management of HIV Disease*, 7: 8–11.

BURCHAM, JOYCE, et al. (1991). CD4 % is the best predictor of development of AIDS in a cohort of HIV-infected homosexual men. *AIDS*, 5:365–372.

CAO, YUNZHEN, et al. (1995). Virologic and immunologic characterization of long-term survivors of human immunodeficiency virus type 1 infection. *N. Engl. J. Med.*, 332:201–208.

CATALAN, JOSÉ, et al. (2001). The changing picture of HIV: Achronic illness, again? *FOCUS*, 16:1–4.

Centers for Disease Control and Prevention. (2001). Report of NIH panel to define principles of therapy of HIV infection and guidelines for the use of antiretroviral agents in HIV infected adults and adolescents. Updated February 5, as a living document: www.hivatis.org.

CHUN, TAE-WOOK, et al. (1998). Early establishment of a pool of latently infected, resting CD4+ T cells during primary HIV-1 infection. *PNAS*, 95:8869–8873.

COCCHI, FIORNZA, et al. (1995). Identification of RANTES, MIP-1a and MIP-1b as the major HIV-suppressive factors produced by CD8+ T cells. *Science*, 270:1811–1815.

COFFIN, JOHN M. (1995). HIV population dynamics in vivo: Implications for genetic variation, pathogenesis and therapy. *Science*, 267:483–489.

COHEN, JON. (1993). Keystone's blunt message: It's the virus stupid. *Science*, 260:292–293.

COHEN, JON. (1995). High turnover of HIV in blood revealed by new studies. *Science*, 267:179.

COLLMAN, RONALD. (1997). Effect of CCR2 and CCR5 variants on HIV disease. *JAMA*, 278:2113–2114.

CONANT, MARCUS. (1995). The current face of the AIDS epidemic. *AIDS Newslink*, 6 (Fall):1–9.

COULIS, PAUL A., et al. (1987). Peptide-based immunodiagnosis of retrovirus infections. *Am. Clin. Prod. Rev.*, 6:34–43.

DAVIS, SUSAN, et al. (1995). Prevalence and incidence of vertically acquired HIV infection in the U.S.A. *JAMA*, 274:952–955.

DEACON, NICHOLAS, et al. (1995). Genomic structure of an attenuated quasi species of HIV from a blood transfusion donor and recipients. *Science*, 270:988–991.

ENSOLI, F., et al. (1990). Proviral sequences detection of human immunodeficiency virus in seronegative subjects by polymerase chain reaction. *Mol. Cell Probes*, 4:153–161.

ENSOLI, F., et al. (1991). Plasma viraemia in seronegative HIV-1 infected individuals. *AIDS*, 5:1195–1199.

ESCAICH, SONIA, et al. (1991). Plasma viraemia as a marker of viral replication in HIV-infected individuals. *AIDS*, 5:1189–1194.

FAUCI, ANTHONY S. (1988). The scientific agenda for AIDS. *Issues Sci. Technol.*, 4:33–42.

FENG, YU, et al. (1996). HIV-1 entry cofactor: Functional cDNA cloning of a seven-transmembrane, G protein-coupled receptor. *Science*, 272:872–877.

FREED, ERIC, et al. (1994). HIV infection of non-dividing cells. *Nature*, 369:107–108.

FRENKEL, LISA, et al. (1998). Genetic evaluation of suspected cases of transient HIV infection of infants. *Science*, 280:1073–1077.

GEGNEY, THOMAS. (2000). Long term nonprogressors: The study of HIV infection without progression to AIDS. Research Initiative Treatment Alert (RITA), 6: No. 2. June 2000. http://www.aegis.org/pubs/rita/ 2000/RI00064.html

GOLDSCHMIDT, RONALD, et al. (1997). Treatment of AIDS and HIV-related conditions—1997. *J. Am. Board Fam. Pract.*, 10:144–167.

GRUBMAN, SAMUEL, et al. (1995). Older children and adolescents living with perinatally acquired HIV infection. *Pediatrics*, 95:657–663.

HAAS, DAVID, et al. (2000). Evidence of a source of HIV-1 within the central nervous system by ultraintensive sampling of cerebrospinal fluid and plasma. *AIDS Res. Hum.Retroviruses*, 16: 1491–1502.

HANLEY, DANIEL F., et al. (1988). When to suspect viral encephalitis. *Patient Care*, 22:77–99.

HAY, CHRISTINE. (1998). Immunologic response to HIV. *AIDS Clinical Care*, 10:1–3.

HAYNES, BARTON, et al. (1996). Toward an understanding of the correlates of protective immunity to HIV infection. *Science*, 271:324–328.

HENRARD, DENIS, et al. (1995). Natural history of HIV cell-free viremia *JAMA*, 274:554–558.

HO, DAVID, et al. (1995). Rapid turnover of plasma virons and CD4 lymphocytes in HIV infection. *Nature*, 373:123–126.

HO, DAVID. (1996). HIV pathogenesis. *Improv. Manage. HIV Dis.*, 4:4–6.

HORSBURG, C.R., et al. (1989). Duration of HIV infection before detection of antibody. *Lancet*, ii:637–639.

IMAGAWA, D.T., et al. (1989). Human immunodeficiency virus type I infection in homosexual men who remain seronegative for prolonged periods. *N. Engl. J. Med.*, 320:1458–1462.

Italian Register for HIV Infection in Children. (1994). Lancet, 343:191–195.

JOHNSON, RICHARD, et al. (1996). Quantitation of human immunodeficiency virus in brains of demented and nondemented patients with acquired immunodeficiency syndrome. *Ann. Neurol.* 39:392–395.

KATZENSTEIN, TERESE, et al. (1996). Longitudinal Serum HIV RNA quantification: Correlation to viral phenotype at seroconversion and clinical outcome. *AIDS*, 10:167–173.

KELLY, MAUREEN, et al. (1991). Oral manifestations of human immunodeficiency virus infection. *Cutis*, 47:44–49.

KIRCHHOFF, FRANK, et al. (1995). Brief report: Absence of intact NEF sequences in a long-term survivor with nonprogressive HIV-1 infection. *N. Engl. J. Med.*, 332:228–232.

KLINE, MARK. (1995). Long-term survival in vertically acquired HIV infection. *AIDS Reader*, 5:153.

LEARMONT, JENNIFER, et al. (1999). Immunological and virologic status after 14 to 18 years of infection with an attenuated strain of HIV-1. *N. Engl. J. Med.*, 340: 1715–1722.

LEVY, JAY. (1995). HIV and long-term survival. *Int. AIDS Soc. USA*, 3:10–12.

LIPTON, STUART. (1997). Treating AIDS dementia. *Science*, 276:1629–1630.

MCARTHUR, JUSTIN. (1999). Declining incidence of neurologic complications of HIV disease. *Hopkins HIV Report*, 11:8.

MCGUIRE, DAWN. (1993). Pathogenesis of brain injury in HIV disease. *Clin. Notes*, 7:1–11.

MERIGAN, THOMAS, et al. (1996). The prognostic significance of viral load, codon 215-reverse transcriptase mutation and CD4+ T cells on HIV Disease Progression. *AIDS*, 10:159–165.

MIGUELES, STEPHEN, et al. (2000). HLA B5701 is highly associated with restriction of virus replication in a subgroup of HIV infected long term nonprogressors. *Pro. Natl. Acad. Sci USA*, 97: 2709–2714.

MISHRAHI, MICHELINE, et al. (1998). CCR5 chemokine receptor variant in HIV-1 mother to child transmission and disease progression. *JAMA*, 279:277–280.

Morbidity and Mortality Weekly Report. (1996). Persistent lack of detectable HIV-antibody in a person with HIV-infection—Utah, 1995. 45:181–185.

Morbidity and Mortality Weekly Report. (1997). Revised guidelines for performing CD4+ T-cell determinations in persons infected with HIV. 46:1–4.

NATIONAL INSTITUTE OF ALLERGY AND INFECTION DISEASES. (1989). Tests confirm lack of mental impairment in asymptomatic HIV-infected homosexual men. June: 1–2.

NEWELL, MARIE, et al. (1996). Detection of virus in vertically exposed HIV-antibody-negative children. *Lancet*, 347:213–215.

NIELSON, CLAUS, et al. (1993). Biological properties of HIV isolates in primary HIV infection: Consequences for the subsequent course of infection. *AIDS*, 7: 1035–1040.

NOWAK, M.A., et al. (1990). The evolutionary dynamics of HIV-1 quasispecies and the development of immunodeficiency disease. *AIDS*, 4:1095–1103.

PANTALEO, GUISEPPE, et al. (1993). The immunopathogenesis of HIV infection. *N. Engl. J. Med.*, 328:327–335.

PANTALEO, GUISEPPE, et al. (1995). Studies in subjects with long-term nonprogressive human immunodeficiency virus infection. *N. Engl. J. Med.*, 332:209–216.

PEDERSEN, C., et al. (1989). Clinical course of primary HIV infection: Consequences for subsequent course of infection. *Br. Med. J.*, 299:154–157.

PERELSON, ALAN, et al. (1996). HIV dynamics in vivo: Viron clearance rate, infected cell life-span and viral generation time. *Science*, 271:1582–1586.

PHILLIPS, ANDREW N., et al. (1991a). p24 Anti-genaemia, CD4 lymphocyte counts and the development of AIDS. *AIDS*, 5:1217–1222.

PHILLIPS, ANDREW N., et al. (1991b). Serial CD4 lymphocyte counts and development of AIDS. *Lancet*, 337:389–392.

PHILLIPS, ANDREW, et al. (1994). A sex comparison of rates of new AIDS-defining disease and death in 2554 AIDS cases. *AIDS*, 8:831–835.

PRICE, RICHARD W. (1988). The brain in AIDS: Central nervous system HIV infection and AIDS dementia complex. *Science*, 239:586–593.

QUINN, THOMAS. (1997). Acute primary HIV infection. *JAMA*, 278:58–62.

RANKI, A., et al. (1987). Long latency precedes overt seroconversion in sexually transmitted human immunodeficiency virus infection. *Lancet*, ii:589–593.

RANKI, ANNAMARI, et al. (1995). Abundant expression of HIV NEF and Rev proteins in brain astrocytes *in vivo* is associated with dementia. *AIDS*, 9:1001–1008.

REYNES, JACQUES, et al. (2001). CD4 T cell surface CCR5 density as a host factor in HIV-1 disease progression. *AIDS*, 15:1627–1634.

RICHMAN, DOUGLAS. (1995). Antiretroviral resistance and HIV dynamics. *Int. AIDS Soc.*, 3:15–16.

ROQUES, PIERRE, et al. (1995). Clearance of HIV infection in 12 perinatally infected children: Clinical, virological and immunological data. *AIDS*, 9: F19–F26.

ROSENBERG, PHILIP, et al. (1994). Declining age at HIV infection in the United States. *N. Engl. J. Med.*, 330: 789–790.

ROYCE, RACHEL A., et al. (1991). The natural history of HIV-1 infection: Staging classifications of disease. *AIDS*, 5:355–364.

SAX, PAUL, et al. (1995). Potential clinical implications of inter-laboratory variability in CD4+ T-lymphocyte counts of patients infected with human immunodeficiency virus. *Clin. Infect. Dis.*, 21:1121–1125.

SCHONNING, KRISTIAN, et al. (1998). Chemokine receptor polymorphism and autologous neutralizing antibody response in long-term HIV infection. *J. Acquired Immune Deficiency Syndrome and Human Retrovirology*, 18:195–202.

SHERNOFF, MICHAEL. (1997). A history of hope: The HIV roller coaster. *Focus*, 12:5–7.

SKURNICK, JOAN, et al. (2002). Correlates of nontransmission in US women at high risk of HIV-1 infection through sexual exposure. *J Infect. Diseases*, 185:428–438.

SOLOWAY, BRUCE, et al. (2000). Antiretroviral failure: A biopsychosocial approach. *AIDS Clinical Care*, 12:23–25, 30.

STRAMER, SUSAN L., et al. (1989). Markers of HIV infection prior to IgG antibody seropositivity. *JAMA*, 262:64–69.

THE EUROPEAN COLLABORATIVE STUDY. (1994). *Pediatrics*, 94:815–819.

VANHEMS, PHILLIPPE, et al. (1999). Recognizing primary HIV infection. *Infections in Medicine*, 16:104–108, 110.

VOELKER, REBECCA. (1995). New studies say viral burden tops CD4 as a marker of HIV-disease progression. *JAMA*, 275:421–422.

WAIN-HOBSON, SIMON. (1995). Virological mayhem. *Nature*, 373:102.

WEI, XIPING, et al. (1995). Viral dynamics in HIV type 1 infection. *Nature*, 373:117–122.

WINKLER, CHERYL, et al. (1998). Genetic restriction of AIDS pathogenesis by an SDF-1 chemokine gene variant. *Science*, 279:389–393.

YU, KALVIN, et al. (2000). Primary HIV infection. *Postgraduate Medicine*, 107: 114–122.

CHAPTER 8

ABBOTT, ALISON. (1995). Murder charges brought in German HIV blood products case. *Nature*, 376:628.

ABBOTT, ALISON. (1996). Japan agrees to pay HIV-blood victims. *Nature*, 380:278.

ALDHOUS, PETER. (1991). France will compensate. *Nature*, 353:425.

AMIRKHANIAN, YURI, et al. (2001). AIDS knowledge, attitudes and behavior in Russia: Results of a population based, random-digit telephone survey in St. Petersburg. *Int. J. STD AIDS*, 12:50–57.

ARCHIBALD, D.W., et al. (1990). *In vitro* inhibition of HIV-1 infectivity by human salivas. *AIDS Res. Human Viruses*, 6:1425–1431.

BAGASRA, OMAR, et al. (1994). Detection of HIV proviral DNA in sperm from HIV-infected men. *AIDS*, 8:1669–1674.

BARON, SAMUEL, et al. (1999). Why is HIV Rarely Transmitted by Oral Secretions? Saliva Can Disrupt Orally Shed, Infected Leukocytes. *Archives of Internal Medicine*, 159:303–310.

BENNETT, AMANDA, et al. (1996). AIDS fight is skewed by Federal campaign exaggerating risks. *Wall Street Journal*, May 1, A1.

BOBKOV, ALEKSEI. (1994). Molecular epidemiology of HIV in the former Soviet Union: Analysis of ENV-3 sequences and their correlation with epidemologic data. *AIDS*, 8:619–624.

BOLLING, DAVID R. (1989). Anal intercourse between women and bisexual men. *Med. Asp. Human Sexuality*, 23:34.

BOYER, PAMELA J., et al. (1994). Factors predictive of maternal-fetal transmission of HIV. *JAMA*, 271:1925–1930.

BREO, DENNIS L. (1991). The two major scandals in France's AIDSGATE. *JAMA*, 266:3477–3482.

BURKETT, ELINOR. (1995). The gravest show on earth: America in the age of AIDS. Houghton Miflin: Boston.

BUTLER, DECLAN. (1994a). Allain freed to face new charges? *Nature*, 370:404.

BUTLER, DECLAN. (1994b). Blood scandal raises spectre of Dreyfus case. *Nature*, 371:548.

CAMERON, WILLIAM D. (1989). Female to male transmission of human immunodeficiency virus type 1: risk factors for sercoconversion in men. *Lancet*, 2:403–407.

CAMERON, WILLIAM D., et al. (1990). Sexual transmission of HIV and the epidemiology of other STDs. *AIDS*, 4:S99–S103.

CDC (Centers for Disease Control and Prevention). (1990). *HIV/AIDS Surveillance Report*, Oct.: 1–18.

CENTERS FOR DISEASE CONTROL AND PREVENTION. AIDS among persons aged >50 years—US 1991–1996. *MMWR Morb Mort Wkly*, 47:21–27.

CHU, S.Y., et al. (1990). Epidemiology of reported cases of AIDS in lesbians, United States 1980–89. *Am. J. Public Health*, 80:1380.

COHEN, J.B., et al. (1989). Heterosexual transmission of HIV. *Immunol. Ser.*, 44:135–137.

COHEN, JON. (1995). Bringing AZT to poor countries. *Science*, 269:624–626.

CONANT, MARCUS. (1995). The current face of the AIDS epidemic. *AIDS Newslink*, 6:14–18.

CONNER, EDWARD, et al. (1994). Reduction of maternal-infant transmission of HIV with zidovudine treatment. *N. Engl. J. Med.*, 331:1173–1180.

COOMBS, ROBERT, et al. (1998). Association between culturable HIV in semen and HIV RNA levels in semen and blood: Evidence for compartmentalization of HIV between semen and blood. *J. Infect. Dis.*, 117:320–323.

COOMBS, ROBERT W., et al. (1989). Plasma viremia in HIV infection. *N. Engl. J. Med.*, 321:1526.

COTTONE, JAMES A., et al. (1990). The Kimberly Bergalis case: An analysis of the data suggesting the possible transmission of HIV infection from a dentist to his patient. *Phys. Assoc. AIDS Care*, 2:267–270.

COUTSOUDIS, ANNA, et al. (1999). Influence of infant-feeding patterns on early mother-to-child transmission of HIV-1 in Durban, South Africa: a prospective cohort study. *The Lancet*, 354:9177, 9471.

COUTSOUDIS, ANNA, et al. (2001). Method of feeding and transmission of HIV-1 from mothers to children by 15 months of age: prospective cohort study from Durban, South Africa. *AIDS*, 15:379–387.

CROMBIE, RENE, et al. (1998). Identification of a CD36-related Thrombospondin 1-binding domain in HIV envelope glycoprotein gp120: Relationship to HIV specific inhibitory factors in human saliva. *J. Exp. Med*, 187:25–35.

CURRAN, JAMES W., et al. (1988). Epidemiology of HIV infection and AIDS in the United States. *Science*, 239:610–616.

DEL ROMERO, JEORGE et al. (2002). Evaluating the risk of HIV transmission through unprotected sex. *AIDS*, 16:1296–1297.

DEMARTINO, MAURIZIO, et al. (1992). HIV-1 transmission through breast-milk: Appraisal of risk according to duration of feeding. *AIDS*, 6:991–997.

DES JARLAIS, DON C., et al. (1989). AIDS and IV drug use. *Science*, 245:578.

DES JARLAIS, DON, et al. (1995). Maintaining low HIV-seroprevalence in populations of injecting drug users. *JAMA*, 274:1226–1231.

DES JARLAIS, DON, et al. (2000). HIV incidence among injection drug users in New York City, 1992–1997; Evidence for a declining epidemic. *Am J. Public Health*, 90:352–359.

DEVINCENZI, I., et al. (1989). Risk factors for male to female transmission of HIV. *Br. Med. J.*, 298:411–415.

DILLON, BETH, et al. (2000). Primary HIV infections associated with oral transmission. Program and abstracts of the 7th Conference on Retroviruses and Opportunistic Infections; January 30–February 2; San Francisco, Calif. Abstract 473.

DORFMAN, ANDREA. (1991). Bad blood in France. *Time*, 138:48.

DROTMAN, PETER. (1996). Professional boxing, bleeding, and HIV testing. *JAMA*, 276:193.

EDWARDS, SARA, et al. (1998). Oral sex and the transmission of viral STD's. *J. Infect. Dis.*, 74:6–10.

ELSON, JOHN. (1991). The dangerous world of wannabes. *Time*, 138:77–80.

Emergency Cardiac Care Committee, American Heart Association. (1990). Risk of infection during CPR training and rescue: Supplemental guidelines. *JAMA*, 262:2714–2715.

European Mode of Delivery Collaboration, The (1999). Elective Caesarean section versus vaginal delivery in prevention of vertical HIV-1 transmission: A randomized clinical trial. *The Lancet*, 353:1035–1039.

FOX, PHILIP. (1991). Saliva and salivary gland alterations in HIV infection. *J. Am. Dental Assoc.*, 122:46–48.

FRIEDLAND, GERALD H. (1991). HIV transmission from health care workers. *AIDS Clin. Care*, 3:29–30.

GAUTHIER, DEANN et al. (1999). Bareback sex, bugchasers and the gift of death. *Deviant Behavior*, 20:85–100.

GIBBONS, MARY. (1994). Childhood sexual abuse. *Am. Fam. Phys.*, 49:125–136.

Global AIDSNEWS. (1994). A new approach to STD control and AIDS prevention. 4:13–14, 20.

GODDARD, JEROME. (1997). Why mosquitoes cannot transmit the AIDS virus. *Infect, Med.*, 14:353–354.

GOLDSCHMIDT, RONALD, et al. (1995). Antiretroviral strategies revisited. *J. Am. Board Fam. Pract.*, 8:62–69.

GOSTIN, Lawrence. (1994). HIV testing, counseling and prophylaxis after sexual assault. *JAMA*, 271:1436–1444.

GOTO, Y., et al. (1991). Detection of proviral sequences in saliva of patients infected with human immunodeficiency virus type 1. *AIDS Res. Hum. Retroviruses*, 7:343–347.

GROSSKURTH, HEINER, et al. (1995). Impact of improved treatment of sexually transmitted diseases on HIV infection in rural Tanzania. *Lancet*, 346:530–536.

GUINAN, MARY. (1995). Artificial insemination by donor: Safety and secrecy. *JAMA*, 273:890–891.

HARRISON, LEE, et al.(2000). Drugs cut HIV in semen: Safe sex still crucial. *Ann. Int. Med.*, 133: 280–284.

HAWTHORNE, PETER. (1999). An epidemic of rapes. *Time*, (11/1/99) 154, No. 18, p. 59.

HEARST, NORMAN, and HULLEY, STEPHEN B. (1988). Preventing the heterosexual spread of AIDS: Are we giving our patients the best advice? *JAMA*, 259:2428.

HECHT, FREDERICK, et al. (1998). Sexual transmission of an HIV-1 variant resistant to multiple reverse-transcriptase and protease inhibitors. *N. Eng. J. Med.*, 339:307–311.

HELPERIN, DANIEL, et al. (1999). Viewpoint: male circumcision and HIV infection: 10 years and counting. *Lancet*, 354(9192):1813–1815.

HEREK, GREGORY, et al. (2002). HIV related stigma and knowledge in the United States: Prevalence and trends, 1991–1999. *Am J. Public Health*, 92:371–377.

HEYMANN, DAVID, et al. (1994). The laboratory, epidemiology, nosocomial infection and HIV. *AIDS*, 8:705–706.

HIV/AIDS Surveillance Report. (1996). December 8:1–39.

HIV/AIDS Surveillance Report. (1997). December 9:1–43.

HIV/AIDS Surveillance Report. (1999). December 10:1–44.

HIV/AIDS Surveillance Report. (2001). June 13:1–41.

HOLDEN, CONSTANCE. (1994). Switzerland has its own blood scandal. *Science*, 264:1254.

HOLMSTROM, PAUL, et al. (1992). HIV antigen detected in gingival fluid. *AIDS*, 6:738–739.

HOOKER, TRACEY. (1996). HIV/AIDS: Facts to consider: 1996 National Conference of State Legislators, Denver, Colorado, February. 1–64.

HORN, TIM. (2001). Safety and efficacy of solid organ transplantation in HIV positive patients. *PRN Notebook*, 6:19–24.

HU, DALE J., et al. (1992). HIV infection and breastfeeding: Policy implications through a decision analysis model. *AIDS*, 6:1505–1513.

JACKSON, BROOKS. (1999). Progress in reducing mother-to-infant HIV transmission. *The Hopkins Report*, 11:2–3.

JAYARAMAN, KRISHNAMURTHY. (1995). HIV scandal hits Bombay blood centre. *Nature*, 376:285.

JOSEPH, STEPHEN C. (1993). Dragon within the gates: The once and future AIDS epidemic. *Med. Doctor*, 37:92–104.

JOVAISAS, E., et al. (1985). LAV/HTLV III in 20-week fetus. *Lancet*, 2:1129.

KAHN, JAMES, et al. (1998). Acute HIV-1 Infection. *N. Eng. J. Med.*, 339:33–40.

KAISER, JOCELYN. (1996). Pasteur implicated in blood scandal? *Science*, 272:185.

KATNER, H.P., et al. (1987). Evidence for a Euro-American origin of human immunodeficiency virus. *J. Natl. Med. Assoc.*, 79:1068–1072.

KATZ, MITCHELL, et al. (2002). Impact of HAART on HIV seroincidence among men who have sex with men: San Francisco. *Am J. Public Health*, 92:388–394.

KIESSLING, ANN. (1999). HIV-1 semen: Risks for transmission, disease progression and reproduction. *Physician's Research Network NYC*. NY: http//www.prn.org/prn_nb_cntnt/vol4/numl/article2_cntnt.com

KIND, CHRISTIAN, et al. (1998). Prevention of Vertical HIV Transmission: Additive Protective Effect of Elective Caesarean Section and Zidovudine Prophylaxis. *AIDS*, 12:205–210.

KINGSLEY, L.A., et al. (1990). Sexual transmission efficiency of hepatitis B virus and human immunodeficiency virus among homosexual men. *JAMA*, 264:230–234.

KLEIN, HARVEY. (2000). Will blood transfusion ever be safe enough? *JAMA*, 284:238–240.

KOSS, M.P., et al. (1991). Deleterious effects of criminal victimization on women's health and medical utilization. *Arch. Intern. Med.*, 151:342–347.

KRIEGER, JOHN, et al. (1998). Risk of sexual transmission of HIV unaffected by vasectomy. *J. of Urology*, 159:820–825.

KUHN, LOUISE, et al. (1994). Maternal-infant HIV transmission and circumstances of delivery. *Am. J. Public Health*, 84:1110–1115.

LACAYO, RICHARD. (1997). Assault with a deadly virus. *Time Magazine*, 149:82.

LAGA, MARIE. (1991). HIV infection and sexually transmitted diseases. *Sexually Transmitted Dis. Bull.*, 10:3–10.

LAGA, MARIE, et al. (1993). Non-ulcerative STDs as risk factors for HIV transmission in women: Results from a cohort study. *AIDS*, 7:95–102.

LEWIS, S.H., et al. (1990). HIV-1 introphoblastic villous Hofbauer cells and haematological precursors in eight-week fetuses. *Lancet*, 335:565.

LICHTMAN, STUART M., et al. (1991). Greater attention urged for HIV in older patients. *Infect. Dis. Update*, 2:5.

MARLINK, RICHARD, et al. (1994). Reduced rate of disease development after HIV infection as compared to HIV-1. *Science*, 265:1587–1590.

MIIKE, LAWRENCE. (1987). Do insects transmit AIDS? Office of Technological Assessment, Sept. 1:43.

MONZON, O.T., et al. (1987). Female to female transmission of HIV. *Lancet*, 2:40–41.

Morbidity and Mortality Weekly Report. (1988a). Update: Universal precautions for prevention of transmission of human immunodeficiency virus, hepatitis B virus, and other bloodborne pathogens in healthcare settings. 37:377–382, 387–388.

Morbidity and Mortality Weekly Report. (1990a). Possible transmission of HIV to a patient during an invasive dental procedure. 39:489–493.

Morbidity and Mortality Weekly Report. (1990b). HIV infection and artificial insemination with processed semen. 39:249–256.

Morbidity and Mortality Weekly Report. (1991a). Update: Transmission of HIV infection during an invasive dental procedure—Florida. 40:21–27, 33.

Morbidity and Mortality Weekly Report. (1991b). Drug use and sexual behaviors among sex partners of injecting-drug users—U.S. 40:855–860.

Morbidity and Mortality Weekly Report. (1992). Childbearing and contraceptive-use plans among women at high risk for HIV infection—Selected U.S. sites, 1989–1991. 41:135–144.

Morbidity and Mortality Weekly Report. (1994a). Human immunodeficiency virus transmission in household settings—United States. 43:347, 353–357.

Morbidity and Mortality Weekly Report. (1994b). Guidelines for preventing transmission of HIV through transplantation of human tissue and organs. 43:1–15.

Morbidity and Mortality Weekly Report. (1994c). Medical-care expenditures attributable to cigarette smoking—United States, 1993. 43:469–472.

Morbidity and Mortality Weekly Report. (1994d). Zidovudine for the prevention of HIV transmission from mother to infant. 43:285–287.

Morbidity and Mortality Weekly Report. (1995). Use of AZT to prevent perinatal transmission (ACTG 076): Workshop on implications for treatment, counseling, and HIV testing. 44:1–12.

Morbidity and Mortality Weekly Report. (1997). Transmission of HIV possibly associated with exposure of mucous membrane to contaminated blood. 46:620–623.

Morbidity and Mortality Weekly Report. (1998). AIDS among people aged 50 years—United States, 1991–1996. 47:21–27.

MUNZER, ALFRED. (1994). The threat of secondhand smoke. *Menopause Manage.*, 3:14–17.

NAFTALIN, RICHARD J. (1992). Anal sex and AIDS. *Nature*, 360:10.

NEWELL, Marie-LOUISE, et al. (1990). HIV-1 infection in pregnancy: Implications for women and children. *AIDS*, 4:S111–S117.

NOWAK, RACHEL. (1995). Rockefeller's big prize for STD test. *Science*, 269:782.

OLESKE, JAMES M. (1994). The many needs of HIV-infected children. *Hosp Pract.* 29:81–87.

OMETTO, LUCIA et al. (1995) Viral phenotype and host-cell susceptibility to HIV infection as risk factors for mother-to-child HIV transmission. *AIDS*, 9:427–434.

PADIAN, NANCY S., et al. (1991). Female to male transmission of HIV. *JAMA*, 266:1664–1667.

PADIAN, NANCY, et al. (1997). Heterosexual transmission of HIV in northern California: Results from a ten-year study. *Am. J. Epidemiol.*, 146:350–357.

PATTERSON, JULIE, et al. (1995). Basic and clinical considerations of HIV infection in the elderly. *Infect. Dis.*, 3:21–34.

PECKHAM, CATHERINE, et al. (1995). Mother-to-child transmission of HIV. *N. Engl. J. Med.*, 333:298–302.

PETERMAN, THOMAS A., et al. (1988). Risk of human immunodeficiency virus transmission from heterosexual adults with transfusion-associated infections. *JAMA*, 259:55–58.

PETO, RICHARD. (1992). Statistics of chronic disease control. *Nature*, 356:557–558.

POURTOIS, M., et al. (1991). Saliva can contribute in quick inhibition of HIV infectivity. *AIDS*, 5:598–599.

QUINN, THOMAS, et al. (2000). Viral load and heterosexual transmission of human HIV-1. *NEJM*, 342: 921–929.

READ, JENNIFER. (1999). The Mode of Delivery and the Risk of Vertical Transmission of Human Immunodeficiency Virus Type 1—A Meta-Analysis of 15 Prospective Cohort Studies. *N. Eng. J. Med.*, 340:977–987.

REICHHARDT, TONY. (1995). Top aide to face charges in French HIV blood scandal. *Nature*, 375:349.

RILEY, LAURA, et al. (1999). Elective caesarean delivery to reduce the transmission of HIV. *N. Eng. J. Med.*, 13:1032–1033.

ROGERS, DAVID, et al. (1993). AIDS policy: Two divisive issues. *JAMA*, 270:494–495.

ROTHENBERG, RICHARD, et al. (1998). Oral Transmission of HIV. *AIDS*, 12:2095–2105.

ROZENBAUM, W. et al. (1988). HIV transmission by oral sex. *Lancet*, 1:1395.

SCHACKER, TIMOTHY, et al. (1998). Frequent recovery of HIV from genital herpes simplex virus lesions in HIV infected men. *JAMA*, 280:61–66.

Science in California. (1993). AIDS: I want a new drug. *Nature*, 362:396.

SCOTT, G.B., et al. (1985). Mothers of infants with the acquired immunodeficiency syndrome: Evidence for both symptomatic and asymptomatic carriers. *JAMA*, 253:363–366.

SEGARS, JAMES H. (1989). Heterosexual anal sex. *Med. Asp. Human Sexuality*, 23:6.

SELWYN, PETER A. (1986). AIDS: What is now known. *Hosp. Pract.*, 21:127–164.

SHERNOFF, MICHAEL. (1988). Integrating safer-sex counseling into social work practice. *Social Casework: J. Contemp. Social Work*, 69:334–339.

SPITZER, P.G., et al. (1989). Transmission of HIV infection from a woman to a man by oral sex. *N. Engl. J. Med.*, 320:251.

SPURGEON, DAVID. (1994). Canadian AIDS suit raises hope for HIV-blood victims. *Nature*, 281.

SPURGEON, DAVID. (1996). Canadian inquiry points the finger. *Nature*, 663.

ST. LOUIS, MICHAEL E., et al. (1993). Risk for perinatal HIV transmission according to maternal immunologic, virologic and placental factors. *JAMA*, 269:2853–2860.

ST. LOUIS, MICHAEL E., et al. (1997). Editorial: Janus considers the HIV pandemic—harnessing recent advances to enhance AIDS prevention. *Am. J. Public Health*, 87:10–11.

STRYKER, JEFF, et al. (1993). AIDS policy: Two divisive issues. *JAMA*, 270:2436–2437.

SWENSON, ROBERT M. (1988). Plagues, History and AIDS. *Am. Scholar*, 57:183–200.

SWINBANKS, DAVID. (1993). American witnesses: Testify in Japan about AIDS risks. *Nature*, 364:181.

UNAIDS. (1997). Implications of HIV variability for transmission: Scientific and policy issues. *AIDS*, 11:S1–S15.

VAN DE PERRE, PHILIPPE, et al. (1993). Infective and anti-infective properties of breast milk from HIV-infected women. *Lancet*, 341:914–918.

VITTECOQ, D., et al. (1989). Acute HIV infection after acupuncture treatments. *N. Engl. J. Med.*, 320:250–251.

VOELKER, REBECCA. (1996). HIV guide for primary care physicians stresses patient-centered prevention. *JAMA*, 276:85–86.

WEBB, PATRICA, et al. (1989). Potential for insect transmission of HIV: Experimental exposure of *Cimex hemipterous* and *Toxorhynchites amboinensis* to human immunodeficiency virus. *J. Infect. Dis.*, 160:970–977.

WILL, GEORGE F. (1991). Foolish choices still jeopardize public health. *Private Pract.*, 24:46–48.

Women's AIDS Network. (1988). Lesbians and AIDS: What's the connection? San Francisco AIDS Foundation, 333 Valencia St., 4th Floor, P.O. Box 6182, San Francisco, CA 94101-6182.

WOOLLEY, ROBERT J. (1989). The biologic possibility of HIV transmission during passionate kissing. *JAMA*, 262:2230.

ZHANG, HUI, et al. (1998). HIV-1 in the semen of men receiving HAART. *N. Eng. J. Med.*, 339:1803–1810.

ZIELER, SALLY, et al. (2001). Violence and HIV: Strategies for primary and secondary prevention. *Focus*, 16: 1–4.

ZIGLER, J.B., et al. (1985). Postnatal transmission of AIDS-associated retrovirus from mother to infant. *Lancet*, 1:896–897.

CHAPTER 9

ABDALA, NADIA, et al. (1999). HIV-1 can survive in syringe for more than 4 weeks. *J. Acq. Imm. Def. Syndromes*, 20:73–80.

ANDERSON, FRANK W.J. (1993). Condoms: A technical guide. *Female Patient*, 18:21–26.

ANDERSON, JOHN, et al. (1998). Needle hygiene and sources of needles for injection drug users: Data from a National Survey. *J. Acq. Imm. Def. Syndromes*, 18:S147

BARBER, HUGH R.K. (1990). Condoms (not diamonds) are a Girl's best friend. *Female Patient*, 15:14–16.

BAROUCH, DAN, et al. (2000). Control of viremia and prevention of clinical AIDS in Rhesus monkeys by cytokine-augmented DNA vaccination. *Science*, 290:486–492.

BAYER, RONALD, et al. (1992). HIV Prevention and the two faces of partner notification. *Am. J. Public Health*, 82:1158–1164.

BOLOGNESI, DANIEL, et al. (1998). Viral envelope fails to deliver? *Nature*, 391:638–639.

BURNETT, JOSEPH. (1995). Fundamental basic science of HIV. *Cutis*, 55:84.

BURRIS, SCOTT, et al. (1996). Legal strategies used in operating syringe-exchange programs in the United States. *Am. J. Public Health*, 86:1161–1166.

BURRIS, SCOTT, et al. (2000). Physician prescribing of sterile injection equipment to prevent HIV infection: Time for action. *Ann. Intern. Med.*, 133: 218–226.

CALAROTA, SANDRA, et al. (1998). Cellular cytotoxic response induced by DNA vaccination in HIV infected patients. *Lancet*, 351:1320–1325.

CHRISTENSEN, DAMARIS. (1994a). A shot in time: The technology behind new vaccines. *Science News*, 145:344–345.

CLEMENT, MICHAEL J. (1993). HIV disease: Are we going anywhere? *Patient Care*, 27:13.

Cohen, Jon. (2001). Long-lasting immunity conferred in monkeys. *Science*, 291: 1879–1881.

Cohen, Jon. (1994a). Bumps on the vaccine road. *Science*, 265:1371–1372.

Cohen, Jon. (1994b). Are researchers racing toward success, or crawling? *Science*, 265:1373–1374.

Consumer Reports. (1989). Can you rely on condoms? 54:135–141.

De Vincenzi, Isabelle. (1994). A longitudinal study of HIV transmission by heterosexual partners. *N. Engl. J. Med.*, 331:341–347.

Drucker, Lurie, et al. (1997). An opportunity lost: HIV infection associated with lack of a national needle-exchange program in the USA. *Lancet*, 349:604–608.

Etzioni, Amitai. (1993). HIV sufferers have a responsibility. *Time*, 142:100.

Ezzell, Carol. (1987). Hospital workers have AIDS virus. *Nature*, 227:261.

Farr, Gaston, et al. (1994). Contraceptive efficacy and acceptability of the female condom. *Am. J. Public Health*, 84:1960–1964.

Fenton, Kevin, et al. (1997). HIV partner notification: Taking a new look. *AIDS*, 11:1535–1546.

Findlay, Steven. (1991). AIDS: The second decade. *U.S. News World Rep.*, 110:20–22.

Fisher, Peter. (1990). A report from the underground. *International Working Group on AIDS and IV Drug Use*, 5:15–17.

Francis, Donald, P., et al. (1987). The prevention of acquired immunodeficiency syndrome in the United States. *JAMA*, 257:1357–1366.

Frezieres, Ron, et al. (1999). Evaluation of the efficacy of a polyurethane condom: Results from a randomized, controlled clinical trial. *Family Planning Perspectives*, 31: 81–87.

Gerberding, Julie Louise. (1991). Reducing occupational risk of HIV infection. *Hosp. Pract.*, 26:103–118.

Gibson, David, et al. (2001). Effectiveness of syringe exchange programs in reducing HIV risk behavior and HIV seroconversion among injecting drug users. *AIDS*, 15:1329–1341.

Gostin, Lawrence, et al. (1998). HIV infection and AIDS in the public health and health care systems: The role of law and litigation. *JAMA*, 279:1108–1113.

Grimes, David A.(1992). Contraception and the STD epidemic: Contraceptive methods for disease prevention. *The Contraception Report: The Role of Contraceptives in the Prevention of Sexually Transmitted Diseases*, III:1–15.

Guttmacher, Sally, et al. (1997). Condom availability in New York City public high schools: Relationships to condom use and sexual behavior. *Am. J. Public Health*, 87:1427–1433.

Hagen, Holly. (1991). Studies support syringe exchange. *FOCUS*, 6:5–6.

Hearst, Norman, et al. (1995). Collaborative AIDS prevention research in the developing world: The CAPS experience. *AIDS*, 9 (suppl 1):51–55.

Homsy, Jacques, et al. (1989). The Fe and not CD4 receptor mediates antibody enhancement of HIV infection in human cells. *Science*, 244: 1357–1359.

Hooker, Tracey. (1996). HIV/AIDS: Facts to consider, 1996. *National Conference of State Legislature*. Denver, February, 1–64.

Judson, Franklyn N. (1989). Condoms and spermicides for the prevention of sexually transmitted diseases. *Sexually Transmitted Dis. Bull.*, 9:3–11.

Kaplan, Edward, et al. (1993). Let the needles do the talking! Evaluating the New Haven needle exchange. *Interfaces*, 23:7–26.

Kirby, Douglas, et al. (1998). The impact of condom distribution in Seattle schools on sexual behavior and condom use. *Am. J. Public Health*, 89:182–187.

Koff, Wayne C. (1988). Development and testing of AIDS vaccines. *Science*, 241:426–432.

Lackritz, Eve, et al. (1995). Estimated risk of transmission of HIV by screened blood in the United States. *N. Engl. J. Med.*, 333:1721–1725.

Levy, Jay A. (1989). Human immunodeficiency viruses and the pathogenesis of AIDS. *JAMA*, 261:2997–3006.

Lewis, David. (1995). Resistance of microorganisms to disinfection in dental and medical devices. *Nature Med.*, 1:956–958.

Lurie, Peter, et al. (1998). A sterile syringe for every drug user injection: how many injections take place annually and how might pharmacists contribute to syringe distribution? *J. Acquired Immune Defic. Syndr. Hum. Retrovirol*, 18:545–551.

Lurie, Peter, et al. (1994). Ethical behavioral and social aspects of HIV vaccine trials in developing countries. *JAMA*, 271:295–302.

Mandell, Wallace, et al. (1994). Correlates of needle sharing among injection drug users. *Am. J. Public Health*, 84:920–923.

Morbidity and Mortality Weekly Report. (1988). Partner notification for preventing human immunodeficiency virus (HIV) infection—Colorado, Idaho, South Carolina, Virginia. 37:393–396; 401–402.

Morbidity and Mortality Weekly Report. (1989). Guideline for prevention of transmission of HIV and hepatitis B virus to health care workers. 38:3–17.

Morbidity and Mortality Weekly Report. (1992). Sexual behavior among high school students—United States, 1990. 40:885–888.

Morbidity and Mortality Weekly Report. (1993a). Update: Barrier protection against HIV infection and other sexually transmitted diseases. 42:589–591.

Morbidity and Mortality Weekly Report. (1993). Impact of new legislation on needle and syringe purchases and possession—Connecticut 1992. 42:145–147.

Morbidity and Mortality Weekly Report. (1995). Notification of syringe-sharing and sex partners of HIV-infected persons—Pennsylvania, 1993–1994. 44:202–204.

Morbidity and Mortality Weekly Report. (1996). School-based HIV-prevention education—United States, 1994. 45:760–764.

Morbidity and Mortality Weekly Report. (1997). Update: Syringe-exchange programs—United States, 1996. 46:565–568.

Morbidity and Mortality Weekly Report. (2000). Cluster of HIV-Infected adolescents and young adults—Mississippi, 1999. 49: 861–864.

Morbidity and Mortality Weekly Report. (2000). Notice to readers: CDC statement on study results of product containing nonoxynol-9. 49:717.

Office Nurse. (1995). Contraception: how today's options stack up. 8:13–14.

PARRAN, THOMAS, P. (1937). *Shadow on the Land: Syphilis.* New York: Reynal and Hitchcock.

RAMOS, ARTUR, et al. (2002). Intersubtype human immunodeficiency virus Type 1 superinfection following seroconversion to primary infection in two injection drug users. *J Virol,* 76:7444–7452.

RAYMOND, CHRIS ANNE. (1988). U.S. cities struggle to implement needle exchanges despite apparent success in European cities. *JAMA,* 260:2620–2621.

ROPER, WILLIAM L., et al. (1993). Commentary: Condoms and HIV/STD prevention—clarifying the message. *Am. J. Public Health,* 83:501–503.

ROTHENBERG, KAREN, et al. (1995). The risk of domestic violence and women with HIV infection: Implications for partner notification, public policy, and the law. *Am. J. Public Health,* 85: 1569–1576.

RUTHERFORD, GEORGE W. (1988). Contact tracing and the control of human immunodeficiency virus infection. *JAMA,* 259:3609–3670.

SATTAR, SYED, A., et al. (1991). Survival and disinfectant inactivation of HIV: A critical review. *Rev. of Infect. Dis.,* 13:430–447.

SELLERS, DEBORAH, et al. (1994). Does the promotion and distribution of condoms increase teen sexual activity? Evidence from an HIV prevention program for Latino youth. *Am. J. Public Health,* 84:1952–1958.

SHEN, XUEFEI, et al. (2000). Preventing AIDS but not HIV-I infection with a DNA vaccine. *Science,* 290: 463–465.

SPRUYT, ALAN, et al. (1998). Identifying condom users at risk for breakage and slippage; Findings from three International Sites. *Am. J. Public Health,* 88:239–240.

STIMSON, GERRY V., et al. (1989). Syringe exchange. *International Working Group on AIDS and IV Drug Use,* 4:15.

STRATHDEE, STEFFANIE, et al. (2002). Sex differences in risk factors for HIV seroconversion among injection drug users: A 10-year perspective. *Archives of Internal Medicine,* 161:1281–1288.

STOVER, JOHN, et al. (2002). Can we reverse the HIV/AIDS pandemic with an expanded response. *Lancet,* 360:73–77.

STRATTON, P., et al. (1993). Prevention of sexually transmitted infections: Physical and Chemical barrier methods. *Infect. Dis. Clin. North Am.,* 7(4):841–859.

STRAUS, STEPHEN, et al. (1994). Placebo-controlled trial of vaccination with recombinant glycoprotein D of herpes simplex virus type 2 for immunotherapy of genital herpes. *Lancet.* 343:1460.

Time. (1992). Closed: Needle Park. 139:53.

U.S. Public Health Service. (1994). Counseling to prevent unintended pregnancy. *Am. Fam. Phys.,* 50(5):971.

VOELKER, REBECCA. (1995). Lessons from cat virus. *JAMA,* 273:910.

WEINSTEIN, STEPHEN P., et al. (1990). AIDS and cocaine: A deadly combination facing the primary care physician. *J. Fam. Prac.,* 31:253–254.

WELLER, SUSAN. (1993). A meta-analysis of condom effectiveness in reducing sexually transmitted HIV. *Soc. Sci. Med.* 36:1635–1644.

WHITE, NICK, et al. (1988). Dangers of lubricants used with condoms. *Nature,* 335:19.

WODAK, ALEX. (1990). Australia smashes international needle and syringe exchange record. *International Working Group on AIDS and IV Drug Use,* 5:28–29.

CHAPTER 10

AIKEN, LINDA, et al. (1997). Hospital nurses' occupational exposure to blood: Prospective, retrospecture and institutional reports. *AM. J. Public Health,* 87:103–107.

BELL, DAVID. (1996). Occupational risk of HIV infection in health care workers. *Improv. Manage. HIV Dise.,* 4:7–9.

BOOTH, WILLIAM. (1988). CDC paints a picture of HIV infection in U.S. *Science,* 242:53.

BOOTH, WILLIAM. (1989). Asking America about its sex life. *Science,* 243:304.

CATANIA, JOSEPH, et al. (2001). The continuing HIV epidemic among gay men. *Am. J. Pub. Health,* 91:907:914.

CHIN, J., et al. (1990). Projections of HIV infections and AIDS cases to the year 2000. *Bull. WHO,* 68:1–11.

COLFAX, GRANT, et al. (1998). Health benfits and risks of reporting HIV-infected individuals by name. *Am J. Public Health,* 88:876–879.

COUTINHO, ROEL, et al. (1996). Summary of Track C: Epidemiology and public health. *AIDS* 10 (suppl. 3):S115–S121.

DE GROOT, ANNE, et al. (1996). Barriers to care of HIV-infected inmates: A public health concern. *AIDS Reader*, 6:78–87.

DOLAN, KATE, et al. (1995). AIDS behind bars: Preventing HIV spread among incarcerated drug infections. *AIDS*, 9:825–832.

EISENBERG, MARLA. (2001). Differences in sexual risk behaviors between college students with same-sex and opposite-sex experience: Results from a national survey. *Archives of Sexual Behavior*, 30:575–589.

EL-SADR, WAFFA, et al. (1994). *Managing Early HIV Infection: Quick Reference Guide for Clinicians.* Agency for Health Care Policy and Research. Publication #94-0573, Rockville, MD.

EL-SADR, WAFFA, et al. (1995). Unrecognized human HIV infection in the elderly. *Arch. Intern. Med.*, 155:184–186.

FAY, ROBERT E., et al. (1989). Prevalence and patterns of same-gender sexual contact among men. *Science*, 243:338–348.

FELDMAN, MITCHELL, et al. (1994). The growing risk of AIDS in older patients. *Patient Care*, 28:61–72.

FILLIT, HOWARD, et al. (1989). AIDS in the elderly: A case and its implications. *Geriatrics*, 44:65–70.

FRANCIS, DONALD P. (1987). The prevention of acquired immunodeficiency syndrome in the United States. *JAMA*, 257:1357–1366.

GAYLE, HELENE. (1988). Demographic and sexual transmission differences between adolescent and adult AIDS patients, U.S.A. *4th International Conference on AIDS.*

GORDON, STEVEN, et al. (1995). The changing epidemiology of HIV infection in older persons. *J. Am. Geriatr. Soc.*, 43:7–9.

GOSTIN, LAWRENCE, et al. (1997). National HIV case reporting for the United States. *N. Engl. J. Med.*, 337:1162–1167.

HENDERSON, DAVID, et al. (1990). Risk for occupational transmission of human immunodeficiency virus type 1 (HIV-1) associated with clinical exposures. *Ann. Intern. Med.*, 113:740.

HIRSCHHORN, LISA. (1995). HIV infection in women: Is it different? *AIDS Reader*, 5:99–105.

HIV/AIDS Surveillance Report. (December 1996). 8:1–36.

HIV/AIDS Surveillance Report. (December 1997). 9:1–43.

HIV/AIDS Surveillance Report. (December 1999). 11:1–45.

HOGG, ROBERT, et al. (1997). HIV disease shortens life expectancy of gay men by up to 20 years. *Inter. J. Epidemiol.* 26:657–661.

HOOKER, TRACEY. (1996). HIV/AIDS: Facts to consider—1996. National Conference of State Legislatures, Denver. pp. 1–64.

KAO, HELEN. (1999). Leaders unite on HIV in the Latino community. *Harvard AIDS Review Women and AIDS.* Spring: 13–15.

KARON, JOHN, et al. (1996). Prevalence of HIV infection in the United States, 1984 to 1992. *JAMA*, 276:126–130.

LEMP, GEORGE. (1991). The young men's survey: Principal findings and results. A presentation to the San Francisco Health Commission, June 4.

LEMP, GEORGE, et al. (1994). Seroprevalence of HIV and risk behaviors among young homosexual and bisexual men. *JAMA*, 272:449–454.

MAHON, NANCY. (1996). New York inmates' HIV risk behaviors: The implications for prevention policy and programs. *Am. J. Public Health*, 86:1211–1215.

MARCUS, R., et al. (1988). AIDS: Health care workers exposed to it seldom contract it. *N. Engl. J. Med.*, 319:1118–1123.

MARTORELL, REYNALDO, et al. (1995). Vitamin A supplementation and morbidity in children born to HIV-infected women. *Am. J. Public Health*, 85: 1049–1050.

MICHAELS, DAVID, et al. (1992). Estimates of the number of motherless youth orphaned by AIDS in the United States. *JAMA*, 268:3456–3461.

MILLER, PATTI, et al. (1997). Compensation for occupationally acquired HIV needs revamping. *Am. J. Public Health*, 87:1558–1562.

Morbidity and Mortality Weekly Report. (1990). HIV prevalence, projected AIDS case estimates. Workshop, Oct. 31–Nov. 1, 1989. 39:110–119.

Morbidity and Mortality Weekly Report. (1991). The HIV/AIDS epidemic: The first 10 years. 40: 357–368.

Morbidity and Mortality Weekly Report. (1992a). HIV prevention in the U.S. correctional system, 1991. 41:389–391, 397.

Morbidity and Mortality Weekly Report. (1992b). Surveillance for occupationally acquired HIV infection—United States, 1981–1992. 41:823–824.

Morbidity and Mortality Weekly Report. (1993). Update: Mortality attributable to HIV infection among persons aged 25–44 years—United States, 1991 and 1992. 42:869–873.

Morbidity and Mortality Weekly Report. (1994a). Heterosexually acquired AIDS-United States, 1993. 43:155–160.

Morbidity and Mortality Weekly Report. (1995a). Update: Trends in AIDS among men who have sex with men—United States, 1989–1994. 44: 401–404.

Morbidity and Mortality Weekly Report. (1995b). First 500,000 AIDS cases—United States, 1995. 44: 849–853.

Morbidity and Mortality Weekly Report. (1996a). AIDS associated with injection drug use—United States, 1995. 45:392–398.

Morbidity and Mortality Weekly Report. (1996b). Case central study of HIV seroconversion in health-care workers after percutaneous exposure to HIV-infected blood—France, United Kingdom, and United States, January 1988–August 1994. 44: 929–933.

Morbidity and Mortality Weekly Report. (1996c). HIV/AIDS education and prevention programs for adults in prisons and jails and juveniles in confinement facilities—United States, 1994. 45:268–271.

Morbidity and Mortality Weekly Report. (1996d). Update: Mortality attributable to HIV infection among persons aged 25–44 years—United States, 1994. 45:121–125.

Morbidity and Mortality Weekly Report. (2000). HIV/AIDS among racial/ethnic minority men who have sex with men—United States, 1989–1998.

Morbidity and Mortality Weekly Report. (2001). HIV incidence among young men who have sex with men—seven U.S. cities, 1994–2000. 50:440–444.

MORGAN, DILYS, et al. (2002). HIV-1 Infection in rural Africa: Is there a difference in median time to AIDS and survival compared with that in industralized countries? *AIDS,* 16:597–603.

Nations Health Report. (1995). Women learn of progress, share deep concerns on HIV/AIDS issues. XXV:10.

OSBORNE, JUNE E. (1993). AIDS policy advisor foresees a new age of activism. *Fam. Prac. News,* 23:1, 45.

OSTROW, DAVID. (2001). HIV incidence trends among gay and bisexual men. *FOCUS,* 16:1–4.

REISMAN, JUDITH. (1990). *Kinsey, Sex and Fraud: The Indoctrination of a People.* Lafayette, LA: Huntington House Press.

ROSENBERG, PHILIP. (1995). Scope of the AIDS epidemic in the United States. *Science,* 270: 1372–1376.

RUBEL, JOHN, et al. (1997). HIV-related mental health in correctional settings. *FOCUS,* 12:1–4.

RYDER, ROBERT, et al. (1994). AIDS orphans in Kinshasa, Zaire: Incidence and socioeconomic consequences. *AIDS,* 8:673–679.

SHIP, J.A., et al. (1991). Epidemiology of AIDS in persons aged 50 years or older. *J. Acquired Immune Deficiency Syndrome,* 4(1):84–88.

SLACK, JAMES D. (1991). *AIDS and the Public Workforce: Local Government Preparedness in Managing the Epidemic.* Tuscaloosa: The University of Alabama Press.

STALL, R., et al. (1990). Relapse from safer sex: The next challenge for AIDS prevention efforts. *J. Acquired Immune Deficiency Syndrome,* 3:1181.

TOUFEXIS, ANASTASIA. (1991). When the doctor gets infected. *Time,* 137:57.

UNAIDS. (1997). The HIV/AIDS situation in 1997: Global and regional highlights, Geneva 27, Switzerland, pp. 1–14.

VALLEROY, LINDA, et al. (2001). High HIV and risk behavior prevalence among 23–29-year-old men who have sex with men in six U.S. cities [Abstract 211]. *8th Conference on Retroviruses and Opportunistic Infections,* Chicago.

VLAHOV, D., et al. (1991). Prevalence of antibody to HIV-1 among entrants to U.S. correctional facilities. *JAMA,* 265:1129.

WEISFUSE, ISAAC C., et al. (1991). HIV-1 infection among New York City inmates. *AIDS,* 5:1133–1138.

WILSON, J., et al. (1990). Keeping your cool in a time of fear. *Emergency Medical Services,* 19:30–32.

WOLITSKI, RICHARD, et al. (2001). Are we headed for a resurgence of the HIV epidemic among gay men? *Am. J Pub. Health,* 91:883–888.

CHAPTER 11

AGGLETON, PETER, et al. (1994). Risking everything? Risk behavior, behavior change, and AIDS. *Science,* 265:341–345.

ALLEN, J. R., et al. (1988). Prevention of AIDS and HIV infection: Needs and priorities for epidemiologic research. *Am. J. Public Health,* 78:381–386.

BARDEGUEZ, ARLENE. (1995). Managing HIV infection in women. *AIDS Reader, Suppl.,* Nov/Dec, pp. 2–3.

BECKERMAN, KAREN. (2002). Mothers, orphans and prevention of pediatric AIDS. *The Lancet,* 359:1168–1169.

BESSINGER, RUTH, et al. (1997). Pregnancy is not associated with the progression of HIV disease in women attending an HIV outpatient program. *Am J. Epidemiol.,* 147:434–440.

Bloomberg School of Public Health and Johns Hopkins University. (2001). Youth and HIV/AIDS: Can We Avoid Catastrophe? http://www.jhuccp.org/pr/112/112print.shtml

BUTLER, DECLAN. (1993). Whose side is focus of AIDS research? *Nature,* 366:293.

California Department of Health Services, STD Control Branch. (1995). Sexually transmitted diseases in California. *Surveillance Report.*

CHU, SUSAN, et al. (1994). Female-to-female sexual contact and HIV transmission. *JAMA,* 272:433.

COHEN, JON. (1995). Women: Absent term in the AIDS research equation. *Science,* 269:777–780.

COLLINS, CHRIS, et al. (1997). Outside the prevention vacuum: Issues in HIV prevention for youth in the next decade. *AIDS Reader,* 7:149–154.

COTTON, PAUL. (1994). U.S. sticks head in sand on AIDS prevention. *JAMA,* 272:756–757.

CU-RIN, SUSAN. (1999). Antiretroviral treatment during pregnancy. *Improving Management of HIV Disease,* 7:14–18.

CURRAN, JAMES W., et al. (1988). Epidemiology of HIV infection and AIDS in the United States. *Science,* 239:610–616.

DARROW, W.W., et al. (1989). HIV antibody in 640 U.S. prostitutes with no evidence of intravenous (IV) drug abuse. *Fourth International Conference on AIDS.* Bio-Data Publishers: Washington, DC.

DIAZ, LESLIE, et al. (1996). Factors influencing mother-child transmission of HIV. *J. Fla. Med. Assoc.,* 83:244–248.

DICKINSON, GORDON M. (1988). Epidemiology of AIDS. *Int. Ped.*, 3:30–32.

DICLEMENTE, RALPH. (1998). Preventing sexually transmitted infections among adolescents: A clash of ideology and science. *JAMA*, 279: 1574–1575.

EHRHARDT, ANKE A. (1992). Trends in sexual behavior and the HIV pandemic. *Am. J. Public Health*, 82:1459–1464.

FARZADEGAN, HOMAYOON, et al. (1998). Sex differences in HIV-1 viral load and progression to AIDS. *Lancet*, 352:1510–1514.

FELMAN, YEHUDI M. (1990). Recent developments in sexually transmitted diseases: Is heterosexual transmission of HIV a major epidemiologic in the spread of AIDS? III: AIDS in Sub-Saharan Africa. *Cutis*, 46:204–206.

FUTTERMAN, DONNA, et al. (1992). Medical care of HIV-infected adolescents. *AIDS Clin. Care*, 4:95–98.

GARCIA, PATRICIA, et al., (2001). Assessing the teratogenic potential of antiretroviral drugs: Data from the Antiretroviral Pregnancy Registry (APR). 41st Interscience Conference on Anti-microbial Agents and Chemotherapy, Chicago, December. Abstract 1325.

Hader, Shannon, et al. (2001). HIV infection in women in the United States. *JAMA*, 285: 1186–1192.

HEALTH. (1966). AIDS still spreading rapidly among young gay men. *Am. Med. News*, 39:30 (March issue).

HIV/AIDS Surveillance Report. (1995). Year end, 7:1–36.

HIV/AIDS Surveillance Report. (1996). Year end, 8: 1–39.

HIV/AIDS Surveillance Report. (1997). December, 9: 1–34.

HOLDEN, CONSTANCE. (1998). World-AIDS The worst is yet to come. *Science*, 278:1715.

IOANNIDIS, JOHN, et al. (1999). Maternal viral load and the risk of perinatal transmission of HIV-1. *NEJM*, 341:1698.

JEMMOT, JOHN, et al. (1998). Abstinence and safer sex high risk-reduction interventions for African American adolescents: A randomized controlled trial. *JAMA*, 279:1529–1536.

JOHNSON, TIMOTHY, et al. (1995). Current issues in the primary care of women with HIV. *Female Patient*, 20:51–58.

JOSEPH, STEPHEN C. (1993). The once and future AIDS epidemic. *Med. Doctor*, 37:92–104.

KATZENSTEIN, MICHAEL, et al. (1999). Serum level of maternal HIV-RNA, infant mortality and vertical transmission of HIV in Zimbabwe. *J. Infectious Diseases*, 179:1382–1387.

KIRBY, DOUGLAS, et al. (1997). The impact of the Postponing Sexual Involvement Curriculum among youths in California. *Fam. Plann. Perspect.*, 29:100–108.

LEMP, GEORGE, et al. (1995). HIV seroprevalence and risk behaviors among lesbians and bisexual women in San Francisco and Berkley, California. *Am. J. Public Health*, 85:1549–1552.

MANDELBROT, LAURENT, et al. (1997). Natural conception in HIV-negative women with HIV-infected partners. *Lancet*, 349:850–851.

MANDELBROT, LAURENT, et al. (1998). Perinatal HIV-1 Transmission. *J. Am Med Assoc*, 280:55–60.

MIOTTI, PAOLO, et al. (1999). HIV transmission through breastfeeding. *JAMA*, 282:744–749.

Morbidity and Mortality Weekly Report. (1992). Selected behaviors that increase risk for HIV infection among high school students—United States, 1990. 41:236–240.

Morbidity and Mortality Weekly Report. (1993). Update: Acquired immunodeficiency syndrome—United States, 1992. 42:547–557.

Morbidity and Mortality Weekly Report. (1994). Update: Impact of the expanded AIDS surveillance case definition for adolescents/adults on case reporting—United States, 1993. 43:160–170.

Morbidity and Mortality Weekly Report. (1996a). HIV testing among women aged 18–44 years—United States, 1991 and 1993. 46:733–736.

Morbidity and Mortality Weekly Report. (1996b). Update: Mortality attributable to HIV infection among persons aged 25–44 years—United States, 1994. 45:121–125.

Morbidity and Mortality Report. (1999). Surveillance for AIDS-defining opportunistic illnesses, 1992–1997. 48:1–20.

NEWELL, MICHAEL, et al. (1997). Immunological markers in HIV-infected pregnant women: The European Collaborative Study and the Swiss HIV Pregnancy Cohort. *AIDS*, 11:1859–1865.

Office of National AIDS Policy. (1996). Youth and HIV/AIDS: An American agenda. *Report to the President*, pp. 1–14.

PARKER–BUSH, TRACEY. (2000). Perinatal HIV: Children with HIV grow up. *FOCUS*, 15:1–4.

PFEIFFER, NAOMI. (1991). AIDS risk high for women; care is poor. *Infect. Dis. News*, 4:1, 18.

PLAEGER, SUSAN, et al. (1999). Decreased CD8 Cell-mediated viral suppression and other immunologic characteristics of women who transmit HIV to their infants. *J. Infectious Diseases*, 1388–1394.

RODRIGUEZ, ZOE, et al. (1996). Medical care and management of infants born to women infected with HIV. *J. Fla. Med. Assoc.*, 83:255–261.

ROTHERAM-BORUS, M., et al. (1991). Sexual risk behaviors, AIDS knowledge, and beliefs about AIDS among runaways. *Am. J. Public Health*, 81: 208–210.

SCHABLE, BARBARA, et al. (1996). Characteristics of women 50 years of age or older with heterosexually acquired AIDS. *Am. J. Public Health*, 86:1616–1618.

SELLS, WAYNE, et al. (1996). Morbidity and mortality among US adolescents: An overview of data and trends. *Am. J. Public Health*, 86:513–519.

SELWYN, PETER A., et al. (1989). Knowledge of HIV antibody status and decisions to continue or terminate pregnancy among intravenous drug users. *JAMA*, 261:3567–3571.

STERLING, TIMOTHY, et al. (2001). Initial plasma HIV-1 RNA levels and progression to AIDS in women and men. *N. Engl J. Med*, 344: 720–725.

TAHA & TAHA, et al. (2000). Morbidity among HIV-1 infected and uninfected African children. *Pediatrics*, 106: http://www.pediatrics.org/cgi/content/full/106/6/e77

THOMAS, PATRICIA. (1988). Official estimates of epidemic's scope are grist for political mill. *Med. World News*, 29:12–13.

THOMAS, PATRICIA. (1989). The epidemic. *Med. World News*, 30:41–49.

TUOMALA, RUTH, et al. (2002). Antiretroviral therapy during pregnancy and the risk of an adverse outcome. *N Engl J Med*, 346:1863–70.

UNAIDS, (1997). Global summary of the HIV/AIDS epidemic. *Report on the global HIV/AIDS epidemic.* December 1997:1–25.

VAN BENTHEM, BIRGIT, et al. (2002). The impact of pregnancy and menopause on CD4 lymphocyte counts in HIV infected women. *AIDS*, 16:919–924.

Women's AIDS Network. (1988). Lesbians and AIDS: What's the connection? *San Francisco AIDS Foundation*, 333 Valencia St., 4th Floor, P.O. Box 6182, San Francisco, CA 94101-6182.

World Health Organization, Geneva. (1994). *Women's Health*, p. 18.

WORTLEY, PASCALE, et al. (1997). AIDS in women in the United States. *JAMA*, 278:911–916.

YAO, FAUSTIN K. (1992). Youth and AIDS: A priority for prevention education. *AIDS Health Promotion Exchange No. 2*, Royal Tropical Institute, The Netherlands: 1–3.

ZIERLER, SALLY, et al. (2000). Violence victimization after HIV infection in a US probability sample of adult patients in primary care. *Am. J. Pub. Health*, 90: 208–215.

CHAPTER 12

AIDS, Health and Human Rights. (1995). Francois-Xavier Bagnoud Center for Health and Human Rights–Harvard School of Public Health, pp. 1–162.

ALLEN, BRADY. (1991). The role of the primary care physician in HIV testing and early stage disease management. *Fam. Pract. Recert.*, 13:30–49.

ANDERSON, JOHN, et al. (1992). HIV antibody testing and post-test counseling in the United States: Data from the 1989 National Health Interview Study. *Am J Public Health*, 82:1533–1535.

ANGELL, MARCIA. (1991). A dual approach to the AIDS epidemic. *N. Engl. J. Med.*, 324:1498–1500.

BAYER, RONALD, et al. (1995). Testing for HIV infection at home (Sounding Board). *N. Engl. J. Med.*, 332:1296–1299.

BELONGIA, EDWARD A., et al. (1989). Premarital HIV screening. *JAMA*, 261:2198.

CARLSON, DESIREE A., et al. (1989). Testing for HIV risk from therapeutic blood products. *Pathology and Pathophysiology of AIDS and HIV Related Diseases* (Eds. Jami J. Harawi and Carl J. O'Hara), St. Louis: C.V. Mosby Co.

CONSTANTINE, NIEL T. (1993). Serologic tests for the retroviruses: Approaching a decade of evolution. *AIDS*, 7:1–13.

CORDES, ROBERT, et al. (1995). Pitfalls in HIV testing. *Postgrad. Med.*, 98:177–189.

DEWAR, ROBIN, et al. (1994). Application of branched DNA signal amplification to monitor HIV-I type burden in human plasma. *J. Infect. Dis.*, 170: 1172–1179.

El-SADR, WAFAA, et al. (1994). Managing early HIV infection: Agency for Health Care Policy and Research. *Clinical Practice Guideline on Evaluation and Management of Early HIV Infection.* January, 7:1–37.

EL-SAHR, W., et al. (1994). *Managing Early HIV Infection: Quick Reference Guide for Clinicians.* AHCPR Publication No. 94-0573. Rockville, MD.

FANG, CHYANG T., et al. (1989). HIV testing and patient counseling. *Patient Care*, 23:19–44.

FRERICHS, RALPH R., et al. (1994). Saliva-based HIV-antibody testing in Thailand. *AIDS*, 8:885–894.

GALLO, DANA, et al. (1997). Testing oral secretions for HIV. *AIDS Clin. Care*, 9:26.

GOSTIN, LAWRENCE, et al. (1997). National HIV case surveillance is urged. *N. Engl. J. Med.*, 337:1162–1167.

HARTLAUB, PAUL, et al. (1993). Obtaining informed consent: It is not simply asking "do you understand?" *J. Fam. Pract.*, 36:383–384.

HEGARTY, J.D., et al. (1988). The medical care costs of human immunodeficiency virus infected children in Harlem. *JAMA*, 260:1901–1905.

HOOKER, TRACEY. (1996). HIV/AIDS: Facts to consider—1996. Natural conference of State Legislatures, February, pp. 1–64.

HORN, THOMAS, et al. (1989). Forks and combs and DNA: The synthesis of branched oligodeoxyribonucleotides. *Nucleic Acids Res.* 17:6959–67.

Intergovernmental AIDS Report.(1989). Illinois court overrules mandatory HIV testing for prostitutes and sex offenders, 2:1–18.

JANSSEN, ROBERT, et al. (1998). New testing strategy to detect early HIV-1 infection for use in incidence estimates and for clinical and prevention purposes. *JAMA*, 280:42–48.

JENNY-AVITAL, ELIZABETH, et al. (2001). Erroneously low or undetectable plasma HIV-1 RNA load, determined by PCR, in West African and American patients with non-B subtype HIV infection. *Clinical Infectious Diseases*, 32:1227–1230.

JOHNSON, CHRISTINE. (2000). Factors known to cause false positive HIV antibody test results. In *Alive and Well* [online] Available: http://www.aliveandwell.org.

KELLER, G.H., et al. (1988). Identification of HIV sequences using nucleic acid probes. *Am. Clin. Lab.*, 7:10–15.

KRAMER, F.R., et al. (1989). Replicatable RNA reporters. *Nature*, 339:401–402.

MACKENZIE, WILLIAM R., et al. (1992). Multiple false positive serologic tests for HIV, HTLV-1 and hepatitis C following influenza vaccination, 1991. *JAMA*, 268:1015–1017.

MCFARLAND, WILLIAM, et al. (1999). Detection of early HIV infection and estimation of incidence using a sensitive/less sensitive enzyme immunoassay testing strategy at anonymous counseling and testing sites in San Francisco. *JAIDS*, 22:484–489.

Medical Tribune. (1991). Beware of blanket AIDS solutions. June:14.

MERCOLA, JOSEPH M. (1989). Premarital HIV screening. *JAMA*, 261:2198.

MIIKE, LAWRENCE. (1987). *AIDS Antibody Testing.* Office of Technological Assessment Testimony To The U.S. Congress. Oct.:1–21.

MILES, STEVEN A., et al. (1993). Rapid serologic testing with immune-complex-dissociated HIV p24 antigen for early detection of HIV infection in neonates. *N. Engl. J. Med.*, 328:297–302.

Morbidity and Mortality Weekly Report. (1988a). Update: Serologic testing for antibody to human immunodeficiency virus. 36:833–840.

Morbidity and Mortality Weekly Report. (1992). Testing for antibodies to HIV-2 in the United States. 41:1–9.

Morbidity and Mortality Weekly Report. (2001) Revised U.S. Public Health Service recommendations for HIV counseling and voluntary testing for pregnant women. 50:59–85.

Morbidity and Mortality Weekly Report. (1996). U.S. Public Health Service Guidelines for testing and counseling blood and plasma donors for HIV type I antigen. 45:1–9.

Morbidity and Mortality Weekly Report. (1998a). Diagnosis and reporting of HIV and AIDS in the Unites States with integrated HIV and AIDS surveillance—United States January 1994–June 1997, 47:309–314.

Morbidity and Mortality Weekly Report. (1998b). Update: Counseling and testing using rapid tests—United States, 1995, 47:211–215.

Morbidity and Mortality Weekly Report (1999). HIV Testing—United States, 1996. 48:52–55.

MOSER, MICHAEL, (1998). Anonymous HIV testing. *Am. J. Pub. Health*, 88:683.

MORE, DANIEL, et al. (2000). Utility of an HIV-1 RNA assay in the diagnosis of acute retroviral syndrome. *Southern Medical Journal*, 93: 1004–1006.

MULLIS, KARY B., et al. (1987). Process for amplifying, detecting, and/or cloning nucleic acid sequences. (U.S. Patent No. 4,683,195). *Official Gazette of the U.S. Patient and Trademark Office*, Volume 1080, Issue 4, July.

NASH, GRANT, et al. (1998). Health benefits and risks of reporting HIV-infected individuals by name. *Am. J. Pub. Health*, 88:876–879.

PASSANNANTE, MARIAN R., et al. (1993). Responses of health care professionals to proposed mandatory HIV testing. *Arch. Fam. Med.*, 2:38–44.

PHILLIPS, KATHRYN, et al. (1995a). Potential use of home HIV testing. *N. Engl. J. Med.*, 332:1308–1310.

PHILLIPS, KATHRYN, et al. (1995b).Who plans to be tested for HIV or would get tested if no one could find out the results? *Am. J. Prevent. Med.*, 11(3):156.

REIMER, LARRY, et al. (1997). Undetectable antibody reported in a patient with typical HIV. *Clin. Infect. Dis.* 25:98–103.

RHAME, FRANK S., et al. (1989). The case for wider use of testing for HIV infection. *N. Engl. J. Med.*, 320:1242–1254.

RICH, JOSIAH, et al. (1999). Misdiagnosis of HIV infection by HIV-1 Plasma Viral load testing: A case series. *Annals of Internal Medicine*, 130:37–39.

ROGERS, MARTHA F., et al. (1989). Use of the polymerase chain reaction for early detection of the proviral sequences of human immunodeficiency virus in infants born to seropositive mothers. *N. Engl. J. Med.*, 320:1649–1654.

SAMET, JEFFREY, et al. (1998). Trillion Niron delay: Time from testing positive for HIV to presentation for primary care. *Arch. Int. Med.*, 158:734–740.

SAX, PAUL, et al. (1997). Novel approaches to HIV antibody testing. *AIDS Clin. Care*, 9:1–5.

SCHEFFEL, J.W. (1990). Retrocell HIV-1 passive haemagglutination assay for HIV-1 antibody screening. *J. Acquired Immune Deficiency Syndromes*, 3:540–545.

SCHOPPER, DORIS, et al. (1996). Testing for HIV at home: What are the issues? *AIDS*, 10:1455–1465.

STEIN, MICHAEL, et al. (1998). Sexual ethics: Disclosure of HIV-positive status to partners. *Arch. Int. Med.*, 158:253–257.

URDEA, MICKEY. (1993). Synthesis and characterization of branched DNA (bDNA) for the direct and quantitative detection of CMV, HBV, HCV, and HIV. *Clin. Chem.*, 39:725–726.

WAKE, WILLIAM T. (1989). How many patients will die because we fear AIDS? *Med. Econ.*, 66:24–30.

WOFOY, C. B. (1987). HIV infection in women. *JAMA*, 257:2074–2076.

CHAPTER 13

American Medical Association News. (1991). Ruling fuels debate over HIV-infected doctors. May:1, 41–43.

AOUN, HACIB. (1990). A handful helped us. *Medical Doctor*, 34:31–32.

BURRIS, SCOTT. (1996). Human immunodeficiency virus-infected health care workers. *Arch. Fam. Med.*, 5:102–106.

CRAVEN, DONALD, et al. (1994). Factitious HIV Infection. *Ann. Intern. Med.*, 121:763–766.

DANIELS, NORMAN. (1992). HIV-infected professionals, patient rights and the 'switching dilemma.' *JAMA*, 267:1368–1371.

EICKHOFF, THEODORE C. (1989). Public perceptions about AIDS and HIV infection. *Infect. Dis. News*, 2:6.

FISHER, J.D., et al. (1992). Changing AIDS risk behavior. *Psychol. Bull.*, 111:455–474.

FOURNIER, A.M., et al. (1989). Preoperative screening for HIV infection. *Arch. Surg.*, 124:1038–1040.

FULTON, ROBERT, et al. (1988). AIDS: Seventh rank absolute. In *AIDS: Principles, Practices and Politics.*, Inge B. Corliss, et al., eds. Bristol, PA: Hemisphere.

GERBERT, BARBARA, et al. (1988). Why fear persists: Health care professionals and AIDS. *JAMA*, 260:3481–3483.

GOSTIN, LAWRENCE, et al. (1998). HIV infection and AIDS in the public health and health care systems: The role of law and litigation. *JAMA*, 279:1108–1113.

GOUJAN, CHRISOPHE, et al. (2000). Phylogenetic analysis indicates an atypical nurse to patient transmission of HIV-1. *J. Virology*, 74:2525–2532.

HAGEN, M.D., et al. (1988). Routine preoperative screening for HIV: Does the risk to the surgeon outweigh the risk to the patient? *JAMA*, 259:1357–1359.

HEGARTY, JAMES D., et al. (1988). The medical care costs of HIV-infected children in Harlem. *JAMA*, 260:1901–1909.

HEREK, GREGORY M., et al. (1993). Public reaction to AIDS in the United States: A second decade of stigma. *Am. J. Public Health*, 83:574–577.

J. Virology 74:2525–2534.

JAPENGA, ANN. (1992). The secret. *Health*, 6:43–52.

KIRBY, D. (1988). The effectiveness of educational programs to help prevent school-age youth from contracting AIDS: A review of relevant research. United States Congress.

LEFKOWITZ, MATHEW. (1990). A health care system in crisis: The possible restriction against HIV-infected health care workers. *PAACNOTES*, 2:175–176.

LEWIS, C.E., et al. (1992). Primary care physicians' refusal to care for patients infected with HIV. *West. J. Med.*, 156:36–38.

LO, BERNARD et al. (1992). Health care workers infected with HIV. *JAMA*, 267:1100–1105.

MANDELBAUM-SCHMID, JUDITH. (1990). AIDS and MDs. *Medical Doctor*, 34:33–40.

MCCARTHY, GILLIAN, et al. (1999). Factors associated with refusal to treat HIV infected patients: The results of a National Survey of Dentists in Canada. *Am. J. of Public Health*, 89:541–545.

MCNEILL, WILLIAM H. (1976). *Plagues and People*, Garden City: Anchor Press.

MICHAELS, DAVID, et al. (1992). Estimates of the number of youth orphaned by AIDS in the United States. *JAMA*, 268:3456–3461.

Morbidity and Mortality Weekly Report. (1990). HIV-related knowledge and behavior among high school students—Selected U.S. cities, 1989. 39: 385–396.

NARY, GORDON. (1990). An editorial. *PAACNOTES*, 2:170.

PHILLIPS, KATHRYN A. (1993). Subjective knowledge of AIDS and Use of HIV testing. *Am. J. Public Health*, 83:1460–1462.

POLDER, JACQUELYN A., et al. (1989). AIDS precautions for your office. *Patient Care*, 23:161–171.

POWELL, JOHN H. (1965). *Bring Out Your Dead.* New York: Time-Life Inc.

RHAME, FRANK S., et al. (1989). The case for wider use of testing for HIV infection. *N. Engl. J. Med.*, 320:1242–1254.

ROWE, MONA, et al. (1987). *A Public Health Challenge: State Issues, Policies and Programs, Volume 2.* Intergovernmental Health Policy Project, George Washington University.

STRYKER, JEFF, et al. (1995). Prevention of HIV infection. *JAMA*, 273:1143–1148.

VOELKER, REBECCA. (1989). No uniform policy among states on HIV/AIDS education. *Am. Med. News*, Sept. 3: 28–29.

WEISS, RICK. (1999). Thousands of deaths linked to medical errors. [online] Available: http://www. washingtonpost. com (November 30)

ZUGER, ABIGAIL. (1995). The high cost of living. *Sci. Am.* 273:108.

Index

progression to. *See* Progression to AIDS (PTA)

protection against. *See* Prevention

public opinion concerning, 11, 288–89, 440–42, 443–44, 445–49, 485

risk groups for. *See* Behavioral risk groups

surveillance, 30–32, 147, 330–31, 333, 397, 423

AIDS ACTION, or AIDS advocacy organization, 259

AIDS Care Center (Syracuse, NY), 163

AIDS cases, 389. *See also specific risk and demographic categories*

by age. *See* Age/age groups

estimates of, 309, 330–38

by exposure category, 315t. *See also specific exposure category*

by gender, 316f. *See also* Men; Women

by geographic region, 319f

global statistics, 3t, 69f, 309, 322–24, 339f, 339–40, 340f, 342, 343

pediatric cases, 372–73, 374, 379f

by race/ethnicity, 316f, 317t, 317–19, 318f, 322

reporting of, 330–32

by transmission category, 200f

in U.S., 3t, 17t, 28–29, 31–32, 171f, 199, 243f, 249, 252, 261, 309, 314–22, 315t, 316f, 317t, 318f, 319f, 325f, 333–43, 335f, 338t

among women, 319, 321, 322, 356, 359, 360t, 362, 364, 389

AIDS Clinical Trial Group (ACTG), 35, 77, 150, 246, 379–80

AIDS Coalition to Unleash Power (ACT UP), 33, 241

AIDS Dementia Complex (ADC), 170, 184t, 194, 195f, 196, 430

"AIDS Dilemma: Drug Diseases Blamed on a Passenger Virus, The" (Duesberg and Rasnick), 35

AIDS Drug Assistance Program, 478

AIDS Healthcare Foundation, 225

AIDS Health Project, University of California-San Francisco, 477–78

AIDS industry, 472–78

AIDS Memorial Quilt, 18–20

"AIDS Programs: An Epidemic of Waste," 477–78

AIDS Project Los Angeles, 333

AIDS Quarterly Report, 327

AIDS to Unleash Power (ACT UP), 241, 438

AIDSVAX, 255, 299, 303–4, 305, 307

AIDS wasting. *See* Wasting syndrome

Air Force, 326

Alabama, 327, 332t, 430, 461, 463

Alan Guttmacher Institute survey, 389

Alaska, 282, 332t

Alcohol, 457

Alcoholic hepatitis, 403

Alive & Well, 33

Allain, Jean-Pierre, 214

Allen family, 447

Alum, 304

Alvarez, Marina, 323

Alzheimer's disease, 6

AMD-3100, 133f

American Airlines, 443

American Association of Blood Banks (AABB), 215, 216, 287

American Association of Retired Persons, 329

American Bar Association, 285

American Civil Liberties Union, 333

American Civil War, 2

American College Health Association, 326, 353

American Foundation for AIDS Research (AMFAR), 462

American Health Organization, 260

American Heart Association, 199

American Indians/Alaskan Natives, 8, 318f, 322, 360f

American Medical Association (AMA), 271, 285, 369, 396, 432, 466, 469, 486

American Public Health Association, 285, 385

American Red Cross, 215, 216, 288, 404, 409, 410

Americans with Disabilities Act (ADA), 443, 460, 467–68, 486

Amikacin, 151t

Amirkhanian, Uri, 250

Amniotic fluid, 291t

Amphotericin B, 73, 151t, 152, 157

AMPLICOR HIV-1 MONITOR UltraSensitive viral load test, 95, 98, 396, 397, 419

Amprenavir (Agenerase), 78t, 79f, 83f, 85

Amsterdam, 262, 281

Amyl nitrate, 28

Anal cancer, 161t

Anal intercourse, 141, 210, 211, 212–22, 223t, 230t, 253, 270, 271, 275, 324, 390, 424, 457

bareback sex, 221

prevention of transmission during, 264t

Anderson, Jack, 441

Anemia, 81, 155, 173f

Anergy, 140

Angola, 68, 347

Anilingus, 158

Animal model, need for small, 195

Annan, Kofi, 481–84, 486

Annual HIV Vaccine Awareness Day, 294

Annual Vaccine Day in America, 294

Anonymous testing, 432, 433

Anorexia, 158, 160, 167, 175t

Ansett, Australia, 286

Anthrax, 9, 50

Antibodies, 125, 126–31, 296

definition, 123

HIV-antibody testing, 397–422, 402–3f, 406f

HIV-specific, 130–31, 143f, 172, 173f, 176, 176f, 184–87, 185f, 208, 245, 300, 302, 377, 411, 412

Antibody-mediated antibody-dependent cell cytotoxicity (ADCC), 139

Antigenemia, 173f, 178f, 184

Antigenic variation, 67

Antigen-presenting cell (APC), 120–21, 124, 126, 127, 139, 140, 295

Antigens, 117, 118, 122, 124, 127, 142

definition, 123

p24, 59, 173f, 178f, 184–85, 187–88, 403, 402, 421

Anti-hemolytic factor (AHF), 215

Anti-HIV therapy. *See* Drug therapy
Antiretroviral drug war of 2001, 485
Antiretroviral therapy (ART), 76, 83. *See also* Combination
    drug therapy; Non-nucleoside reverse transcriptase in-
    hibitors; Nucleoside analogs; Protease inhibitors
    attitudes toward condom usage and, 276
    economic of producing drugs, 102
    guidelines, 99, 177
    highly active (HAART), 88–89, 97, 99, 100, 101, 102–6,
      108, 144, 146, 175, 177, 181, 186, 246, 261, 299
    latent HIV in patients on, 108
    for post-exposure prevention (PEP), 109–10
    during pregnancy, 109–10, 112, 246, 380–83
    in South Africa, 312
Apollon, Inc., 300
Apoptosis, 116, 140, 177
Appendix, 120*f*
Appetite, loss of, 177
Aqualube, 279*t*
Arap Moi, Daniel, 388
Arbovirus, 3*t*
Archibald, David, 207
Argentina, 68, 231
Arizona, 227, 332*t*, 430
Arkansas, 238, 294, 332*t*, 377, 431
Armed Forces Institute of Pathology, 9
Army, 326
Arthralgia, 175*t*
Artificial insemination, 207, 208, 234, 264*t*, 363
Ashe, Arthur, 11, 11*f*, 158, 459
Ashkenazi Jews, 164
Asia, 3*t*, 68, 232*f*, 233–34, 267, 306, 322, 324*f*, 339*f*, 340*f*, 357*f*,
    372*f*, 373*f*, 374, 384, 392*f*, 424
Asians/Pacific Islanders, 318*f*, 322, 360*f*
Aspartyl, 83
Assault with HIV, 237–40. *See also* Sexual assault
Association of State and Territorial Health Officers, 410
Astroglide, 279*t*
Asymptomatic stage of HIV/AIDS, 15
Atherosclerosis, 6
Athletes, 197, 224–27
Athlete's foot, 148*f*
Atlanta, GA, 331*t*, 429
Attitudes, 11, 288–89, 440–42, 443–44, 445–49, 485
    adult perceptions, 458
Australasia, 324*f*
Australia, 160, 208, 232*f*, 238, 274, 283–86, 339*f*, 340*f*, 357*f*,
    372*f*, 373*f*, 469
Austria, 283
Autocatalysis, 83
Autoimmune disorders, 403
Autoimmune response, 140
Autologous transfusion, 287, 288, 307
Autopsy diagnoses of diseases in AIDS patients, 167
Azithromycin (Zithromax), 151*t*
AZT. *See* Zidovudine (AZT, ZDV, Retrovir)

Aztecs, smallpox among, 2

"Baby AIDS" bill, 432
Bacillus anthracis, 9
Bacterial diseases/infections, 2, 31*t*, 148*f*, 173*f*, 196
    opportunistic, 151*t*, 159–60
Bactrim, 151*t*
Bagasra, Omar, 206, 208
Bagnoud, Francois-Xavier, 381
Bahamas, 234
Bailey, Robert, 211
Balance problems, 194
Balm in Gilead, 427
Baltimore, David, 132, 192, 192*f*
Baltimore, MD, 220, 306, 380
Barbados, 234
Bardeguez, Arlene, 366
Bareback sex, 221
Baron, Samuel, 207–8
Barrier methods, 265–79. *See also* Condoms; Dental dams
Barthwell, Andrea, 103
Bass, Thomas A., 74
Bathhouses, 222
Baudry, Patrick, 214
B cell differentiating factor, 123
B-cell lymphoma, 6, 151*t*, 166, 167
B cells, 116, 118, 120–21, 122*t*, 122–26, 125, 127, 141, 141*f*,
    295, 296
B cell stimulating factor, 123
Beckerman, Karen, 381
Beckhols, Dawn, 455
Bedbugs, 201
Behavior, AIDS education and, 449–60
Behavioral change, prevention and, 262–65
Behavioral risk groups, 14, 202, 220, 229*f*, 229–30, 230*t*, 309,
    347. *See also specific groups*
    statistical evaluation of, 316–30, 317*t*
Bell's palsy, 180
Benadryl, 157
Benzamide-disulfide, 78*t*
Beral, Valerie, 164
Bergalis, Kimberly, 209*f*, 209–10
Berger, Edward, 134, 135*f*
Bergeron, Michael, 275
Beta-2 microglobulin (B-2M), 173*f*, 175*t*, 188
Biaxin, 151*t*
Bilateral aid, 482
Bill and Melinda Gates Foundation, 263, 301
Bioavailability, 83
Biocine Inc., 303
Bioelectrical impedance analysis (BIA), 179
Biological latency, 177, 184
Biological warfare, 43
Biology, HIV disease and male vs. female, 366. *See also* Men;
    Women
Bioterrorism, 9

Bird flu virus, 10
Birth control pills, 200
Bisexual males, 197, 200*f*, 204*t*, 210, 229*f*, 287, 309, 317, 343, 353, 390, 425, 433, 456, 458
  HIV/AIDS statistics on, 315*t*, 317, 317*t*, 321, 330, 334, 342
Bites, infection via, 236, 240
Black Death (Black Plague, bubonic plague). *See* Plague
Blackliners, 428
Blacks, 224–26, 332, 333, 334
  adolescent cases, 389, 390
  beliefs about HIV/AIDS, 441
  bisexual, 321
  cases among women, 162–64, 319, 337*f*, 339, 342, 356, 358–59, 360*f*, 361, 362, 367, 390
  HIV/AIDS statistics on, 31, 32, 246, 247, 258, 280, 289, 316*f*, 317*t*, 317–19, 318*f*, 321, 322, 337*f*, 339, 342, 353, 435, 453
  ministers, 427
  pediatric cases, 380
Blame, placing, 440
Blastomycosis, 152
Bleach, 262, 265*t*, 280, 281, 284–85
Bleomycin, 151*t*
Blinded testing, 433–34
Blindness, 155, 156, 157. *See also* Vision, changes in
Blood and blood products
  autologous transfusions, 287, 307
  contaminated, 214–19
  donation of, 286–87, 289
  HIV transmission via, 40–41, 141, 183–84, 189, 192–93, 197, 198, 200*f*, 202–3, 205, 206, 244, 245, 246, 250, 253, 262, 286–92, 307, 371, 372
  prevention of transmission via, 286–92
  screening of, 255, 326, 353, 396, 397, 399–401, 403, 411*t*, 436. *See also* ELISA HIV test; Testing
  statistics on cases related to, 309, 315*t*, 317, 317*t*, 330, 353, 363, 380
  transfusions, 14, 27, 183–84, 189, 202–3, 204*t*, 205*t*, 207, 213, 230*t*, 244, 246, 247, 264*t*, 286, 287, 289, 290, 307, 344, 424
Blood and body substance isolation (BBSI), 255, 291–92
Blood Factor 8, 215
Blood Transfusion Organization (Iran), 219
Blood Transfusion Services Board (Ireland), 219
Bluette, William "Skip," 24*f*, 73*f*, 75*f*, 76*f*
B lymphocytes. *See* B cells
BMS805, 110
Body fluids, 155
  HIV transmission via, 14, 126, 197, 198, 203, 205–8, 251, 262, 291*t*, 353
  universal precautions in dealing with, 255, 288–91, 291*t*, 307, 353
Bolivia, 392
Bolognesi, Dani, 184
Bombay, 217
Bone marrow, 120*f*, 185*f*
Bone marrow transplant, 155

Borrowed Time: AN AIDS Memoir (Monette), 156, 157
Botswana, 341*f*, 344, 346–47, 348*f*, 349, 358, 381, 392
Bovine spongiform encephalopathy agent, 4
Bowen, Otis, 330, 441
Boxing, 225, 226, 430
Brachioproctic activities (anal fisting), 223*t*
Brachiovaginal activities (fisting), 223*t*
Bradbury, Ray, 211
Bragdon, Dr. Randon, 467
Bragdon v. *Abbott*, 467–68
Brain, 142, 151*t*, 155, 193–94
Brain-blood barrier, 142
Branched-chain DNA (bDNA), 94, 98, 396, 397, 419, 420*f*, 436
Brandner, Gerhard, 50
Brands, Martien, 34
Brazil, 7, 68, 231, 260, 348*f*, 357–58
Breakbone fever (dengue fever), 4, 301
Breastfeeding, 198, 204*t*, 205, 208, 209, 244, 245, 247, 250, 253, 368, 375–79, 457
  conflicting reports on, 382–83
Bridges, Fabian, 237
Bring Out Your Dead (Powell), 466
Britain. *See* United Kingdom
Brown, Willie, 239
Brucellosis, 50
Brundtland, Gro Harlem, 20
Bubonic plague. *See* Plague
Buchbinder, Susan, 190, 222
Budding, 61*f*
Budget, AIDS costs as percentage of national health care, 474–77
Buffalo hump, 105, 105*f*
BufferGel, 280
"Bug chasing," 221
Burden of a Secret: A Story of Truth and Mercy in the Face of AIDS (Allen), 447
Burials in Africa, 350–51
Burkitt's lymphoma, 161*t*, 179*t*
Burman, William, 102
Burnet, MacFarlane, 6
Burnett, Joseph, 262
Bush, George, 17, 444
Bush, George W., 74, 257*f*, 259, 260, 377–78, 484

Cabbage baths, 10
Calcutta, India, 445–46
California, 208, 239, 246, 282–83, 327, 331*t*, 332*t*, 362, 372, 380, 386, 388, 390, 425, 430, 447–48, 458, 464
California Medical Association, 333
Callen, Michael, 139
Cameron, William, 211, 244
Cameroon, 69, 70, 306, 358
Campo, Rafel, 323
Campylobacter, 159*t*
Camus, Albert, 444, 487
Canada, 208, 216–17, 256, 271, 283, 466

Nucleic Acid Test, 288
Nucleocapsid, 60*t*
Nucleoside analogs, 72, 76, 78, 78*t*, 79*f*, 79–82, 80*f*, 379
    action of, 79–81, 82
    in combination therapy, 85
    HIV resistance to, 67
    side effects of, 81–82
Nucleotide deletion-32, 136–38
Nukes. *See* Nucleoside analogs
Null (natural killer) cells, 122*t*, 124–25, 126, 127
Numbness, 158
Nurses. *See* Health care workers
Nutrition, 140, 145
Nystatin, 151*t*

Oasis, 394
O'Brien, Stephen, 65, 138
O'Connor, Justice Sandra Day, 468, 469
Of Feigned and Fictitious Diseases (Gavin), 462
Office of National AIDS Policy, 257*f*
Office of Technology Assessment, 201
Ohio, 208, 238, 332*t*, 430, 447
Oils, 279*t*
Oklahoma, 332*t*
Older people, 146, 159, 247, 249, 328, 329, 361, 398
Oncogene (onc), 59
Oncoviruses, 54
O'Neill, Joseph, 257*f*
O'Neill, Paul, 478
Opportunistic infections (OIs), 27, 30, 96*f*, 122, 127, 130,
       146–61, 167, 173*f*, 180, 181, 185, 185*f*, 187, 192, 196,
       199, 330, 344
    bacterial, 151*t*, 159–60
    causes of, 30, 73
    in children, 196
    defined, 146
    fungal, 151*t*, 152–55, 172
    hemophiliacs with, 40–41
    memory T4 cell pool and, 132
    prevalence of, 146–47
    projected resurgence of, 150
    protozoal, 151*t*, 156–58
    treatment of, 147, 151*t*
    viral, 125, 151*t*, 155–56
Oral candidiasis. *See* Candidiasis; Thrush
Oral polio vaccines, 49–50
Oral sex, 109, 208, 209, 210, 220, 222, 223*t*, 252, 389, 441, 450
OraSure, 417, 418*f*
Oregon, 227, 327, 332*t*, 432, 457
Organization of Petroleum Exporting Countries (OPEC)
    Fund for International Development, 485
Organon, 419
Orogenital sex. *See* Oral sex
Orphans, 323, 343, 346, 373–75, 376, 378, 381, 382–83, 394
Osmond, Dennis, 165
Osterhaus, Albert, 45, 46
Ottawa, Canada, 216, 283

Outbreak (film), 12
Owen, Greg, 465
Oxford University, 304

Pacific Islands, 330
Padian, Nancy, 229
Pain, 177
Pakistan, 219
Palacio, Ruben, 430
Palsies, 151*t*
Pan Africanist Congress, 241
Pan American Health Organization, 482
Pancreatitis, 81
Pandemics, fear and ignorance about, 6–10
Pan troglodytes, 45, 45*f*, 46, 46*f*, 47
Papilloma virus, 275. *See also* Genital warts
    human (HGPV), 6, 161, 210
Papovavirus (Jamestown Canyon virus, JCV), 151*t*, 159*t*, 166
Paralysis, 172
Paramyxovirus, 3*t*
Paraphernalia laws, 282, 284
Parasites, viruses as, 53
Parker, Jon, 281
Parolees, 327
Parran, Thomas, 292
Partner notification, 255, 265*t*, 292–94, 307, 434–35
Partners, number of sexual, 213–22, 233
Passive hemagglutination assay (PHA), 418
Pasteur Institute, 214, 299
Pasteur-Merieux, 303
Pataki, George E., 431
Paterson, Floyd, 226
Patients' rights, 470
Patterson, Bruce, 40
PBS, 237
Peace Corps, 482
Pediatric AIDS Foundation, 372, 429
Pediatric HIV/AIDS, 31*t*, 72, 194–96, 319, 356. *See also*
    Children; Infants/newborns; Perinatal transmission
    cost of care for, 372, 429
    drug therapy for, 41, 112, 246
    global estimates (2000 and 2001), 372*f*, 373*f*
    nosocomial transmission, 241
    resources, 383
    statistics on, 31–32, 194–96, 244–46, 356, 371–82
    in U.S., 196, 231, 368, 371–73
Pelvic inflammatory disease (PID), 243, 365, 366
Pennsylvania, 227, 282, 331*t*, 332*t*, 333, 372
Pentafuside, 78*t*
Pentafuside (fuzeon), 110
Pentagon, 9/11 terrorist attack on, 309–10
Pentamidine, 151*t*, 154
People with AIDS Coalition Newsline, 327
Peptides, 118, 125, 126. *See also* Antigens
Perception of personal risk, 271, 385, 387
Perelson, Alan, 182
Perez, Colleen, 106

via CPR, 199
of drug-resistant HIV, 90–91
factors facilitating, 344
female-to-female, 251–52, 364–65
in health care settings. *See* Dentistry; Health care workers;
   Needlestick injuries
heterosexual. *See* Heterosexuals
homosexual. *See* Homosexuals
in household settings, 202–3
among injection drug users. *See* Injection drug users
insects and, 201
via kissing, 197, 199, 207–9, 223*t*, 265*t*
male-to-female, 13, 14, 212, 229, 358
noncasual, 203–30
nosocomial, 241, 292
perinatal. *See* Perinatal transmission
prenatal, 197
probability of, 250
via sexual intercourse/contact, 136*f*, 197, 198, 204*t*, 205*t*,
   206, 210–11, 236–40, 250, 252, 265*t*. *See also specific*
   type of contact
sexually transmitted disease and, 15, 211, 241–44, 243*f*,
   245*f*
T4 cell count and, 181
in U.S., 197, 199, 205*t*, 222, 230–31, 234–41, 280
vertical, 194–96, 244–46, 375–77, 393–94. *See also* Perinatal
   transmission
Transmission cycle, 182
Transplantation antigens, 118
Transplants, 118, 240–41, 315*t*
Travel, 2, 205, 234, 427–28
Treatment. *See* Combination drug therapy; Drug therapy
Treatment Action Group (TAG), 111
Treatment failure, 92, 111–12
   clinical, 183
   immunologic, 183
   virologic, 183
Treponema pallidum, 159*t*
Trichomonas vaginalis (trichomoniasis), 244, 245*f*
Trimethoprim-sulfamethoxazole (Bactrim, Septra), 151*t*
Trimetrexate, 151*t*
Trinidad, 256
Trizivir, 85
Tropism, 64, 67, 136*f*, 170
TRUGENE HIV-1 Genotyping Kit and OpenGene DNA Se-
   quencing System, 93
Tsg101 protein, 52
Tshabalala-Msimang, Manto, 38, 312, 485
T-20 (enfuvirtide), 110–11, 133*f*
T20 (Pentafuside), 78*t*
Tuberculosis (TB; *Mycobacterium tuberculosis*), 3*t*, 4, 10, 50,
   146, 148*f*, 151*t*, 159*t*, 160, 296, 327, 343, 344, 426
   AIDS diagnosis and, 160
   deaths from, 3*t*, 10, 311
   extrapulmonary, 31*t*, 150, 160, 179*t*, 366*t*
   pulmonary, 31, 147, 173*f*, 179*t*, 184*t*
Tumor cells, 129

Tumor-necrosis factor alpha, 177
Tuomala, Ruth, 380
Tutu, Desmond, 479
Twins, 245
Twin State Women's Network (TSWN), 371, 477
Typhoid fever, 5–6, 138
"Typhoid Mary," 5–6
Typhus, 2, 3*t*

UB Plasma, 214–15
Uganda, 8, 104, 260, 349, 357, 358, 379, 384, 464–65
Ukraine, 231, 392
Ulcerations, 175*t*
UNAIDS (United Nations Program on AIDS), 21, 232, 233,
   234, 260, 263, 270, 276, 310, 311, 312, 313, 314, 322,
   324*f*, 343, 346, 349, 357, 358, 381, 382, 384, 480, 482
UNICEF, 368, 385, 392, 398
"Unique identifier" system, 333
United Kingdom, 3*t*, 222, 250, 267, 274, 428
United Nations Children's Fund, 233
United Nations Convention on the Rights of the Child, 373
United Nations General Assembly Special Session on AIDS
   (UNGASS), 368, 398, 483
   declaration on HIV/AIDS, 311–12
United States
   AIDS cases in, 199
   blood screening in, 215–16
   Caribbean connection to, 234
   condom usage rate in, 267
   deaths from AIDS in, 14
   diseases and epidemics in, 7, 14
   drug/syringe laws and programs in, 281–83, 284, 285–86
   expenditures on HIV/AIDS, 15
   foreign monetary and other assistance for HIV/AIDS, 482,
      483–84
   geographic distribution of HIV/AIDS in, 319*f*, 322, 362
   HIV/AIDS-experienced physicians in, 101
   HIV/AIDS immigration laws, 205
   HIV/AIDS pyramid for, 171*f*
   HIV transmission in, 197, 199, 205*t*, 222–24, 230–31,
      234–41, 280
   Kaposi's sarcoma in, 164
   number of cases of HIV/AIDS in, 3*t*, 17*t*, 28–29, 31–32,
      199, 200*f*, 211, 243*f*, 252, 261, 267–68, 309, 314–22,
      315*t*, 316*f*, 317*t*, 318*f*, 319*f*, 325*f*, 333–43, 337*f*. *See also*
      specific risk and demographic categories
   opportunistic infections in, 150–52
   pediatric HIV-positive and AIDS cases in, 196, 368, 371–73
   prevention in, 267–68
   prostitution in, 222–24
   sexually transmitted diseases in, 242
   shape of HIV epidemic in, 335–38, 336*f*
   subtypes of HIV/AIDS in, 68, 69*f*, 70, 137
   women with HIV/AIDS in, 332–33, 356, 358–71, 360*t*
U.S. Bureau of Justice Statistics, 326
U.S. Census Bureau, 263, 381
U.S. Conference of Mayors, 285

World TB Day, 160
World Trade Center, 9/11 terrorist attack on, 309–10
Wound exudates, 291*t*
Wound to wound contact, 251
Wu, Yuntao, 62–63
Wulfsohn, Adrienne, 110
Wyatt, Richard, 132
Wyoming, 332*t*, 430

YBF30, 70–71
Yeast, 163
Yebga, Jean-Emil, 428
Yecs, John, 210
Yellow fever, 3*t*, 4, 68, 201, 301, 465–66
Yerkes Primate Center, 65
Yersinia pestis, 3*t*
Yoder, Michael, 256
"Youth and HIV/AIDS: Can We Avoid Catastrophe?," 391
YX-478, 78*t*

Zaire, 6, 7, 45, 46, 48, 201
Zalcitabine (ddc, Hivid, dideoxycytosine), 79*f*, 80*f*, 81, 81*f*

cost of, 78*t*
side effects of, 81, 367
Zambia, 260, 344, 348*f*, 349, 350, 358, 375, 384
ZDV. *See* Zidovudine (AZT, ZDV, Retrovir)
Zerit. *See* Stavudine (d4T, Zerit)
Zidovudine (AZT, ZDV, Retrovir), 35, 36, 73, 81, 102, 106, 157, 167, 196, 368, 377, 381, 382
action and structure of, 79*f*, 80*f*
cost of, 78*t*, 379
incorporation into HIV DNA, 81*f*
during pregnancy, 109, 112, 197, 246, 248, 379–80, 429
side effects of, 81, 157, 367, 400
Zierler, Solley, 365
Zimbabwe, 248, 274, 322, 344, 347, 348*f*, 351, 357, 358, 359, 368, 381, 398, 465
Zinc Finger Inhibitors, 78*t*
Zintevir, 78*t*
Zithromax, 151*t*
Zovirax. *See* Acyclovir
Zurich, Switzerland, 285